Acta Neurochirurgica Supplement 134

Series Editor

Hans-Jakob Steiger
Department of Neurosurgery
Heinrich Heine University
Düsseldorf, Nordrhein-Westfalen
Germany

ACTA NEUROCHIRURGICA's Supplement Volumes provide a unique opportunity to publish the content of special meetings in the form of a Proceedings Volume. Proceedings of international meetings concerning a special topic of interest to a large group of the neuroscience community are suitable for publication in ACTA NEUROCHIRURGICA. Links to ACTA NEUROCHIRURGICA's distribution network guarantee wide dissemination at a comparably low cost. The individual volumes should comprise between 120 and max. 250 printed pages, corresponding to 20-50 papers. It is recommended that you get in contact with us as early as possible during the preparatory stage of a meeting. Please supply a preliminary program for the planned meeting. The papers of the volumes represent original publications. They pass a peer review process and are listed in PubMed and other scientific databases. Publication can be effected within 6 months. Hans-Jakob Steiger is the Editor of ACTA NEUROCHIRURGICA's Supplement Volumes. Springer Verlag International is responsible for the technical aspects and calculation of the costs. If you decide to publish your proceedings in the Supplements of ACTA NEUROCHIRURGICA, you can expect the following: • An editing process with editors both from the neurosurgical community and professional language editing. After your book is accepted, you will be assigned a developmental editor who will work with you as well as with the entire editing group to bring your book to the highest quality possible. • Effective text and illustration layout for your book. • Worldwide distribution through Springer-Verlag International's distribution channels.

More information about this series at http://www.springer.com/series/4

Victor E. Staartjes • Luca Regli • Carlo Serra
Editors

Machine Learning in Clinical Neuroscience

Foundations and Applications

Springer

Editors
Victor E. Staartjes
Machine Intelligence in Clinical Neuroscience (MICN) Laboratory, Department of Neurosurgery
Clinical Neuroscience Center, University Hospital Zurich, University of Zurich
Zurich
Switzerland

Luca Regli
Machine Intelligence in Clinical Neuroscience (MICN) Laboratory, Department of Neurosurgery
Clinical Neuroscience Center, University Hospital Zurich, University of Zurich
Zurich
Switzerland

Carlo Serra
Machine Intelligence in Clinical Neuroscience (MICN) Laboratory, Department of Neurosurgery
Clinical Neuroscience Center, University Hospital Zurich, University of Zurich
Zurich
Switzerland

ISSN 0065-1419 ISSN 2197-8395 (electronic)
Acta Neurochirurgica Supplement 134
ISBN 978-3-030-85291-7 ISBN 978-3-030-85292-4 (eBook)
https://doi.org/10.1007/978-3-030-85292-4

This Springer imprint is published by the registered company Springer Nature Switzerland AG
The registered company address is: Gewerbestrasse 11, 6330 Cham, Switzerland

Contents

Machine Intelligence in Clinical Neuroscience: Taming the Unchained Prometheus

1

Victor E. Staartjes, Luca Regli, and Carlo Serra

1.1 Preface

The question is not whether intelligent machines can have any emotions, but whether machines can be intelligent without any emotions — Marvin Minsky [1]

Advances in both statistical modeling techniques as well as in computing power over the last few decades have enabled the rapid rise of the field of data science, including artificial intelligence (AI) and machine learning (ML) [2]. While AI can be defined as a goal—the goal to emulate human, "wide" intelligence with the ability to solve a range of different complex tasks with one brain or algorithm—ML deals with learning problems by inductively and iteratively learning from experience (in the form of data) without being explicitly programmed, as a form of "narrow" AI (focused on just one specific task). Along with the broader application of epidemiological principles and larger sample sizes ("big data"), this has led to broad adoption of statistical prediction modeling in clinical practice and research. Clinical prediction models integrate a range of input variables to predict a specific outcome in the future and can aid in evidence-based decision-making and improved patient counseling [3–6].

Even in the field of clinical neuroscience—including neurosurgery, neurology, and neuroradiology—ML has been increasingly applied over the years, as evidenced by the sharp rise in publications on machine learning in clinical neuroscience indexed in PubMed/MEDLINE since the 2000s (Fig. 1.1). While the history of ML applications to the field of neurosurgery is rather compressed into the past two decades, some early efforts have been made as early as the late 1980s. Disregarding other uses of AI and ML—such as advanced histopathological or radiological diagnostics—and focusing on predictive analytics, in 1989 Mathew et al. [7] published a report in which they applied a fuzzy logic classifier to 150 patients, and were able to predict whether disc prolapse or bony nerve entrapment were present based on clinical findings. In 1998, Grigsby et al. [8] were able to predict seizure freedom after anterior temporal lobectomy using neural networks based on EEG and MRI features, using data from 87 patients. Similarly, in 1999, Arle et al. [9] applied neural networks to 80 patients to predict seizures after epilepsy surgery. Soon, and especially since 2010, a multitude of publications followed, applying ML to clinical outcome prediction in all subspecialties of the neurosurgical field [10–11]. The desire to model reality to better understand it and in this way predict its future behavior has always been a goal of scientific thought, and "machine learning," if not just for the evocative power of the term, may appear under this aspect at first sight as a resolutive tool. However, if on one hand there cannot be any doubt that predicting the future will always remain a chimera, on the other hand it is true that machine learning tools can improve our possibilities to analyze and thus understand reality. But while clinical prediction modeling has certainly been by far the most common application of ML in clinical neuroscience, other applications such as, e.g. in image recognition [12, 13], natural language processing [14], radiomic feature extraction [15, 16], EEG classification [17], and continuous data monitoring [18] should not be disregarded and probably constitute the most interesting fields of application.

Today, ML and other statistical learning techniques have become so easily accessible to anyone with a computer and internet access, that it has become of paramount importance to ensure correct methodology. Moreover, there has been a major "hype" around the terms ML and AI in recent years. Because of their present-day low threshold accessibility, these techniques can easily be misused and misinterpreted, without intent to do so. For example, it is still common to see highly complex and "data-hungry" algorithms such as deep

V. E. Staartjes (✉) · L. Regli · C. Serra
Machine Intelligence in Clinical Neuroscience (MICN) Laboratory, Department of Neurosurgery, Clinical Neuroscience Center, University Hospital Zurich, University of Zurich, Zurich, Switzerland
e-mail: victoregon.staartjes@usz.ch; https://micnlab.com/

V. E. Staartjes et al. (eds.), *Machine Learning in Clinical Neuroscience*, Acta Neurochirurgica Supplement 134,
https://doi.org/10.1007/978-3-030-85292-4_1

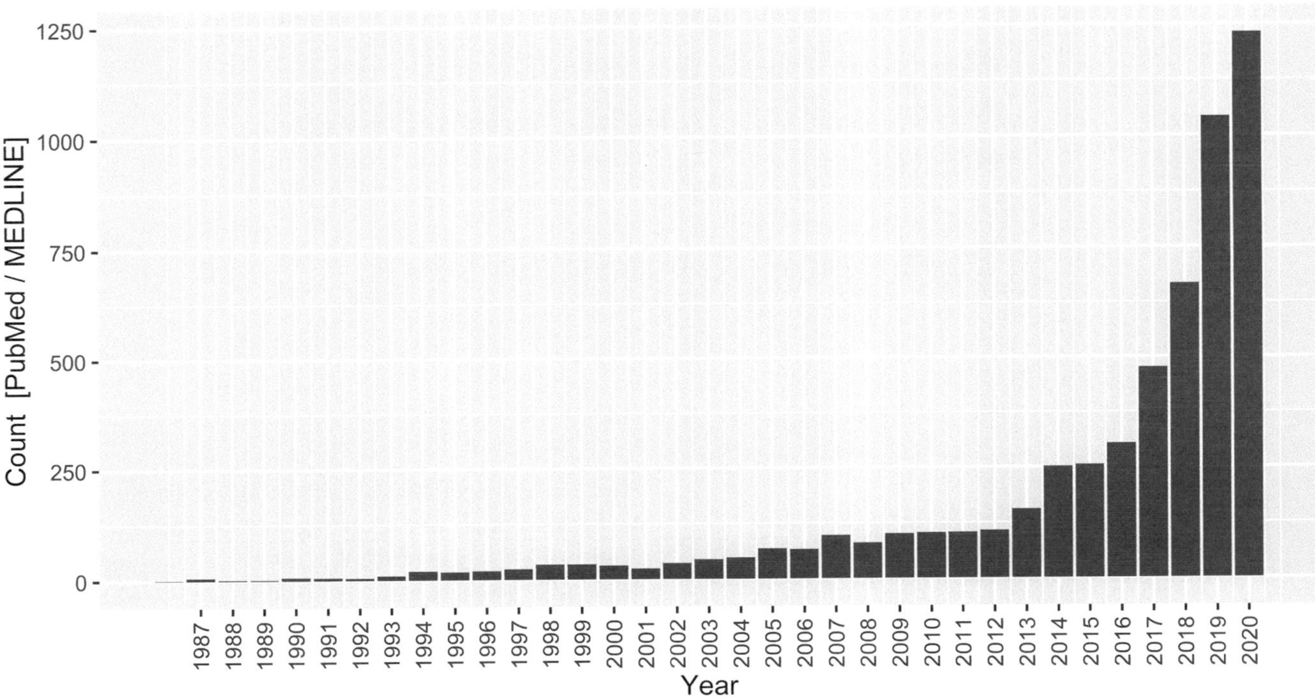

Fig. 1.1 Development of publication counts on machine learning in neurosurgery over the years. Counts were arrived at by searching "*(neurosurgery OR neurology OR neuroradiology) AND (machine learning OR artificial intelligence)*" on PubMed/MEDLINE

neural networks applied to very small datasets, to see overtly overfitted or imbalanced models, or models trained for prediction that are then used to "identify risk factors" (prediction vs. explanation/inference). Especially in clinical practice and in the medico-legal arena, it is vital that clinical prediction models intended to be implemented into clinical practice are developed with methodological rigor, and that they are well-validated and generalizable.

Some efforts such as, e.g. the EQUATOR Network's "Transparent reporting of a multivariable prediction model for individual prognosis or diagnosis" (TRIPOD) statement [19] have led to improved methodological quality and standardized reporting throughout the last 5 years [20]. Still, it is a fact that ML is often poorly understood, and that the methodology has to be well-appreciated to prevent publishing flawed models—standardized reporting is valuable, but not enough. Open-source ML libraries like Keras [21] and Caret [22] have truly democratized ML. While this fact—combined with the steadily increasing availability of large amounts of structured and unstructured data in the "big data" era—has certainly provided leverage to the whole field of ML, putting so much analytical power into anyone's hands without clear methodological foundations can be risky.

The immense technological progress during the past century has certainly sparked reflection on the responsibilities of humanity regarding limitations, safe use, fair distribution, and consequences of these advances.

Progress can be risky. As a matter of fact, ML tools are increasingly being used to aid in decision-making in several domains of human society. The lack of profound understanding of the capabilities and, most importantly, of the limitations of ML may lead to the erroneous assumption that ML may overtake, and not just aid, the decision-making capacity of the human mind. Needless to say, this attitude can have serious practical and most importantly ethical consequences. Today's greater power of humanity in controlling nature means that we must also realize their limitations and potential dangers, and to consequently limit our applications of those technologies to avoid potential disaster—this has become the most popular topic of modern philosophy on artificial intelligence [23].

Today, every scientific study is subject to ethical review and approval, but potential long-term sequelae of ML studies are seldomly considered. ML in medicine has great potential, but both doctors applying these technologies in clinical practice as well as those researchers developing tools based on these technologies must be acutely aware of their limitations and their ramifications. Further unsolved ethical issues regarding the use of ML and AI in clinical medicine pertain to protecting *data integrity*, ensuring *justice* in the distribution of ML-based resources, and maintaining *accountability*—Could algorithms learn to assign values and become independent moral agents? While some progress has been made in protecting data integrity, such as the use of *federated learning*, developments in other ethical issues remain less predictable [24].

Therefore, ML and AI must remain tools adjunctive to our own mind, tools that we should be able to master, control, and apply to our advantage—and that should not take over our minds. For example, it is inconceivable and even potentially dangerous to fully rely on predictions made by a ML algorithm in clinical practice, currently. The future cannot be easily predicted by machines, or by anyone for that matter—And even if near-perfect predictions were theoretically possible, our intuition would tell us that the mere knowledge of what is very likely going to happen in the future may lead us to change events, not dissimilar to *Heisenberg's uncertainty principle*. While our mind can recognize, abstract, and deal with the many uncertainties in clinical practice, algorithms cannot. Among many others, concepts such as *Turing's Test* [25] underline the importance of appreciating the limits of ML and AI: They are no alchemy, no magic. They do not make the impossible possible. They merely serve to assist and improve our performance on certain very specific tasks.

For these reasons, we embarked on a journey to compile a textbook for clinicians that demystifies the terms "machine learning" and "artificial intelligence" by illustrating their methodological foundations, as well as some specific applications throughout the different fields of clinical neuroscience, and its limitations. Of note, this book has been inspired and conceived by the group of machine learning specialists that also contributed to the *1st Zurich Machine Intelligence in Clinical Neuroscience Symposium* that took place on January 21st 2021 with presentations on their respective book chapters which we encourage readers to consider watching (the recorded contributions are available on: www.micnlab.com/symposium2021).

The book is structured in five major parts:

1. The first part deals with the methodological foundations of clinical prediction modeling as the most common clinical application of ML [4]. The basic workflow for developing and validating a clinical prediction model is discussed in detail in a five-part series, which is followed by spotlights on certain topics of relevance ranging from feature selection, dimensionality reduction techniques as well as Bayesian, deep learning, and clustering techniques, to how to deploy, update, and interpret clinical prediction models.
2. Part II consists of a brief *tour de force* through the domain of ML in neuroimaging and its foundational methods. First, the different applications and algorithms are laid out in detail, which is then followed by specific workflows including radiomic feature extraction, segmentation, and brain imaging classification.
3. The next part provides a glimpse into the world of natural language processing (NLP) and time series analysis (TSA), going through the algorithms used for such analyses, as well as workflows for both domains.
4. The fourth part of this book handles the various ethical implications of applying ML in clinical practice—From general ethical considerations on AI, to ways in which ML can assist doctors in daily practice and the limitations of predictive analytics. In addition, a brief history of ML in neurosurgery is provided, too.
5. The fifth and final part is targeted to demonstrating an overview over the various clinical applications that have already been implemented in clinical neuroscience, covering neuroimaging, neurosurgery, neurology, and ophthalmology.

Our hope is that this book may inspire and instruct a generation of physician-scientists to continue to grow and develop the seeds that have been planted for machine intelligence in clinical neuroscience, and to discover the limits of the clinical applications therein.

References

1. Minsky M. The Society of Mind. Simon and Schuster. 1986.
2. Kononenko I. Machine learning for medical diagnosis: history, state of the art and perspective. Artif Intell Med. 2001;23:89. https://doi.org/10.1016/S0933-3657(01)00077-X.
3. Senders JT, Staples PC, Karhade AV, Zaki MM, Gormley WB, Broekman MLD, Smith TR, Arnaout O. Machine learning and neurosurgical outcome prediction: a systematic review. World Neurosurg. 2018;109:476. https://doi.org/10.1016/j.wneu.2017.09.149.
4. Staartjes VE, Stumpo V, Kernbach JM, et al. Machine learning in neurosurgery: a global survey. Acta Neurochir. 2020;162(12):3081–91.
5. Saposnik G, Cote R, Mamdani M, Raptis S, Thorpe KE, Fang J, Redelmeier DA, Goldstein LB. JURaSSiC: accuracy of clinician vs risk score prediction of ischemic stroke outcomes. Neurology. 2013;81:448. https://doi.org/10.1212/WNL.0b013e31829d874e.
6. Steyerberg EW. Clinical prediction models: a practical approach to development, validation, and updating. New York, NY: Springer Science & Business Media; 2008.
7. Mathew B, Norris D, Mackintosh I, Waddell G. Artificial intelligence in the prediction of operative findings in low back surgery. Br J Neurosurg. 1989;3:161. https://doi.org/10.3109/02688698909002791.
8. Grigsby J, Kramer RE, Schneiders JL, Gates JR, Smith WB. Predicting outcome of anterior temporal lobectomy using simulated neural networks. Epilepsia. 1998;39:61. https://doi.org/10.1111/j.1528-1157.1998.tb01275.x.
9. Arle JE, Perrine K, Devinsky O, Doyle WK. Neural network analysis of preoperative variables and outcome in epilepsy surgery. J Neurosurg. 1999;90:998. https://doi.org/10.3171/jns.1999.90.6.0998.
10. Azimi P, Mohammadi HR, Benzel EC, Shahzadi S, Azhari S, Montazeri A. Artificial neural networks in neurosurgery. J Neurol

Neurosurg Psychiatry. 2015;86:251. https://doi.org/10.1136/jnnp-2014-307807.
11. Senders JT, Zaki MM, Karhade AV, Chang B, Gormley WB, Broekman ML, Smith TR, Arnaout O. An introduction and overview of machine learning in neurosurgical care. Acta Neurochir. 2018;160:29. https://doi.org/10.1007/s00701-017-3385-8.
12. Swinburne NC, Schefflein J, Sakai Y, Oermann EK, Titano JJ, Chen I, Tadayon S, Aggarwal A, Doshi A, Nael K. Machine learning for semi-automated classification of glioblastoma, brain metastasis and central nervous system lymphoma using magnetic resonance advanced imaging. Ann Transl Med. 2019;7(11):232.
13. Titano JJ, Badgeley M, Schefflein J, et al. Automated deep-neural-network surveillance of cranial images for acute neurologic events. Nat Med. 2018;24(9):1337–41.
14. Senders JT, Karhade AV, Cote DJ, et al. Natural language processing for automated quantification of brain metastases reported in free-text radiology reports. JCO Clin Cancer Inform. 2019;3:1–9.
15. Chang K, Bai HX, Zhou H, et al. Residual convolutional neural network for the determination of IDH status in low- and high-grade gliomas from MR imaging. Clin Cancer Res. 2018;24(5):1073–81.
16. Kernbach JM, Yeo BTT, Smallwood J, et al. Subspecialization within default mode nodes characterized in 10,000 UK Biobank participants. Proc Natl Acad Sci U S A. 2018;115(48):12295–300.
17. Varatharajah Y, Berry B, Cimbalnik J, Kremen V, Van Gompel J, Stead M, Brinkmann B, Iyer R, Worrell G. Integrating artificial intelligence with real-time intracranial EEG monitoring to automate interictal identification of seizure onset zones in focal epilepsy. J Neural Eng. 2018;15(4):046035.
18. Schwab P, Keller E, Muroi C, Mack DJ, Strässle C, Karlen W. Not to cry wolf: distantly supervised multitask learning in critical care. ArXiv. 2018:1802.05027. [cs, stat].
19. Collins GS, Reitsma JB, Altman DG, Moons KGM. Transparent reporting of a multivariable prediction model for individual prognosis or diagnosis (TRIPOD): the TRIPOD statement. BMJ. 2015;350:g7594.
20. Zamanipoor Najafabadi AH, Ramspek CL, Dekker FW, Heus P, Hooft L, Moons KGM, Peul WC, Collins GS, Steyerberg EW, van Diepen M. TRIPOD statement: a preliminary pre-post analysis of reporting and methods of prediction models. BMJ Open. 2020;10(9):e041537.
21. Chollet F. Keras: deep learning library for Theano and TensorFlow. 2015. https://keras.io/k.
22. Kuhn M, Wing J, Weston S, Williams A, et al. caret: classification and regression training. 2019.
23. Jonas H. Das Prinzip Verantwortung: Versuch einer Ethik für die technologische Zivilisation. Berlin: Suhrkamp; 2003.
24. Yang Q, Liu Y, Chen T, Tong Y. Federated machine learning: concept and applications. ArXiv. 2019:1902.04885. [cs].
25. Oppy G, Dowe D. The turing test. Stanford, CA: The Stanford Encyclopedia of Philosophy; 2020.

Part I

Clinical Prediction Modeling

Foundations of Machine Learning-Based Clinical Prediction Modeling: Part I—Introduction and General Principles

2

Julius M. Kernbach and Victor E. Staartjes

2.1 Introduction

Although there are many applications of machine learning (ML) in clinical neuroscience, including but not limited to applications in neuroimaging and natural language processing, classical predictive analytics still form the majority of the body of evidence that has been published on the topic.

When reviewing or working on research involving ML-based predictive analytics—which is becoming increasingly common—it is important to do so with a strong methodological basis. Especially considering the "democratization" of ML methods through libraries and the increasing computing power, as well as the exponentially increasing influx of ML publications in the clinical neurosciences, methodological rigor has become a major issue. This chapter and in fact the entire five-part series (cite Chaps. 3–6) is intended to convey that basic conceptual and programming knowledge to tackle ML tasks with some basic prerequisite R knowledge, with a particular focus on predictive analytics.

At this point, it is important to stress that the concepts and methods presented herein are intended as an entry-level guide to ML for clinical outcome prediction, presenting one of many valid approaches to clinical prediction modeling, and thus does not encompass all the details and intricacies of the field. Further reading is recommended, including but not limited to Max Kuhn's "Applied Predictive Modeling" [1] and Ewout W. Steyerberg's "Clinical Prediction Models" [2].

This first part focuses on defining the terms ML and AI in the context of predictive analytics, and clearly describing their applications in clinical medicine. In addition, some of the basic concepts of machine intelligence are discussed and explained. Part II goes into detail about common problems when developing clinical prediction models: What overfitting is and how to avoid it to arrive at generalizable models, how to select which input features are to be included in the final model (feature selection) or how to simplify highly dimensional data (feature reduction). We also discuss how data splits and resampling methods like cross-validation and the bootstrap can be applied to validate models before clinical use. Part III touches on several topics including how to prepare your data correctly (standardization, one-hot encoding) and evaluate models in terms of discrimination and calibration, and points out some recalibration methods. Some other points of significance and caveats that the reader may encounter while developing a clinical prediction model are discussed: sample size, class imbalance, missing data and how to impute it, extrapolation, as well as how to choose a cutoff for binary classification. Parts IV and V present a practical approach to classification and regression problems, respectively. They contain detailed instructions along with a downloadable code for the R statistical programming language, as well as a simulated database of Glioblastoma patients that allows the reader to code in parallel to the explanations. This section is intended as a scaffold upon which readers can build their own clinical prediction models, and that can easily be modified. Furthermore, we will not in detail explain the workings of specific ML algorithms such as generalized linear models, support vector machines, neural networks, or stochastic gradient boosting. While it is certainly important to have a basic understanding of the specific

J. M. Kernbach and V. E. Staartjes have contributed equally to this series, and share first authorship.

J. M. Kernbach
Neurosurgical Artificial Intelligence Laboratory Aachen (NAILA), Department of Neurosurgery, RWTH Aachen University Hospital, Aachen, Germany

V. E. Staartjes (✉)
Machine Intelligence in Clinical Neuroscience (MICN) Laboratory, Department of Neurosurgery, Clinical Neuroscience Center, University Hospital Zurich, University of Zurich, Zurich, Switzerland
e-mail: victoregon.staartjes@usz.ch; https://micnlab.com/

V. E. Staartjes et al. (eds.), *Machine Learning in Clinical Neuroscience*, Acta Neurochirurgica Supplement 134,
https://doi.org/10.1007/978-3-030-85292-4_2

algorithms one applies, these details can be looked up online [3] and detailed explanations of these algorithms would go beyond the scope of this guide. The goal is instead to convey the basic concepts of ML-based predictive modeling, and how to practically implement these.

2.2 Machine Learning: Definitions

As a field of study, ML in medicine is positioned between statistical learning and advanced computer science, and typically evolves around *learning problems*, which can be conceptually defined as optimizing a performance measure on a given task by learning through training experience on prior data. A ML algorithm inductively learns to automatically extract patterns from data to generate insights [4, 5] without being explicitly programmed. This makes ML an attractive option to predict even complex phenomena without prespecifying an a priori theoretical model. ML can be used to leverage the full granularity of the data richness enclosed in the *Big Data* trend. Both the complexity and dimensionality of modern medical data sets are constantly increasing and nowadays comprise many variables per observation, much so that we speak of "wide data" with generally more variables (in ML lingo called *features*) than observations (samples) [6, 7]. This has given rise to the so-called *omics* sciences including radiomics and genomics [8–10]. The sheer complexity and volume of data ranging from hundreds to thousands of variables at times exceeds human comprehension, but combined with increased computational power enables the full potential of ML [3, 11].

With the exponential demand of AI and ML in modern medicine, a lot of confusion was introduced regarding the separation of these two terms. AI and ML are frequently used interchangeably. We define ML as subset of AI—to quote Tom Mitchell—ML "is the study of computer algorithms that allow computer programs to automatically improve through experience" [12], involving the concept of "learning" discussed earlier. In contrast, AI is philosophically much vaster, and can be defined as an ambition to enable computer programs to behave in a human-like nature. That is, showing a certain human-like intelligence. In ML, we learn and optimize an algorithm from data for maximum performance on a certain learning task. In AI, we try to emulate natural intelligence, to not only learn but also apply the gained knowledge to make elaborate decisions and solve complex problems. In a way, ML can thus be considered a technique towards realizing (narrow) AI. Ethical considerations on the "AI doctor" are far-reaching [13, 14], while the concept of a clinician aided by ML-based tools is well accepted.

The most widely used ML methods are either supervised or unsupervised learning methods, with the exceptions of semi-supervised methods and reinforcement learning [6, 15]. In supervised learning, a set of input variables are used as training set, e.g. different meaningful variables such as age, gender, tumor grading, or functional neurological status to predict a known target variable ("label"), e.g. overall survival. The ML method can then learn the pattern linking input features to target variable, and based on that enable the prediction of new data points—hence, *generalize* patterns beyond the present data. We can train a ML model for survival prediction based on a retrospective cohort of brain tumor patients, since we know the individual length of survival for each patient of the cohort. Therefore, the target variable is *labeled*, and the machine learning-paradigm *supervised*. Again, the actually chosen methods can vary: Common models include support vector machines (SVMs), as example of a *parametric* approach, or *the k*-nearest neighbor (KNN) algorithm as a *non-parametric* method [16]. On the other hand, in *unsupervised* learning, we generally deal with *unlabeled* data with the assumption of the structural coherence. This can be leveraged in clustering, which is a subset of unsupervised learning encompassing many different methods, e.g. hierarchical clustering or *k*-means clustering [4, 17]. The observed data is partitioned into clusters based on a measure of similarity regarding the structural architecture of the data. Similarly, dimensionality reduction methods—including principal component analysis (PCA) or autoencoders—can be applied to derive a low-dimensional representation explicitly from the present data [4, 18].

A multitude of diverse ML algorithms exist, and sometimes choosing the "right" algorithm for a given application can be quite confusing. Moreover, based on the so-called *no free lunch theorem* [19] no single statistical algorithm or model can generally be considered superior for all circumstances. Nevertheless, ML algorithms can vary greatly based on the (a) representation of the candidate algorithm, (b) the selected performance metric, and (c) the applied optimization strategy [4, 5, 20]. Representation refers to the learner's hypothesis space of how they formally deal with the problem at hand. This includes but is not limited to instance-based learners, such as KNN, which instead of performing explicit generalization compares new observations with similar instances observed during training [21]. Other representation spaces include hyperplane-based models, such as logistic regression or naïve Bayes, as well as rule-based learners, decision trees or complex neural networks, all of which are frequently leveraged in various ML problems across the neurosurgical literature [22, 23]. The evaluated performance metrics can vary greatly, too. Performance evaluation and reporting play a pivotal role in predictive analytics (c.f. cite Chap. 4). Lastly, the applied ML algorithm is *optimized* by a so-called objective function such as greedy search or unconstrained continuous optimization options, including different choices of gradient descent [24, 25]. Gradient descent represents the most common optimization strategy for neural networks and can take different forms, e.g. batch- ("vanilla"), stochastic- or mini-batch gradient descent [25]. We delve deeper into optimization to illustrate how it is used in learning.

2.3 Optimization: The Central Dogma of Learning Techniques

At the heart of nearly all ML and statistical modeling techniques used in data science lies the concept of *optimization.* Even though optimization is the backbone of algorithms ranging from linear and logistic regression to neural networks, it is not often stressed in the non-academic data science space. Optimization describes the process of iteratively adjusting parameters to improve performance. Every optimization problem can be decomposed into three basic elements: First, every algorithm has *parameters* (sometimes called *weights*) that govern how the values of the input variables lead to a prediction. In linear and logistic regression, for example, these parameters include the coefficients that are multiplied with the input variable values, as well as the intercept. Second, there may be realistic *constraints* within which the parameters, or their combinations, must fall. While simple models such as linear and logistic regression often do not have such constraints, other ML algorithms such as support vector machines or *k*-means clustering do. Lastly and importantly, the optimization process is steered by evaluating a so-called *objective function* that assesses how well the current iteration of the algorithm is performing. Commonly, these objective functions are *error* (also called *loss*) functions, describing the deviation of the predicted values from the true values that are to be predicted. Thus, these error functions must be *minimized.* Sometimes, you may choose to use indicators of performance, such as accuracy, which conversely need to be *maximized* throughout the optimization process.

The optimization process starts by randomly *initializing* all model parameters—that is, assigning some initial value for each parameter. Then, predictions are made on the training data, and the error is calculated. Subsequently, the parameters are adjusted in a certain direction, and the error function is evaluated again. If the error increases, it is likely that the direction of adjustment of the parameters was awry and thus led to a higher error on the training data. In that case, the parameter values are adjusted in different directions, and the error function is evaluated again. Should the error decrease, the parameter values will be further modified in these specific directions, until a *minimum* of the error function is reached. The goal of the optimization process is to reach the *global minimum* of the error function, that is, the lowest error that can be achieved through the combination of parameter values within their constraints. However, the optimization algorithm must avoid getting stuck at *local minima* of the error function (see Fig. 2.1).

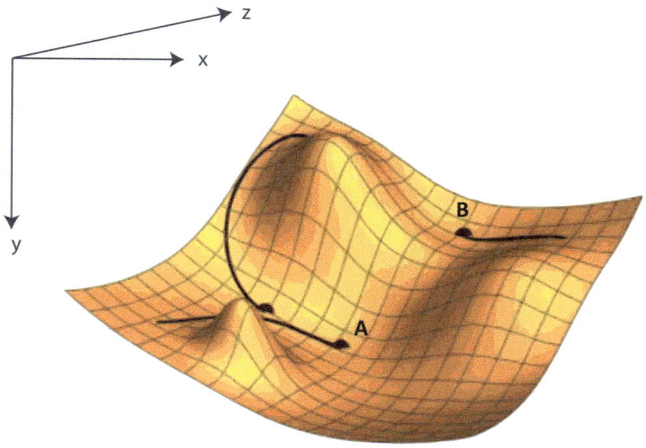

Fig. 2.1 Illustration of an optimization problem. In the *x* and *z* dimension, two parameters can take different values. In the *y* dimension, the error is displayed for different values of these two parameters. The goal of the optimization algorithm is to reach the *global minimum* (**A**) of the error through adjusting the parameter values, without getting stuck at a *local minimum* (**B**). In this example, three models are initialized with different parameter values. Two of the models converge at the global minimum (**A**), while one model gets stuck at a local minimum (**B**). Illustration by Jacopo Bertolotti. (This illustration has been made available under the Creative Commons CC0 1.0 Universal Public Domain Dedication)

The way in which the parameters are adjusted after each iteration is governed by an *optimization algorithm,* and approaches can differ greatly. For example, linear regression usually uses the ordinary least square (OLS) optimization method. In OLS, the parameters are estimated by solving an equation for the minimum of the sum of the square errors. On the other hand, *stochastic gradient descent*—which is a common optimization method for many ML algorithms—iteratively adjusts parameters as described above and as illustrated in Fig. 2.1. In stochastic gradient descent, the amount by which the parameters are changed after each iteration (also called *epoch*) is controlled by the calculated derivative (i.e. the slope or *gradient*) for each parameter with respect to the error function, and the *learning rate.* In many models, the learning rate is an important hyperparameter to set, as it controls how much parameters change in each iteration.

On the one hand, small learning rates can take many iterations to converge and make getting stuck at a local minimum more likely—on the other hand, a large learning rate can overshoot the global minimum. As a detailed discussion of the mathematical nature behind different algorithms remains beyond the scope of this introductory series, we refer to popular standard literature such as "Elements of Statistical Learning" by Hastie and Tibshirani [4], "Deep Learning" by Goodfellow et al. [26], and "Optimization for Machine Learning" by Sra et al. [27].

2.4 Explanatory Modeling Versus Predictive Modeling

The "booming" of applied ML has generated a methodological shift from *classical statistics* (experimental setting, hypothesis testing, group comparison, inference) to data-driven *statistical learning* (empirical setting, algorithmic modeling comprising ML, AI, pattern recognition) [28]. Unfortunately, the two statistical cultures have developed separately over the past decades [29] leading to incongruent evolved terminology and misunderstandings in the absence of an agreed-upon technical theorem (Table 2.1). This already becomes evident in the basic terminology describing model inputs and outputs: *predictors* or *independent variables* refer to model inputs in classical statistics, while *features* are the commonly used term in ML; outputs, known as *dependent variable* or *response*, are often labeled *target variable* or *label* in ML instead [30]. The duality of language has led to misconceptions regarding the fundamental difference between inference and prediction, as the term *prediction* has frequently been used incompatibly as in-sample correlation instead of out-of-sample generalization [31, 32]. The variation of one variable with a subsequent correlated variable later in time, such as the outcome, in the same group (in-sample correlation) does not imply prediction, and failure to account for this distinction can lead to false clinical decision-making [33, 34]. Strong associations between variables and outcome in a clinical study remain averaged estimates of the evaluated patient cohort, which does not necessarily enable predictions in unseen new patients. To shield clinicians from making wrong interpretations, we clarify the difference between explanatory modeling and predictive modeling, and highlight the potential of ML for strong predictive models.

Table 2.1 A comparison of central concepts in classical/inferential statistics versus in statistical/machine learning

Classical/inferential statistics	Statistical/machine learning
Explanatory modeling	**Predictive modeling**
An a priori chosen theoretical model is applied to data in order to test for causal hypotheses.	The process of applying a statistical model or data mining algorithm to data for the purpose of predicting new or future observations.
Focus on in-sample estimates	**Focus on out-of-sample estimates**
Goal: to confirm the existence of an effect in the entire data sample. Often using significance testing.	Goal: Use the best performing model to make new prediction for single new observations. Often using resampling techniques.
Focus on model interpretability	**Focus on model performance**
The model is chosen a priori, while models with intrinsic means of interpretability are preferred, e.g. a GLM, often parametric with a few fixed parameters.	Different models are applied and the best performing one is selected. Models tend to be more flexible and expressive, often non-parametric with many parameters adapting to the present data.
Experimental data	**Empirical data**
Long data (*n* samples > *p* variables)	**Wide data (*n* samples ≪ *p* variables)**
Independent variables	**Features**
Dependent variable	**Target variable**
Learn deductively by model testing	**Learn a model from data inductively**

Knowledge generation in clinical research has nearly exclusively been dominated by classical statistics with the focus on *explanatory modeling* (EM) [32]. In carefully designed experiments or clinical studies, a constructed theoretical model, e.g. a regression model, is applied to data in order to test for causal hypotheses. Based on theory, a model is chosen a priori, combining a fixed number of experimental variables, which are under the control of the investigator. Explicit model assumptions such as the Gaussian distribution assumption are made, and the model, which is believed to represent the true *data generating process*, is evaluated for the entire present data sample based on hypothesis and significance testing ("inference"). In such association-based modeling, a set of independent variables (X) are assumed to behave according to a certain mechanism ("theory") and ultimately cause an effect measured by the dependent variable (Y). Indeed, the role of *theory* in explanatory modeling is strong and is always reflected in the applied model, with the aim to obtain the most accurate representation of the underlying theory (technically speaking, classical statistics seeks to minimize *bias*). Whether *theory* holds true and the effect actually exists is then confirmed in the data, hence the overall analytical goal is *inference*.

Machine learning-based *predictive modeling* (PM) is defined as the process of applying a statistical model or data mining algorithm to data for the purpose of predicting future observations. In a heuristic approach, ML or PM is applied to *empirical data* as opposed to experimentally controlled data.

As the name implies, the primary focus lays on optimizing the prediction of a target variable (Y) for new observations given their set of features (X). As opposed to explanatory modeling, PM is *forward looking* [32] with the intention of predicting new observations, and hence *generalization beyond the present data* is the fundamental goal of the analysis. In contrast to EM, PM seeks to minimize both *variance* and *bias* [35, 36], occasionally sacrificing the theoretical interpretability for enhanced predictive power. Any underlying method can constitute a predictive model ranging from parametric and rigid models to highly flexible non-parametric and complex models. With a minimum of a priori specifications, a model is then heuristically derived from the data [37, 38]. The true data generating process lays in the data, and is inductively learned and approximated by ML models.

2.5 Workflow for Predictive Modeling

In clinical predictive analytics, *generalization* is our ultimate goal. To answer different research objectives, we develop, test, and evaluate different models for the purpose of clinical application (for an overview see https://topepo.github.io/caret/available-models.html). Many research objectives in PM can be framed either as the prediction of a continuous endpoint (regression) such as progression-free survival measured in months or alternatively as the prediction of a binary endpoint (classification), e.g. survival after 12 months as a dichotomized binary. Most continuous variables can easily be reduced and dichotomized into binary variables, but as a result data granularity is lost. Both regression and classification share a common analytical workflow with difference in regard to model evaluation and reporting (c.f. *cite* Chap. 5 *Classification problems* and *cite* Chap. 6 *Regression problems* for a detailed discussion). An adaptable pipeline for both regression and classification problems is demonstrated in Parts IV and V. Both sections contain detailed instructions along with a simulated dataset of 10,000 patients with glioblastoma and the code based on the statistical programming language R, which is available as open-source software.

For a general overview, a four-step approach to PM is proposed (Fig. 2.2): First and most important (1) all data needs to be pre-processed. ML is often thought of as *letting data do the heavy lifting*, which in part is correct, however, the raw data is often not suited to learning well in its current form. A lot of work needs to be allocated to preparing the input data including data cleaning and pre-processing (imputation, scaling, normalization, encoding) as well as *feature engineering* and *selection*. This is followed by using (2) resampling techniques such as *k*-fold cross-validation (c.f. cite Chap. 3 *generalization and overfitting*) to train different models and perform hyperparameter tuning. In a third step (3), the different models are compared and evaluated for generalizability based on a chosen out-of-sample performance measure in an independent testing set. The best performing model is ultimately selected, the model's out-of-sample calibration assessed (c.f. cite Chap. 4 *Evaluation and points of significance*), and, in a fourth step (4) the model is externally validated—or at least prospectively internally validated—to ensure clinical usage is safe and generalizable across locations, different populations and end users (c.f. *cite* Chap. 3 *Generalization and overfitting*). The European Union (EU) and the Food and Drug Administration (FDA) have both set standards for classifying machine learning and other software for use in healthcare, upon which the extensiveness of validation that is required before approved introduction into clinical practice is based. For example, to receive the CE mark for a clinical decision support (CDS) algorithm—depending on classification—the EU requires compliance with ISO 13485 standards, as well as a clinical evaluation report (CER) that includes a literature review and clinical testing (validation) [39].

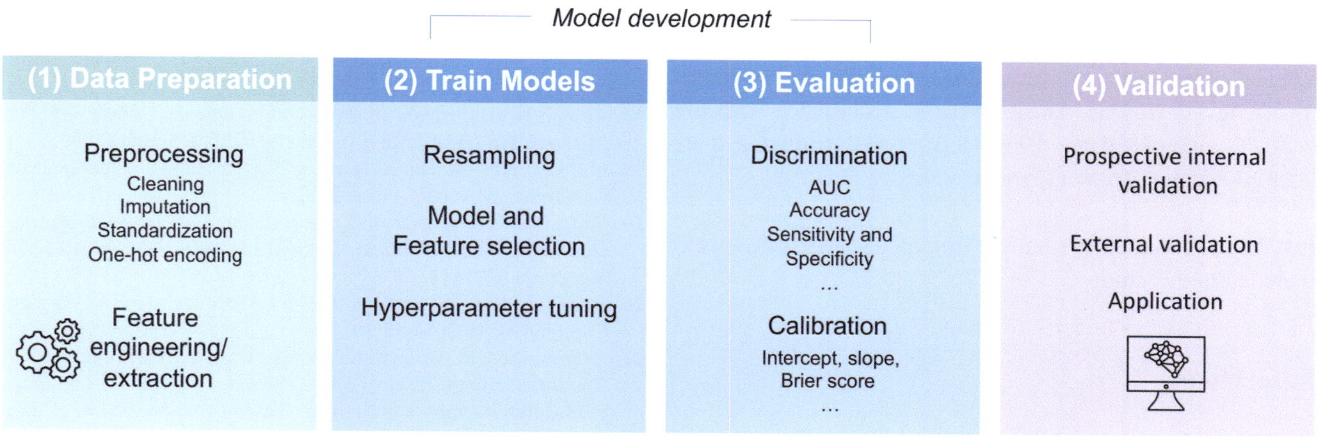

Fig. 2.2 A four-step predictive modeling workflow. (1) Data preparation includes cleaning and featurization of the given raw data. Data preprocessing combines cleaning and outlier detection, missing data imputation, the use of standardization methods, and correct feature encoding. The pre-processed data is further formed into features—manually in a process called *feature engineering* or automatically deduced by a process called *feature extraction*. In the training process (2) resampling techniques such as *k*-fold cross-validation are used to train and tune different models. Most predictive features are identified in a *feature selection* process. (3) Models are compared and evaluated for generalizability in an independent testing set. The best performing model is selected, and out-of-sample discrimination and calibration are assessed. (4) The generalizing model is prospectively internally and externally validated to ensure safe clinical usage across locations and users

2.6 Conclusion

We appear to be at the beginning of an accelerated trend towards data-driven decision-making in biomedicine enabled by a transformative technology—machine learning [5]. Given the ever-growing and highly complex "big data" biomedical datasets and increases in computational power, machine learning approaches prove to be highly successful analytical strategies towards a patient-tailored approach regarding diagnosis, treatment choice, and outcome prediction. Going forward, we expect that training neuroscientists and clinicians in the concepts of machine learning will undoubtably be a corner stone for the advancement of individualized medicine in the realm of precision medicine. With the series "*Machine learning-based clinical prediction modeling*," we aim to provide both a conceptual and practical guideline for predictive analytics in the clinical routine to strengthen every clinician's competence in modern machine learning techniques.

Disclosures

Funding No funding was received for this research.

Conflict of Interest All authors certify that they have no affiliations with or involvement in any organization or entity with any financial interest (such as honoraria; educational grants; participation in speakers' bureaus; membership, employment, consultancies, stock ownership, or other equity interest; and expert testimony or patent-licensing arrangements), or non-financial interest (such as personal or professional relationships, affiliations, knowledge or beliefs) in the subject matter or materials discussed in this manuscript.

Ethical Approval All procedures performed in studies involving human participants were in accordance with the ethical standards of the 1964 Helsinki declaration and its later amendments or comparable ethical standards.

Informed Consent No human or animal participants were included in this study.

References

1. Kuhn M, Johnson K. Applied predictive modeling. New York, NY: Springer Science & Business Media; 2013.
2. Steyerberg EW. Clinical prediction models: a practical approach to development, validation, and updating. New York, NY: Springer Science & Business Media; 2008.
3. Senders JT, Zaki MM, Karhade AV, Chang B, Gormley WB, Broekman ML, Smith TR, Arnaout O. An introduction and overview of machine learning in neurosurgical care. Acta Neurochir. 2018;160:29. https://doi.org/10.1007/s00701-017-3385-8.
4. Hastie T, Tibshirani R, Friedman J. The elements of statistical learning: data mining, inference, and prediction. New York, NY: Springer Science & Business Media; 2013.
5. Jordan MI, Mitchell TM. Machine learning: trends, perspectives, and prospects. Science. 2015;349:255. https://doi.org/10.1126/science.aaa8415.
6. Hastie T, Tibshirani R, Wainwright M. Statistical learning with sparsity: the lasso and generalizations. New York, NY: Chapman and Hall; 2015. https://doi.org/10.1201/b18401.
7. Tibshirani R. Regression shrinkage and selection via the Lasso. J R Stat Soc Ser B Methodol. 1996;58:267. https://doi.org/10.1111/j.2517-6161.1996.tb02080.x.
8. Aerts HJWL, Velazquez ER, Leijenaar RTH, et al. Decoding tumour phenotype by noninvasive imaging using a quantitative radiomics approach. Nat Commun. 2014;5:4006. https://doi.org/10.1038/ncomms5006.
9. Li H, Zhu Y, Burnside ES, et al. Quantitative MRI radiomics in the prediction of molecular classifications of breast cancer subtypes in the TCGA/TCIA data set. NPJ Breast Cancer. 2016;2:16012. https://doi.org/10.1038/npjbcancer.2016.12.
10. Thawani R, McLane M, Beig N, Ghose S, Prasanna P, Velcheti V, Madabhushi A. Radiomics and radiogenomics in lung cancer: a review for the clinician. Lung Cancer. 2018;115:34. https://doi.org/10.1016/j.lungcan.2017.10.015.
11. Weng SF, Vaz L, Qureshi N, Kai J. Prediction of premature all-cause mortality: a prospective general population cohort study comparing machine-learning and standard epidemiological approaches. PLoS One. 2019;14(3):e0214365.
12. Mitchell TM. The discipline of machine learning. Mach Learn. 2006;17:1. https://doi.org/10.1080/026404199365326.
13. Keskinbora KH. Medical ethics considerations on artificial intelligence. J Clin Neurosci. 2019;64:277. https://doi.org/10.1016/j.jocn.2019.03.001.
14. Shortliffe EH, Sepúlveda MJ. Clinical decision support in the era of artificial intelligence. JAMA. 2018;320:2199. https://doi.org/10.1001/jama.2018.17163.
15. Grigsby J, Kramer RE, Schneiders JL, Gates JR, Smith WB. Predicting outcome of anterior temporal lobectomy using simulated neural networks. Epilepsia. 1998;39:61. https://doi.org/10.1111/j.1528-1157.1998.tb01275.x.
16. Bzdok D, Krzywinski M, Altman N. Points of significance: machine learning: supervised methods. Nat Methods. 2018;15:5. https://doi.org/10.1038/nmeth.4551.
17. Altman N, Krzywinski M. Points of significance: clustering. Nat Methods. 2017;14:545. https://doi.org/10.1038/nmeth.4299.
18. Murphy KP. Machine learning: a probabilistic perspective. Cambridge, MA: MIT Press; 2012.
19. Wolpert DH. The lack of a priori distinctions between learning algorithms. Neural Comput. 1996;8:1341. https://doi.org/10.1162/neco.1996.8.7.1341.
20. Domingos P. A few useful things to know about machine learning. Commun ACM. 2012;55(10):78.
21. Armañanzas R, Alonso-Nanclares L, DeFelipe-Oroquieta J, Kastanauskaite A, de Sola RG, DeFelipe J, Bielza C, Larrañaga P. Machine learning approach for the outcome prediction of temporal lobe epilepsy surgery. PLoS One. 2013;8:e62819. https://doi.org/10.1371/journal.pone.0062819.
22. Bydon M, Schirmer CM, Oermann EK, Kitagawa RS, Pouratian N, Davies J, Sharan A, Chambless LB. Big data defined: a practical review for neurosurgeons. World Neurosurg. 2020;133:e842. https://doi.org/10.1016/j.wneu.2019.09.092.
23. Senders JT, Staples PC, Karhade AV, Zaki MM, Gormley WB, Broekman MLD, Smith TR, Arnaout O. Machine learning and neurosurgical outcome prediction: a systematic review.

World Neurosurg. 2018;109:476. https://doi.org/10.1016/j.wneu.2017.09.149.
24. Bottou L. Large-scale machine learning with stochastic gradient descent. In: Proc COMPSTAT2010; 2010. https://doi.org/10.1007/978-3-7908-2604-3_16.
25. Ruder S. An overview of gradient descent optimization algorithms. ArXiv. 2017:160904747. Cs.
26. Goodfellow I, Bengio Y, Courville A. Deep learning. Cambridge, MA: MIT Press; 2016.
27. Sra S, Nowozin S, Wright SJ. Optimization for machine learning. Cambridge, MA: MIT Press; 2012.
28. Gravesteijn BY, Nieboer D, Ercole A, Lingsma HF, Nelson D, van Calster B, Steyerberg EW, CENTER-TBI Collaborators. Machine learning algorithms performed no better than regression models for prognostication in traumatic brain injury. J Clin Epidemiol. 2020;122:95–107.
29. Breiman L. Statistical modeling: the two cultures (with comments and a rejoinder by the author). Stat Sci. 2001;16(3):199–231.
30. Bzdok D. Classical statistics and statistical learning in imaging neuroscience. Front Neurosci. 2017;11:543. https://doi.org/10.3389/fnins.2017.00543.
31. Gabrieli JDE, Ghosh SS, Whitfield-Gabrieli S. Prediction as a humanitarian and pragmatic contribution from human cognitive neuroscience. Neuron. 2015;85:11. https://doi.org/10.1016/j.neuron.2014.10.047.
32. Shmueli G. To explain or to predict? Stat Sci. 2011;25(3):289–310.
33. Whelan R, Garavan H. When optimism hurts: inflated predictions in psychiatric neuroimaging. Biol Psychiatry. 2014;75:746. https://doi.org/10.1016/j.biopsych.2013.05.014.
34. Yarkoni T, Westfall J. Choosing prediction over explanation in psychology: lessons from machine learning. Perspect Psychol Sci. 2017;12:1100. https://doi.org/10.1177/1745691617693393.
35. Domingos P. A unified bias-variance decomposition and its applications. In: Proc 17th Int. Conf Mach. Learn. San Francisco, CA: Morgan Kaufmann; 2000. p. 231–8.
36. James G, Hastie T. Generalizations of the bias/variance decomposition for prediction error. Stanford, CA: Department of Statistics, Stanford University; 1997.
37. Abu-Mostafa YS, Malik M-I, Lin HT. Learning from data: a short course. Chicago, IL: AMLBook; 2012. https://doi.org/10.1108/17538271011063889.
38. Van der Laan M, Hubbard AE, Jewell N. Learning FROM DATA. Epidemiology. 2010;21:479. https://doi.org/10.1097/ede.0b013e3181e13328.
39. Harvey H. How to get clinical AI tech approved by regulators. Medium; 2019. https://towardsdatascience.com/how-to-get-clinical-ai-tech-approved-by-regulators-fa16dfa1983b. Accessed 3 May 2020.

Foundations of Machine Learning-Based Clinical Prediction Modeling: Part II—Generalization and Overfitting

3

Julius M. Kernbach and Victor E. Staartjes

3.1 Introduction

In the first part of this review series, we have discussed general and important concepts of machine learning (ML) and presented a four-step workflow for machine learning-based predictive pipelines. However, many regularly faced challenges, which are well-known within the ML community, are less established in the clinical community. One common source of trouble is *overfitting*. It is a common pitfall in predictive modeling, whereby the model not only fits the true underlying relationship of the data but also fits the individual biological or procedural noise associated with each observation. Dealing with overfitting remains challenging in both regression and classification problems. Erroneous pipelines or ill-suited applied models may lead to drastically inflated model performance, and ultimately cause unreliable and potentially harmful clinical conclusions. We discuss and illustrate different strategies to address overfitting in our analyses including *resampling methods*, regularization and penalization of model complexity [1]. In addition, we discuss *feature selection* and *feature reduction*. In this section, we review overfitting as potential danger in predictive analytic strategies with the goal of providing useful recommendations for clinicians to avoid flawed methodologies and conclusions (Table 3.1).

3.2 Overfitting

Overfitting occurs when a given model adjusts too closely to the training data, and subsequently demonstrates poor performance on the testing data (Fig. 3.1). While the model's goodness of fit to the present data sample seems impressive, the model will be unable to make accurate predictions on new observations. This scenario represents a major pitfall in ML. At first, the performance within the training data seems excellent, but when the model's performance is evaluated on the hold-out data ("out-of-sample error") it generalizes poorly. There are various causes of overfitting, some of which are intuitive and easily mitigated. Conceptually, the easiest way to overfit is simply by memorizing observations [2–4].

We simply remember all data patterns, important patterns as well as unimportant ones. For our training data, we will get an exceptional model fit, and minimal training error by recalling the known observations from memory—implying the illusion of success. However, once we test the model's performance on independent test data, we will observe predictive performance that is no better than random. By overtraining on the present data, we end up with a too close fit to the training observations. This fit only partially reflects the underlying true data-generating process, but also includes random noise specific to the training data. This can either be sample-specific noise, both procedural as well as biological, but also the hallucination of unimportant patterns [5]. Appling the overfitted model to new observations will out itself as an out-of-sample performance that is massively worse than the training performance. In this way, the amount of overfitting can be defined as the difference among discriminatory training and testing performance—while it is

J. M. Kernbach and V. E. Staartjes have contributed equally to this series, and share first authorship.

J. M. Kernbach
Neurosurgical Artificial Intelligence Laboratory Aachen (NAILA), Department of Neurosurgery, RWTH Aachen University Hospital, Aachen, Germany

V. E. Staartjes (✉)
Machine Intelligence in Clinical Neuroscience (MICN) Laboratory, Department of Neurosurgery, Clinical Neuroscience Center, University Hospital Zurich, University of Zurich, Zurich, Switzerland
e-mail: victoregon.staartjes@usz.ch; https://micnlab.com/

V. E. Staartjes et al. (eds.), *Machine Learning in Clinical Neuroscience*, Acta Neurochirurgica Supplement 134,
https://doi.org/10.1007/978-3-030-85292-4_3

Table 3.1 Concept summaries

Concept	Explanation
Noise	Noise is unexplained and random variation inherent to the data (biological noise) or introduced by variables of no interest (procedural noise, including measurement errors, site variation).
Overfitting	Over-learning of random patterns associated with noise or memorization in the training data. Overfitting leads to a drastically decreased ability to generalize to new observations.
Bias	Bias quantifies the error term introduced by approximating highly complicated real-life problems by a much simpler statistical model. Models with high bias tend to underfit.
Variance	Variance refers to learning random structure irresponsible of the underlying true signal. Models with high variance tend to overfit.
Data Leakage/ Contamination	Or the concept of "looking at data twice". Overfitting is introduced when observations used for testing also re-occur in the training process. The model then "remembers" instead of learning the underlying association.
Model Selection	Iterative process using resampling such as *k*-fold cross-validation to fit different models in the training set.
Model Assessment	Evaluation of a model's out-of-sample performance. This should be conducted on a test set of data that was set aside and not used in training or model selection. The use of multiple measures of performance (AUC, F1, etc.) is recommended.
Resampling	Resampling methods fit a model multiple times on different subsets of the training data. Popular methods are *k*-fold cross-validation and the bootstrap.
k-Fold Cross-Validation	Data is divided in *k* equally sized folds/sets. Iteratively, $k - 1$ data is used for training and evaluated on the remaining unseen fold. Each fold is used for testing once.
LOOCV	LOOCV (leave-one-out cross-validation) is a variation of cross-validation. Each observation is left out once, the model is trained on the remaining data, and then evaluated on the held-out observation.
Bootstrap	The bootstrap allows to estimate the uncertainty associated with any given model. Typically, in 1000–10,000 iterations bootstrapped samples are repetitively drawn with replacement from the original data, the predictive model is iteratively fit and evaluated.
Hyperparameter Tuning	Hyperparameters define how a statistical model learns and need to be specified before training. They are model specific and might include regularization parameters penalizing model's complexity (ridge, lasso), number of trees and their depth (random forest), and many more. Hyperparameters can be tuned, that is, iteratively improved to find the model that performs best given the complexity of the available data.

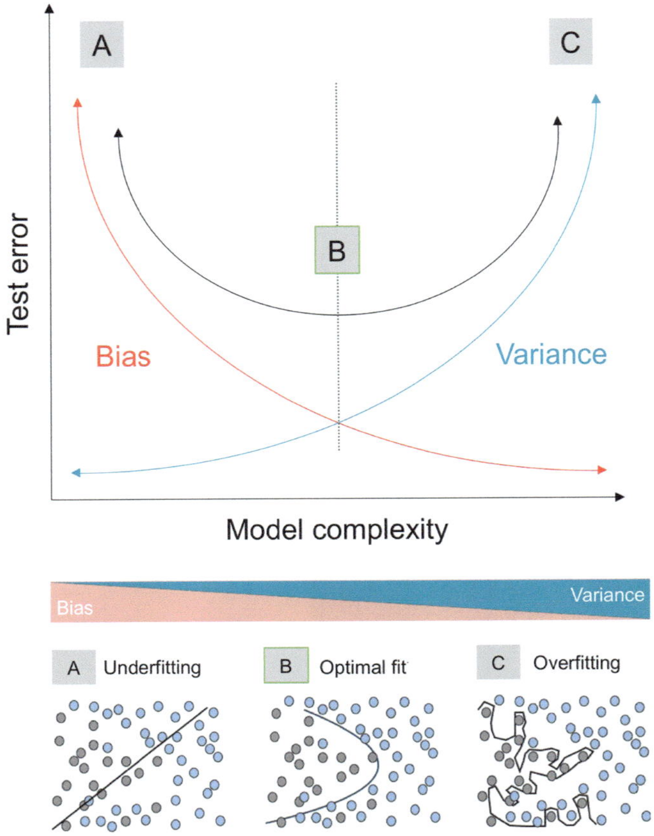

Fig. 3.1 Conceptual visualization of the bias-variance trade-off. A predictive model with *high bias* and *low variance* (**A**), consistently approximates the underlying data-generating process with a much simpler model (here a hyperplane), and hence result in an underfit solution. (**B**) A U-shaped decision boundary represents the optimal solution in this scenario, here, both bias and variance are low, resulting in the lowest test error. (**C**) Applying an overly flexible model results in overfitting. Data quirks and random non-predictive structures that are unrelated to the underlying signal are learned

normal that out-of-sample performance is equal to or ever so slightly worse than training performance for any adequately fitted model, a massive difference suggests relevant overfitting. This is one reason why in-sample model performance should never be reported as evidence for predictive performance. Instead model training and selection should always be performed on a separate train set, and only in the final step should the final model be evaluated on an independent test set to judge true out-of-sample performance.

The Bias-Variance Trade-Off

In ML we opt to make accurate and generalizable predictions. When the test error is significantly higher than the training error, we can diagnose overfitting. To understand what is going on we can decompose the predictive error into its essential parts *bias* and *variance* [6, 7]. Their competing nature, commonly known under the term *bias-variance trade-off*, is very important and notoriously famous in the machine learning community. Despite its fame and importance, the concept is less prominent within the clinical community. *Bias* quantifies the error term introduced by approximating highly complicated real-life problems by a much simpler statistical model, that is underfitting the complexity of the data-generating process. In other words, a model with high bias tends to consistently learn the wrong response. That by itself does not necessarily need to be a problem, as simple models were often found to perform very well sometimes even better than more sophisticated ones [8]. However, for maximal predictive compacity we need to find the perfect balance between bias and variance. The term *variance* refers to learning random structure irresponsible of the underlying true signal. That is, models with high variance can hallucinate patterns that are not given by the reality of the data. Figure 3.1 illustrates this in a classification problem. A linear model (Fig. 3.1a, high bias and low variance) applied to class data, in which the frontier between the two classes is not a hyperplane, is unable to induce the underlying true boundary. It will consistently learn the wrong response, that is a hyperplane, despite the more complex true decision boundary and result into "underfitting" the true data-generating process. On the other extreme, an excessively flexible model with high variance and low bias (Fig. 3.1c) will learn random non-predictive structure that is unrelated to the underlying signal. Given minimally different observations, the overly flexible model fit could drastically change in an instance. The latter complex model would adapt well to all training observations but would ultimately fail to generalize and predict new observations in an independent test set. Neither the extremely flexible nor the insufficiently flexible model is capable of generalizing to new observations.

Combatting Overfitting: Resampling

We could potentially collect more data for an independent cohort to test our model, but this would be highly time-consuming and expensive. In rich data situations, we can alternatively split our sample into a data set for training and a second set for testing (or hold-out set) to evaluate the model's performance in new data (i.e., the model's out-of-sample performance) more honestly. We would typically use a random 80%/20% split for training and testing (while remaining class balance within the training set, see Chap. 4). Because we often lack a sufficiently large cohort of patients to simply evaluate generalization performance using data splits, we need to use a less data-hungry but equally efficient alternatives. The gold standard and popular approach in machine learning to address overfitting is to evaluate the model's generalization ability via *resampling methods* [9]. Some of these resampling methods—particularly the bootstrap—have already long been used in inferential statistical analysis to generate measures of variance [10]. Resampling methods are an indispensable tool in today's modern data science and include various forms of *cross-validation* [3, 11]. All forms have a common ground: they involve splitting the available data iteratively into a non-overlapping train and test set. Our statistical model is then refitted and tested for each subset of the train and test data to obtain an estimate of generalization performance. Most modern resampling methods have been derived from the jackknife—a resampling technique developed by Maurice Quenouille in 1949 [12]. The simplest modern variation of cross-validation—also based on the jackknife—is known as leave-one-out cross-validation (LOOCV). In LOOCV, the data (n) is iteratively divided into two unequal subsets with the train set of $n - 1$ observations and the test set containing the remaining one observation. The model is refitted and evaluated on the excluded held-out observation. The procedure is then repeated n times and the test error is then averaged over all iterations. A more popular alternative to LOOCV and generally considered the gold standard is k-fold cross-validation (Fig. 3.2). The k-fold approach randomly divides the available data into a k amount of non-overlapping groups, or folds, of approximately equal size. Empirically, $k = 5$ or $k = 10$ are preferred and commonly used [13]. Each fold is selected as test set once, and the model is fitted on the remaining $k - 1$ folds. The average over all fold-wise performances estimates the generalizability of a given statistical model. Within this procedure, importantly, no observation is selected for both training and testing. This is essential, because, as discussed earlier, predicting an observation that was already learned during training equals memorization, which in turn leads to overfitted conclusions.

Cross-validation is routinely used in both model selection and model assessment. Yet another extremely powerful and popular resampling strategy is the *bootstrap* [14, 15], which allows for the estimation of the accuracy's uncertainty applicable to nearly any statistical method. Here, we obtain new bootstrapped sets of data by repeatedly sampling observations from the original data set *with replacement*, which means any observation can occur more than once in the bootstrapped data sample. Thus, when applying the bootstrap, we repeatedly randomly select n patients from an n-sized training dataset, and model performance is evaluated after every iteration. This process is repeated many times—usually with 25–1000 repetitions.

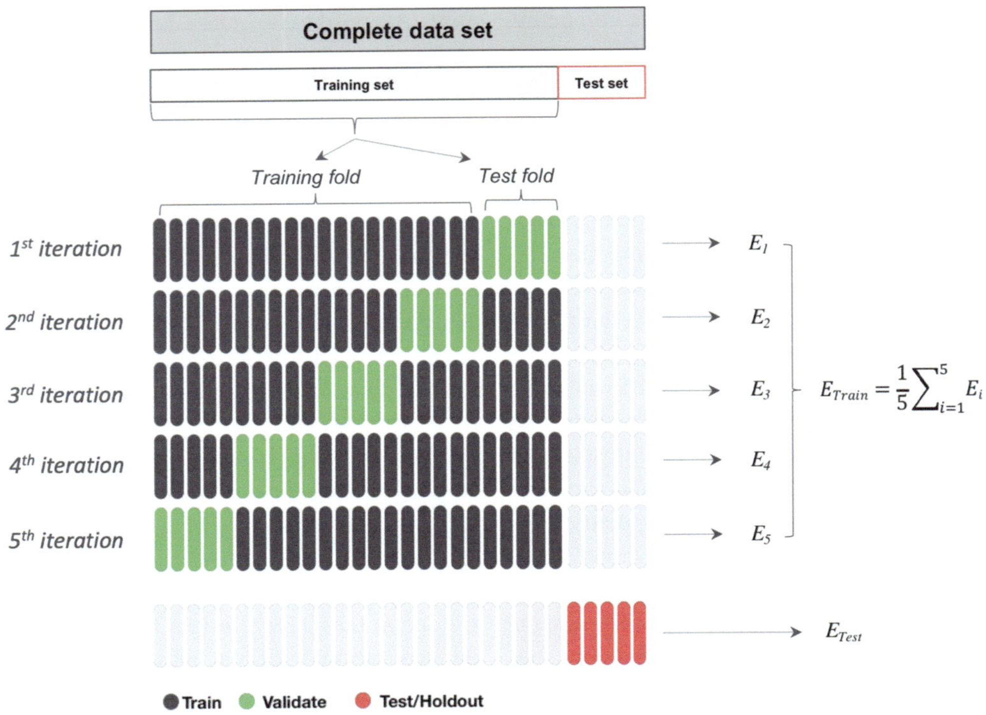

Fig. 3.2 *k*-fold cross-validation with an independent hold-out set. The complete dataset is portioned into training data (~80%) and testing data (~20%) before any resampling is applied. Within the training set, *k*-fold cross-validation is used to randomly divide the available data into $k = 5$ equally sized folds. Iteratively, $k - 1$ folds are used to train a chosen model, and the fold-wise performance (E_k) is evaluated on the remaining unseen validation fold. These fold-wise performances are averaged, and together, the out-of-sample performance is estimated as E_{Train}. When different models are trained, the best performing one is selected and tuned (model selection, hyperparameter tuning) and evaluated on the independent hold-out set (or "test set"). The resulting performance E_{Test} is reported and estimates the predictive performance beyond the present data

Considerations on Algorithm Complexity

To avoid over- or underfitting, an appropriate level of model complexity is required [11, 16]. Modulating complexity can be achieved by adding a regularization term, which can be used with any type of predictive model. In that instance, the regularization term is added to favor less-complex models with less room to overfit. As complexity is intrinsically related to the number and magnitude of parameters, we can add a regularization or penalty term to control the magnitude of the model parameters, or even constrain the number of parameters used. There are many different penalties specific to selected models. In a regression setting, we could add either a *L1 penalty* (LASSO, least absolute shrinkage and selection operator), which selectively removes variables form the model, a *L2 penalty* (Ridge or Tikhonov regularization), which shrinks the magnitude of parameters but never fully removes them from the model or an *elastic net* (combination of L1 and L2) [13, 17, 18]. For neural networks, *dropout* is a very efficient regularization method [19]. Finding the right balance based on regularization, that is, to define how complex a model can be, is controlled by the model's hyperparameters (L1 or L2 penalty term in regression, and many more). Restraining model complexity by adding a regularization term is an example of a model hyperparameter. Typically, hyperparameters are *tuned*, which means that the optimal level is evaluated during model training. Again, it is important to respect the distinction of train and test data. As a simple guideline, we recommend to automate all necessary pre-processing steps including hyperparameter tuning within the chosen resampling approach to ensure none of the above are performed on the complete data set before cross-validation [20]. Otherwise, this would result in circularity and inflate the overall predictive performance [21].

Data Leakage

Whenever resampling techniques are applied, the investigator has to ensure that *data leakage* or *data contamination* is not accidently introduced. From the standpoint of ML, data contamination—part of the test data leaking into the model-fitting procedure—can have severe consequences, and lead to drastically inflated predictive performance. Therefore, caution needs to be allocated to the clean isolation of train and test data. As a general rule-of-thumb, no feature selection or dimensionality reduction method that involves the outcome measure should be performed on the complete data set before cross-validation or splitting. This would open doors for procedural bias, and raise concerns regarding model validity. Additionally, nested cross-validation should be used in model selection and hyperparameter tuning. The nestedness adds an additional internal cross-validation loop to guarantee clean distinction between the "test data" for model selection and tuning and ultimately the "test data" used for model performance assessment.

Usually the data splits are then named "train"—"test"—"(external) validation," however, different nomenclatures are frequently used.

While resampling techniques can mitigate overfitting, they can also lead to manual overfitting when too many hyperparameter choices are made in the process [22]. Another consideration to keep in mind is that whenever a random data split is selected, it is with the assumption that each split is representative of the full data set. This can become problematic in two cases: (1) When data is dependent, data leakage occurs when train and test data share non-independent observations, such as the inclusion of both the index and revision surgery of patients. Both observations are systematically similar, induce overfitting and ultimately undermine the validity of the resulting model performance. (2) When data is not identically distributed: this is a serious problem in small sample scenarios, where splits are drawn out of a highly variable set of observations. Depending on which of the patients end up in the train or test data, the model performance can greatly fluctuate, and can be an overly optimistic estimate of predictive performance. Generally, less inflated predictive performance can be observed as the sample size increases [23]. As studies based on small sample sizes can generate highly variable estimates, conclusions may often be exaggerated or even invalid. Hence, predictive modeling should be restricted or used with caution when only small amounts of data are available. Considerations regarding sample size are discussed in *Part III*.

3.3 Importance of External Validation in Clinical Prediction Modeling

External validation of clinical prediction models represents an important part in their development and rollout [24, 25]. In order to generalize, the input data, i.e. the training sample, needs to be *representative*. However, without external validation, the *site bias* or *center bias*, which includes variations in treatment protocols, surgical techniques, level of experience between departments and clinical users, as well as the so-called *sampling/selection bias*, which refers to systematically different data collection in regard to the patient cohort, cannot be detected. For these reasons, an empirical assessment of model performance on an unrelated, "external" data-set is required before an application can publicly be released. Erroneous or biased predictions can have severe sequelae for patients and clinicians alike, if misjudgments are made based upon such predictions. As a gold standard, external validation enables *unbiased testing* of model performance in a new cohort with different demographics. If a clinical prediction model shows comparable discrimination and calibration performance at external validation, generalizability may be confirmed. Then, it may be safe to release the model into the clinical decision-making progress. As an alternative to external validation—certainly the gold standard to ensure generalizability of a clinical prediction model—one might consider prospective internal validation (i.e. validation on a totally new sample of patients who are, however, derived from the same center with the same demographics, surgeons, and treatment protocols as the originally developed model). While prospective internal validation will also identify any overfitting that might be present, and will enable safe use of the prediction model at that specific center, this method does not allow ruling out center bias, i.e. does not ensure the safe use of the model in other populations.

3.4 Feature Reduction and Selection

In overtly complex and high-dimensional data with too many parameters, we find ourselves in an over-parameterized analytical setting. However, due to 'the curse of dimensionality'—a term famously coined by Richard Bellmann in 1961—generalization becomes increasingly more difficult in high dimensions. The approach to avoid "the curse" has been to find lower representation of the given feature space [26]. If there were too many features or variables present, *feature reduction* or *feature selection* methods can be applied. In *feature reduction*, methods are applied to simplify the complexity of the given high-dimensional data while retaining important and innate patterns of the data. Principal component analysis (PCA) is a popular illustration [27]. As an unsupervised ML method PCA is conceptually similar to clustering, and learns from data without any reference or a priori knowledge of the predicted outcome. Analytically, PCA reduces high-dimensional data by projecting them onto the so-called principal components, which represent summaries of the data in fewer dimensions. PCA can hence be used as a strong statistical tool to reduce the main axis of variance within a given feature space. *Feature selection* refers to a similar procedure, which is also applied to initially too large feature spaces to reduce the number of input features. The key in feature selection is not to summarize data into lower dimensions as in feature reduction, but to actually reduce the number of included features to end up with only the "most useful" ones—and eliminate all non-informative ones. Naturally, if certain domain knowledge is present, vast sets of features can be constructed to a better set of informative features. For instance, in brain imaging, voxels of an MRI scan can either be considered individually or can be summarized into functionally or anatomically homogenous areas—a concept of topographical segregation that dates back to Brodmann [28, 29]. The problem of feature selection is well-known in the ML community and has generated a vast body of literature early on [30, 31]. A common pruning technique to select features that together maximize, e.g. classification performance is *recursive feature elimination* (RFE) [32, 33]. In RFE, a given classifier or regressor is iteratively trained, and a ranking criterion for all features is estimated. The feature with the smallest respective ranking criterion is then eliminated. Introduced by Guyon and colleagues [32], RFE was initially used to extract small subsets of highly discriminant genes in DNA arrays and build reliable cancer classifiers. As an instance of backward elimination—that is, we start with the complete set of variables and progressively eliminate the least informative features—RFE can be used both in classification and regression settings with any given learner, but remains computationally greedy ("brute force"), as many different, e.g. classifiers on feature subsets of decreasing size are revisited. As an important consideration, RFE selects *subsets* of variables based on an optimal *subset* ranking criterion. Consequently, a group of features combined may lead to optimal predictive performance, while the individual features included do not necessarily have to be the most important. Embedded in the process of model training, variable selection procedures such as RFE can improve performance by selecting subsets of variables that together maximize predictive power. Importantly, resampling methods should be applied when using RFE to factor in the variability caused by feature selection when calculating performance.

3.5 Conclusion

Overfitting is a multifactorial problem, and there are just as many possible approaches to reduce its negative impact. We encourage the use of resampling methods such as cross-validation in every predictive modeling pipeline. While there are various options to choose from, we recommend the usage of k-fold cross-validation or the bootstrap. Nested loops may be used for hyperparameter tuning and model selection. While the use of resampling does not solve overfitting, it helps to gain a more representative understanding of the predictive performance, especially of out-of-sample error. Feature reduction and selection methods, such as PCA and RFE are introduced for handling high-dimensional data. A potential pitfall along the way is *data contamination*, which occurs when data leaks from the resampled test to train set and hence leads to overconfident model performance. We encourage the use of standardized pipelines (see Chaps. 5 and 6 here for examples), which include feature engineering, hyperparameter tuning and model selection within one loop to minimize the risk of unintentionally leaking test data. Finally, we recommend including a regularization term as hyperparameter and to restrict extensive model complexity, which will avoid overfitted predictive performance.

Disclosures

Funding No funding was received for this research.

Conflict of Interest All authors certify that they have no affiliations with or involvement in any organization or entity with any financial interest (such as honoraria; educational grants; participation in speakers' bureaus; membership, employment, consultancies, stock ownership, or other equity interest; and expert testimony or patent-licensing arrangements), or non-financial interest (such as personal or professional relationships, affiliations, knowledge or beliefs) in the subject matter or materials discussed in this manuscript.

Ethical Approval All procedures performed in studies involving human participants were in accordance with the ethical standards of the 1964 Helsinki declaration and its later amendments or comparable ethical standards.

Informed Consent No human or animal participants were included in this study.

References

1. Domingos P. Process-oriented estimation of generalization error. In: IJCAI Int. Jt. Conf. Artif. Intell; 1999. p. 714–9.
2. Arplt D, Jastrzebskl S, Bailas N, et al. A closer look at memorization in deep networks. In: 34th Int. Conf. Mach. Learn. ICML 2017; 2017.
3. Goodfellow I, Yoshua Bengio AC. Deep learning book. In: Deep learn. Cambridge, MA: MIT Press; 2015. https://doi.org/10.1016/B978-0-12-391420-0.09987-X.
4. Zhang C, Vinyals O, Munos R, Bengio S. A study on overfitting in deep reinforcement learning. ArXiv. 2018:180406893.
5. Domingos P. A few useful things to know about machine learning. Commun ACM. 2012;55(10):78.
6. Domingos P. A unified bias-variance decomposition and its applications. In: Proc 17th Int. Conf Mach. Learn. San Francisco, CA: Morgan Kaufmann; 2000. p. 231–8.
7. James G, Hastie T. Generalizations of the bias/variance decomposition for prediction error. Stanford, CA: Department of Statistics, Stanford University; 1997.
8. Holte RC. Very simple classification rules perform well on most commonly used datasets. Mach Learn. 1993;11:63. https://doi.org/10.1023/A:1022631118932.
9. Staartjes VE, Kernbach JM. Letter to the editor regarding "Investigating risk factors and predicting complications in deep brain stimulation surgery with machine learning algorithms". World Neurosurg. 2020;137:496.
10. Davison AC, Hinkley DV. Bootstrap methods and their application. Cambridge: Cambridge University Press; 1997.
11. Gravesteijn BY, Nieboer D, Ercole A, Lingsma HF, Nelson D, van Calster B, Steyerberg EW, CENTER-TBI Collaborators. Machine

learning algorithms performed no better than regression models for prognostication in traumatic brain injury. J Clin Epidemiol. 2020;122:95–107.
12. Quenouille MH. Notes on bias in estimation. Biometrika. 1956;43(3–4):353–60.
13. Hastie T, Tibshirani R, Friedman J. The elements of statistical learning: data mining, inference, and prediction. New York, NY: Springer Science & Business Media; 2013.
14. Efron B, Tibshirani RJ. An introduction to the bootstrap. New York, NY: Chapman and Hall; 1993. https://doi.org/10.1007/978-1-4899-4541-9.
15. Hastie T, Tibshirani R, James G, Witten D. An introduction to statistical learning. New York, NY: Springer; 2006. https://doi.org/10.1016/j.peva.2007.06.006.
16. Staartjes VE, Kernbach JM. Letter to the editor. Importance of calibration assessment in machine learning-based predictive analytics. J Neurosurg Spine. 2020;32:985–7.
17. Lever J, Krzywinski M, Altman N. Points of significance: regularization. Nat Methods. 2016;13:803. https://doi.org/10.1038/nmeth.4014.
18. Zou H, Hastie T. Regularization and variable selection via the elastic net. J R Stat Soc Ser B Stat Methodol. 2005;67:301. https://doi.org/10.1111/j.1467-9868.2005.00503.x.
19. Srivastava N, Hinton G, Krizhevsky A, Sutskever I, Salakhutdinov R. Dropout: a simple way to prevent neural networks from overfitting. J Mach Learn Res. 2014;15(1):1929–58.
20. Poldrack RA, Huckins G, Varoquaux G. Establishment of best practices for evidence for prediction: a review. JAMA Psychiatry. 2019;77:534. https://doi.org/10.1001/jamapsychiatry.2019.3671.
21. Kriegeskorte N, Simmons WK, Bellgowan PS, Baker CI. Circular analysis in systems neuroscience: the dangers of double dipping. Nat Neurosci. 2009;12:535. https://doi.org/10.1038/nn.2303.
22. Ng AY. Preventing "overfitting" of cross-validation data. CEUR Workshop Proc. 2015;1542:33. https://doi.org/10.1017/CBO9781107415324.004.
23. Varoquaux G. Cross-validation failure: small sample sizes lead to large error bars. NeuroImage. 2018;180:68. https://doi.org/10.1016/j.neuroimage.2017.06.061.
24. Collins GS, Ogundimu EO, Le Manach Y. Assessing calibration in an external validation study. Spine J. 2015;15:2446. https://doi.org/10.1016/j.spinee.2015.06.043.
25. Staartjes VE, Schröder ML. Class imbalance in machine learning for neurosurgical outcome prediction: are our models valid? J Neurosurg Spine. 2018;26:736. https://doi.org/10.3171/2018.5.SPINE18543.
26. Breiman L. Statistical modeling: the two cultures (with comments and a rejoinder by the author). Stat Sci. 2001;16(3):199–231.
27. Lever J, Krzywinski M, Altman N. Points of significance: principal component analysis. Nat Methods. 2017;14:641. https://doi.org/10.1038/nmeth.4346.
28. Amunts K, Zilles K. Architectonic mapping of the human brain beyond brodmann. Neuron. 2015;88:1086. https://doi.org/10.1016/j.neuron.2015.12.001.
29. Glasser MF, Coalson TS, Robinson EC, et al. A multi-modal parcellation of human cerebral cortex. Nature. 2016;536:171. https://doi.org/10.1038/nature18933.
30. Blum AL, Langley P. Selection of relevant features and examples in machine learning. Artif Intell. 1997;97:245. https://doi.org/10.1016/s0004-3702(97)00063-5.
31. Kohavi R, John GH. Wrappers for feature subset selection. Artif Intell. 1997;97:273. https://doi.org/10.1016/s0004-3702(97)00043-x.
32. Guyon I, Weston J, Barnhill S, Vapnik V. Gene selection for cancer classification using support vector machines. Mach Learn. 2002;46:389. https://doi.org/10.1023/A:1012487302797.
33. Iguyon I, Elisseeff A. An introduction to variable and feature selection. J Mach Learn Res. 2003;3:1157. https://doi.org/10.1162/153244303322753616.

Foundations of Machine Learning-Based Clinical Prediction Modeling: Part III—Model Evaluation and Other Points of Significance

4

Victor E. Staartjes and Julius M. Kernbach

4.1 Introduction

Once a dataset has been adequately prepared and a training structure (e.g. with a resampling method such as *k*-fold cross validation, see Chap. 3) has been set up, a model is ready to be trained. Already during training and the subsequent model tuning and selection, metrics to evaluate model performance become of central importance, as the hyperparameters and parameters of the models are tuned according to one or multiple of these performance metrics. In addition, after a final model has been selected based on these metrics, internal or external validation should be carried out to assess whether the same performance metrics can be achieved as during training. This section walks the reader through some of the common performance metrics to evaluate the discrimination and calibration of clinical prediction models based on machine learning (ML). We focus on clinical prediction models for continuous and binary endpoints, as these are by far the most common clinical applications of ML in neurosurgery. Multiclass classification—thus, the prediction of a categorical endpoint with more than two levels—may require other performance metrics.

Second, when developing a new clinical prediction model, there are several caveats and other points of significance that the readers should be aware of. These include what sample size is necessary for a robust model, how to pre-process data correctly, how to handle missing data and class imbalance, how to choose a cutoff for binary classification, and why extrapolation is problematic. In the second part of this section, these topics are sequentially discussed.

J. M. Kernbach and V. E. Staartjes have contributed equally to this series, and share first authorship.

V. E. Staartjes (✉)
Machine Intelligence in Clinical Neuroscience (MICN) Laboratory, Department of Neurosurgery, Clinical Neuroscience Center, University Hospital Zurich, University of Zurich, Zurich, Switzerland
e-mail: victoregon.staartjes@usz.ch; https://micnlab.com/

J. M. Kernbach
Neurosurgical Artificial Intelligence Laboratory Aachen (NAILA), Department of Neurosurgery, RWTH Aachen University Hospital, Aachen, Germany

4.2 Evaluation of Classification Models

The Importance of Discrimination and Calibration

The performance of classification models can roughly be judged along two dimensions: Model discrimination and calibration [1]. The term *discrimination* denotes the ability of a prediction model to correctly classify whether a certain patient is going to or is not going to experience a certain outcome. Thus, discrimination described the accuracy of a binary prediction—yes or no. *Calibration*, however, describes the degree to which a model's predicted probabilities (ranging from 0% to 100%) correspond to the actually observed incidence of the binary endpoint (true posterior). Many publications do not report calibration metrics, although these are of central importance, as a well-calibrated predicted probability (e.g. your predicted probability of experiencing a complication is 18%) is often much more valuable to clinicians—and patients!—than a binary prediction (e.g. you are likely not going to experience a complication) [1].

There are other factors that should be considered when selecting models, such as complexity and interpretability of the algorithm, how well a model calibrates out-of-the-box, as well as e.g. the computing power necessary [2]. For instance, choosing an overly complex algorithm for relatively simple data (i.e. a deep neural network for tabulated medical data) will vastly increase the likelihood of overfitting with only negligible benefits in performance. Similarly, even though discrimination performance may be ever so slightly better with a more complex model such as a neural network, this

V. E. Staartjes et al. (eds.), *Machine Learning in Clinical Neuroscience*, Acta Neurochirurgica Supplement 134,
https://doi.org/10.1007/978-3-030-85292-4_4

comes at the cost of reduced interpretability ("black box" models) [3]. The term "black box" model denotes a model for which we may know the input variables are fed into it and the predicted outcome, although there is no information on the inner workings of the model, i.e. why a certain prediction was made for an individual patient and which variables were most impactful. This is often the case for highly complex models such as deep neural networks or gradient boosting machines. For these models, usually only a broad "variable importance" metric that described a ranking of the input variables in order of importance can be calculated and should in fact be reported. However, how exactly the model integrated these inputs and arrived at the prediction cannot be comprehended in highly complex models [3]. In contrast, simpler ML algorithms, such as generalized linear models (GLMs) or generalized additive models (GAMs), which often suffice for clinical prediction modeling, provide interpretability in the form of odds ratios or partial dependence metrics, respectively. Lastly, highly complex models often exhibit poorer calibration out-of-the-box [2].

Consequently, the single final model to be internally or externally validated, published, and readied for clinical use should not only be chosen based on resampled training performance [4]. Instead, the complexity of the dataset (i.e. tabulated patient data versus a set of DICOM images) should be taken into account. Whenever suitable, highly interpretable models such as generalized linear models or generalized additive models should be used. Overly complex models such as deep neural networks should generally be avoided for basic clinical prediction modeling.

Model Discrimination

For a comprehensive assessment of model discrimination, the following data are necessary for each patient in the sample: A true outcome (also called "label" or "true posterior"), the predicted probabilities produced by the model, and the classification result based on that predicted probability (predicted outcome). To compare the predicted outcomes and the true outcomes, a confusion matrix (Table 4.1) can be generated. Nearly all discrimination metrics can then be derived from the confusion matrix.

Area Under the Curve (AUC)

The only common discrimination metric that cannot be derived directly from the confusion matrix is the area under the receiver operating characteristic curve (AUROC, commonly abbreviated to AUC or ROC, also called c-statistic). For AUC, the predicted probabilities are instead contrasted with the true outcomes. The curve (Fig. 4.1) shows the performance of a classification model at all binary classification cutoffs, plotting the true positive rate (Sensitivity) against the false positive rate (1—Specificity). Lowering the binary classification cutoff classifies more patients as positive, thus increasing both false positives and true positives. It follows that AUC is the only common discrimination metric that is uniquely not contingent upon the chosen binary classification cutoff. The binary classification cutoff at the top left point of the curve, known as the "closest-to-(0,1)-criterion," can even be used to derive an optimal binary classification cutoff, which is explained in more detail further on [5]. Models are often trained and selected for AUC, as AUC can give a relatively broad view of a model's discriminative ability. An AUC value of 1.0 indicates perfect discrimination, while an AUC of 0.5 indicates a discriminative performance not superior to random prediction. Usually, a model is considered to perform well if an AUC of 0.7 or 0.8 is achieved. An AUC above 0.9 indicated excellent performance.

Table 4.1 A confusion matrix

	Negative label	Positive label
Predicted Negative	800 (*True Negative*)	174 (*False Negative*)
Predicted Positive	157 (*False Positive*)	869 (*True Positive*)

Accuracy

$$\text{Accuracy} = \frac{\text{TP} + \text{TN}}{P + N}$$

Based on the confusion matrix, a model's accuracy equals the total proportion of patients who were correctly classified as either positive or negative cases. While accuracy can give

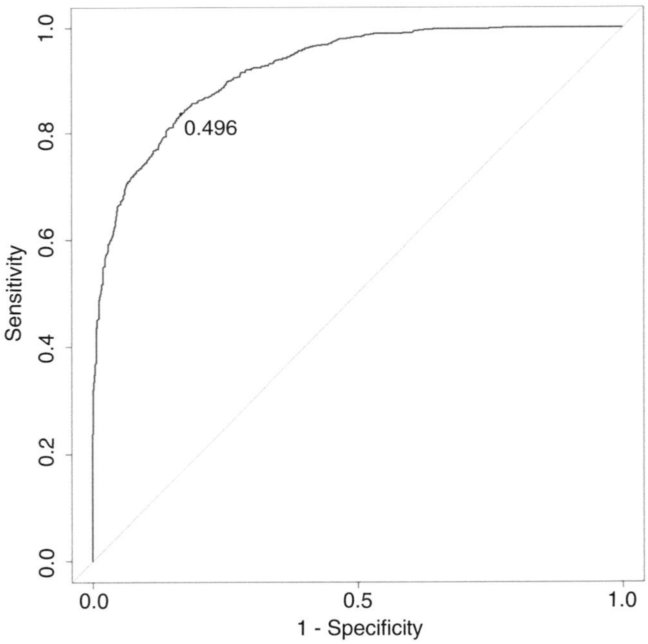

Fig. 4.1 Area under the receiver operating characteristic curve (AUC) plot demonstrating an AUC of 0.922. The plot also indicated that, according to the "closest-to-(0,1)-criterion", 0.496 is the optimal binary classification cutoff that balances sensitivity and specificity perfectly

a broad overview of model performance, it is important to also consider sensitivity and specificity, as accuracy can be easily skewed by several factors including class imbalance (a caveat discussed in detail later on). An accuracy of 100% is optimal, while an accuracy of 50% indicates a performance that is equal to random predictions. The confusion matrix in Table 4.1 gives an accuracy of 83.5%.

Sensitivity and Specificity

$$\text{Sensitivity} = \frac{\text{TP}}{P}$$

$$\text{Specificity} = \frac{\text{TN}}{N}$$

Sensitivity denotes the proportion of patients who are positive cases and who were indeed correctly predicted to be positive. Conversely, specificity measures the proportion of patients who are negative cases, and who were correctly predicted to be negative. Thus, a prediction model with high sensitivity generates only few false negatives, and the model can be used to "rule-out" patients if the prediction is negative. A model with high specificity, however, can be used to "rule-in" patients if positive, because it produces only few false positives. In data science, sensitivity is sometimes called "recall." The confusion matrix in Table 4.1 gives a sensitivity of 83.3% and a specificity of 83.6%.

Positive Predictive Value (PPV) and Negative Predictive Value (NPV)

$$\text{PPV} = \frac{\text{TP}}{\text{TP} + \text{FP}}$$

$$\text{NPV} = \frac{\text{TN}}{\text{TN} + \text{FN}}$$

PPV is defined as the proportion of positively predicted patients who are indeed true positive cases. Conversely, NPV is defined as the proportion of negatively predicted patients who turn out to be true negatives. PPV and NPV are often said to be more easily clinically interpretably in the context of clinical prediction modeling than sensitivity and specificity, as they relate more directly to the prediction itself: For a model with a high PPV, a positive prediction is very likely to be correct, and for a model with a high NPV, a negative prediction is very likely to be a true negative. In data science, PPV is sometimes called "precision." The confusion matrix in Table 4.1 gives a PPV of 84.7% and a NPV of 82.1%.

F1 Score

$$\text{F1} = 2 \times \frac{\text{PPV} \times \text{Sensitivity}}{\text{PPV} + \text{Sensitivity}}$$

The F1 score is a composite metric popular in the ML community, which is mathematically defined as the harmonic mean of PPV and sensitivity. Higher values represent better performance, with a maximum of 1.0. The F1 score is also commonly used to train and select models during training. The confusion matrix in Table 4.1 gives a F1 score of 0.840.

Model Calibration

Calibration Intercept and Slope

As stated above, calibration describes the degree to which a model's predicted probabilities (ranging from 0% to 100%) correspond to the actually observed incidence of the binary endpoint (true posterior). Especially for clinically applied models, a well-calibrated predicted probability (e.g. your predicted probability of experiencing a complication is 18%) is often much more valuable to clinicians and patients alike than a binary prediction (e.g. you are likely not going to experience a complication) [1]. A quick overview of a model's calibration can be gained from generating a calibration plot (Fig. 4.2), which we recommend to include for every published clinical prediction model. In a calibration plot, the patients of a certain cohort are stratified into g equally-sized groups ranked according to their predicted probabilities. If you have a large cohort available, opt for $g = 10$; if you have only few patients you may opt for $g = 5$ to smooth the calibration curve to a certain degree. On the y axis, for each of the g groups, the observed proportion of positive cases is

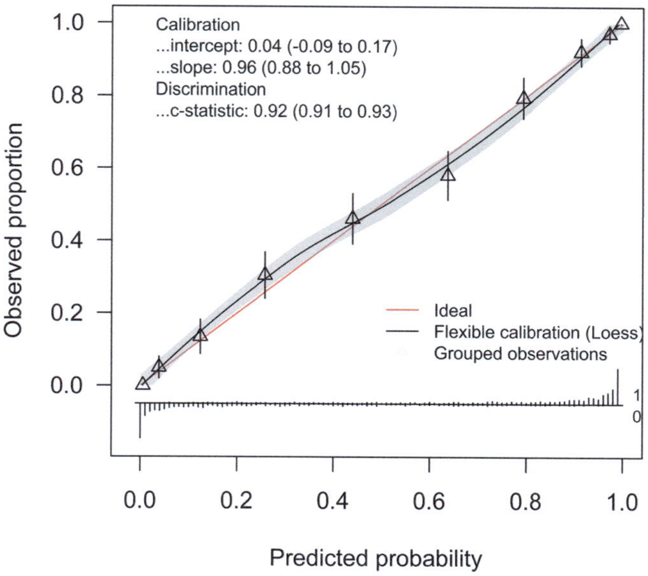

Fig. 4.2 Calibration plot comparing the predicted probabilities—divided into ten bins—of a binary classification model to the true observed outcome proportions. The diagonal line represents the ideal calibration curve. A smoother has been fit over the ten bins. This model achieved an excellent calibration intercept of 0.04, with a slope of 0.96

plotted, while the mean predicted probability for each group is plotted on the x-axis. A model with perfect calibration will have a calibration curve closely resembling a diagonal line. A poorly calibrated model will deviate in some way from the ideal diagonal line, or simply show an erratic form. From the predicted probabilities and the true posteriors, the two major calibration metrics can be derived: Calibration intercept and slope [6].

The calibration intercept, also called "calibration-in-the-large," is a measure of overall calibration—A perfectly calibrated model has an intercept of 0.00. A model with a calibration intercept much larger than 0 generally puts out too high predicted probabilities—and thus overestimates the likelihood of a positive outcome. Likewise, a model with a negative intercept systematically underestimates probabilities. The model depicted in Fig. 4.1 sports an intercept of 0.04.

The calibration slope quantifies the increase of true risk compared to predicted risk. A perfectly calibrated model has an intercept of 1.00. If a model has a calibration slope that is much larger than 1, the increase of the predicted probabilities on the calibration curve is too steep, and vice versa.

Brier Score

The Brier score [7] measures overall calibration and is defined as the average squared difference between predicted probabilities and true outcomes. It takes on values between 0 and 1, with lower values indicating better calibration. As a proper scoring rule, the Brier score simultaneously captures calibration itself as well as sharpness: A property that measures how much variation there is in the true probability across predictions. When assessing the performance of different binary classification models, the Brier score is mainly used to compare model performances, and—being mainly a relative measure—the actual value of the score is only of limited value. As a caveat, the Brier score only inaccurately measures calibration for rare outcomes.

Other Calibration Metrics

Various other calibration metrics have been developed, of which the following three are more commonly used. First, the expected/observed ratio, or E/O-ratio, describes the overall calibration of a prediction model, and is defined as the ratio of expected positive (predicted positive) cases and observed positive (true positive) cases [8]. A value of 1 is optimal. Second, the Estimated Calibration Index (ECI) [9] is a measure of overall calibration, and is defined as the average squared difference of the predicted probabilities with their grouped estimated observed probabilities. It can range between 0 and 100, with lower values representing better overall calibration. Lastly, the Hosmer-Lemeshow goodness-of-fit test can be applied to assess calibration, and is based on dividing the sample up according to g groups of predicted probabilities, with $g = 10$ being a common value [10]. The test then compares the distribution to a chi-square distribution. A $p > 0.2$ is usually seen as an indication of a good fit, i.e. fair calibration.

Recalibration Techniques

Should you have arrived at a robustly validated model with high performance in discrimination but poor calibration, there are several methods available to recalibrate the model to fit a population with a knowingly different incidence of the endpoint, or to even out a consistent deformation of the calibration curve [1]. These scenarios are explained in some more detail below. Also, if a study reports development of a model as well as external validation of that model in a different population for which the model is recalibrated, both the recalibrated as well as the uncalibrated performance of the model in the external validation cohort have to be reported, as the uncalibrated performance is the only representative and unbiased measure of generalizability available. In the first case, a model may have been developed in a certain country in which the incidence of a certain outcome is 10%. If other authors want to apply the same exact model in a different country with a known incidence of this outcome that is higher at e.g. 20%, the model will systematically underestimate predicted probabilities—and thus have a negative intercept, while maintaining a calibration slope of around 1.0. To adjust for the difference in outcome incidence, the intercept of the model can be updated to recalibrate the model [11]. In the second case, calibration curves may consistently show a sigmoid or other reproducible deviation from the ideal diagonal calibration curve. Two commonly applied methods to improve the calibration of the predicted probabilities are logistic regression and isotonic regression. Logistic regression can be used to train a wrapper model that learns to even out the deviation. This technique is called logistic recalibration of Platt scaling [12]. Second, isotonic regression can be applied to recalibrate the model [12]. Isotonic (also called monotonic) regression is a nonparametric technique that for fitting a free-form line (such as a calibration plot) to a series of reference values (such as a perfect diagonal line), under the constraints that the fitted line has to be monotonically increasing and must lie as close to the reference values as feasible [12].

It is important to stress here that we recommend recalibration only in these two cases listed above: On the other hand, if the calibration curve is erratic or a deformation of the calibration curve (e.g. sigmoid deformation) is not consistent among resamples or validation cohorts, we do not recommend recalibration.

4.3 Evaluation of Regression Models

For regression problems, performance can only be evaluated by comparing the predicted value and the true value directly. There are three major performance metrics that are used to evaluate the performance of regressors: First, root mean square error (RMSE), defined as the standard deviation of the differences between the predicted and true values (residuals), explains the distribution of the residuals around the perfect predictions. A perfect RMSE would be 0.00, with lower values indicating better performance. Similarly, mean absolute error (MAE) measures the difference among the predicted and the true values directly. Thus, a MAE of 0.00 would indicate no error at all, with deviations from 0 indicating overall over- or underestimation of values. Lastly, the R^2 value, defined as the square of the of the correlation coefficient among predicted and true values, discloses what proportion of the variation in the outcome is explained by the model. Consequently, a R^2 value of 1.0 would indicate perfect explanatory power, and 0.00 would indicate zero explanatory power of the model. For regression models, a quantile–quantile plot can optionally be included to illustrate the relationship among predicted and true values over the entire dataset (see Chap. 6).

4.4 Points of Significance

Choosing a Cutoff for Binary Classification

For binary classifiers which produce predicted probabilities, a cutoff (or threshold) has to be set to transform the predicted probabilities—ranging from 0.00 to 1.00—to a binary classification (i.e. yes/no or positive/negative or 1/0). While it might be tempting and often adequate to simply always use a cutoff of 0.50 for binary classification, in many cases different cutoffs will produce more accurate results in general, and the cutoff should also be chosen depending on the intended application of a given model.

One quantitative method to calculate a cutoff for binary classification that optimizes both sensitivity and specificity is the AUC-based "closest-to-(0,1)-criterion" or Youden's index [5]. Using packages in R such as pROC [13], this can be done easily. This technique will lead to the most balanced estimation of a binary classification cutoff, and can be chosen on a model with generally high performance measures that is aimed at achieving maximum classification *accuracy* overall. However, in many cases, models are clinically intended to *rule-in* or *rule-out* critical events. In these cases, the binary classification cutoff may be adjusted to achieve high specificity or sensitivity, respectively. For example, a rule-in model requires a high specificity, whereas sensitivity is of secondary importance. In other words, if a model with high specificity (>90%) makes a positive prediction, this rules in true case positivity, while a negative prediction will have rather little value. To increase specificity, the cutoff for binary classification can be adjusted *upwards* (e.g. to 75%). This can be seen as a "higher burden of proof" for a positive case. Inversely, a rule-out model will require high sensitivity and a negative result to rule-out an event, in which case the cutoff for binary classification can be adjust *downwards*. Whether a clinical prediction model is laid out as a neutral model (cutoff 0.50 or calculated using the "closest-to-(0,1)-criterion"), rule-in model (cutoff adjusted upwards), or rule-in model (cutoff adjusted downwards) will depend on the clinical question.

Again, it is important to stress at this point that the selection of a cutoff for binary classification must occur using exclusively training data. Based on the (resampled) training performance, a cutoff should be chosen using one of the methods described above. Only one final, fully trained model and its determined cutoff should then be tested on the internal or external validation data, which will confirm the generalizability of both the model parameters and the cutoff that was chosen. If the cutoff is post-hoc adjusted based on the internal or external validation data, which are intended to provide an assessment of likely "real-world" performance, this evaluation of generalizability becomes rather meaningless and generalizability cannot be assessed in an unbiased way. Lastly, the threshold for binary classification should be reported when publishing a clinical prediction model.

Sample Size

While even the largest cohort with millions of patients is not guaranteed to result in a robust clinical prediction model if no relevant input variables are included ("garbage in, garbage out"—do not expect to predict the future from age, gender, and body mass index), the relationship among predictive performance and sample size is certainly directly proportional, especially for some data-hungry ML algorithms. To ensure generalizability of the clinical prediction model, the sample size should be both representative enough of the patient population, and should take the complexity of the algorithm into account. For instance, a deep neural network—as an example of a highly complex model—will often require thousands of patients to converge, while a logistic regression model may achieve stable results with only a few hundreds of patients. In addition, the number of input variables plays a role. Roughly, it can be said that a bare minimum of ten positive cases are required per included input variable to model the relationships. Often, erratic behavior of the models and high variance in performance among splits is observed when sample sizes are smaller than calculated with this rule of thumb. Of central importance is also the proportion of patients who experience the outcome. For very rare events, a much larger total sample size is consequentially needed. For instance, a prediction based on ten input features for an outcome occurring in only 10% of cases would require at least 1000 patients including at least 100 who experienced the outcome, according to the above rule of thumb. In general and from personal experience, we do not recommend developing ML models on cohorts with less than 100 positive cases and reasonably more cases in total, regardless of the rarity of the outcome. Also, one might consider the available literature on risk factors for the outcome of interest: If epidemiological studies find only weak associations with the outcome, it is likely that one will require more patients to arrive at a model with good predictive performance, as opposed to an outcome which has several highly associated risk factors, which may be easier to predict. Larger sample sizes also allow for more generous evaluation through a larger amount of patient data dedicated to training or validation, and usually results in better calibration measures. Lastly, some more nuanced and protocolized methods to arrive at a sample size have been published, such the Riley et al. expert's consensus on deriving a minimum sample size for generating clinical prediction models, which can also be consulted [14, 15].

Standardization

In clinical predictive modeling, the overall goal is to get the best discriminative performance from your ML algorithm, and some small steps to optimize your data before training may help to increase performance. In general, ML algorithms benefit from standardization of data, as they may perform more poorly if individual features to not appear more or less like normally distributed, e.g. representing Gaussian data with a mean value of 0 and a variance of 1. While most algorithms handle other distributions with ease, some (e.g. support vector machines with a radial basis function) assume centered and scaled data. If one input feature is orders of magnitude larger than all others, this feature may predominantly influence predictions and may decrease the algorithm's ability to learn from the other input data. In data science, centering and scaling are common methods of standardizing your data. To center continuous variables, means are subtracted from each value to arrive at a mean of 0. Scaling occurs through dividing all variables through their standard deviation, after which you end up with z scores (the number of standard deviations a value is distanced from the mean). As an alternative to this *standardization* approach, data can also be *normalized*. This means that data are rescaled between their minimum and maximum (also called Min-Max Scaling) to take on values from 0 to 1, which is particularly useful when data do not approximately follow a Gaussian distribution, in which case standardization based on standard deviations could lead to skewed results. Sometimes it can also be advantageous to transform i.e. logarithmically distributed variables. These steps are well-integrated into R through the caret package (see Chaps. 5 and 6) [16]. There are many other methods to pre-process data, which are also partially discussed in Part II and below. At this point, it is important to stress that all pre-processing steps should take place after data splitting into training and testing sets, as data leakage can occur (see Chap. 3).

One-Hot Encoding

In many cases, dealing with categorical data as opposed to continuous data is challenging in data science. Especially when categorical variables are not ordinal, handling them similarly to continuous data can lead to wrong assumptions as to relationships among variables. In addition, some algorithms cannot work with categorical data directly and require numerical inputs instead, often rather due to their specific implementation in statistical programming languages like R and not due to hard mathematical limitations of the algorithm itself. Take the variable "Histology," with the levels "Glioblastoma," "Low-grade Glioma," "Meningioma," and "Ependymoma" as an example of a non-ordinal feature. In the "Histology" variable, the encoding of the four levels in numerical form as "1" to "4" (simple *integer* encoding) would yield catastrophic results, as the four levels would be interpreted as a continuous variable and the level encoded as "4" is not necessarily graded higher as the level encoded as "1." This may lead to poorer performance and unanticipated results. In addition, any explanatory power, such as derived from measures of variables importance, will no longer be correct and would lead to clinical misinterpretation.

Instead, categorical variables with more than two levels should be *one-hot encoded*. This means that the original variable is removed, and that for each unique level of this categorical variable, a new dichotomous variable is created with the values "0" and "1." Thus, for the above "Histology" example, four new dichotomous variables will be created, namely "Glioblastoma [0,1]," "Low-grade Glioma [0,1]," and so forth. One-hot encoding ensures that the influence of each individual level of a categorical variable on the dependent variable can be accurately represented.

Missing Data and Imputation

There are also other considerations in pre-processing other than centering and scaling, including the handling of missing data. In ideal circumstances, we would prefer to only work with complete datasets, but we are mostly faced with various amount of missing values. To deal with missing values is a science on its own, which has generated a vast body of literature [17, 18] and analytical strategies, broadly classified in either deletion ("complete case analysis") or imputation. In cases, in which values are missing at random (MAR) or completely at random (MCAR), it is safe to discard single observations with missing values or even complete feature columns when, e.g. more than >50% of the column's observations are unaccounted for. When values are systematically missing instead, dropping features or observations subsequently introduces bias. In this case, imputation might yield better results. Strategies can range from simple approaches such as mean, mode, or median imputation, which, however, defeat the purpose of imputation for clinical prediction modeling since they do not factor in correlations between variables and do not work well with categorical variables, to more complex algorithmic imputation techniques. Any applied imputation method should however be used with care, and its necessity should be carefully considered especially when the fraction of missing data is substantial. The best approach will always be to keep missing data at a minimum.

There are also situations when imputing missing data may not be strictly necessary. First, some implementations of certain algorithms—for example, the popular XGBoost [19] implementation of boosted decision trees—can handle missing data natively by treating empty fields as a unique value. However, the majority of algorithms will simply throw out any patients with missing data or impute automatically. An additional point to consider is that, while some algorithms may be theoretically able to handle missing data natively, there is no reason that they should be made to do so. One of the cases in which imputing data is not strictly necessary is when an abundance of data is available with only few fields missing, or when data is missing for only a certain few patients—in which case it may be more convenient to simply delete the missing observations. Deleting larger amounts of data—as stated above—is not recommended because it may introduce systematic bias. More importantly, when data is clearly missing not at random (MNAR), imputation and deletion both will lead to inaccurate results, and the missingness must be explicitly modeled [20]. MNAR occurs when missingness depends on specific values of the data, e.g. when there is a systematic bias such as when certain populations are much less likely to return for follow-up visits due to geographical distance, or when obese patients are much less likely to report their weight. In cases with data that is MNAR, simple imputation will not yield correct results.

However, in the majority of cases it is advisable to co-train an imputer with the actual clinical prediction model, even if there is no missing data in the training set. This will allow for easy handling of missing data that the model may come across in the future, e.g. in an external validation set. Again, it is important to stress that as with all pre-processing steps, the co-trained imputer should only ever be trained on the training dataset of the prediction model—and should never see the validation data. Otherwise, data leakage may occur (see Chap. 3). Several simple packages for imputation exist in R, including algorithmic imputation using the k-nearest neighbor (kNN) algorithm [21]. In this approach, the missing datapoint is imputed by the average of k-nearest neighboring datapoints based on a chosen distance metric. In addition, single imputation can be achieved by simple regression models and predictive mean matching (PMM) [22]. This approach works for both continuous and categorical variables, as a regressor predicts the missing value from the other available patient data, and then subsequently imputes the most closely matching value from the other patients without missing values. The advantage here is avoidance of imputation of extreme or unrealistic values, especially for categorical variables. This approach can also be extended to the state of the art of multiple imputation through multivariate imputation based on chained equations (MICE) [23], which is harder to implement but depicts the uncertainty of the missing values more accurately.

While imputation can be achieved using many different algorithms including the methods described, we selected the nonparametric kNN method for internal consistency in both regression and classification (see Chaps. 5 and 6) in our practical examples, and because there is some evidence that kNN-based imputation may outperform some other imputation methods [24]. In addition, kNN imputers are highly computationally efficient.

Class Imbalance

Class imbalance is evident when one class—the minority class (i.e. patients who experienced a rare complication)—is much rarer than the majority class (i.e. patients who did not experience this rare complication) [25]. In clinical neurosciences, class imbalance is a common caveat, and many published models do not adjust for it. Because ML models extract features better and are most robust if all classes are approximately equally distributed, it is important to know how to diagnose and counteract class imbalance. If a considerable amount of class imbalance is present, ML models will often become "lazy" in learning how to discriminate between classes and instead choose to simply vote for the majority class. This bias provides synthetically high AUC, accuracy, and specificity. However, sensitivity will be near zero, making the model unemployable. This "accuracy paradox" denotes the situation when synthetically high accuracy only reflects the underlying class distribution in unbalanced data. For instance, if sensitivity and specificity are not reported, class imbalance can still be spotted if the model accuracy is virtually identical to the incidence of the majority class. In general, if class imbalance is present, care should be taken to weight classes or to under- or oversample using data science techniques. Accuracy and AUC alone do not always give a full representation of an ML model's performance. This is why reporting a minimum of sensitivity and specificity is crucial [25].

As an example, one might want to predict complications from a cohort containing 90% of patients without complications. By largely voting for the majority class (no complication), the model would achieve an accuracy and specificity of around 90% and very low sensitivity without actually learning from the data. This can be countered by adjusting class weights within the model, by undersampling and thus removing observations from the majority class or by oversampling the minority class [26]. Specifically, the synthetic minority oversampling technique (SMOTE) has been validated, shows robust performance, and is easy to employ [27]. SMOTE simulates new observations for the minority class by using *k*-means clustering, thus generating "synthetic" patients that have realistic characteristics derived from similar patients already present in the dataset. However, conventional upsampling—the simple copying of randomly selected patients of the minority class until class balance is achieved—often works similarly well. When training models, the method of handling class imbalance (i.e. none, conventional upsampling, or SMOTE) may be regarded as a hyperparameter.

Extrapolation

The vast majority of ML models are only capable of interpolating data—thus, making predictions on cases similar to the ones available in the training data—and are incapable of extrapolating—making predictions on situations that are relevantly different. This can be seen similarly to trying to apply the results of a randomized controlled drug trial to patients who were excluded from the study. For example, a model that predicts neurological impairment after brain tumor surgery that has been trained and externally validated on a large cohort of patients from 30 to 90 years of age should not be expected to make accurate predictions for pediatric brain tumor patients. Although the goal when developing algorithms is generalization to slightly other demographics, most algorithms learn to fit the training data as closely as possible locally, regardless of potential other situations not included in the training dataset (see Chap. 3). Thus, caution must be taken when making predictions outside the bounds of the type of patients included in the training data. Some algorithms are considered as being more prone to extrapolation errors, such as GAMs based on locally estimated scatterplot smoothing (LOESS) due to their reliance on local regression. In conclusion, trained models should not be clinically expected to extrapolate to patients with vastly differing characteristics.

4.5 Conclusion

Various metrics are available to evaluate the performance of clinical prediction models. A suggested minimum set of performance metrics includes AUC, accuracy, sensitivity, specificity, PPV, and NPV along with calibration slope and intercept for classification models, or RMSE, MAE, and R^2 for regression models. These performance metrics can be supplemented by a calibration plot or a quantile–quantile plot, respectively. Furthermore, there are some common caveats when developing clinical prediction models that readers should be aware of: Sample sizes must be sufficiently large to allow for adequate extraction of generalizable interactions among input variables and outcome and to allow for suitable model training and validation. Class imbalance has to be recognized and adjusted for. Missing data has to be reported and, if necessary, imputed using the state-of-the-art methods. Trained models should not be clinically expected to extrapolate to patients with vastly differing characteristics. Finally, in binary classification problems, the cutoff to transform the predicted probabilities into a dichotomous outcome should be reported and set according to the goal of the clinical prediction model.

Disclosures

Funding No funding was received for this research.

Conflict of Interest All authors certify that they have no affiliations with or involvement in any organization or entity with any financial interest (such as honoraria; educational grants; participation in speakers' bureaus; membership, employment, consultancies, stock ownership, or other equity interest; and expert testimony or patent-licensing arrangements), or non-financial interest (such as personal or professional relationships, affiliations, knowledge or beliefs) in the subject matter or materials discussed in this manuscript.

Ethical Approval All procedures performed in studies involving human participants were in accordance with the ethical standards of the 1964 Helsinki declaration and its later amendments or comparable ethical standards.

Informed Consent No human or animal participants were included in this study.

References

1. Staartjes VE, Kernbach JM. Letter to the editor. Importance of calibration assessment in machine learning-based predictive analytics. J Neurosurg Spine. 2020;32:985–7.
2. Guo C, Pleiss G, Sun Y, Weinberger KQ. On calibration of modern neural networks. ArXiv. 2017:170604599. Cs.
3. Rudin C. Stop explaining black box machine learning models for high stakes decisions and use interpretable models instead. Nat Mach Intell. 2019;1(5):206.
4. Staartjes VE, Kernbach JM. Letter to the editor regarding "Investigating risk factors and predicting complications in deep brain stimulation surgery with machine learning algorithms". World Neurosurg. 2020;137:496.
5. Perkins NJ, Schisterman EF. The inconsistency of "optimal" cutpoints obtained using two criteria based on the receiver operating characteristic curve. Am J Epidemiol. 2006;163(7):670–5.
6. Steyerberg EW, Vickers AJ, Cook NR, Gerds T, Gonen M, Obuchowski N, Pencina MJ, Kattan MW. Assessing the performance of prediction models: a framework for some traditional and novel measures. Epidemiology. 2010;21(1):128–38.
7. Brier GW. Verification of forecasts expressed in terms of probability. Mon Weather Rev. 1950;78(1):1–3.
8. Riley RD, Ensor J, Snell KIE, Debray TPA, Altman DG, Moons KGM, Collins GS. External validation of clinical prediction models using big datasets from e-health records or IPD meta-analysis: opportunities and challenges. BMJ. 2016;353:i3140.
9. Van Hoorde K, Van Huffel S, Timmerman D, Bourne T, Van Calster B. A spline-based tool to assess and visualize the calibration of multiclass risk predictions. J Biomed Inform. 2015;54:283–93.
10. Hosmer DW, Lemeshow S, Sturdivant RX. Assessing the fit of the model. In: Applied logistic regression. New York, NY: John Wiley & Sons; 2013. p. 153–225.
11. Janssen KJM, Moons KGM, Kalkman CJ, Grobbee DE, Vergouwe Y. Updating methods improved the performance of a clinical prediction model in new patients. J Clin Epidemiol. 2008;61(1):76–86.
12. Niculescu-Mizil A, Caruana R. Predicting good probabilities with supervised learning. In: Proc. 22Nd Int. Conf. Mach. Learn. New York, NY: ACM; 2005. p. 625–32.
13. Robin X, Turck N, Hainard A, Tiberti N, Lisacek F, Sanchez J-C, Müller M. pROC: an open-source package for R and S+ to analyze and compare ROC curves. BMC Bioinformatics. 2011;12:77.
14. Riley RD, Snell KIE, Ensor J, Burke DL, Harrell FE, Moons KGM, Collins GS. Minimum sample size for developing a multivariable prediction model: Part I – continuous outcomes. Stat Med. 2019;38(7):1262–75.
15. Riley RD, Snell KI, Ensor J, Burke DL, Harrell FE Jr, Moons KG, Collins GS. Minimum sample size for developing a multivariable prediction model: PART II - binary and time-to-event outcomes. Stat Med. 2019;38(7):1276–96.
16. Kuhn M. Building predictive models in *R* using the **caret** package. J Stat Softw. 2008;28:1. https://doi.org/10.18637/jss.v028.i05.
17. Little RJA, Rubin DB. Statistical analysis with missing data. New York, NY: John Wiley & Sons; 2019.
18. Rubin DB. Inference and missing data. Biometrika. 1976;63(3):581–92.
19. Chen T, Guestrin C. XGBoost: a scalable tree boosting system. ArXiv. 2016:160302754. Cs 785–794.
20. Molenberghs G, Beunckens C, Sotto C, Kenward MG. Every missingness not at random model has a missingness at random counterpart with equal fit. J R Stat Soc Ser B Stat Methodol. 2008;70(2):371–88.
21. Templ M, Kowarik A, Alfons A, Prantner B. VIM: visualization and imputation of missing values. 2019.
22. Landerman LR, Land KC, Pieper CF. An empirical evaluation of the predictive mean matching method for imputing missing values. Sociol Methods Res. 1997;26(1):3–33.
23. van Buuren S, Groothuis-Oudshoorn CGM. mice: multivariate imputation by chained equations in R. J Stat Softw. 2011;45:1. https://doi.org/10.18637/jss.v045.i03.
24. Batista GEAPA, Monard MC. An analysis of four missing data treatment methods for supervised learning. Appl Artif Intell. 2003;17(5–6):519–33.
25. Staartjes VE, Schröder ML. Letter to the Editor. Class imbalance in machine learning for neurosurgical outcome prediction: are our models valid? J Neurosurg Spine. 2018;29(5):611–2.
26. Batista GEAPA, Prati RC, Monard MC. A study of the behavior of several methods for balancing machine learning training data. SIGKDD Explor Newsl. 2004;6(1):20–9.
27. Chawla NV, Bowyer KW, Hall LO, Kegelmeyer WP. SMOTE: synthetic minority over-sampling technique. J Artif Intell Res. 2002;16:321–57.

Foundations of Machine Learning-Based Clinical Prediction Modeling: Part IV—A Practical Approach to Binary Classification Problems

5

Victor E. Staartjes and Julius M. Kernbach

5.1 Introduction

Predictive analytics are currently by far the most common application of machine learning in neurosurgery [1–4], although the potential of machine learning techniques for other applications such as natural language processing, medical image classification, radiomic feature extraction, and many more should definitely not be understated [5–13]. The topic of predictive analytics also uniquely lends itself to introducing machine learning methods due to its relative ease of implementation. Thus, we chose to specifically focus on predictive analytics as the most popular application of machine learning in neurosurgery. This section of the series is intended to demonstrate the programming methods required to train and validate a simple, machine learning-based clinical prediction model for any binary endpoint. Prediction of continuous endpoints (regression) will be covered in Part V of this series (see Chap. 6).

J. M. Kernbach and V. E. Staartjes have contributed equally to this series, and share first authorship.

Supplementary Information The online version contains supplementary material available at (https://doi.org/10.1007/978-3-030-85292-4_5).

V. E. Staartjes (✉)
Machine Intelligence in Clinical Neuroscience (MICN) Laboratory, Department of Neurosurgery, Clinical Neuroscience Center, University Hospital Zurich, University of Zurich, Zurich, Switzerland
e-mail: victoregon.staartjes@usz.ch; https://micnlab.com/

J. M. Kernbach
Neurosurgical Artificial Intelligence Laboratory Aachen (NAILA), Department of Neurosurgery, RWTH Aachen University Hospital, Aachen, Germany

We focus on the statistical programming language R [14], as it is freely available and widely regarded as the state of the art in biostatistical programming. Other programming languages such as Python are certainly equally suited to the kind of programming introduced here. While we elucidate all necessary aspects of the required code, a basic understanding of R is thus required. Basic R courses are offered at many universities around the world, as well as through numerous media online and in print. We highly recommend that users first make themselves familiar with the programming language before studying this section. Python is another programming language often used in machine learning. The same general principles and pipeline discussed here can be applied in Python to arrive at a prediction model.

At this point we again want to stress that this section is not intended to represent a single perfect method that will apply to every binary endpoint, and to every data situation. Instead, this section represents one possible, generalizable methodology, that incorporates most of the important aspects of machine learning and clinical prediction modeling.

To illustrate the methods applied, we supply a simulated database of 10,000 glioblastoma patients who underwent microsurgery, and predict the occurrence of 12-month survival. Table 5.1 provides an overview over the glioblastoma database. We walk the reader through each step, including import, checking, splitting, imputation, and pre-processing of the data, as well as variable selection, model selection and training, and lastly correct evaluation of discrimination and calibration. Proper visualization and reporting of machine learning-based clinical prediction models for binary endpoints are also discussed.

The centerpiece of this section is the provided R code (Supplement 5.1), which is intended to be used in combination with the provided glioblastoma database (Supplement 5.2). When executed correctly and in parallel with this section's

V. E. Staartjes et al. (eds.), *Machine Learning in Clinical Neuroscience*, Acta Neurochirurgica Supplement 134,
https://doi.org/10.1007/978-3-030-85292-4_5

Table 5.1 Structure of the simulated glioblastoma dataset. The number of included patients is 10,000. Values are provided as means and standard deviations or as numbers and percentages

Variable name	Description	Value
Survival	Overall survival from diagnosis in months	12.1 ± 3.1
TwelveMonths	Patients who survived 12 months or more from diagnosis	5184 (51.8%)
IDH	IDH mutation present	4136 (41.4%)
MGMT	MGMT promoter methylated	5622 (56.2%)
TERTp	TERTp mutation present	5108 (51.1%)
Male	Male gender	4866 (48.7%)
Midline	Extension of the tumor into the midline	2601 (26.0%)
Comorbidity	Presence of any systemic comorbidity such as diabetes, coronary heart disease, chronic obstructive pulmonary disease, etc.	5135 (51.4%)
Epilepsy	Occurrence of an epileptic seizure	3311 (33.1%)
PriorSurgery	Presence of prior cranial surgery	5283 (52.8%)
Married	Positive marriage status	5475 (54.8%)
ActiveWorker	Patient is actively working, i.e. not retired, student, out of work, etc.	5459 (54.6%)
Chemotherapy	Patients who received chemotherapy for glioblastoma	4081 (40.8%)
HigherEducation	Patients who received some form of higher education	4209 (42.1%)
Caseload	Yearly glioblastoma microsurgery caseload at the treating center	165.0 ± 38.7
Age	Patient age at diagnosis in years	66.0 ± 6.2
RadiotherapyDose	Total radiotherapy absorbed dose in Gray	24.8 ± 6.7
KPS	Karnofsky Performance Scale	70.5 ± 8.0
Income	Net yearly household income in US dollars	268,052 ± 62,867
Height	Patient body height in cm	174.6 ± 6.7
BMI	Deviation of body mass index from 25; in kg/m^2	0.02 ± 1.0
Size	Maximum tumor diameter in cm	2.98 ± 0.55

contents, the code will output the same results as those achieved by the authors, which allows for immediate feedback. The R code itself is numbered in parallel to this section, and also contains abundant explanations which enable a greater understanding of the functions and concepts that are necessary to succeed in generating a robust model. Finally, the code is intended as a scaffold upon which readers can build their own clinical prediction models for binary classification, and can easily be modified to do so for any dataset with a binary outcome.

5.2 Setup and Pre-processing Data

R Setup and Package Installation

Installing the most recent version of R (available at https://cran.r-project.org/) as well as the RStudio graphic user interface (GUI) (available at https://rstudio.com/products/rstudio/download/) is recommended [14]. A core strength of the R programming language is its wide adoption, and thus the availability of thousands of high-end, freely downloadable software packages that facilitate everything from model training to plotting graphs. Running the "*pacman*" [15] codes in section 1.1 will automatically ensure that all packages necessary for execution of this code are installed and loaded into the internal memory. You will require an internet connection to download these packages. If you have a clean R installation and have no installed any of the packages yet, it might take multiple minutes to download and install all necessary data. The script also gives you the option to update your R installation, should you desire to do so.

Importing Data

Generally, it is easiest to prepare your spreadsheet in the following way for machine learning: First, ensure that all data fields are in numerical form. That is, both continuous and categorical variables are reported as numbers. We recommend formatting binary (dichotomous) categorical variables (i.e. male gender) as 0 and 1, and categorical variables with multiple levels (i.e. tumor type [Astrocytoma, Glioblastoma, Oligodendroglioma, etc.]) as 1, 2, 3, and so forth, instead of as strings (text). Second, we recommend always placing your endpoint of interest in the last column of your spreadsheet. The Glioblastoma dataset that is provided is already correctly formatted. To import the data from the Glioblastoma database in Microsoft Excel (Supplement 5.2), run the code in section 1.2. For R to find the Glioblastoma database on your computer, you can either store the .xlsx file in the same folder as the R script or you have to manually enter the path to the .xlsx file, as demonstrated in Fig. 5.1. You could also use RStudio's GUI to import the dataset.

```
#Import the dataset from the downloaded Excel using the RStudio GUI, OR runt this code:
#A - Store the .xlsx file in the same folder as the script
df <- as.data.frame(read_excel("GlioblastomaData.xlsx"))
#B - Alternatively, you may have to enter the path to the .xlsx. file. For example:
df <- as.data.frame(read_excel("C:/Machine Learning/Folder/GlioblastomaData.xlsx")) #Replace this string (" ") with the path to the downloaded Glioblastoma dataset!!!
```

Fig. 5.1 Code section 1.2: You can either import the Glioblastoma database by keeping its .xlsx file in the same folder as the R script (A). Alternatively, you may have to find the path (e.g. "C:/Desktop/database.xlsx") to the .xlsx file and enter it as a string, i.e. between quotes (B). Lastly, you could also use the graphic user interface of RStudio to import the file

Check the Imported Data

Run "str(df)" to get an overview of the imported data's structure. We see that all 22 variables are correctly imported, but that they are all currently handled by R as numerical ("num") variables, whereas some of them are categorical and should thus be handled in R as "factor" variables. An overview of the variables in the Glioblastoma database is provided in Table 5.1.

Reformat Categorical Variables

To reformat all categorical variables to "factor" variables in R, allocate them to the "cols" object. Subsequently, we apply the "factor" function to all columns of the database using the "lapply" function. Lastly, the binary endpoint of interest ("TwelveMonths") should be internally labeled as "yes" and "no," again using the "factor" function. Lastly, "str(df)" is used again to confirm the correct reformatting.

Remove Unnecessary Columns

Your imported data may contain extra columns with variables that are irrelevant to the current classification problem, such as patient numbers, names, or other endpoints. The latter is the case in the Glioblastoma database: The 21st column contains the variable "Survival," which is a continuous form of our binary endpoint of interest "TwelveMonths." Leaving this redundant variable in would lead to data leakage—the model could simply take the continuous "Survival" variable and extrapolate our endpoint "TwelveMonths" from it, without actually learning any features. Columns can be removed from a R dataframe by specifying the column number to be removed. "Survival" is situated in the 21st column of the database, and can thus be removed by applying the function "df <- df[,-21]."

Enable Multicore Processing

If you are working on a machine with multiple central processing unit (CPU) cores, you can enable parallel computing for some functions in R. Using the code in section 1.6, create a computational cluster by entering the number of cores you want to invest into model development [16]. The default is set to 4, which is nowadays a common number of CPU cores.

Partition the Data for Training and Testing

Figure 5.2 illustrates the procedure. To randomly split the data into 80% for training an 20% for testing (internal validation), we first set a random seed, such as "set.seed(123)," although you could choose any number. Setting seeds initializes random functions in a constant way, and thus enables reproducibility. Subsequently, we randomly sample 80% of patients and allocate them to the training set ("train"), and do the same for the test set ("test"). Then, the rows of the two newly partitioned sets are shuffled, and the two sets are checked for an approximately equal distribution of the binary endpoint using the "prop.table()" function. Both sets contain around 52% of patients who survived for at least 12 months.

Impute Missing Data

The glioblastoma database contains no missing data, as the function "VIM::kNN" [17] will let you know. However, should you encounter missing data, this code block should automatically impute missing data using a *k*-nearest neighbor (KNN) algorithm [18]. It is important only to impute missing data within the training set, and to leave the test set alone. This is to prevent data leakage. Also, imputation can be achieved using many different algorithms. We elected to use a KNN imputer for reasons of consistency—during model training, a separate KNN imputer will be co-trained with the prediction model to impute any future missing data.

Variable Selection Using Recursive Feature Elimination

Recursive Feature Elimination (RFE) is just one of various methods for variable selection (see Chap. 7 for further explanation). In this example, we apply RFE (Fig. 5.3) due to its relative simplicity, generalizability, and reproducibility.

```
#1.7 Split training and testing set. Here, we choose a 80%/20% random split ----
set.seed(123)   #Setting seeds allows reproducibility
dt = sort(sample(nrow(df), nrow(df)*.80)) #Allocate 80% split
train <-df[dt,] #Split
test <-df[-dt,]
train <- train[sample(nrow(train)),] #Shuffle
test <- test[sample(nrow(test)),]
#Check approximate equal distribution of the endpoint - Here we see that 12-month survival was virtually equal in training and testing sets
prop.table(table(train$TwelveMonths))
prop.table(table(test$TwelveMonths))
```

Fig. 5.2 Code section 1.7: This section illustrates how to partition a database into training and test (internal validation) sets

```
#1.9 Variable Selection using Recursive Feature Elimination ----
set.seed(123) #Set a seed
rfecontrol <- rfeControl(functions=nbFuncs, method = "boot", number = 25, rerank = F, verbose = T, allowParallel = T) #RFE using naive Bayes classifier, in 25-fold bootstrap
set.seed(123)
RFE <- rfe(x = train[,1:(ncol(train)-1)], y = train[,ncol(train)], sizes=c(10:(ncol(train)-1)), rfeControl=rfecontrol) #Run the RFE algorithm
print(RFE) #Results
plot(RFE, type=c("g", "o")) #Plot performance over #vars
predictors(RFE) #Variables to be kept
#Apparently, this combination of 13 selected variables explains the highest amoung of variance in our endpoint.
#Thus, we should keep only these 13 independent variables, and our dependent variable, and remove the 7 "garbage"/"low-impact"/"multicollinear" independent variables that were not selected by RFE
#Keep only the RFE-selected 13 variables & our endpoint "TwelveMonths"
keepvars <- c(predictors(RFE), "TwelveMonths")
train <- train[keepvars]
```

Fig. 5.3 Code Sect. 1.9: This section illustrates the recursive feature elimination (RFE) procedure. A naïve Bayes classifier is chosen, along with bootstrap resampling with 25 repetitions

Because random functions are involved, seeds need to be set. A naïve Bayes classifier is selected, and bootstrap resampling with 25 repetitions is used to ensure generalizability of the results. Suing the "sizes" argument in the "rfe" function [19], the number of combined variables that are to be assessed can be limited. As we have 20 independent variables, we choose to limit the search for the optimal number and combination of variables to between 10 and 20. The "rfe()" function is executed, which may take some minutes. Using "plot()", the results of the RFE procedure can be illustrated (Fig. 5.4), and it is clear that a combination of 13 variables led to the highest performance. The selected variables are stored in "predictors(RFE)." These 13 selected variables, plus the endpoint "TwelveMonths" are stored in "keepvars," and the training set is subsequently reduced to 14 columns.

Get a Final Overview of the Data

Before diving directly into model training, it is advisable to look over the training and test set using the "summary()" function to assess the correctness of the independent variables and the endpoint.

5.3 Model Training

Setting Up the Training Structure

Now that the data are prepared, training of the different models can be initiated. In this example, we elected to train five different algorithms to predict binary 12-month survival: Logistic regression [20] (generalized linear models, GLM), random forests [21] (RF), stochastic gradient boosting machines [22] (GBM), generalized additive models [23] (GAM), and naïve Bayes classifiers [24] (NB). A brief overview of the five different models is provided in Table 5.2. We specifically refrained from using more complex models, such as neural networks, due to their inherently decreased interpretability and because they are more prone to overfitting on the relatively simple, clinical data used in this example [25]. All five models are trained sequentially and in a similar way using a universal wrapper that executes training, the "caret" package [19]. Hyperparameters—if available—are tuned automatically. To prevent overfitting, bootstrap resampling with 25 repetitions is chosen in this example (Fig. 5.5) [26]. However, fivefold cross validation could also easily be implemented (see Chap. 6). To adjust for any potential class imbalance (see Chap. 4), random upsampling is implemented by choosing "sampling = "up"", although synthetic minority oversampling (SMOTE) could also be used (sampling = "smote") [27, 28]. The current Glioblastoma dataset is, however, without class imbalance, as short-term and longer-term survivors are approximately equally common.

Model Training

The procedure (Fig. 5.5) is equivalent for all five models (Sections 2.2.1–2.2.5). First, a seed is set to initialize the random number generator in a reproducible way. Subsequently, the algorithm to be used is specified in the "method" argument—the first model to be trained is a logistic GLM, so "method = "glm"" is chosen. The "tuneLength" argument depends on the complexity and of the hyperparameters: GLM has no hyperparameters, so a low value is specified. We specify that the parameters and hyperparameters are to be optimized according to area under the curve (AUC, metric = "ROC"), and that a KNN imputer is co-trained for future missing data (preProcess = "knnImpute"). The inputs are automatically centered and scaled by the "caret" package. After running the fully specified "caret::train" function, it may take some minutes for all resamples to finish training. The red "STOP" dot at the top right of the RStudio console will be present for as long as the model is training. Subsequently, a confusion matrix (conf) is generated, along with some other metrics that allow evaluation of the model's discrimination. Now, calibration is assessed and a calibration plot is generated using the "val.prob()" function [29]. Finally, the model specifications and resampled training performance are printed, and the model can be saved using the "save()" function for potential further use.

After completion of training the GLM (Section 2.2.1), the same procedure is repeated for the RF (Section 2.2.2), GBM (Section 2.2.3), GAM (Section 2.2.4), and NB (Section 2.2.5) models.

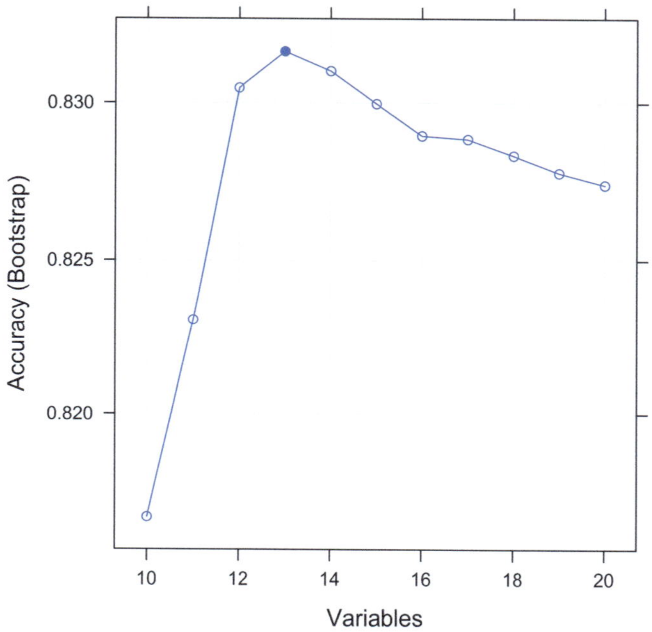

Fig. 5.4 Results of the recursive feature elimination (RFE) variable election procedure. It was determined that using 13 variables explained the highest amount of variance, as seen in the superior accuracy that was achieved with this number and combination of variables

5.4 Model Evaluation and Selection

Model Training Evaluation

As soon as all five models have been trained, their performance on the training data can be compared. The final model should be selected based upon training data only. Criteria for clinical prediction model selection may include discrimination and calibration on the training set, as well as the degree of interpretability of the algorithm. Section 3.1 compiles the results of all five models, and allows their comparison in terms of discrimination (AUC, accuracy, sensitivity, specificity, positive predictive value (PPV), negative predictive value (NPV), F1 score) and calibration

Table 5.2 Overview of the five models that were employed

Model	caret::train() input	Package	Suitability	Hyperparameters
Generalized Linear Model	glm	stats	Classification, Regression	None
Random Forest	rf	randomForest	Classification, Regression	mtry (number of variables at each tree node)
Stochastic Gradient Boosting	gbm	gbm	Classification	n.trees (number of trees), interaction.depth (maximum nodes per tree), shrinkage (learning rate), n.minobsinnode (minimum number of patients per terminal node)
Generalized Additive Model	gamLoess	gam	Classification, Regression	span (smoothing span width), degree (degree of polynomial)
Naïve Bayes Classifier	nb	klaR	Classification	fL (Laplace correction factor), usekernel (normal or kernel density estimate), adjust

```
#2.1 Set Up the Training and Resampling Structure ----
#As a standard, we choose bootstraping with replacement as the resampling method, with 25 repeats.
#We also choose random upsampling as a standard to adjust for class imbalance if present. Alternatively, sampling =
"smote" could be used for SMOTE upsampling.
ctrl <- trainControl(method = "boot", number = 25, classProbs = T, summaryFunction = twoClassSummary, allowParallel
= T, sampling = "up", returnResamp = "all")

#2.2.1 Train Model #1: GLM (Logistic Regression) ----
set.seed(123)
lrfit <- caret::train(TwelveMonths ~ ., data = train, method = "glm", trControl = ctrl, tuneLength = 5, metric =
"ROC", preProcess = "knnImpute", na.action = na.pass)
#We automatically tune our models based on AUC (=ROC), and co-train a KNN imputer that then automatically imputes
any potential missing data for future samples
#Assess Discrimination
conf <- print(confusionMatrix.train(lrfit, norm = "none", positive = "yes")[1])[[1]]; tp <- conf[2,2]; tn <-
conf[1,1]; fp <- conf[2,1]; fn <- conf[1,2]; sens <- tp/(tp+fn); spec <- tn/(tn+fp); prev <-
as.numeric(prop.table(table(train[,ncol(train)])))[2]
#Assess Calibration
prob <- predict(lrfit, train, type="prob", na.action = na.pass)
calLogReg <- val.prob(prob[,2], as.numeric(train$TwelveMonths)-1, ylab = "Observed Frequency", xlab = "Predicted
Probability", g = 10)
LogReg <- as.data.frame(cbind(max(lrfit$results$ROC), sens * prev + spec * (1-prev), sens, spec,
(sens*prev)/(sens*prev+(1-spec)*(1-prev)), (spec*(1-prev))/((1-sens)*prev+spec*(1-prev)), (2*
((sens*prev)/(sens*prev+(1-spec)*(1-prev)))*(sens))/(((sens*prev)/(sens*prev+(1-spec)*(1-prev)))+sens)))
LogReg <- as.data.frame(cbind(LogReg, calLogReg[12], calLogReg[13]))
colnames(LogReg)  <- c("AUC", "Accuracy", "Sensitivity", "Specificity", "PPV", "NPV", "F1 Score", "Intercept",
"Slope")

#Summary
print(lrfit)
print(LogReg)
#Save Model File
save(lrfit, file= "GLM.Rdata")
```

Fig. 5.5 Code sections 2.1 and 2.2: First, the training structure is established: Bootstrap resampling with 25 repetitions is used. As a standard, random upsampling is applied to adjust for class imbalance if present. Subsequently, a logistic regression model (generalized linear model, GLM) is trained. All predictor variables are provided to the model, and it is automatically tuned for AUC. A *k*-nearest neighbor imputer is co-trained to impute any potential missing data in future predictions. Subsequently, discrimination and calibration are assessed, and the final model information and resampled training performance are printed

(intercept and slope) metrics [30]. The code in this section will also open a new plot viewer window using "dev.new()", that allows graphical comparison of the five models. If you have executed all parts of the script correctly up to this point, you will be presented with a plot that is identical to Fig. 5.6. In this plot, we see that—while all models performed admirably—the GLM and GAM had the highest discrimination metrics. Models perform well if these discrimination measures approach 1. In addition, while all absolute values of intercept were very low, not all models had excellent calibration slopes. A perfectly calibrated model has an intercept of 0.0 and a slope of 1.0. Only the GLM and GAM had virtually perfect slopes. As both algorithms are highly interpretable, the GLM and the GAM both would make fine options for a final model. In this example, we elected to carry on with the GAM.

Select the Final Model

The fully trained GAM model was previously stored as "gamfit," and its resampled training evaluation as "GAM" in section 2.2.4. Now, as the GAM model is selected as the final model, it is renamed "finalmodel," and its training evaluation is renamed "finalmodelstats." You can choose any other model by replacing these two terms with the corresponding objects from section 2.2.

Internal Validation on the Test Set

For the first time since partitioning the original Glioblastoma database, the 20% of patients allocated to the test set are now used to internally validate the final model. First, a prediction is made on the test set using "finalmodel" and the "predict()"

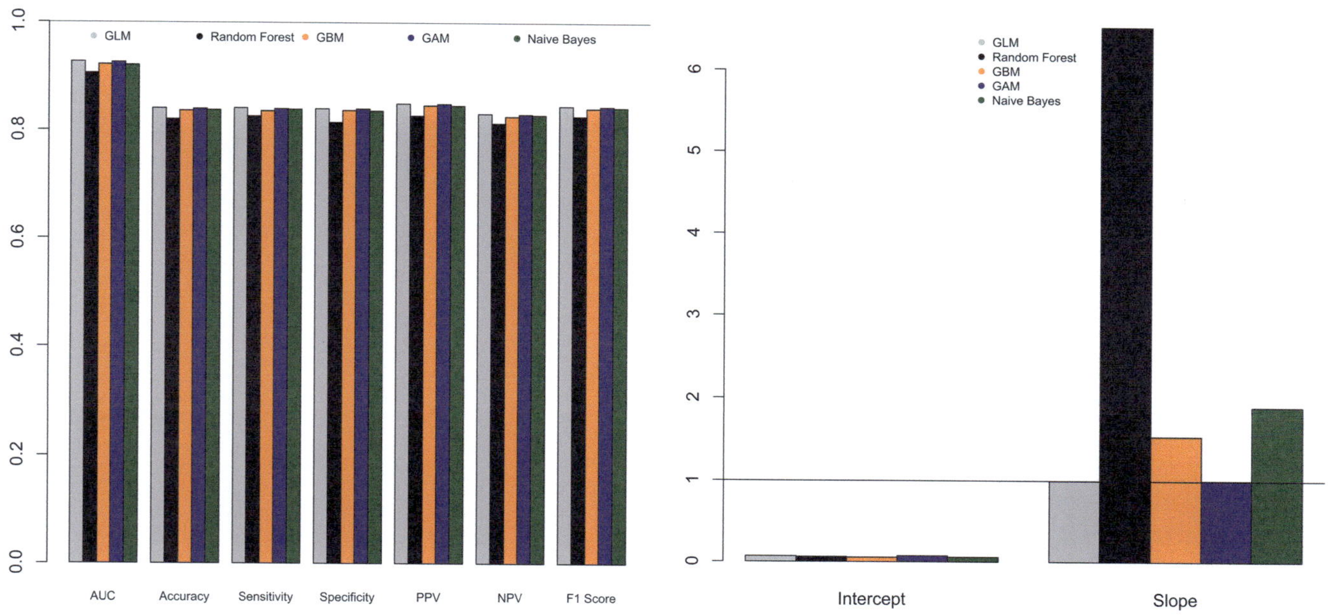

Fig. 5.6 Graphical comparison of discrimination (left) and calibration (right) metrics (Code section 3.1). The GLM and GAM both exhibited the highest discrimination measures, with very low absolute intercept values and almost perfect slopes approaching 1

function. Of note, during prediction with the GAM on the test set, you will encounter warning messages indicating that extrapolation took place. These warning messages are not to be considered as errors, but as informative warnings indicating that some patients in the test set had characteristics that were outside of the bounds encountered by the GAM during training. GAMs rely on local regression, which makes extrapolation to extreme input values problematic. This is discussed in some more detail in Part III.

The predicted probabilities for the entire test set are then contrasted with the actual class labels from the endpoint (test$TwelveMonths) to arrive at an AUC value [31]. Subsequently, the predicted probabilities are converted into binary predictions using "factor(ifelse(prob$yes > 0.50, "yes", "no"))." Thus, predicted probabilities over 0.50 are counted as positive predictions (yes), and vice versa. This cutoff for binary classification can be changed to different values, changing sensitivity and specificity of the clinical prediction model. However, the decision to do so must be based solely on the training data, and thus already be taken before evaluation of the test set—otherwise, a clean assessment of out-of-sample error through internal validation is not possible anymore. This is discussed in some more detail in Part III. However, in most cases and especially with well-calibrated models, a standard cutoff of 0.50 is appropriate.

Subsequently, discrimination and calibration are calculated in the same way as previously. Using "print(Final)," the internal validation metrics can be viewed. Performance that

Table 5.3 Performance metrics of the binary classification model (generalized additive model; GAM) for 12-month glioblastoma survival. The difference in performance among training and testing is minimal, demonstrating a lack of overfitting at internal validation

	Cohort	
	Training	Internal validation
Metric	(n = 8000)	(n = 2000)
Discrimination		
AUC	0.926	0.922
Accuracy	0.839	0.847
Sensitivity	0.839	0.848
Specificity	0.839	0.846
PPV	0.849	0.848
NPV	0.830	0.826
F1 score	0.844	0.843
Calibration		
Intercept	0.074	0.039
Slope	1.004	0.961

is on par with or slightly worse than the training performance usually indicates a robust, generalizable model. Performance that is relevantly worse than the training performance indicates overfitting during training. These problems are discussed in detail in Part II. The final model can be saved, and will be available as "FINALMODEL.Rdata" in the same folder as the R script. Using the "load()" function, models can be imported back into R at a later date.

If you end up with the same performance metrics for the final GAM as in Table 5.3, you have executed all steps correctly.

5.5 Reporting and Visualization

When generating clinical prediction models and publishing their results, there is a minimum set of information that ought to be provided to the reader. First, the training methods and exact algorithm type should be reported, if possible along with the code that was used for training. Second, the characteristics of the cohort that was used for training should be provided, such as in Table 5.1. If multiple cohorts are combined or used for external validation, the patient characteristics should be reported in separate. Discrimination and calibration must be reported. There are countless metrics to describe calibration and discrimination of prediction models. The bare minimum that should be reported for a binary prediction model probably consists of AUC, accuracy, sensitivity, specificity, PPV, and NPV, along with calibration intercept and slope. The F1 score can also be provided. A calibration plot should also be provided for binary prediction models. Lastly, whenever feasible, an attempt at interpreting the model should be made. For example, logistic regression (GLM) models produce odds ratios, and GAMs can produce partial dependence values. However, there are also universal methods to generate variable importance measures that can apply to most binary prediction models, usually based on AUC, which we present below. To simplify reporting, this final section helps compile all these data required for publication of clinical prediction models. For further information on reporting standards, consult the transparent reporting of a multivariable prediction model for individual prognosis or diagnosis (TRIPOD) checklist [32].

Compiling Training Performance

The resampled training performance in terms of discrimination and calibration can be printed using "print(finalmodelstats)." The metrics that are produced include AUC, accuracy, sensitivity (recall), specificity, PPV (precision), NPV, F1 score, intercept, and slope. Subsequently, a calibration plot is generated for the training set using the "val.prob()" function.

Compiling Internal Validation Performance

Similarly, the performance on the test set (internal validation) can be recapitulated, and a calibration plot produced (analogous to Fig. 5.7).

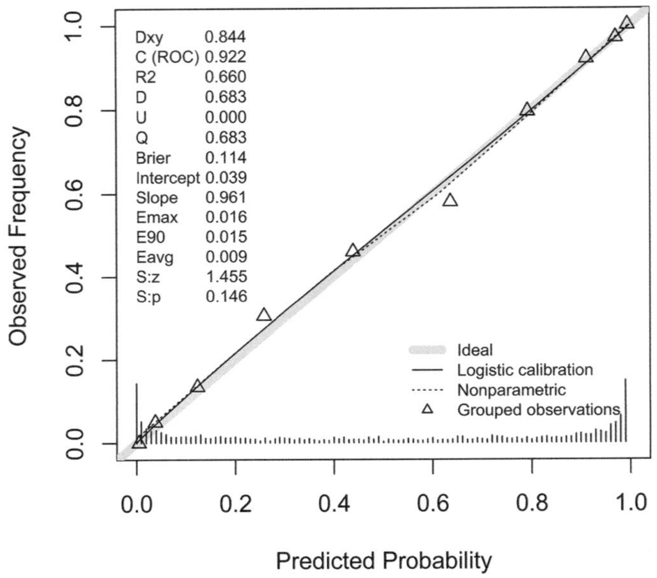

Fig. 5.7 Calibration plot for the final GAM, demonstrating its calibration on the test set (internal validation). The calibration curve closely approximates the diagonal line, indicating excellent calibration

Assessing Variable Importance

By using "varImp(finalmodel)," a universal method for estimation of variable importance based on AUC is executed, and results in a list of values ranging from 0 to 100, with 100 indicating the variable that contributed most strongly to the predictions, and vice versa. Finally, "plot(imp)" generates a variable importance plot that can also be included in publication of clinical prediction models (see Chap. 6).

5.6 Conclusion

This section presents one possible and standardized way of developing clinical prediction models for binary endpoints. Proper visualization and reporting of machine learning-based clinical prediction models for binary endpoints are also discussed. We provide the full, structured code, as well as the complete Glioblastoma survival database for the readers to download and execute in parallel to this section. The methods presented can and are in fact intended to be extended by the readers to new datasets, new endpoints, and new algorithms.

Disclosures

Funding No funding was received for this research.

Conflict of Interest All authors certify that they have no affiliations with or involvement in any organization or entity with any financial interest (such as honoraria; educational grants; participation in speakers' bureaus; membership, employment, consultancies, stock ownership, or other equity interest; and expert testimony or patent-licensing arrangements), or non-financial interest (such as personal or professional relationships, affiliations, knowledge or beliefs) in the subject matter or materials discussed in this manuscript.

Ethical Approval All procedures performed in studies involving human participants were in accordance with the ethical standards of the 1964 Helsinki declaration and its later amendments or comparable ethical standards.

Informed Consent No human or animal participants were included in this study.

References

1. Brusko GD, Kolcun JPG, Wang MY. Machine-learning models: the future of predictive analytics in neurosurgery. Neurosurgery. 2018;83(1):E3–4.
2. Celtikci E. A systematic review on machine learning in neurosurgery: the future of decision making in patient care. Turk Neurosurg. 2017;28:167. https://doi.org/10.5137/1019-5149.JTN.20059-17.1.
3. Senders JT, Staples PC, Karhade AV, Zaki MM, Gormley WB, Broekman MLD, Smith TR, Arnaout O. Machine learning and neurosurgical outcome prediction: a systematic review. World Neurosurg. 2018;109:476–486.e1.
4. Senders JT, Zaki MM, Karhade AV, Chang B, Gormley WB, Broekman ML, Smith TR, Arnaout O. An introduction and overview of machine learning in neurosurgical care. Acta Neurochir. 2018;160(1):29–38.
5. Djuric U, Zadeh G, Aldape K, Diamandis P. Precision histology: how deep learning is poised to revitalize histomorphology for personalized cancer care. NPJ Precis Oncol. 2017;1(1):22.
6. Kernbach JM, Yeo BTT, Smallwood J, et al. Subspecialization within default mode nodes characterized in 10,000 UK Biobank participants. Proc Natl Acad Sci U S A. 2018;115(48):12295–300.
7. Rajkomar A, Dean J, Kohane I. Machine learning in medicine. N Engl J Med. 2019;380(14):1347–58.
8. Rajkomar A, Oren E, Chen K, et al. Scalable and accurate deep learning with electronic health records. NPJ Digit Med. 2018;1(1):1–10.
9. Senders JT, Karhade AV, Cote DJ, et al. Natural language processing for automated quantification of brain metastases reported in free-text radiology reports. JCO Clin Cancer Inform. 2019;3:1–9.
10. Swinburne NC, Schefflein J, Sakai Y, Oermann EK, Titano JJ, Chen I, Tadayon S, Aggarwal A, Doshi A, Nael K. Machine learning for semi-automated classification of glioblastoma, brain metastasis and central nervous system lymphoma using magnetic resonance advanced imaging. Ann Transl Med. 2019;7(11):232.
11. Titano JJ, Badgeley M, Schefflein J, et al. Automated deep-neural-network surveillance of cranial images for acute neurologic events. Nat Med. 2018;24(9):1337–41.
12. Weng SF, Vaz L, Qureshi N, Kai J. Prediction of premature all-cause mortality: a prospective general population cohort study comparing machine-learning and standard epidemiological approaches. PLoS One. 2019;14(3):e0214365.
13. Zlochower A, Chow DS, Chang P, Khatri D, Boockvar JA, Filippi CG. Deep learning AI applications in the imaging of glioma. Top Magn Reson Imaging. 2020;29(2):115–0.
14. R Core Team. R: a language and environment for statistical computing. Vienna: R Foundation for Statistical Computing; 2020.
15. Rinker T, Kurkiewicz D, Hughitt K, Wang A, Aden-Buie G, Wang A, Burk L. pacman: package management tool. 2019.
16. Ooi H, Microsoft Corporation, Weston S, Tenenbaum D. doParallel: foreach parallel adaptor for the "parallel" package. 2019.
17. Templ M, Kowarik A, Alfons A, Prantner B. VIM: visualization and imputation of missing values. 2019.
18. Batista GEAPA, Monard MC. An analysis of four missing data treatment methods for supervised learning. Appl Artif Intell. 2003;17(5–6):519–33.
19. Kuhn M. Building predictive models in *R* using the **caret** package. J Stat Softw. 2008;28:1. https://doi.org/10.18637/jss.v028.i05.
20. Hosmer DW, Lemeshow S. Applied logistic regression. 2nd ed. New York, NY: Wiley; 2000.
21. Breiman L. Random forests. Mach Learn. 2001;45(1):5–32.
22. Greenwell B, Boehmke B, Cunningham J. Developers. GBM (2019) gbm: generalized boosted regression models. 2020. https://github.com/gbm-developers.
23. Hastie T. gam: generalized additive models. 2019.
24. Roever C, Raabe N, Luebke K, Ligges U, Szepannek G, Zentgraf M. klaR: classification and visualization. 2018.
25. Gravesteijn BY, Nieboer D, Ercole A, Lingsma HF, Nelson D, van Calster B, Steyerberg EW, CENTER-TBI Collaborators. Machine learning algorithms performed no better than regression models for prognostication in traumatic brain injury. J Clin Epidemiol. 2020;122:95–107.
26. Staartjes VE, Kernbach JM. Letter to the editor regarding "Investigating risk factors and predicting complications in deep brain stimulation surgery with machine learning algorithms". World Neurosurg. 2020;137:496.
27. Chawla NV, Bowyer KW, Hall LO, Kegelmeyer WP. SMOTE: synthetic minority over-sampling technique. J Artif Intell Res. 2002;16:321–57.
28. Staartjes VE, Schröder ML. Letter to the editor. Class imbalance in machine learning for neurosurgical outcome prediction: are our models valid? J Neurosurg Spine. 2018;29(5):611–2.
29. Harrell FE. rms: regression modeling strategies. 2019.
30. Staartjes VE, Kernbach JM. Letter to the editor. Importance of calibration assessment in machine learning-based predictive analytics. J Neurosurg Spine. 2020;32:985–7.
31. Robin X, Turck N, Hainard A, Tiberti N, Lisacek F, Sanchez J-C, Müller M, S Siegert, M Doering, Z Billings. pROC: display and analyze ROC curves. 2021.
32. Collins GS, Reitsma JB, Altman DG, Moons KGM. Transparent reporting of a multivariable prediction model for individual prognosis or diagnosis (TRIPOD): the TRIPOD statement. BMJ. 2015;350:g7594.

Foundations of Machine Learning-Based Clinical Prediction Modeling: Part V—A Practical Approach to Regression Problems

6

Victor E. Staartjes and Julius M. Kernbach

6.1 Introduction

In the neurosurgical literature, applications of machine learning for clinical prediction modeling are by far the most common [1–4]. The topic of predictive analytics also uniquely lends itself to introducing machine learning methods due to its relative ease of implementation. Still, we chose to specifically focus on predictive analytics as the most popular application of machine learning in neurosurgery. Nonetheless, the great potential of machine learning methods in fields other than prediction modeling, such as, e.g. natural language processing, medical image classification, radiomic feature extraction, and many more must not go unmentioned [5–13]. In clinical predictive analytics, those models concerned with prediction of continuous endpoints (e.g. survival in months) as opposed to binary endpoints (e.g. occurrence of a complication) are coined regressors. Regression problems, in contrast to classification problems, require different methodology, different algorithms, and different evaluation and reporting strategies.

J. M. Kernbach and V. E. Staartjes have contributed equally to this series, and share first authorship.

Supplementary Information The online version contains supplementary material available at (https://doi.org/10.1007/978-3-030-85292-4_6).

V. E. Staartjes (✉)
Machine Intelligence in Clinical Neuroscience (MICN) Laboratory, Department of Neurosurgery, Clinical Neuroscience Center, University Hospital Zurich, University of Zurich, Zurich, Switzerland
e-mail: victoregon.staartjes@usz.ch; https://micnlab.com/

J. M. Kernbach
Neurosurgical Artificial Intelligence Laboratory Aachen (NAILA), Department of Neurosurgery, RWTH Aachen University Hospital, Aachen, Germany

Whereas Part IV laid out the details of generating binary prediction models, this chapter of the series is intended to demonstrate the programming methods required to train and validate a simple, machine learning-based clinical prediction model for any continuous endpoint. Many concepts and parts of the code have already been discussed in more detail in Part IV, and this part will focus on the differences to predicting binary endpoints. For a better understanding of the methods presented herein, Part IV should thus be studied first.

We focus on the statistical programming language R [14], as it is freely available and widely regarded as the state of the art in biostatistical programming. While we elucidate all necessary aspects of the required code, a basic understanding of R is thus required. Basic R courses are offered at many universities around the world, as well as through numerous media online and in print. We highly recommend that users first make themselves familiar with the programming language before studying this section.

At this point we again want to stress that this section is not intended to represent a single perfect method that will apply to every continuous endpoint, and to every data situation. Instead, this section represents one possible, generalizable methodology, that incorporates most of the important aspects of machine learning and clinical prediction modeling.

To illustrate the methods applied, we supply a simulated database of 10,000 glioblastoma patients who underwent microsurgery, and predict the occurrence of 12-month survival. Table 6.1 provides an overview over the glioblastoma database. We walk the reader through each step, including import, checking, splitting, imputation, and pre-processing of the data, as well as variable selection, model selection and training, and lastly correct evaluation of the regression model. Proper reporting is also discussed.

The centerpiece of this section is the provided R code (Supplement 6.1), which is intended to be used in combination with the provided glioblastoma database containing 10,000 simulated patients (Supplement 6.2). When exe-

V. E. Staartjes et al. (eds.), *Machine Learning in Clinical Neuroscience*, Acta Neurochirurgica Supplement 134,
https://doi.org/10.1007/978-3-030-85292-4_6

Table 6.1 Structure of the simulated glioblastoma dataset. The number of included patients is 10,000. Values are provided as means and standard deviations or as numbers and percentages

Variable name	Description	Value
Survival	Overall survival from diagnosis in months	12.1 ± 3.1
TwelveMonths	Patients who survived 12 months or more from diagnosis	5184 (51.8%)
IDH	IDH mutation present	4136 (41.4%)
MGMT	MGMT promoter methylated	5622 (56.2%)
TERTp	TERTp mutation present	5108 (51.1%)
Male	Male gender	4866 (48.7%)
Midline	Extension of the tumor into the midline	2601 (26.0%)
Comorbidity	Presence of any systemic comorbidity such as diabetes, coronary heart disease, chronic obstructive pulmonary disease, etc.	5135 (51.4%)
Epilepsy	Occurrence of an epileptic seizure	3311 (33.1%)
PriorSurgery	Presence of prior cranial surgery	5283 (52.8%)
Married	Positive marriage status	5475 (54.8%)
ActiveWorker	Patient is actively working, i.e. not retired, student, out of work, etc.	5459 (54.6%)
Chemotherapy	Patients who received chemotherapy for glioblastoma	4081 (40.8%)
HigherEducation	Patients who received some form of higher education	4209 (42.1%)
Caseload	Yearly glioblastoma microsurgery caseload at the treating center	165.0 ± 38.7
Age	Patient age at diagnosis in years	66.0 ± 6.2
RadiotherapyDose	Total radiotherapy absorbed dose in Gray	24.8 ± 6.7
KPS	Karnofsky Performance Scale	70.5 ± 8.0
Income	Net yearly household income in US dollars	268,052 ± 62,867
Height	Patient body height in cm	174.6 ± 6.7
BMI	Deviation of body mass index from 25; in kg/m^2	0.02 ± 1.0
Size	Maximum tumor diameter in cm	2.98 ± 0.55

cuted correctly and in parallel with this section's contents, the code will output the same results as those achieved by the authors, which allows for immediate feedback. The R code itself is numbered in parallel to this section, and also contains abundant explanations which enable a greater understanding of the functions and concepts that are necessary to succeed in generating a robust model. Finally, the code is intended as a scaffold upon which readers can build their own clinical prediction models for regression, and can easily be modified to do so for any dataset with a continuous outcome.

6.2 Setup and Pre-processing Data

Sections 1.1–1.3 are identical to those required for classification problems, and are thus covered in Part IV [15]. Thus, we kindly ask the reader to consult Part IV for further clarification on R setup, package loading, importing data, and checking the formatting of the imported data.

Reformat Categorical Variables

To reformat all categorical variables to "factor" variables in R, allocate them to the "cols" object. Subsequently, we apply the "factor" function to all columns of the database using the "lapply" function. Lastly, "str(df)" is used again to confirm the correct reformatting.

Remove Unnecessary Columns

Your imported data may contain extra columns with variables that are irrelevant to the current regression problem, such as patient numbers, names, or other endpoints. The latter is the case in the Glioblastoma database: The 22nd column contains the variable "TwelveMonths," which is a binary form of our continuous endpoint of interest "Survival." Leaving this redundant variable in would lead to data leakage—the model could simply take the binary "TwelveMonths" variable and extrapolate some parts of our endpoint "Survival" from it, without actually learning any features. Columns can be removed from a R dataframe by specifying the column number to be removed. "TwelveMonths" is situated in the 22nd column of the database, and can thus be removed by applying the function "df <- df[,-22]."

Enable Multicore Processing

If you are working on a machine with multiple central processing unit (CPU) cores, you can enable parallel computing for some functions in R. Using the code in section 1.6, create a computational cluster by entering the number of cores (= number of separate R instances) you want to invest into model development [16]. The default is set to 4, a common number of CPU cores in 2021.

Partition the Data for Training and Testing

Figure 6.1 illustrates the procedure. To randomly split the data into 80% for training an 20% for testing (internal validation), we first set a random seed, such as "set.seed(123)," although you could choose any number. Setting seeds initializes random functions in a constant way, and thus enables reproducibility. Subsequently, we randomly sample 80% of patients and allocate them to the training set ("train"), and do the same for the test set ("test"). Then, the rows of the two newly partitioned sets are shuffled, and the two sets are checked for an approximately equal distribution of the continuous endpoint using "hist(train$Survival)." The histograms show a very similar distribution, both with mean survival of around 12 months.

Impute Missing Data

The glioblastoma database contains no missing data, as the function "VIM::kNN" [17] will let you know. However, should you encounter missing data, this code block should automatically impute missing data using a *k*-nearest neighbor (KNN) algorithm [18]. It is important only to impute missing data within the training set, and to leave the test set alone. This is to prevent data leakage. Also, imputation can be achieved using many different algorithms. We elected to use a KNN imputer for reasons of consistency—during model training, a separate KNN imputer will be co-trained with the prediction model to impute any future missing data.

Variable Selection using Recursive Feature Elimination

Recursive Feature Elimination (RFE) is just one of various methods for variable selection (see Chap. 7 for further explanation). In this example, we apply RFE (Fig. 6.2) due to its relative simplicity, generalizability, and reproducibility. Because random functions are involved, seeds need to be set. A linear model is selected as the regressor, and bootstrap resampling with 25 repetitions is used to ensure generalizability of the results. Using the "sizes" argument in the "rfe" function [19], the number of combined variables that are to be assessed can be limited. As we have 20 independent variables, we choose to limit the search for the optimal number and combination of variables to between 10 and 20. The "rfe()" function is executed, which may take some minutes. Using "plot()", the results of the RFE procedure can be illustrated (Fig. 6.3), and it is clear that a combination of 16 variables led to the highest performance. The selected variables are stored in "predictors(RFE)." These 16 selected variables, plus the endpoint "Survival" are stored in "keepvars," and the training set is subsequently reduced to 17 columns.

Get a Final Overview of the Data

Before diving directly into model training, it is advisable to look over the training and test set using the "summary()" function to assess the correctness of the independent variables and the endpoint.

```
#1.7 Split training and testing set. Here, we choose a 80%/20% random split ----
set.seed(123)   #Setting seeds allows reproducibility
dt = sort(sample(nrow(df), nrow(df)*.80)) #Allocate 80% split
train <-df[dt,] #Split
test <-df[-dt,]
train <- train[sample(nrow(train)),]  #Shuffle
test <- test[sample(nrow(test)),]
#Check approximate equal distribution of the endpoint - Here we see that survival was virtually equal in training
and testing sets
hist(train$Survival)
hist(test$Survival)
```

Fig. 6.1 Code section 1.7: This section illustrates how to partition a database into training and test (internal validation) sets

```
#1.9 Variable Selection using Recursive Feature Elimination ----
set.seed(123) #Set a seed
rfecontrol <- rfeControl(functions = caretFuncs, method = "boot", number = 25, rerank = F,
                         verbose = T, allowParallel = T)
#RFE using generalized linear models (GLM), in 25-fold bootstrap
set.seed(123)
RFE <- rfe(Survival ~ ., data = train, sizes=c(10:ncol(train)-1), rfeControl=rfecontrol,
           method = "glm", trControl = trainControl(method = "boot"))
print(RFE) #Results
plot(RFE, type=c("g", "o")) #Plot performance over #vars
predictors(RFE) #Variables to be kept
```

Fig. 6.2 Code section 1.9: This section illustrates the recursive feature elimination (RFE) procedure. A generalized linear model (GLM) is chosen as the regressor, along with bootstrap resampling with 25 repetitions

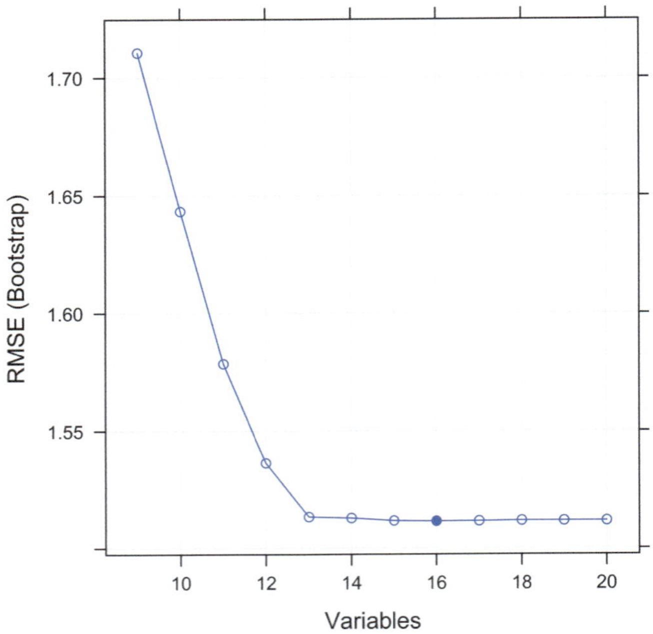

Fig. 6.3 Results of the recursive feature elimination (RFE) variable election procedure. It was determined that using 16 variables explained the highest amount of variance, as seen in the low RMSE that was achieved with this number and combination of variables

6.3 Model Training

Setting Up the Training Structure

Now that the data are prepared, training of the different models can be initiated. In this example, we elected to train five different algorithms to predict continuous survival in months: Linear regression using a generalized linear model (GLM), random forests [20] (RF), generalized additive models [21] (GAM), Least Absolute Shrinkage and Selection Operator (Lasso) regression [22], and ridge regression [22]. A brief overview of the five different models is provided in Table 6.2. We specifically refrained from using more complex models, such as neural network regressors, due to their inherently decreased interpretability and because they are more prone to overfitting on the relatively simple, clinical data used in this example [23]. All five models are trained sequentially and in a similar way using a universal wrapper that executes training, the "caret" package [19]. Hyperparameters—if available—are tuned automatically. To prevent overfitting, fivefold cross validation was chosen as resampling technique in this example (Fig. 6.4) [24]. However, bootstrap resampling with 25 repetitions could also easily be implemented (see Chap. 5).

Model Training

The procedure (Fig. 6.4) is equivalent for all five regressors (Sections 2.2.1–2.2.5). First, a seed is set to initialize the random number generator in a reproducible way. Subsequently, the algorithm to be used is specified in the "method" argument—the first model to be trained is a linear GLM, so "method = "glm"" is chosen. The "tuneLength" argument depends on the complexity and of the hyperparameters: GLM has no hyperparameters, so a low value is specified. We specify that the parameters and hyperparameters are to be optimized according to root mean square error (RMSE, metric = "RMSE"), and that a KNN imputer is co-trained for future missing data (preProcess = "knnImpute"). The inputs are automatically centered and scaled by the "caret" package. After running the fully specified "caret::train" function, it may take some minutes for all resamples to finish training. The red "STOP" dot at the top right of the RStudio console will be present for as long as the model is training. Subsequently, the resampled performance metrics RMSE, mean average error (MAE), and R^2 are calculated. Finally,

Table 6.2 Overview of the five models that were employed

Model	caret::train() input	Package	Suitability	Hyperparameters
Generalized Linear Model	glm	stats	Classification, Regression	None
Random Forest	rf	randomForest	Classification, Regression	mtry (number of variables at each tree node)
Least Absolute Shrinkage and Selection Operator (Lasso)	lasso	elasticnet	Regression	fraction (sum of absolute values of the regression coefficients)
Ridge Regression	ridge	elasticnet	Regression	lambda (shrinkage factor)
Generalized Additive Model	gamLoess	gam	Classification, Regression	span (smoothing span width), degree (degree of polynomial)

```
#2.1 Set Up the Training and Resampling Structure ----
#As a standard, we choose 5-fold cross validation as the resampling method.
ctrl <- trainControl(method = "cv", number = 5, allowParallel = T, returnResamp = "all")

#2.2.1 Train Model #1: (Generalized) Linear Model (LM) ----
set.seed(123)
lmfit <- caret::train(Survival ~ ., data = train, method = "glm", trControl = ctrl, tuneLength = 25, metric =
"RMSE", preProcess = "knnImpute", na.action = na.pass)
#We automatically tune our models based on RMSE, and co-train a KNN imputer that then automatically imputes any
potential missing data for future samples.
LM <- as.data.frame(cbind(min(lmfit$results$RMSE), min(lmfit$results$MAE), max(lmfit$results$Rsquared)))
colnames(LM)  <- c("RMSE", "MAE", "R2")

#Summary
print(lmfit)
print(LM)
#Save Model File
save(lmfit, file= "LM.Rdata")
```

Fig. 6.4 Code sections 2.1 and 2.2: First, the training structure is established: fivefold cross validation is used. Subsequently, a linear regression model (generalized linear model, GLM) is trained. All predictor variables are provided to the model, and it is automatically tuned for root mean square error (RMSE). A *k*-nearest neighbor imputer is co-trained to impute any potential missing data in future predictions. Subsequently, performance is assessed, and the final model information and resampled training performance are printed

the model specifications and resampled training performance are printed, and the model can be saved using the "save()" function for potential further use.

After completion of training the GLM (Section 2.2.1), the same procedure is repeated for the GAM (Section 2.2.2), Lasso regressor (Section 2.2.3), ridge regressor (Section 2.2.4), and RF (Section 2.2.5) models.

6.4 Model Evaluation and Selection

Model Training Evaluation

As soon as all five models have been trained, their performance on the training data can be compared. The final model should be selected based upon training data only. Criteria for clinical prediction model selection may include discrimination and calibration on the training set, as well as the degree of interpretability of the algorithm. Section 3.1 compiles the results of all five models, and allows their comparison in terms of RMSE, MAE, and R^2.

The code in this section will also open a new plot viewer window using "dev.new()", that allows graphical comparison of the five models. If you have executed all parts of the script correctly up to this point, you will be presented with a plot that is identical to Fig. 6.5. In this plot, we see that—while all models performed admirably—the GLM (linear model), GAM, and ridge regressor had the lowest error values (RMSE and MAE). Models perform well if these error values approach 0. In addition, all models except for the RF had very high R^2 values, indicating high correlation of predicted with actual survival values. The R^2 value, taken together with quantile–quantile plots that will be demonstrated further on, can serve a role similar to calibration measures in binary classification models—namely, as an indication of how well the predicted values correspond to the actual values over the spectrum of survival lengths [25]. As all of the best-performing algorithms are highly interpretable, the GLM, GAM, and ridge regressor would all make fine options for a final model. In this example, we elected to carry on with the ridge regressor.

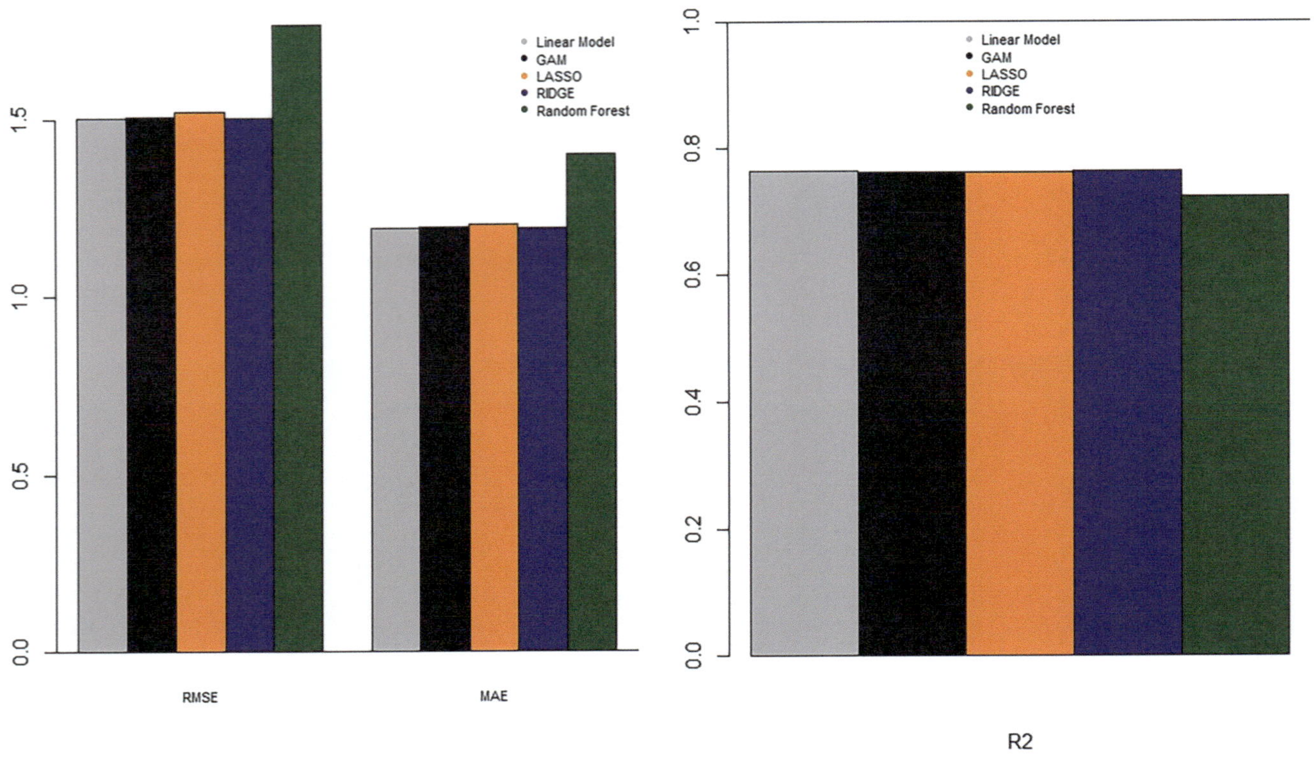

Fig. 6.5 Graphical comparison of root mean square error (RMSE) and mean average error (MAE) to the left, and R^2 to the right (Code section 3.1). The linear model, the LASSO model, and the ridge regressor all exhibited similarly low error values (RMSE and MAE), and all three achieved high R^2 values

Select the Final Model

The fully trained ridge regressor was previously stored as "ridgefit," and its resampled training evaluation as "RIDGE" in section 2.2.4. Now, as the ridge regressor model is selected as the final model, it is renamed "finalmodel," and its training evaluation is renamed "finalmodelstats." You can choose any other model by replacing these two terms with the corresponding objects from section 2.2.

Table 6.3 Performance metrics of the final regression model (ridge regression) for glioblastoma survival in months. The difference in performance among training and testing is minimal, demonstrating a lack of overfitting at internal validation

	Cohort	
	Training	Internal validation
Metric	(n = 8000)	(n = 2000)
Root mean square error (RMSE)	1.504	1.515
Mean absolute error (MAE)	1.191	1.211
R^2	0.763	0.759

Internal Validation on the Test Set

For the first time since partitioning the original Glioblastoma database, the 20% of patients allocated to the test set are now used to internally validate the final model. First, a prediction is made on the test set using "finalmodel" and the "predict()" function. The predicted survival values for the entire test set are then contrasted with the actual survival values from the endpoint (test$Survival) to arrive at error values. Using "print(Final)," the internal validation metrics can be viewed. Performance that is on par with or slightly worse than the training performance usually indicates a robust, generalizable model. Performance that is relevantly worse than the training performance indicates overfitting during training. These problems are discussed in detail in Part II. The final model can be saved, and will be available as "FINALMODEL.Rdata" in the same folder as the R script. Using the "load()" function, models can be imported back into R at a later date.

If you end up with the same performance metrics for the final ridge regressor as in Table 6.3, you have executed all steps correctly.

6.5 Reporting and Visualization

When generating clinical prediction models and publishing their results, there is a minimum set of information that ought to be provided to the reader. First, the training methods and exact algorithm type should be reported, if possible along with the code that was used for training. Second, the characteristics of the cohort that was used for training should be provided, such as in Table 6.1. If multiple cohorts are combined or used for external validation, the patient characteristics should be reported in separate. For regression models, a minimum of RMSE, MAE, and R^2 should be reported for both training and testing performance. There are countless other metrics to describe regression performance of clinical prediction models. Lastly, whenever feasible, an attempt at interpreting the model should be made. For example, logistic regression (GLM) models produce odds ratios, and GAMs can produce partial dependence values. However, there are also universal methods to generate variable importance measures that can apply to most regression models, which we present below. To simplify reporting, this final section helps compile all these data required for publication of clinical prediction models. For further information on reporting standards, consult the transparent reporting of a multivariable prediction model for individual prognosis or diagnosis (TRIPOD) checklist [26].

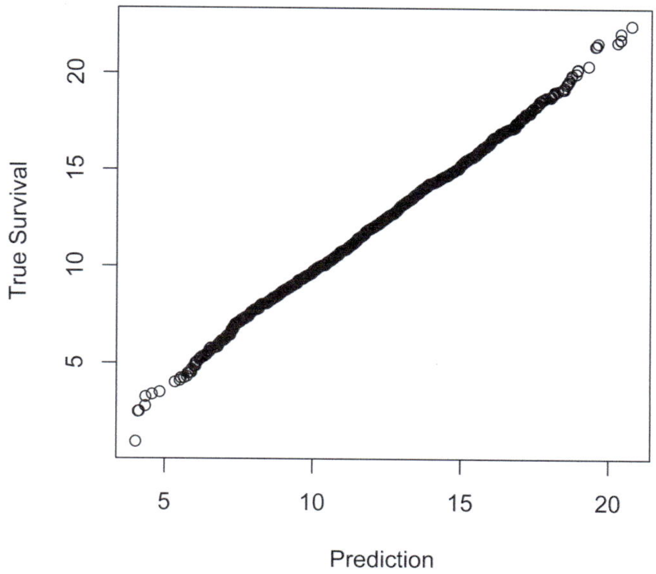

Fig. 6.6 Quantile-Quantile plot for the final ridge regressor, demonstrating the relationship between predicted survival values and actual survival in months on the test set (internal validation). The curve can be interpreted similarly to a calibration curve seen for binary classification models. The curve closely approximates a diagonal line, indicating excellent performance for both short-term and long-term survivors

Compiling Training Performance

The resampled training performance can be printed using "print(finalmodelstats)." The metrics that are produced include RMSE, MAE, and R^2. Subsequently, a quantile–quantile (Q-Q) plot is generated for the training set using the "qqplot()" function. A quantile–quantile plot plots quantiles of predicted values against quantiles of true survival values, and can thus be used to judge how a regressor performs over the wide span of survival values (short-term and long-term survivors).

Compiling Internal Validation Performance

Similarly, the performance on the test set (internal validation) can be recapitulated, and a quantile–quantile plot produced (analogous to Fig. 6.6).

Assessing Variable Importance

By using "varImp(finalmodel)," a universal method for estimation of variable importance based on AUC is executed, and results in a list of values ranging from 0 to 100, with 100 indicating the variable that contributed most strongly to the predictions, and vice versa. Finally, "plot(imp)" generates a variable importance plot that can also be included in publication of clinical prediction models (See Fig. 6.7).

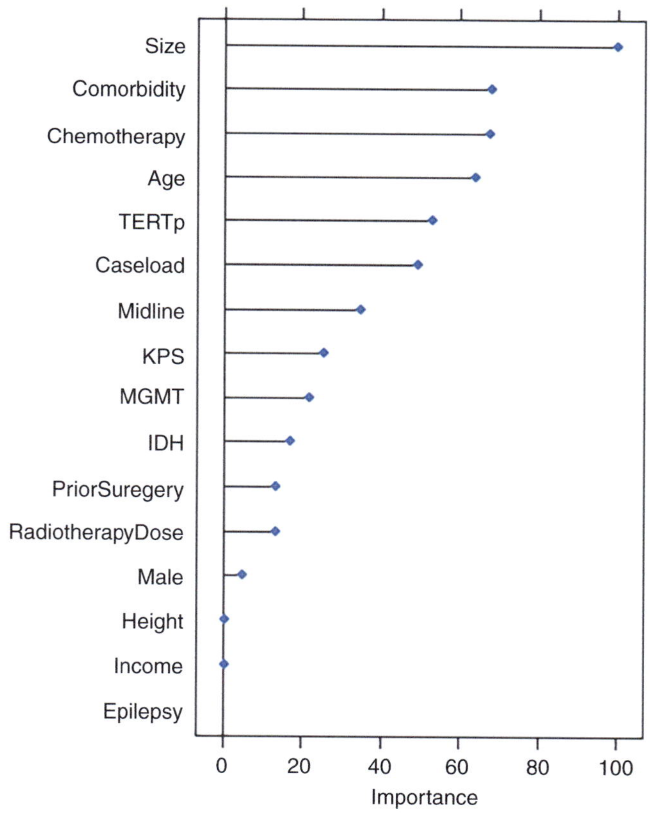

Fig. 6.7 Variable importance of the final model based on a nonparametric, model-independent method. The importance metrics are scaled from 0 to 100

6.6 Conclusion

This section presents one possible and standardized way of developing clinical prediction models for regression problems such as patient survival. Proper visualization and reporting of machine learning-based clinical prediction models for continuous endpoints are also discussed. We provide the full, structured code, as well as the complete Glioblastoma survival database for the readers to download and execute in parallel to this section. The methods presented can and are in fact intended to be extended by the readers to new datasets, new endpoints, and new algorithms.

Disclosures

Funding No funding was received for this research.

Conflict of Interest All authors certify that they have no affiliations with or involvement in any organization or entity with any financial interest (such as honoraria; educational grants; participation in speakers' bureaus; membership, employment, consultancies, stock ownership, or other equity interest; and expert testimony or patent-licensing arrangements), or non-financial interest (such as personal or professional relationships, affiliations, knowledge or beliefs) in the subject matter or materials discussed in this manuscript.

Ethical Approval All procedures performed in studies involving human participants were in accordance with the ethical standards of the 1964 Helsinki declaration and its later amendments or comparable ethical standards.

Informed Consent No human or animal participants were included in this study.

References

1. Brusko GD, Kolcun JPG, Wang MY. Machine-learning models: the future of predictive analytics in neurosurgery. Neurosurgery. 2018;83(1):E3–4.
2. Celtikci E. A systematic review on machine learning in neurosurgery: the future of decision making in patient care. Turk Neurosurg. 2017;28:167. https://doi.org/10.5137/1019-5149.JTN.20059-17.1.
3. Senders JT, Staples PC, Karhade AV, Zaki MM, Gormley WB, Broekman MLD, Smith TR, Arnaout O. Machine learning and neurosurgical outcome prediction: a systematic review. World Neurosurg. 2018;109:476–486.e1.
4. Senders JT, Zaki MM, Karhade AV, Chang B, Gormley WB, Broekman ML, Smith TR, Arnaout O. An introduction and overview of machine learning in neurosurgical care. Acta Neurochir. 2018;160(1):29–38.
5. Djuric U, Zadeh G, Aldape K, Diamandis P. Precision histology: how deep learning is poised to revitalize histomorphology for personalized cancer care. NPJ Precis Oncol. 2017;1(1):22.
6. Kernbach JM, Yeo BTT, Smallwood J, et al. Subspecialization within default mode nodes characterized in 10,000 UK Biobank participants. Proc Natl Acad Sci U S A. 2018;115(48):12295–300.
7. Rajkomar A, Dean J, Kohane I. Machine learning in medicine. N Engl J Med. 2019;380(14):1347–58.
8. Rajkomar A, Oren E, Chen K, et al. Scalable and accurate deep learning with electronic health records. NPJ Digit Med. 2018;1(1):1–10.
9. Senders JT, Karhade AV, Cote DJ, et al. Natural language processing for automated quantification of brain metastases reported in free-text radiology reports. JCO Clin Cancer Inform. 2019;3:1–9.
10. Swinburne NC, Schefflein J, Sakai Y, Oermann EK, Titano JJ, Chen I, Tadayon S, Aggarwal A, Doshi A, Nael K. Machine learning for semi-automated classification of glioblastoma, brain metastasis and central nervous system lymphoma using magnetic resonance advanced imaging. Ann Transl Med. 2019;7(11):232.
11. Titano JJ, Badgeley M, Schefflein J, et al. Automated deep-neural-network surveillance of cranial images for acute neurologic events. Nat Med. 2018;24(9):1337–41.
12. Weng SF, Vaz L, Qureshi N, Kai J. Prediction of premature all-cause mortality: a prospective general population cohort study comparing machine-learning and standard epidemiological approaches. PLoS One. 2019;14(3):e0214365.
13. Zlochower A, Chow DS, Chang P, Khatri D, Boockvar JA, Filippi CG. Deep learning AI applications in the imaging of glioma. Top Magn Reson Imaging. 2020;29(2):115–0.
14. R Core Team. R: a language and environment for statistical computing. Vienna: R Foundation for Statistical Computing; 2020.
15. Rinker T, Kurkiewicz D, Hughitt K, Wang A, Aden-Buie G, Wang A, Burk L. pacman: package management tool. 2019.
16. Ooi H, Microsoft Corporation, Weston S, Tenenbaum D. doParallel: foreach parallel adaptor for the "parallel" package. 2019.
17. Templ M, Kowarik A, Alfons A, Prantner B. VIM: visualization and imputation of missing values. 2019.
18. Batista GEAPA, Monard MC. An analysis of four missing data treatment methods for supervised learning. Appl Artif Intell. 2003;17(5–6):519–33.
19. Kuhn M. Building predictive models in *R* using the **caret** package. J Stat Softw. 2008;28:1. https://doi.org/10.18637/jss.v028.i05.
20. Breiman L. Random forests. Mach Learn. 2001;45(1):5–32.
21. Hastie T. gam: generalized additive models. 2018.
22. Hastie HZ, T Hastie. elasticnet: elastic-net for sparse estimation and sparse PCA. 2018.
23. Gravesteijn BY, Nieboer D, Ercole A, Lingsma HF, Nelson D, van Calster B, Steyerberg EW, CENTER-TBI Collaborators. Machine learning algorithms performed no better than regression models for prognostication in traumatic brain injury. J Clin Epidemiol. 2020;122:95–107.
24. Staartjes VE, Kernbach JM. Letter to the editor regarding "Investigating risk factors and predicting complications in deep brain stimulation surgery with machine learning algorithms". World Neurosurg. 2020;137:496.
25. Staartjes VE, Kernbach JM. Letter to the editor. Importance of calibration assessment in machine learning-based predictive analytics. J Neurosurg Spine. 2020;32:985–7.
26. Collins GS, Reitsma JB, Altman DG, Moons KGM. Transparent reporting of a multivariable prediction model for individual prognosis or diagnosis (TRIPOD): the TRIPOD statement. BMJ. 2015;350:g7594.

Foundations of Feature Selection in Clinical Prediction Modeling

7

Victor E. Staartjes, Julius M. Kernbach, Vittorio Stumpo, Christiaan H. B. van Niftrik, Carlo Serra, and Luca Regli

7.1 Introduction

Most readers are familiar with the concept of "*Occam's Razor*" or termed *Lex Parsimoniae* (Law of Parsimony), arguing that the explanation with the minimum amount of assumptions is often the most reliable choice [1]. This concept transfers relatively well to machine learning (ML)—and especially to clinical prediction modeling, where the goal is also to *explain* the variance of a given dependent variable (clinical endpoint in the future) based on *assumptions* in the form of input variables (features) collected in the present, which are assumed to have certain more or less "generalizable" relationships.

Increasingly often, within the era of "big data," clinical researchers are faced with "wide" datasets (i.e., containing a large number of different features in relation to the amount of observations) for clinical prediction modeling [2]. Due to the increasing availability of data, over-parametrization has become ubiquitous to continually improve performance. However, this also increases the risk of overfitting, and less complex models are often desired in real-world applications [3]. Besides, many of the features may only marginally improve predictive performance, anyway.

There are numerous approaches to select features to arrive at a feature set for a clinical prediction model: First, one could simply include all features—This can certainly be an option when the number of features is small relative to the number of observations ("long" data). However, in most cases, at least some of the features will not, or only to an insignificant extent, contribute to the explaining variance of the clinical endpoint. A more elegant avenue is to base the choice of included features based on prior domain knowledge (biological plausibility): Which factors are known to be associated with a given clinical endpoint? While this approach is certainly more parsimonious and thoughtful than only including all variables, selecting features purely based on prior domain knowledge is limited by the extent of prior research and the analyst's domain knowledge. Various complex interactions among variables may also not be considered. Lastly, remember that prediction is not equal to inference—The parameters of an inferential model may differ from a prediction model based on the same data.

For these reasons, methods for *feature selection* using some sort of objective *algorithm* have been developed. In this chapter, we aim to walk the reader through the foundations of feature selection and demonstrate some of the most popular methods.

7.2 Foundations of Feature Selection

The goals of feature selection can also go beyond simplifying models to facilitate input in a clinical setting or to reduce overfitting by reducing variance. Reduction of the feature space can also ameliorate model interpretation and, therefore,

Supplementary Information The online version contains supplementary material available at (https://doi.org/10.1007/978-3-030-85292-4_7).

V. E. Staartjes (✉) · V. Stumpo · C. H. B. van Niftrik · C. Serra
L. Regli
Machine Intelligence in Clinical Neuroscience (MICN) Laboratory, Department of Neurosurgery, Clinical Neuroscience Center, University Hospital Zurich, University of Zurich, Zurich, Switzerland
e-mail: victoregon.staartjes@usz.ch; https://micnlab.com/

J. M. Kernbach
Neurosurgical Artificial Intelligence Laboratory Aachen (NAILA), Department of Neurosurgery, RWTH Aachen University Hospital, Aachen, Germany

Department of Neurosurgery, Faculty of Medicine, RWTH Aachen University, Aachen, Germany

V. E. Staartjes et al. (eds.), *Machine Learning in Clinical Neuroscience*, Acta Neurochirurgica Supplement 134,
https://doi.org/10.1007/978-3-030-85292-4_7

is one of the cornerstones in the quest for truly explainable ML [4]. In addition, feature selection will yield shorter training times through less complex models and consequently faster computing in the pipeline.

Apart from parsimony, another interesting aspect is that feature selection can even increase model performance. Because most algorithms estimate parameters for each term of the model, non-informative or redundant features can add uncertainty to the predictions and reduce overall performance. Thus, the main goal of feature selection is the removal of non-informative or redundant features [5].

The "*curse of dimensionality*"—a concept coined by Richard Bellman in 1957 [6]—refers to the fact that, with increasing numbers of features, the possible configurations of feature interactions can grow exponentially. In turn, one single observation can cover less of all possible configurations. This translates to a clinical dataset with, e.g., a number of features that could even be higher than the number of observations, leading potentially to *sparsity* of the dataset—if some values of some features are only seldomly encountered in the dataset. In ML specifically, the Hughes phenomenon [7] implies that—as long as the number of observations is stable—a classifier or regressor's expected predictive performance will first increase with an increasing number of features (dimensions). Still, beyond a certain number of features, performance will start deteriorating. Of course, feature selection also helps in tackling the *curse of dimensionality*.

When starting with feature selection, the motto "*garbage in, garbage out*" must be remembered: Features that are known to correlate with the endpoint poorly, that are unreliable in their capturing (e.g., features with very poor interrater reliability), extremely sparse features, and features such as patient ID or names should already be filtered from a dataset in the first place.

Another seemingly minor but critical point is that feature selection should always only be based on the training dataset's observations. The relationships between variables will vary at least slightly among different subsets of the studied patient population (e.g., consider different variable importance and other parameters learned during different bootstrap resamples, demonstrating expected heterogeneity in how features interact when certain patient subgroups are in- or excluded). This means that—as a form of data leakage—performing feature selection with a mix of train and test observations may lead to an overestimation of real-world out-of-sample performance.

When considering feature selection methods, a fundamental classification can consist of supervised selection methods (in which the endpoint is considered) and unsupervised selection methods (in which the endpoint is ignored). Feature selection techniques can be further classified in the following way:

- Supervised Feature Selection Methods
  - Statistical Filtering
    - *Significance testing*
    - *Correlation*
  - Algorithmic Wrappers
    - *Feature importance-based*
    - *Purposeful Variable Selection*
    - *Recursive Feature Elimination (RFE)*
  - Intrinsic Methods
    - *Tree- and rule-based models*
    - *Lasso (least absolute shrinkage and selection operator) regression*
- Unsupervised Feature Selection Methods
  - Correlation

Which method is best for clinical prediction modeling? The short answer is: There is no universally superior method for feature selection. Therefore, like many options that one encounters in practical ML, one must understand the available techniques and their indications and limitations and carefully choose the method that works best for a specific problem using systematic empirical experimentation. In a certain sense, choosing a feature selection method can be seen as a hyperparameter that the human operator needs to determine.

Lastly, remember that *dimensionality reduction*, covered in a separate chapter (see Chap. 8), is a concept related to feature selection and should also be considered for high-dimensional datasets. Dimensionality reduction aims to simplify the dataset by expressing a large amount of the variance in just a few newly generated features.

In this chapter, we will elucidate each method briefly, focusing on feature selection methods in clinical prediction modeling, and provide examples in R for the most salient methods. Code examples are added in the supplementary material, and examples are based on simulated Glioblastoma survival data from the MICN and NAILA laboratories (Supplementary Content 7.1).

7.3 Statistical Filtering Methods

In statistical filtering methods, features are selected based on their direct (univariable) relationship with the endpoint, and some form of numerical cut-off is set to decide whether any feature ought to be included or not. Methods for statistical filtering are based on the type of available data. Continuous and categorical data—both endpoint and features—require different approaches, which will be covered in the following section.

In general, the advantage of statistical filtering methods is that they are easy and quick to implement and that they can provide more clarity than other more complex methods do.

However, they have significant drawbacks that have led to the clinical prediction modeling community moving on towards more integrative feature selection methods. Most importantly, these methods fail to consider the relationship among features and only focus on the univariable relationship among a certain feature and the endpoint. That way, interactions among features are missed. Some features may not correlate very strongly with the endpoint. However, they may still represent significant confounders (i.e., they influence other features in the dataset) and indirectly contribute to generalizability and predictive performance. Furthermore, redundant features are almost always included.

Correlation and Significance Testing

If both the features and the endpoint are continuous, correlation methods such as *Pearson's product-moment correlation* (parametric) or *Spearman's rank correlation* (nonparametric) can be applied, depending on the distribution of the data, for which histograms may be considered. If the endpoint is categorical, then *univariable logistic regression* (binary endpoint) or the *ANOVA correlation coefficient* (categorical endpoint with more than two levels) can be applied if features are continuous, and contingency table analysis such as *Pearson's* χ^2 *test* can be used if features are categorical.

The second step is then to determine a cut-off for the chosen test, above or below, which features are included or not included in model training. Often, p values (statistical significance) are used as a cut-off: Commonly, features with $p < 0.05$ will be included in the model. However, this approach is fundamentally flawed since p values are strictly dependent on sample size and do not necessarily represent the strength of an association. Furthermore, if p values are used, a generous cut-off such as 0.25 should be preferred over 0.05 or other lower cut-offs, since this would allow certain confounding variables to be included, too.

7.4 Algorithmic Wrapper Methods

Feature Importance-Based

Some approaches for feature selection based on feature importance have been developed (REF?). While some models intrinsically generate feature importance information, such as regression coefficients in generalized linear models and partial dependence in generalized additive models (GAMs). Still, generalizable methods that can be applied to virtually any model have also been developed—for example, based on differences in performance (e.g., area under the curve, AUC) calculated by leaving out each of the included features one-by-one [5]. Using these measures of feature importance, features can be ranked.

Feature selection can then be based on, e.g., removing all variables under a certain variable importance threshold or by a stepwise reduction of the variable with the lowest variable importance, which is further explained below. Another option is to add multiple random features to the feature set and evaluating feature importance against these features. If any feature ranks below these random features, it may be removable. An extension of this concept is *Boruta* [8]—A feature selection algorithm commonly applied to tree-based methods. Boruta creates "shadow features" for each feature (i.e., it copies all values of a particular feature but shuffles them among observations so that they are randomly distributed) and running a set number of multiple training iterations while after each set number of iterations, the feature importance is calculated and the features that rank lower than their shadow feature are removed until certain stopping conditions are met. Boruta can be implemented in R using the Boruta package [8].

Purposeful Variable Selection Algorithm

Several methods for stepwise inclusion and exclusion of features have been developed explicitly for generalized linear models (GLMs). Because univariable filtering based on univariable linear or logistic regression—much akin to the filtering methods described above—has become unfavorable due to the mentioned drawbacks, stepwise methods have been developed to allow for multivariable model selection. First, forward stepwise regression—in which features are added one-by-one to an empty model, and those who lead to a statistically significant improvement are retained until the model does not statistically significantly improve any further—and backward stepwise regression—in which all features are initially added to the model, and the model is reduced by deletion of each variable according to significance criteria—have been developed. However, both approaches are based on significance testing. Slightly more elegant methods based on the *Akaike information criterion* (AIC) have also been implemented, which may be more suitable in non-normally distributed data and can be generalized widely to other models [9].

However, all of these approaches fail to consider interactions between features directly. The idea of the Purposeful Variable Selection method, developed by Hosmer and Lemeshow [10, 11], aims to directly assess confounding by looking at change-in-estimate criteria, in addition to pure performance measures or statistical significance. The algorithm has become relatively popular, particularly for logistic regression but also for linear regression.

The authors of the Purposeful Variable Selection algorithm (Bursac et al. [10]) describe the process in this way: "*The purposeful selection process begins by a univariate analysis of each variable. Any variable having a significant univariate test at some arbitrary level is selected as a candidate for the multivariate analysis. We base this on the Wald test from logistic regression and p-value cut-off point of 0.25. More traditional levels such as 0.05 can fail in identifying variables known to be important. In the iterative process of variable selection, covariates are removed from the model if they are non-significant and not a confounder. Significance is evaluated at the 0.1 alpha level and confounding as a change in any remaining parameter estimate greater than, say, 15% or 20% as compared to the full model. A change in a parameter estimate above the specified level indicates that the excluded variable was important in the sense of providing a needed adjustment for one or more of the variables remaining in the model. At the end of this iterative process of deleting, refitting, and verifying, the model contains significant covariates and confounders. At this point any variable not selected for the original multivariate model is added back one at a time, with significant covariates and confounders retained earlier. This step can be helpful in identifying variables that, by themselves, are not significantly related to the outcome but make an important contribution in the presence of other variables. Any that are significant at the 0.1 or 0.15 level are put in the model, and the model is iteratively reduced as before but only for the variables that were additionally added. At the end of this final step, the analyst is left with the preliminary main effects model.*" [10].

Figure 7.1 demonstrates a code example, which is also provided in Supplementary Content 7.2 and can be tested alongside this text on the provided Glioblastoma data (Supplementary Content 7.1) [13].

Briefly, univariable logistic regression for all features is carried out in Step 1. To evaluate Step 1, run *View()* and have a look at the generated p values: Each feature with a $p \leq 0.25$ should be included in the next step.

In Step 2, a multivariable model is fitted. The importance of each feature is assessed to reduce the model to a more parsimonious model with only significant predictors. As "*predictors*," include all features that passed Step 1. The argument "*keep_in_mod*" can be used to mark specific, clinically relevant variables that ought to be included regardless of their significance—These will then stay in the model. To evaluate Step 2, run the *View()* function and inspect the generated p values. This step will choose significant predictors, usually according to a 0.15 or 0.10 level, and create a reduced feature space.

In Step 3, it is assessed whether features removed in the previous steps represent confounders. In "*predictors*,"

```r
#Purposeful Variable Selection - Packages
install.packages("remotes")
library(remotes)
remotes::install_github("emilelatour/purposeful")
library(purposeful)
library(dplyr)

#Step 1
step1 <- purposeful_step_1(data = df,
                    outcome = "TwelveMonths",
                    predictors = c("IDH", "MGMT", "Male", "TERTp", "Midline", "Comorbidity",
                            "Epilepsy", "PriorSurgery", "Married", "ActiveWorker", "Chemotherapy", "HigherEducation"),
                    conf_level = 0.95,
                    format = T,
                    exponentiate = T)
View(step1)

#Step 2
step2 <- purposeful_step_2(data = df,
                   outcome = "TwelveMonths",
                   predictors = c("IDH", "MGMT", "Male", "TERTp", "Midline", "Comorbidity", "Epilepsy", "PriorSurgery",
                           "Chemotherapy"),
                   keep_in_mod = c("PriorSurgery", "Epilepsy"))
View(step2$lrt_full_model)

#Step 3
step3 <- purposeful_step_3(data = df,
                    outcome = "TwelveMonths",
                    predictors = c("IDH", "MGMT", "Male", "TERTp", "Midline", "Comorbidity", "Epilepsy", "PriorSurgery",
                            "Chemotherapy"),
                    potential_confounders = c("Married", "ActiveWorker", "HigherEducation"))
View(step3)

#Create Final GLM
model <- glm(TwelveMonths ~ IDH + MGMT + Male + TERTp + Midline + Comorbidity + Epilepsy + PriorSurgery + Chemotherapy,
          data = df, family = binomial(link = "logit"))
summary(model)
round(exp(cbind(OR = coef(model), confint(model, level = 0.95))),2)
```

Fig. 7.1 Code snippet demonstrating the Purposeful Variable Selection method using the *"purposeful"* package in R [12]

include all features that survived Step 2. In "*potential_confounders*," include all features removed in Steps 1 and 2. To evaluate Step 3, have a look at the *View()* function and specifically the percentage change in estimates: If any change in estimate is larger than 15% or 20%, include this confounding feature in the final model.

Recursive Feature Elimination

Purposeful Variable Selection is a powerful method but is limited to GLMs and still based mainly on statistical significance. In contrast, Recursive Feature Elimination (RFE) is a wrapper method that can be applied to most models, is independent of the data type, and empirically selects the most informative features. In some sense, it is a "brute force" approach for trying out combinations of features in clinical prediction modeling. This is also termed a "greedy" approach in ML linguistics and can be computationally expensive. Nonetheless, RFE is likely the most popular feature selection method in ML. RFE was first introduced in 2002 by Guyon et al. [14]. It works with the following intuition: First, a classifier with all features is trained *more solito* on the training set. Second, a ranking criterion is calculated for each feature, based on an estimation of the effect of removing one feature at a time on an objective function, such as AUC. Lastly, the feature with the smallest ranking criterion is removed [14] (Supplementary Content 7.3).

In this way, RFE starts with all features included and iteratively reduces the model in what is essentially a backwards stepwise selection procedure based on a feature importance criterion, as described above. Thus, RFE recursively considers smaller and smaller subsets of features. When the optimum subset of features has been identified according to a certain performance measure (performance profile, see Fig. 7.2), a full model can be developed on the training data using the identified features.

The human operator needs to set only a few hyperparameters, necessarily: The size or size range of the feature subsets that are tried out, whether re-ranking should be carried out, and what model is to be used.

The size of the subsets that are tried out can vary between 1 and the total number of features. In general, if data sets are not overly large and computational power is provided, we advise studying all feature subset sizes. However, when dealing with large datasets that already require long training times with RFE, one can also consider limiting the number of features to be selected, e.g., empirically between 5 and 10.

Re-ranking can, in some cases, provide a performance benefit. In essence, when re-ranking is enabled, all feature importance rankings are recalculated at every step, leading to a more accurate estimation of feature importance at each step. This is computationally expensive. While in some cases, mainly when highly collinear features are present, re-ranking can provide some performance benefit, it has also been shown that—for random forest—a decrease in performance can also result from re-ranking features [5, 15].

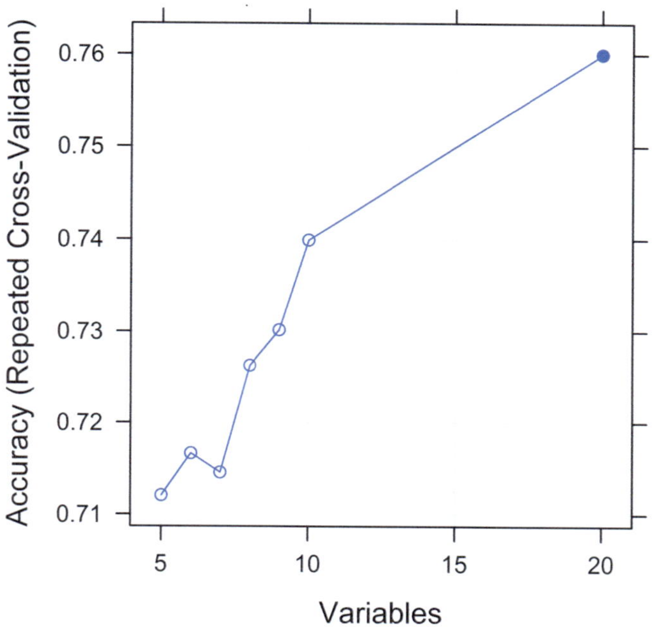

Fig. 7.2 Performance profile using recursive feature elimination: Accuracy is calculated for each optimum subset of features. Apparently, in this example, including all 20 features leads to the best performance

Lastly, many models can, in theory, be used for RFE. However, random forest [16] is the most popular model for feature selection using RFE in regression and classification problems. First, random forest—through its ensemble nature—usually does not exclude any features outright. Second, random forest has an intrinsic method for measuring feature importance [16].

Figure 7.3 demonstrates code in R, demonstrating RFE implemented using *Caret* [17] (Supplementary Content 7.3). Since random functions are used, a seed is first set. The *rfeControl()* function is set with the following arguments: To implement a random forest, *functions = rfFuncs* is chosen. We also specify that *repeated cross-validation* with two repeats as well as *re-ranking* are to be carried out. The *rfe()* function requires an indication of which columns represent features and which column represents the endpoint and a decision on the feature subset sizes that should be evaluated. Running the *rfe()* function may take some time. The results can then be printed, and the performance over the various subsets can be plotted. Finally, the object *predictors(RFE)* contains all selected features and can be used to train a full clinical prediction model.

Fig. 7.3 Code snippet demonstrating recursive feature elimination (RFE) using the *"caret"* package in R [17] (Supplementary Content 7.3)

```
#Recursive Feature Elimination - RFE
library(caret)
set.seed(123)
ctrl <- rfeControl(functions = rfFuncs,
                   method = "repeatedcv",
                   repeats = 2,
                   rerank = T)
RFE <- rfe(df[,1:20], df[[21]],
           sizes = c(1:5),
           rfeControl = ctrl)
print(RFE) #Results
plot(RFE, type=c("g", "o")) #Plot performance over No. of variables
predictors(RFE) #Variables to be kept
```

7.5 Intrinsic Methods

Tree- and Rule-Based Methods

Various tree-based and rule-based models are intrinsically able to exclude less important features during training. The intuition here is that during the optimization of decision trees, the optimal features are selected to split the data based on certain performance metrics. If non-informative features exist in the dataset, they simply will not be included in the final model. This also translates to *random forest* as an extension of decision trees such as *C5.0* [16, 18]. As rule-based systems are commonly derived from decision trees to gain the ability to write specific rules, the same applies to rule-based systems, too.

However, there is some evidence that, at least in some instances, relying only on the intrinsic ability of, e.g., decision trees to select features may be harmful to predictive performance, compared to employing other feature selection methods [19].

C5.0 and random forest can be implemented easily in Caret for R by choosing *method = "C5.0"* or *method = "rf"* in the *train()* function, respectively [16–18].

Lasso

The least absolute shrinkage and selection operator (Lasso) is a regression method useful for tackling regression problems (continuous endpoint) that performs feature selection and regularization intrinsically and is commonly used with linear regression models, although it can also be adapted to GLMs. Lasso regression is also called *L1 regularization*. The idea of the Lasso is similar to *ridge regression (L2 regularization)*, where the sum of the squares of all regression coefficients are shrunk to a value that is below a fixed threshold to reduce overfitting—however, in ridge regression, the regression coefficients cannot become zero, effectively excluding these features. The Lasso forces the sum of the absolute values of all regression coefficients to be lower than a fixed threshold, which in turn will force certain regression coefficients to take on a value of zero, which results in feature selection. The *elastic net* was later introduced as a further extension of Lasso and is more robust when there are large amounts of highly correlated features that may still all be important and should thus not necessarily be excluded from the model [20].

Lasso regression can be implemented easily in Caret for R by choosing *method = "lasso"* in the *train()* function [17, 20].

7.6 Unsupervised Feature Selection Methods

The most common use for unsupervised feature selection methods—thus, methods that do not take the endpoint into consideration—is to eliminate highly correlated features before training using simple correlation. Pearson's product-moment correlation can be applied to create a correlation matrix among all features, and extremely highly correlated variables (multicollinearity) can be removed based upon these correlations. Considering multicollinearity is critical in regression analysis because multicollinearity can change coefficients to make them unsuitable for inference—for example, an increase in one feature that is highly correlated with another may be offset by a decrease in the other, negating each other's effect and making the coefficients unsuitable for inference. Predictions will usually—empirically—remain stable, and this is often enough for ML. However, remember that empirical methods such as *RFE* or intrinsic methods such as the *elastic net* may also be equipped to handle highly correlated variables in a more efficient way.

7.7 Conclusions

Feature selection is a critical step in building clinical prediction models, and there are various pathways to arriving at a parsimonious feature space that explains a high proportion of the variance of the dependent variable. Multiple factors must be considered, such as the size of the dataset, clinical applicability and availability of the potential input features, and the computational power available. Feature selection based on univariable tests and corresponding p values, or correlations, are limited in their capacity to arrive at competitive models because they fail to consider more intricate interactions among features. Instead, wrapper methods, such as RFE, represent a powerful and empiric method for feature selection that can easily be implemented in the most common ML libraries.

Conflict of Interest The authors declare that they have no conflict of interest.

References

1. Crombie AC. Medieval and early modern science. Cambridge, MA: Harvard University Press; 1963.
2. Obermeyer Z, Emanuel EJ. Predicting the future - big data, machine learning, and clinical medicine. N Engl J Med. 2016;375(13):1216–9.
3. Fu Y, Liu C, Li D, Sun X, Zeng J, Yao Y. Parsimonious deep learning: a differential inclusion approach with global convergence. ArXiv. 2019:1905.09449. [cs, math, stat].
4. Rudin C. Stop explaining black box machine learning models for high stakes decisions and use interpretable models instead. Nat Mach Intell. 2019;1(5):206.
5. Kuhn M, Johnson K. Applied predictive modeling. New York, NY: Springer Science & Business Media; 2013.
6. Bellman R, Bellman RE. Dynamic programming. Princeton, NJ: Princeton University Press; 1957.
7. Hughes G. On the mean accuracy of statistical pattern recognizers. IEEE Trans Inf Theory. 1968;14(1):55–63.
8. Kursa MB, Rudnicki WR. Feature selection with the **Boruta** package. J Stat Softw. 2010;36:1. https://doi.org/10.18637/jss.v036.i11.
9. Yamashita T, Yamashita K, Kamimura R. A stepwise AIC method for variable selection in linear regression. Commun Stat Theory Methods. 2007;36(13):2395–403.
10. Bursac Z, Gauss CH, Williams DK, Hosmer DW. Purposeful selection of variables in logistic regression. Source Code Biol Med. 2008;3:17.
11. Hosmer DW, Stanley L, Sturdivant RX. Applied logistic regression. 2013. http://site.ebrary.com/id/10677827.
12. Latour E. emilelatour/purposeful. 2020.
13. Hebbali A. olsrr: tools for building OLS regression models. 2020.
14. Guyon I, Weston J, Barnhill S, Vapnik V. Gene selection for cancer classification using support vector machines. Mach Learn. 2002;46(1):389–422.
15. Svetnik V, Liaw A, Tong C, Wang T. Application of Breiman's random forest to modeling structure-activity relationships of pharmaceutical molecules. Multiple classifier systems. Berlin: Springer; 2004. p. 334–43.
16. Breiman L. Random forests. Mach Learn. 2001;45(1):5–32.
17. Kuhn M, Wing J, Weston S, Williams A, et al. caret: classification and regression training. 2019.
18. Quinlan JR. C4.5: programs for machine learning. Amsterdam: Elsevier; 2014.
19. Wang YY, Li J. Feature-selection ability of the decision-tree algorithm and the impact of feature-selection/extraction on decision-tree results based on hyperspectral data. Int J Remote Sens. 2008;29(10):2993–3010.
20. Zou H, Hastie T. Regularization and variable selection via the Elastic Net. J R Stat Soc Ser B. 2005;67:301–20.

8 Dimensionality Reduction: Foundations and Applications in Clinical Neuroscience

Julius M. Kernbach, Jonas Ort, Karlijn Hakvoort, Hans Clusmann, Daniel Delev, and Georg Neuloh

8.1 Introduction

In the emerging era of big data sciences, the domain of brain sciences and neuroimaging is projected to follow genetics as the next most data-rich biomedical specialty [1, 2]. The complexity of biomedical imaging is rapidly increasing due to the sheer mass of readily-available high-resolution data, including different imaging modalities such as magnetic resonance tomography (MRI), positron emission tomography, or electroencephalography. Considering the vast quantity and granularity of the available data, several large-scale collection initiatives have since emerged. In 2013, the Human Connectome Project (HCP) [3] was established, collecting multimodal high-resolution MRI data of >1000 healthy adults to characterize human brain connectivity and function. Other collaborations, such as the Enhancing NeuroImaging Genetics through Meta-Analysis (ENIGMA) Consortium, emphasized genetic profiling combined with neuroimaging in psychiatric diseases, including schizophrenia, depression, and attention-deficit/hyperactivity disorder [4]. Across disciplines, disease-specific open datasets became widely used. In the field of neurology, the Alzheimer's Disease Neuroimaging Initiative (ADNI) [5, 6] initiated multimodal MRI collection in 2004 and has since been successful in finding predictive phenotypes for the development of Alzheimer's disease [7]. The UK Biobank (UKBB) was recently introduced as the perhaps most compelling data resource for population neuroimaging [8]. Prospective data aggregation was initiated in 2006 to gather various phenotyping descriptors across genetic profiling, environmental data, and electronic health records in 500,000 participants. In 2014, the UKBB brain imaging extension was launched to collect multimodal MRI data across 100,000 participants by 2022 [9]. Various neuroimaging investigations have since successfully targeted major principles of brain organization at the population scale using the UKBB imaging-genetics cohort. These investigations included multimodal examinations of the neural structural-functional integration [10], brain phenotypes of gender differences [11], or the timely investigation of the neural correlates of loneliness amid the COVID-19 crisis [12].

The UKBB brain imaging cohort covers multimodal MRI data, including six different modalities as a raw and preprocessed dataset for 40,000 participants as of the latest release [9, 12]. In the expected full set of 100,000 participants, the amount of raw neuroimaging data alone will result in approximately 20 PB, that is 20,000,000 GB, of data. These numbers immediately illustrate the challenges that come along with big data neuroscience. Data sizes of that amount are hard to manage in terms of storage, computational speed, and memory. Without further processing, they inevitably lead to an over-parameterized setting, where the number of given features massively exceeds the number of samples. As the number of features increases, the applied statistical model becomes more complex and more prone to overfitting (see Chap. 3). Based on the "curse of dimensionality," famously coined by Richard Bellmann in 1961, generalization becomes increasingly difficult in said high dimensions. To work against the curse, the raw data's dimensionality has to be reduced to meaningful and concise information, finding a lower-dimensional representation of the given feature space [13, 14]. Three different methodological approaches can be applied to alleviate the problems that arise in over-parameterized situations: (1) features can manually be designed into new sensible features in the process of *feature engineering* [15], (2) a subset of the original variables can be used within *feature selection* or subset selection using, e.g.,

J. M. Kernbach (✉) · J. Ort · K. Hakvoort · D. Delev
Neurosurgical Artificial Intelligence Laboratory Aachen (NAILA), RWTH Aachen University Hospital, Aachen, Germany

Department of Neurosurgery, Faculty of Medicine, RWTH Aachen University, Aachen, Germany
e-mail: jkernbach@ukaachen.de

H. Clusmann · G. Neuloh
Department of Neurosurgery, Faculty of Medicine, RWTH Aachen University, Aachen, Germany

V. E. Staartjes et al. (eds.), *Machine Learning in Clinical Neuroscience*, Acta Neurochirurgica Supplement 134,
https://doi.org/10.1007/978-3-030-85292-4_8

regularizing penalties to shrink their coefficients toward zero, and (3) dimensionality reduction methods can be applied to simplify the given high-dimensional data's complexity while retaining the underlying patterns of the data.

8.2 Feature Engineering Using Imaging-Derived Phenotypes (IDPs)

A pivotal step in any data analysis regime has been identifying and efficiently encoding the most relevant variables. Using domain knowledge and analytical processing, the vast raw data can be encoded into an informative and concise set of features that allows a research objective to be answered. For example, in the UKBB, the raw imaging recordings are thoroughly preprocessed using a standardized protocol [16], which has already reduced the 20 PB (20,000,000 GB) of unprocessed data to 300 TB (300,000 GB) of high quality preprocessed data [2]. In addition to preprocessing the brain imaging data, approximately 4350 imaging-derived phenotypes (IDPs) are automatically generated, which represent distinct measures of brain structure and function.

Examples of IDPs include volumes of different tissue types, total brain volume and volumetric summaries for cortical and subcortical structures, microstructural parameters of tract-wise diffusion imaging data, or parcellations of resting-state network activity. Based on domain knowledge, the preprocessed data has been further engineered to summaries of relevant regions of interest (ROIs), e.g., derived from anatomical or cyto-architectonic atlas parcellations, to compile structural or functional homogenous cortical areas. Similarly, recorded resting-state MRI time-series can be parcellated into spatially coherent regions of homogenous functional connectivity using a data-driven fashion or established ROI delineations [17]. For instance, in the UKBB, resting-state MRI recordings were summarized using spatial independent component analysis (ICA) at two different dimensionalities resulting in a parcellation of spatial components representing group-average resting-state networks. In contrast to PCA, ICA separates the data into independent and additive subcomponents. Using available dictionaries of, e.g., cortical ROIs or data-driven network parcellations, effectively reduces the raw temporal data into meaningful units. Whenever possible, using domain knowledge can lead to more efficient representations of our data.

8.3 Dimensionality Reduction Using Principal Component Analysis

Another approach to reducing data's complexity is *feature extraction* or *transformation*, where the original features are combined in a certain way to create new, more concise features. While numerous dimensionality reduction methods exist, principal component analysis (PCA) [14, 18] has proven to be a competitive approach to simplify the high-dimensional data while retaining the underlying relevant patterns. PCA is conceptually similar to clustering and a popular illustration of an unsupervised learning method, as it finds trends and patterns without any knowledge of the target variable. When faced with a large-scale set of correlated data, PCA allows us to summarize the features by projecting them onto a smaller number of representative principal components (PC), which are analytically defined as linear combinations of the data's original features. The lower-dimensional representation of the data is maximized to capture as much of the underlying variation in the original data. However, the fundamental idea is that (a) often a small number of PCs sufficiently captures most variability in the original data, and (b) not all PCs are equally important. Based on these implications, PCA can be a powerful statistical tool for data exploration and contribute a sensible reduction of the features' complexity for further analyses.

The resulting PC can be geometrically interpreted. The projected directions of the PCs run along the axis of the highest variability in the original feature space. These projections consequently define lines and subspaces that are as close as possible to the observed data. This notion is appealing since a close relation between the PC and observed data points will likely provide a decent summary measure of the data. Additionally, all PCs must be geometrically orthogonal, meaning that they are uncorrelated with all previous PCs. The constraint of orthogonality explains why the second PC naturally captures far less information than the first PC. Geometrically interpreted, the first PC is defined as the direction along which the observed data varies the most (corresponding to the highest r^2 of explained variance among the PCs). The second PC provides a lower-dimensional linear surface that remains closest to the observed data points. Hence, the intuition that the discovered dimensions correspond closely to the observations extends beyond just the first PC.

In practice, it is sensible to use both approaches, feature engineering and dimensionality reduction methods. In a first step, combining raw data, such as information for every brain voxel in MR imaging, into concise IDPs already reduces the original data's inherent complexity. In Smith et al., the authors investigated the relationship between the functional connectome and 280 behavioral measures in the HCP cohort [19]. First, PCA was applied to the recorded functional MR imaging (4 × 15 min recordings for each participant) using the MIGP algorithm [20], which resulted in a lower-dimensional representation (4500 eigenvectors or PCs) of the original data. The PCs were then fed into group-ICA using the MELODIC tool [21] to further reduce the information into dimensionalities of $D = 100$ distinct spatial components.

Similarly, 158 non-imaging features were reduced to $n \times 100$. Both reduced set of features, the network matrices of the functional connectome and PCs of the non-imaging data, were then jointly analyzed in a canonical correlation analysis. The complexity of the original data was successfully simplified while important patterns were retained, resulting in an interpretable representation of a singular positive–negative mode of population covariation between brain connectivity and demographical data was identified [19].

8.4 Methodological Pitfalls

When appropriately applied, PCA is a powerful tool to handle high-dimensional data, where the number of features p drastically exceeds the available samples n. Choosing a value of M principal components, where $M \ll p$, can reduce the associated coefficient's variance and significantly boost prediction. However, several methodological pitfalls and their consequences for any resulting interpretations should be kept in mind.

Scale Invariance

Standardization or scaling is a pivotal step required for PCA [18]. Quoting Lever et al.: "Scale matters with PCA" [22]. Therefore, we generally recommend standardizing each feature before generating PCs, which ensures that all variables are on the same scale. In the absence of standardization, the features with high variance will play a larger role in the component solution obtained. In a small set of features, e.g., the simulated glioblastoma dataset for 10,000 samples (www.micnlab.com/files), entailing 22 different features, including age (range 40–90, mean 66.0 [standard deviation 6.2], unit in years) and income (range 20,000–500,000, mean 268,052 [62,867], unit in dollars), it is evident that based on different units the respective scales differ. Without standardization, the obtained PCs will be heavily weighted towards the features with a larger magnitude, while the remaining features will be ignored. As a consequence, the PCA results will be strongly biased towards the features with the higher magnitude and will selectively recover the related patterns of the respective features. Therefore, before performing PCA, all features should be standardized. Different scaling or standardization approaches within the same dataset should be avoided. However, in homogenous and already scaled data such as gene expression data, standardization should be treated carefully, as the transformed gene expression data may closely resemble expression owing to noise [22].

The Optimal Number of PCs

Unfortunately, there is no simple solution to find the optimal number of components. The question itself is ill-defined, as the optimal number of components highly depends on the application, specific dataset, and investigated research objective [18]. While an objective approach is lacking, we can revert to a different approach to estimate how many components suffice. Generally, we would like to use the smallest number of PCs while retaining as much variation as possible to understand the data. We can visually investigate a scree plot in an exploratory aim, a graphical illustration of the proportion of variance explained by the principal components (Fig. 8.1). The "elbow" of the plot indicates that the variance explained by each following PC drops off. In the given example (Fig. 8.1), the first and second PC explain a sizable proportion of variation, while the following PC3-10 do not add any additional variation. In this scenario, two PCs can be seen as the optimal number of components based on the scree plot method.

8.5 Conclusion

PCA can serve as an excellent data summary tool. But the underlying assumptions place limitations on its use. First, the structure of the original data is assumed to be linear. As the lower-dimensional PCs resemble linear combinations of the data's original features, non-linear patterns might be missed. Based on the orthogonality constraint, highly correlated trends may unresolved, as all PCs are uncorrelated. Conceptually, PCA is similar to clustering. However, important distinctions should be kept in mind. PCA, generally, finds a low-dimensional representation that explain most of the data's variance, while clustering finds homogenous subgroups so that the observations within each group are similar to each other, while observations across subgroups are maximally different [18]. With the aim of maximizing captured variance, PCA cannot always unmask underlying clusters [22]. Additional caveats, such as standardization and defining the number of components, should be considered when using PCA. When applied correctly, PCA is a competitive approach to simplify high-dimensional data to the main axes of variance.

Further resources There are excellent sources with different in-depth descriptions of PCA. James et al. can be highly recommended [18], which supplies the reader with different applications and provides R code for easy implementation. Further detailed literature can be found in: [14, 23], with additional extensions of sparsity in [24].

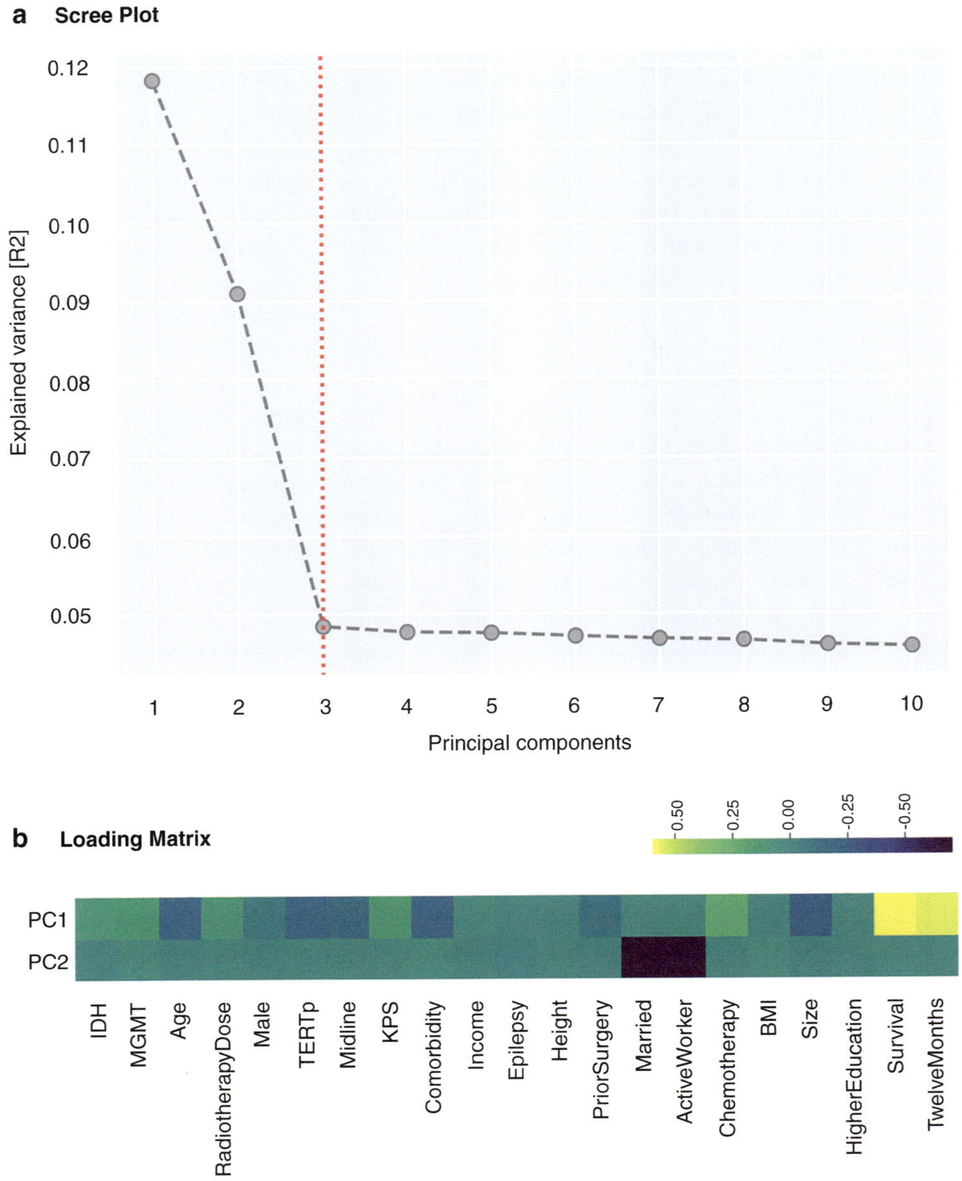

Fig. 8.1 In an example of a simulated dataset (www.micnlab.com/files), the optimal number of principal components (PCs) can visually be determined in a scree plot (**a**) displaying the proportional variance explained by each PC. An "elbow" can be seen after the second PC. Cumulative, PC1 and PC2 explain the most variance, while from PC3 onward, only a minimal amount of variance is subsequently captured. (**b**) The loading matrix can be used to understand how the original features contribute to the PCs' lower-dimensional representation. The axis of variance in PC1 is highly influenced by overall survival (yellow), while, e.g., age and comorbidity show negative weights (purple). PC2 represents a negative socio-economic axis highly influenced by marital status and working status

Acknowledgments and Disclosure

Funding J.M.K. and D.D. are supported by the Bundesministerium für Bildung und Forschung (BMBF COMPLS3-022).

Conflicts of Interest/Competing Interests None of the authors has any conflict of interest to disclose.

References

1. Editorial. Daunting data. Nature. 2016;539:467–8.
2. Smith SM, Nichols TE. Statistical challenges in "big data" human neuroimaging. Neuron. 2018;97:263. https://doi.org/10.1016/j.neuron.2017.12.018.
3. Van Essen DC, Smith SM, Barch DM, Behrens TEJ, Yacoub E, Ugurbil K. The WU-minn human connectome project: an overview. NeuroImage. 2013;80:62. https://doi.org/10.1016/j.neuroimage.2013.05.041.
4. Thompson PM, Stein JL, Medland SE, et al. The ENIGMA Consortium: large-scale collaborative analyses of neuroimaging and genetic data. Brain Imaging Behav. 2014;8:153. https://doi.org/10.1007/s11682-013-9269-5.
5. Jack CR, Barnes J, Bernstein MA, et al. Magnetic resonance imaging in Alzheimer's disease neuroimaging initiative 2. Alzheimers Dement. 2015;11:740. https://doi.org/10.1016/j.jalz.2015.05.002.
6. Weiner MW, Veitch DP, Aisen PS, et al. 2014 Update of the Alzheimer's disease neuroimaging initiative: a review of papers published since its inception. Alzheimers Dement. 2015;11:e1. https://doi.org/10.1016/j.jalz.2014.11.001.
7. Mueller SG, Weiner MW, Thal LJ, Petersen RC, Jack CR, Jagust W, Trojanowski JQ, Toga AW, Beckett L. Ways toward an early diagnosis in Alzheimer's disease: the Alzheimer's Disease Neuroimaging Initiative (ADNI). Alzheimers Dement. 2005;1:55. https://doi.org/10.1016/j.jalz.2005.06.003.
8. Sudlow C, Gallacher J, Allen N, et al. UK Biobank: an open access resource for identifying the causes of a wide range of complex diseases of middle and old age. PLoS Med. 2015;12:e1001779. https://doi.org/10.1371/journal.pmed.1001779.

9. Miller KL, Alfaro-Almagro F, Bangerter NK, et al. Multimodal population brain imaging in the UK Biobank prospective epidemiological study. Nat Neurosci. 2016;19:1523. https://doi.org/10.1038/nn.4393.
10. Kernbach JM, Yeo BTT, Smallwood J, et al. Subspecialization within default mode nodes characterized in 10,000 UK Biobank participants. Proc Natl Acad Sci U S A. 2018;115(48):12295–300.
11. Kiesow H, Dunbar RIM, Kable JW, Kalenscher T, Vogeley K, Schilbach L, Marquand AF, Wiecki TV, Bzdok D. 10,000 social brains: sex differentiation in human brain anatomy. Sci Adv. 2020;6:eaa1170. https://doi.org/10.1126/sciadv.aaz1170.
12. Spreng RN, Dimas E, Mwilambwe-Tshilobo L, et al. The default network of the human brain is associated with perceived social isolation. Nat Commun. 2020;11(1):6393.
13. Breiman L. Statistical modeling: the two cultures. Stat Sci. 2001;16:199.
14. Hastie T, Tibshirani R, Friedman JH. The elements of statistical learning: data mining, inference, and prediction. New York, NY: Springer; 2009.
15. Abu-Mostafa YS, Malik M-I, Lin HT. Learning from data: a short course. Chicago, IL: AMLBook; 2012. https://doi.org/10.1108/17538271011063889.
16. Alfaro-Almagro F, Jenkinson M, Bangerter NK, et al. Image processing and quality control for the first 10,000 brain imaging datasets from UK Biobank. NeuroImage. 2018;166:400. https://doi.org/10.1016/j.neuroimage.2017.10.034.
17. Craddock RC, James GA, Holtzheimer PE, Hu XP, Mayberg HS. A whole brain fMRI atlas generated via spatially constrained spectral clustering. Hum Brain Mapp. 2012;33:1914. https://doi.org/10.1002/hbm.21333.
18. James G, Witten D, Hastie T, Tibshirani R. An introduction to statistical learning with applications in R. New York, NY: Springer; 2013.
19. Smith SM, Nichols TE, Vidaurre D, Winkler AM, Behrens TEJ, Glasser MF, Ugurbil K, Barch DM, Van Essen DC, Miller KL. A positive-negative mode of population covariation links brain connectivity, demographics and behavior. Nat Neurosci. 2015;18:1565. https://doi.org/10.1038/nn.4125.
20. Smith SM, Hyvärinen A, Varoquaux G, Miller KL, Beckmann CF. Group-PCA for very large fMRI datasets. NeuroImage. 2014;101:738. https://doi.org/10.1016/j.neuroimage.2014.07.051.
21. Beckmann CF, Smith SM. Probabilistic independent component analysis for functional magnetic resonance imaging. IEEE Trans Med Imaging. 2004;23:137. https://doi.org/10.1109/TMI.2003.822821.
22. Lever J, Krzywinski M, Altman N. Points of significance: principal component analysis. Nat Methods. 2017;14:641. https://doi.org/10.1038/nmeth.4346.
23. Hastie T, Tibshirani R, James G, Witten D. An introduction to statistical learning. New York, NY: Springer; 2006. https://doi.org/10.1016/j.peva.2007.06.006.
24. Hastie T, Tibshirani R, Wainwright M. Statistical learning with sparsity: the lasso and generalizations. New York, NY: Chapman and Hall; 2015. https://doi.org/10.1201/b18401.

A Discussion of Machine Learning Approaches for Clinical Prediction Modeling

9

Michael C. Jin, Adrian J. Rodrigues, Michael Jensen, and Anand Veeravagu

9.1 Introduction

Machine learning is a domain of artificial intelligence (AI) that involves computer algorithms improving their pattern recognition and predictive ability through experience [1, 2]. Over the past two decades, machine learning techniques have been applied across medical domains, aiding in early diagnosis, patient management, and determining prognosis. As the algorithms have advanced, so too have their predictive capabilities, which sometimes rival or outperform those of experts [2]. In the context of neuro-oncology, neurosurgery, and neurology, machine learning models have accurately classified glioma World Health Organization grades [3], differentiated pediatric posterior fossa tumors based on clinical symptomatology and imaging characteristics [4], and classified spike clusters in epilepsy [5].

Beneath the umbrella of "machine learning" falls a number of distinct approaches, each with relative advantages and disadvantages. The two main paradigms within machine learning involve supervised versus unsupervised learning.[1] While supervised algorithms require the use of a pre-labeled dataset on which to train the model for predictions on future data, thereby simulating "intelligent" behavior, unsupervised approaches detect patterns across unlabeled data. In the following sections, several common supervised and unsupervised machine learning approaches are summarized, with attention to model background and past application in the neurosciences, neurosurgery, and neurology.

9.2 Early Applications of Machine Learning to Clinical Applications

Original explorations of machine learning and artificial intelligence applied to the medical sphere have been documented as early as the mid- to late-1970s. In one of the first demonstrations of computerized decision making, Edward Shortliffe developed MYCIN [6, 7], a rule-based approach to decision analysis purposed to guide antibiotic administration to patients with severe bacterial infections. Created under the tutelage of Bruce G. Buchanan, Stanley N. Cohen, and other faculty mentors at Stanford University, MYCIN was intended to resolve overutilization and inappropriate prescription of antibiotics, which was attributed to either a paucity of or poor accessibility to infectious disease experts [8]. As a relatively primitive rule-based system, MYCIN was bounded by its expansive set of a priori compiled "rules," each of which represented a modular chunk of medical knowledge. Subsequent validation of the MYCIN suggested classification performance rivaling infectious disease subspecialists [9]; however, a number of limitations remained. First, as a rule-based approach, the ceiling of MYCIN's performance was directly proportional to the granularity and breadth of rule set used. Second, while MYCIN's rule set was designed to be modular for subsequent updating, the process for doing so was low throughput and inefficient, essentially requiring both an infectious disease expert and a programmer to manually update MYCIN's knowledge base [6, 7].

Among early endeavors harmonizing machine learning theory with neuroscience applications included explorations into visual processing, rapid automated injury diagnosis, and molecular pathway reconstruction. Original studies exploring image recognition pioneered approaches to edge detection, motion recognition, and lightness perception; however,

[1] Reinforcement learning, a third subcategory, is not discussed here.

M. C. Jin (✉) · A. J. Rodrigues · M. Jensen · A. Veeravagu (✉)
Department of Neurosurgery, Stanford University, Stanford, CA, USA
e-mail: mjin2@stanford.edu; anand.veeravagu@stanford.edu

V. E. Staartjes et al. (eds.), *Machine Learning in Clinical Neuroscience*, Acta Neurochirurgica Supplement 134,
https://doi.org/10.1007/978-3-030-85292-4_9

these models relied heavily on empiric constraints defined by users and developers [10]. Similarly, early attempts to develop automated approaches to nerve injury diagnosis, such as PLEXXUS, were often rule-based expert systems emulating the approach taken by MYCIN over a decade prior [11]. Lastly, SENEX was developed to integrate previously described central nervous system (CNS) signal transduction pathways (specifically those pertinent to aging) under an object-oriented programming framework designed to facilitate inter- and intra-pathway relationship recognition and knowledge retrieval [12]. Since the 1980s and 1990s, however, the rapid expansion of computing capabilities has led to exponential increases in both interest and investigations into leveraging machine learning principles to augment the science and practice of neuroscience, neurology, and neurosurgery. This has led to diversity in not only application but also approach; while the above-mentioned studies pioneered the study of automata in medicine using rule-based and highly constrained expert systems, recent studies have incorporated a broad spectrum of methods for scientific and clinical purposes. The subsequent sections categorize these approaches and highlight exemplar studies contributing to the continued integration of computerized methods in the neurosciences. Emphasis will be placed on supervised machine learning approaches given their prevalence in clinical predictive modeling but a brief exploration of the role of unsupervised learning will also be presented.

9.3 Supervised Machine Learning Approaches

As previously noted, the origins of machine learning approaches in medicine and neuroscience leveraged rule-based supervised expert systems. More broadly, supervised algorithms are designed to learn a systematic approach to classification using a pre-labeled training set with known groupings. Subsequent application of the learned approach would then allow the user to estimate the class of future data that has not yet been classified. Methods such as regression analysis, support vector machines, and neural networks have seen increasingly extensive application for the prediction of clinical outcomes. In this section, we outline the overarching categories of supervised machine learning algorithms. Furthermore, we present notable advantages and limitations inherent to each approach while describing recent examples developed for use in clinical neurology and neurosurgery.

Regression Analysis

Predictive modeling can be summarized as the incorporation of a set of input features that, taken together, can provide an estimate for the likelihood of a particular outcome-of-interest. Yet, beyond accurate prediction and robust classification, understanding the contributions and significance of each feature is also of importance. Regression analysis offers an avenue to pursue both—while it is most frequently used for identification of independently important covariates in multivariable analyses, regression models may also be used for extrapolation and outcome prediction. Though regression analysis has existed since the early nineteenth century [13], their simplicity and reliability has made it foundational to clinical applications of machine learning. Most often, clinical regression models take one of two forms: generalized linear models (GLMs) or proportional hazards models. When applied to machine learning in clinical medicine, the former aims to predict the expected value of a Bernoulli variable (essentially a "yes" or "no" response) by relating the included model features within a logistic function bounded by 0 and 1. In solving the linear combination of features and associated coefficients, the user can estimate the log-odds of the outcome-of-interest. Proportional hazards models, the most popular of which is the Cox model [14], apply the multiplicative effects of model features to a baseline hazard rate to approximate the time-to-event risk that the outcome-of-interest will occur. It is important to recognize that the baseline hazard is assumed and not explicitly parameterized, making the Cox model semiparametric.

In particular, logistic regression remains a steadfast approach for both regression and classification analysis of Bernoulli outcomes (e.g., risk of readmission, presence of complications, poor discharge status, Fig. 9.1a). As such, it remains critical to understand the advantages and disadvantages of logistic regression as well as the contexts to which it is most aptly applied. A major advantage of logistic regression is the ease with which it can be used and interpreted—each included feature is associated with a coefficient which can be subsequently assessed for additive contribution to the likelihood of the outcome-of-interest. Additionally, because it inherently seeks to minimize logistic loss, a logistic regression model that meets all assumptions is generally well-calibrated and does not require subsequent refitting of class outputs as probability distributions (as is often required of SVM, decision trees, and neural networks) [15]. Nonetheless, a major drawback of logistic regression is the need to meet all assumptions, which include presumed linearity between the independent model features and the log-odds of the outcome-of-interest and the absence of multicollinearity between included covariates. Finally, sample size and event rate are important considerations for logistic regression, as an overly complex model trained on an insufficiently large sample is prone to overfitting [16, 17]. To address this last concern, logistic regression models may be penalized to limit complexity and improve generalizability through a process called *regularization*. Regularization comes in three general forms: ridge regression, LASSO, and Elastic Net. Practically, the fundamental difference between ridge

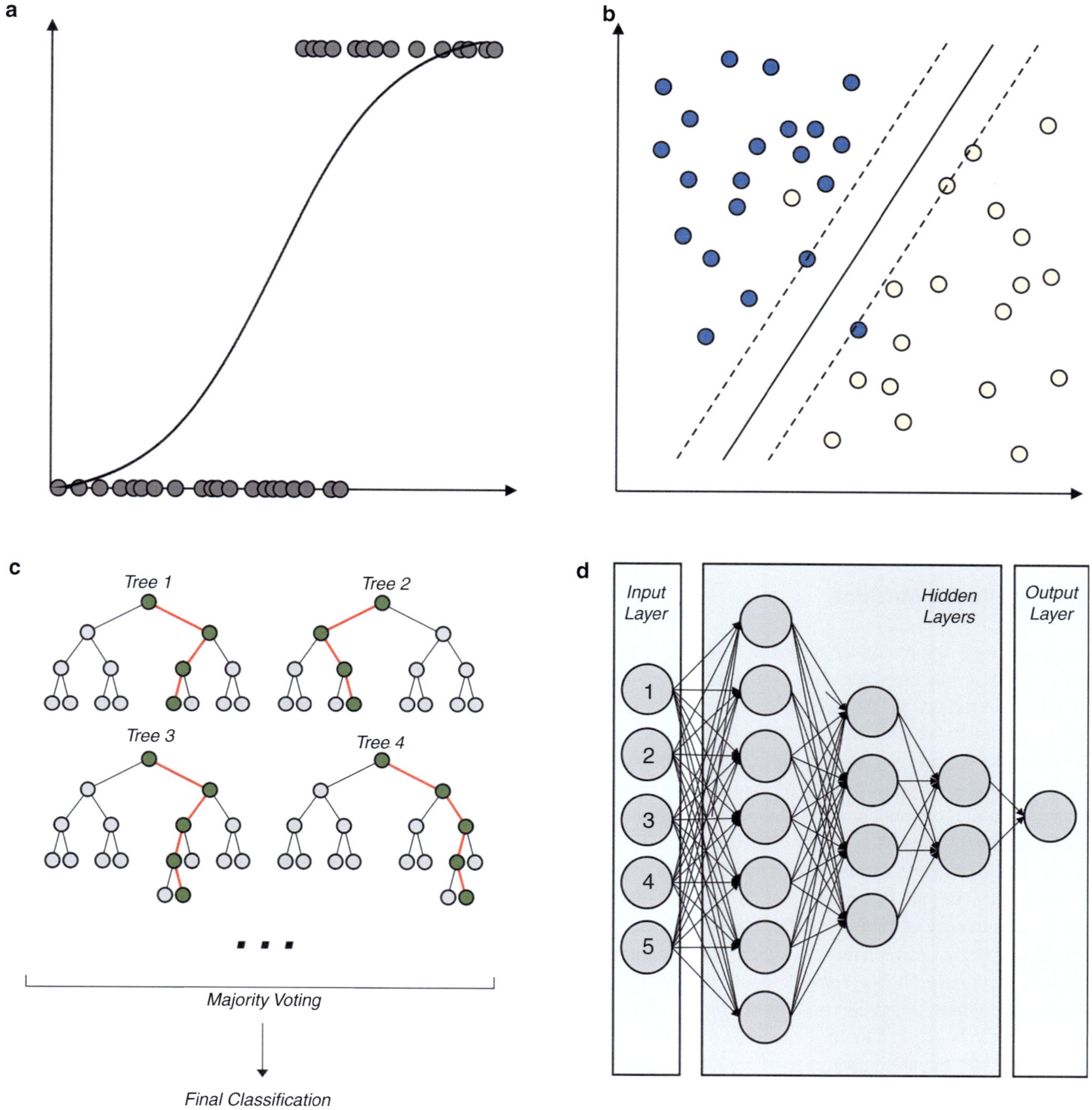

Fig. 9.1 Graphical overview of machine learning archetypes frequently used for clinical predictive modeling. Visual representations of (**a**) logistic regression, (**b**) support vector machine, (**c**) random forest, and (**d**) artificial neural network approaches

regression and LASSO is the ability to perform the *variable selection*; while ridge regression, also called L2 regularization, asymptotically shrinks coefficients of large model coefficients towards zero, no features are actually removed as part of the regularization process [18]. On the other hand, LASSO (L1 regularization) requires that the summed absolute values of model coefficients be restricted, leading to removal of noncontributory features and simplification of the model itself (hence selection of features most important to predicting the outcome-of-interest) [19]. To address concerns with each approach (for ridge regression, the lack of variable selection and for LASSO, model instability), Elastic Net was developed to incorporate both L1 and L2 penalties [20]. More recently, approaches for regularization of Cox models have also been developed [21, 22].

In a study of neurosurgical patients receiving endoscopic transsphenoidal surgery for resection of pituitary tumors, Voglis and Serra developed a boosted GLM model to predict post-operative hyponatremia [23]. *Gradient boosting*, in short, refers to an ensemble method—defined as one that seeks to develop multiple models subsequently combined into a single optimized combined model—that leverages serial sampling and reweighting to optimize the pertinent loss function. A GLM classifier with component-wise boosting, a modification of gradient boosting that allows for variable selection during model construction, outperformed alternative approaches including random forest, Naïve Bayes, and non-boosted GLMs by achieving a sensitivity of 81.8% with a specificity of 77.5%. However, a limitation noted in Voglis et al. was that, while machine learning methods aim to optimize model performance, steps such as coefficient shrinkage and variable selection limit the ability to directly infer clinical benefit from the individual model components. Nonetheless, GLMs do offer easier interpretability than other "black box" models such artificial neural networks and often achieve comparable discriminative ability for prediction of simple binary outcomes.

Support Vector Machine

An alternative approach to supervised machine learning, support vector machine (SVM) is best summarized as a geometric counterpart to the parametric approach taken by regression analysis (Fig. 9.1b). Unlike regression analysis, which seeks to discover underlying relationships explained by a user-defined feature set, SVM leverages the geometric distribution of the input dataset to define an "optimal" hyperplane or hyperplanes by which to discriminate data clusters based on the outcome-of-interest. In the case of linear SVM, these hyperplanes are drawn in $d - 1$ dimensions, where d is the dimensionality of the input data, and are selected to maximize the margin between these clusters. This resultant series of *maximum-margin hyperplanes* could then be used to extrapolate subsequent predictions by defining d-dimensional boundaries to be applied to newly sourced data. In the case of data that is not linearly separable, where a $d - 1$ dimension hyperplane is insufficient to robustly define cluster boundaries, non-linear kernel functions may be applied to map the explicit data onto a higher dimension feature space allowing increasingly complex hyperplanes optimally classifying clusters to be drawn. In theory, and under ideal circumstances governed by limitless time and computational resources, SVMs with non-linear kernels may offer performance improvements compared to their linear counterparts. For example, it has been described that the frequently used Gaussian kernel, also known as the radial basis function (RBF) kernel, offers equal or better discrimination given comprehensive optimization of model hyperparameters [24]. In practice, linear SVM is often sufficient and offers similar classification performance to non-linear SVM while reducing model complexity and, by extension, improving computational scalability; this may be especially true in medical applications, in which information canvassed from the medical history, physical exam, laboratory assessments, and molecular diagnostics is vast and provides an expansive feature set reducing the need for transformation into higher dimension space [25]. In comparison to logistic regression, SVM offers numerous advantages such as the ability to be applied to semi-structured data without a rigidly defined feature set and may be less prone to overfitting (particularly in the case of linear SVM) [26]. However, a major downside of SVM is that subsequent cross-validation is necessary empirically determined class probability estimates [15]; furthermore, users must be deliberate with kernel choice and adequate tuning of model hyperparameters to achieve optimal performance with SVM-based approaches.

SVM-based algorithms have long been used in the neurosciences for classification of disease properties and patient outcomes. In an evaluation of individuals with at-risk mental states (ARMS) with increased risk of progression to clinical psychosis, research led by Koutsouleris and Meisenzahl developed a non-linear SVM approach with an RBF kernel to distinguish between healthy control subjects and patients with early and late stage ARMS (ARMS-E and ARMS-L, respectively) [27]. ARMS-E and ARMS-L were distinguished by the presence of either attenuated psychotic symptoms (e.g. magical thinking, ideas of reference, suspiciousness, paranoid ideation) or brief limited intermittent psychotic symptoms (e.g. hallucinations, delusions, formal thought disorder). Evaluating binary classification of healthy controls versus ARMS-E and ARMS-L, sensitivity was 95% and 76%, respectively, while specificity was 80% for both comparisons. Three-group classification was also robust, with sensitivity ranging between 76% and 90% and specificity ranging from 89% to 92%; overall model accuracy was 81%. Secondary analyses comparing healthy controls to ARMS patients with and without transition to psychosis achieved similar discriminatory performance. While many of the limitations of the study require further external validation, such as evaluation across diverse institutions and a broader subject population, the preliminary results presented in this study indicate a role for machine learning approaches in anticipating presence and progression of neuropsychiatric syndromes.

Decision Trees and Random Forest

Decision trees also seek to identify geometric boundaries with which to best stratify data clusters into classes defined by the outcome-of-interest. Unlike SVM, which in high dimensions and with various kernel transformations applied may be difficult to comprehend and visualize, decision trees are simpler. In the popular approach put forth by Breiman, classification and regression tree (CART) construction is comprised of recursive partitioning of the dataset into progressively smaller subgroups called nodes based on a series of heuristics [28]. This approach, called *binary recursive partitioning*, defines splits that minimize a predefined cost function (frequently the sum of squared errors, entropy, or the Gini index) [29]. Compared to logistic regression and linear SVM, which seek to define an optimal hyperplane with which to stratify data, decision trees are able to define nonlinear boundaries by bisecting the data at each node. Decision trees, compared to logistic regression and linear SVM, offer a number of advantages including improved intuitive interpretability (particularly given visual representation of the full tree) and easier implementation without requiring prior advanced statistical knowledge (given the heuristic-based approach). However, decision trees also harbor disadvantages; namely, developing a robust decision tree requires a significant training cohort as each level of the tree results in an increasingly smaller portion of the original cohort on which the next decision heuristic can be constructed. Poorly constructed decision trees and those predicated upon insufficient data run the risk of overfitting and, although the user can preemptively safeguard against this with either pre-pruning or post-pruning (thereby limiting the complexity of the resultant tree), it remains difficult to balance the desire to maximally improve classification performance with the possibility of an overly complex and overfit model.

An extension of the simple decision tree, random forest refers to the ensemble approach characterized by aggregation of a collection of decision trees trained on random samplings of the training data (Fig. 9.1c) [30–32]. As previously discussed, a major concern with individual trees is the risk of overfitting complex models to the training set [33]; to address this, random forest mirrors a technique called *bootstrap aggregating* (*bagging*), which relies on repeated bootstrap sampling from the training dataset to each create a decision tree. Furthermore, these bagged decision trees are grown with a random subset of the full feature set (*feature bagging*). This is a significant modification to the classical bagging approach as individual decision trees are most frequently constructed using greedy algorithms intended to minimize error at each decision heuristic. In the absence of feature bagging, individual decision trees are likely to be highly correlated with each other, which limits the advantages of ensemble learning, as that relies on the construction of diverse individual models to maximize aggregate model accuracy [34]. In practice, the performance improvements of random forest over alternative approaches are well-recognized [35]. Nonetheless, proper bootstrap sampling and tuning of all model hyperparameters are necessary to achieve optimal classifier performance [36].

A recent study by Audureau et al. evaluated the performance of single decision tree and random forest approaches for predicting post-recurrence survival of glioblastoma patients [37]. Incorporating demographic and clinical features available at the time of disease progression, both approaches narrowly outperformed a Cox regression-based approach by each achieving a Harrell's concordance index of over 70 [38]. Beyond identifying KPS score at progression as the most important predictor of overall post-recurrence survival, they were able to identify four risk groups which drastically differed in survival duration: while patients with highest risk experienced a median survival of less than 3 months post-recurrence, the majority of those classified as lowest risk lived for more than 12 months post-recurrence. Of note, glioblastoma outcomes are known to be strongly associated with genomic and epigenomic features not available in this study [39, 40]; subsequent efforts to improve risk classification may further increase performance by diversifying the feature set included during model construction and training.

Artificial Neural Networks

Artificial neural networks (ANNs) are best explained as a replication of the human brain: a collection of neurons which each modify an input by performing a simple computational task and propagate an output to the next downstream neuron in the chain. These interconnections form a network comprising three flavors of neurons arranged in layers: the input layer, the output layer, and a number of hidden layers responsible for modification of the received input from upstream neurons (in the case of multilayer networks, Fig. 9.1d). More simply, the input layer is defined by the input feature set by defining each feature as an individual neuron while each output class of the model is represented by a neuron in the output layer. Single layer neural networks, known as *perceptrons*, consist only of an input layer and an output layer with interneuron input–output connections serving as a computational layer. The computational layer itself includes an input-specific weight that scales with the contribution of each particular input neuron and an activation function, which transforms the weighted sum of the aggregate input neurons onto a user-defined output distribution. Depending on the intended output, the activation function can take various forms including sigmoid functions or piecewise functions. Sigmoid functions, bounded by 0 and 1, are appropriate when the output of a perceptron is expected to be a probability for a binary outcome (as opposed to a softmax function for multi-class outcomes). A major drawback of sigmoid activation functions is known as the *vanishing gradient*, which describes the tendency of the incremental response variable change to asymptotically approach zero as the magnitude of the input becomes exceedingly large. This means that as the output trends towards the boundaries of the distribution, less learning is possible. This is particularly important in the context of *deep learning* where an increasing number of hidden layers comprising a *multilayer perceptron* (*MLP*) facilitates the detection of non-linear patterns and representations within the data. For applications requiring multilayer neural networks, *ReLUs* (*rectified linear units*, essentially a piecewise linear function expressed as $f(x) = \max(0,x)$) solve the vanishing gradient problem while retaining more complexity than a simple linear function. Furthermore, *ReLUs* allow for zero representations within the model leading to increased model sparsity thereby improving learning speed. This property only becomes more valuable when considering models with a high quantity of hidden layers or neurons and models implementing backpropagation of signals within *convolutional neural networks*.

Oermann and Ewend leveraged ensemble learning and ANNs to develop a method for predicting survival following definitive stereotactic radiosurgery to brain metastases [41]. Features included in ANN construction were ECOG score, primary tumor type, presence of systemic disease, age, and number of brain metastases. Both the single ANN and ensemble ANN approach outperformed multivariable logistic regression, achieving AUROCs of 0.84 and 0.78, respectively. At a fixed sensitivity of 95%, 1-year survival prediction yielded a specificity of 38% for ensemble ANNs and 32% for single ANN (compared to 26% for multivariable logistic regression). While these results are encouraging, a major advantage of the ANNs, particularly MLPs with signal backpropagation, is the ability to explore highly complex, non-linear relationships; by incorporating a more expansive feature set including genomic, epigenomic, and proteomic features known to correlate with patient outcomes, future studies may further harness the flexibility of ANN-based approaches for clinical predictive modeling.

Naïve Bayes

Until now, all approaches discussed have been discriminative models that seek to define a boundary optimally separating classes defined by the outcome-of-interest. An alternative approach to predictive modeling is computing the posterior probability distribution explicitly based on all available information; models that take this approach are referred to as "generative," among which one of the most frequently used is the Naïve Bayes classifier [42]. Briefly, the Naïve Bayes approach applies Bayes' theorem to compute the probability of the outcome-of-interest occurring given a series of available features, each of which are independent of each other given the outcome-of-interest (*conditional independence*). This can be summarized by

$$P\left(O|,x_1|,x_2|,x_3|,\ldots|,x_n\right)=\frac{P\left(x_1,|x_2,|x_3,|\ldots,|x_n,|O\right)P\left(O\right)}{P\left(x_1,x_2,x_3,\ldots,x_n\right)},$$

which given conditional independence, can be expressed as

$$P\left(O|,x_1|,x_2|,x_3|,\ldots|,x_n\right)=\frac{P\left(O\right)\prod_i^n P\left(x_i|O\right)}{P\left(x_1,x_2,x_3,\ldots,x_n\right)}.$$

Under Naïve Bayes assumptions, the denominator is, by definition, a constant, making the posterior probability proportional to $P\left(O\right)\prod_i^n P\left(x_i|O\right)$. Understanding the distribution of $P(x_i|O)$ is important, and continuous and discrete features are frequently modeled as Gaussian and Bernoulli variables, respectively. Another consideration necessary for application of Naïve Bayes for classification is the possibility of features or feature levels absent in the training set but present in future data input into the classifier; to avoid the risk of zeroed probabilities, Laplace smoothing may be applied [43].

Practically, the performance of Naïve Bayes models can be juxtaposed against that of logistic regression models; while the theoretical asymptotic error of the logistic regression is lower under perfect conditions with abundant training data, Naïve Bayes more efficiently approaches the asymptotic error making it an attractive alternative under realistic conditions in which the availability of training data may be limited [44]. However, it is rare to have data that flawlessly fulfills the conditional independence assumption, impacting the accuracy of the posterior probability estimate. Nonetheless, the classification performance of Naïve Bayes remains comparable to that of discriminative models and may offer additional benefits in sample-sparse settings with a limited training cohort.

One example of the Naïve Bayes approach to outcome prediction can be seen in a study conducted by Tunthanathip and Taweesomboonyat assessing risk of surgical site infections following neurosurgical operations [45]. Using features spanning demographics, operation type and course, and other post-operative complications, the authors identified Naïve Bayes as the optimal approach compared to decision tree and ANN-based models. At a specificity of nearly 90%, sensitivity for predicting post-operative surgical site infection was nearly 60%. Among limitations of the study include the low event rate of the outcome-of-interest, which may have contributed to the relatively superior performance of Naïve Bayes compared to discriminative methods. Additionally, it is likely that at least a subset of the features does not satisfy the assumption of conditional independence. However, as previously mentioned, few feature sets exhibit true conditional independence and even imperfect feature choice may offer sufficient performance to be of value.

9.4 Unsupervised Machine Learning Approaches

As previously noted, the vast majority of predictive modeling in medicine has utilized supervised learning approaches; however, it bears noting that unsupervised learning also occupies a critical niche. Unlike supervised learning, which is predicated upon developing a predictive model using a pre-classified training set for classification of future data, unsupervised learning relies on pattern recognition and structure discovery within datasets without prior labels. Though there are many approaches to unsupervised machine learning including signal separation algorithms, such as principal components analysis and singular value decomposition, and outlier detection, via techniques like isolation forests, emphasis will be placed on one of the most common applications in medicine: *cluster analysis*.

Clustering

One of the most well-recognized uses of unsupervised machine learning is for cluster analysis, which refers to the identification of groupings within data comprised of members with higher intra-cluster similarity than inter-cluster similarity [46]. Numerous algorithms exist for clustering but some of the most frequently applied include hierarchical clustering, *k*-means clustering, expectation-maximization, and DBSCAN. Hierarchical clustering can be characterized as either agglomerative (bottom-up starting from *n* clusters each containing a single datapoint) or divisive (top-down starting from a single cluster containing *n* datapoints) and seek to minimize dissimilarity within clusters as usually measured by metric such as Euclidean distance. While hierarchical clustering is highly interpretable given its intuitive nature, it is also computationally inefficient with a run time that scales cubically with dataset size [47]. An alternative approach is *k*-means clustering, which iteratively identifies *k* cluster centroids and categorizing datapoints based on closeness to each centroid [48]. However, application of the *k*-means algorithm requires sufficient prior knowledge of the dataset to intelligently specify the number of centroids. Expectation-maximization, similar to *k*-means, aims to iteratively refine its cluster definition given an expected number of groupings. Unlike *k*-means, however, expectation-maximization takes a putative *mixture model* architecture (e.g. *n* Gaussian distributions) and fits distribution parameters on the input dataset; once the mixture model is fully parameterized, each element in the dataset can be assigned a probability of belonging to each of the clusters [49]. Lastly, DBSCAN (*Density-Based Spatial Clustering of Applications with Noise*) is a nonparametric method for cluster identification based on data density [50, 51].

Applications of clustering algorithms in the neurosciences have led to revolutionary advances in our understanding of disease pathogenesis, furthering physicians' ability to design increasingly accurate and robust predictive models. Agglomerative hierarchical clustering has not only been applied to genomics and transcriptomics to identify molecular subclasses of glioblastoma with differential outcomes [52], but has also been used to deconvolute the single-cell transcriptional microenvironment within glioblastoma tumors [53]. Others have used expectation-maximization for segmentation of brain MRIs, performing comparably to manual alternatives [54]. Finally, DBSCAN has been applied for clustering applications on brain MRI; combining DBSCAN with supervised machine learning, Plant and Ewers were able to both distinguish individuals with Alzheimer's disease (AD) from healthy individuals and predict progression to AD in subjects with mild cognitive impairment [55].

9.5 Conclusion

Probabilistic modeling, risk estimation, and prediction are inherent to the practice of neuroscience, neurosurgery, and neurology. The use of machine learning algorithms to aid those processes will only continue to increase in the coming years as the maintenance of large clinical databases and the digitization of medical records continuously provide rich sources of data. From the early rule-based supervised expert systems, advances in computing have led to a diverse array of machine learning methodologies that allow extensive applications across the neurosciences. While the investigator must recognize the limitations of their data and the constraints inherent to individual models, they are able to tailor their approach given the need for variable selection, exploration of non-linear relationships, pre-labeled training sets, computational scalability, or learning speed, among other considerations. In the preceding sections, six machine learning approaches across two broad learning paradigms were summarized. Though not a comprehensive review, it is hoped the descriptions herein provide an overarching summary of the current landscape of machine learning in the neurosciences as well as an understanding how existing models may be used to answer clinical or experimental questions.

Conflict of Interest Statement The authors report no relevant conflicts of interest or financial relationships.

References

1. Ghahramani Z. Probabilistic machine learning and artificial intelligence. Nature. 2015;521:452–9. https://doi.org/10.1038/nature14541.
2. Senders JT, Arnaout O, Karhade AV, Dasenbrock HH, Gormley WB, Broekman ML, Smith TR. Natural and artificial intelligence in neurosurgery: a systematic review. Neurosurgery. 2018;83:181–92. https://doi.org/10.1093/neuros/nyx384.
3. Zhao ZX, Lan K, Xiao JH, Zhang Y, Xu P, Jia L, He M. A new method to classify pathologic grades of astrocytomas based on magnetic resonance imaging appearances. Neurol India. 2010;58:685–90. https://doi.org/10.4103/0028-3886.72161.
4. Bidiwala S, Pittman T. Neural network classification of pediatric posterior fossa tumors using clinical and imaging data. Pediatr Neurosurg. 2004;40:8–15. https://doi.org/10.1159/000076571.
5. Tankus A, Yeshurun Y, Fried I. An automatic measure for classifying clusters of suspected spikes into single cells versus multiunits. J Neural Eng. 2009;6:056001. https://doi.org/10.1088/1741-2560/6/5/056001.
6. Shortliffe E. Computer-based medical consultations: MYCIN, vol. 2. Amsterdam: Elsevier; 2012.
7. Shortliffe EH, Axline SG, Buchanan BG, Merigan TC, Cohen SN. An artificial intelligence program to advise physicians regarding antimicrobial therapy. Comput Biomed Res. 1973;6:544–60. https://doi.org/10.1016/0010-4809(73)90029-3.
8. Roberts AW, Visconti JA. The rational and irrational use of systemic antimicrobial drugs. Am J Hosp Pharm. 1972;29:828–34.
9. Yu VL, Buchanan BG, Shortliffe EH, Wraith SM, Davis R, Scott AC, Cohen SN. Evaluating the performance of a computer-based consultant. Comput Programs Biomed. 1979;9:95–102. https://doi.org/10.1016/0010-468x(79)90022-9.
10. Ullman S. Artificial intelligence and the brain: computational studies of the visual system. Annu Rev Neurosci. 1986;9:1–26. https://doi.org/10.1146/annurev.ne.09.030186.000245.
11. Fisher WS 3rd. Computer-aided intelligence: application of an expert system to brachial plexus injuries. Neurosurgery. 1990;27:837–43; discussion 843.
12. Ball SS, Mah VH, Miller PL. SENEX: a computer-based representation of cellular signal transduction processes in the central nervous system. Comput Appl Biosci. 1991;7:175–87. https://doi.org/10.1093/bioinformatics/7.2.175.
13. Stigler SM. Gauss and the invention of least squares. Ann Stat. 1981;9:465–74.
14. Cox DR. Regression models and life-tables. J R Stat Soc Ser B Methodol. 1972;34:187–202.
15. Platt J. Probabilistic outputs for support vector machines and comparisons to regularized likelihood methods. In: Advances in large margin classifiers, vol. 10; 1999. p. 61–74.
16. Hsieh FY. Sample size tables for logistic regression. Stat Med. 1989;8:795–802. https://doi.org/10.1002/sim.4780080704.
17. Peduzzi P, Concato J, Kemper E, Holford TR, Feinstein AR. A simulation study of the number of events per variable in logistic regression analysis. J Clin Epidemiol. 1996;49:1373–9. https://doi.org/10.1016/s0895-4356(96)00236-3.
18. Hoerl AE, Kennard RW. Ridge regression: biased estimation for nonorthogonal problems. Technometrics. 1970;12:55–67.
19. Tibshirani R. Regression shrinkage and selection via the lasso. J R Stat Soc Ser B Methodol. 1996;58:267–88.
20. Zou H, Hastie T. Regularization and variable selection via the elastic net. J R Stat Soc Ser B Sstat Methodol. 2005;67:301–20.
21. Simon N, Friedman J, Hastie T, Tibshirani R. Regularization paths for Cox's proportional hazards model via coordinate descent. J Stat Softw. 2011;39:1.
22. Tibshirani R. The lasso method for variable selection in the Cox model. Stat Med. 1997;16:385–95.
23. Voglis S, van Niftrik CHB, Staartjes VE, Brandi G, Tschopp O, Regli L, Serra C. Feasibility of machine learning based predictive modelling of postoperative hyponatremia after pituitary surgery. Pituitary. 2020;23:543–51. https://doi.org/10.1007/s11102-020-01056-w.
24. Keerthi SS, Lin C-J. Asymptotic behaviors of support vector machines with Gaussian kernel. Neural Comput. 2003;15:1667–89.
25. Hsu C-W, Chang C-C, Lin C-J. A practical guide to support vector classification. Taipei: University of National Taiwan; 2003.
26. Pochet N, Suykens J. Support vector machines versus logistic regression: improving prospective performance in clinical decision-making. Ultrasound Obstet Gynecol. 2006;27:607–8.
27. Koutsouleris N, Meisenzahl EM, Davatzikos C, Bottlender R, Frodl T, Scheuerecker J, Schmitt G, Zetzsche T, Decker P, Reiser M, Moller HJ, Gaser C. Use of neuroanatomical pattern classification to identify subjects in at-risk mental states of psychosis and predict disease transition. Arch Gen Psychiatry. 2009;66:700–12. https://doi.org/10.1001/archgenpsychiatry.2009.62.
28. Breiman L, Friedman J, Stone CJ, Olshen RA. Classification and regression trees. Boca Raton, FL: CRC press; 1984.
29. Kingsford C, Salzberg SL. What are decision trees? Nat Biotechnol. 2008;26:1011–3. https://doi.org/10.1038/nbt0908-1011.
30. Amit Y, Geman D. Shape quantization and recognition with randomized trees. Neural Comput. 1997;9:1545–88.
31. Breiman L. Random forests. Mach Learn. 2001;45:5–32.
32. Ho TK. The random subspace method for constructing decision forests. IEEE Trans Pattern Anal Mach Intell. 1998;20:832–44.
33. Hastie T, Tibshirani R, Friedman J. The elements of statistical learning: data mining, inference, and prediction. New York, NY: Springer Science & Business Media; 2009.
34. Kuncheva LI, Whitaker CJ. Measures of diversity in classifier ensembles and their relationship with the ensemble accuracy. Mach Learn. 2003;51:181–207.
35. Fernández-Delgado M, Cernadas E, Barro S, Amorim D. Do we need hundreds of classifiers to solve real world classification problems? J Mach Learn Res. 2014;15:3133–81.
36. Tang C, Garreau D, von Luxburg U. When do random forests fail? In: Advances in neural information processing systems; 2018. p. 2983–93.
37. Audureau E, Chivet A, Ursu R, Corns R, Metellus P, Noel G, Zouaoui S, Guyotat J, Le Reste PJ, Faillot T, Litre F, Desse N, Petit A, Emery E, Lechapt-Zalcman E, Peltier J, Duntze J, Dezamis E, Voirin J, Menei P, Caire F, Dam Hieu P, Barat JL, Langlois O, Vignes JR, Fabbro-Peray P, Riondel A, Sorbets E, Zanello M, Roux A, Carpentier A, Bauchet L, Pallud J, Club de Neuro-Oncologie of the Societe Francaise de N. Prognostic factors for survival in adult patients with recurrent glioblastoma: a decision-tree-based model. J Neuro-Oncol. 2018;136:565–76. https://doi.org/10.1007/s11060-017-2685-4.
38. Harrell FE Jr. Regression modeling strategies: with applications to linear models, logistic and ordinal regression, and survival analysis. New York, NY: Springer; 2015.
39. Brennan CW, Verhaak RG, McKenna A, Campos B, Noushmehr H, Salama SR, Zheng S, Chakravarty D, Sanborn JZ, Berman SH, Beroukhim R, Bernard B, Wu CJ, Genovese G, Shmulevich I, Barnholtz-Sloan J, Zou L, Vegesna R, Shukla SA, Ciriello G, Yung WK, Zhang W, Sougnez C, Mikkelsen T, Aldape K, Bigner DD, Van Meir EG, Prados M, Sloan A, Black KL, Eschbacher J, Finocchiaro G, Friedman W, Andrews DW, Guha A, Iacocca M, O'Neill BP, Foltz G, Myers J, Weisenberger DJ, Penny R, Kucherlapati R, Perou CM, Hayes DN, Gibbs R, Marra M, Mills GB, Lander E, Spellman P, Wilson R, Sander C, Weinstein J, Meyerson M, Gabriel S, Laird PW, Haussler D, Getz G, Chin L, Network TR. The

somatic genomic landscape of glioblastoma. Cell. 2013;155:462–77. https://doi.org/10.1016/j.cell.2013.09.034.
40. Frattini V, Trifonov V, Chan JM, Castano A, Lia M, Abate F, Keir ST, Ji AX, Zoppoli P, Niola F, Danussi C, Dolgalev I, Porrati P, Pellegatta S, Heguy A, Gupta G, Pisapia DJ, Canoll P, Bruce JN, McLendon RE, Yan H, Aldape K, Finocchiaro G, Mikkelsen T, Prive GG, Bigner DD, Lasorella A, Rabadan R, Iavarone A. The integrated landscape of driver genomic alterations in glioblastoma. Nat Genet. 2013;45:1141–9. https://doi.org/10.1038/ng.2734.
41. Oermann EK, Kress MA, Collins BT, Collins SP, Morris D, Ahalt SC, Ewend MG. Predicting survival in patients with brain metastases treated with radiosurgery using artificial neural networks. Neurosurgery. 2013;72:944–51. https://doi.org/10.1227/NEU.0b013e31828ea04b; discussion 952.
42. Duda RO, Hart PE, Stork DG. Pattern classification. New York, NY: John Wiley & Sons; 2012.
43. Manning C, Schutze H. Foundations of statistical natural language processing. Cambridge, MA: MIT press; 1999.
44. Ng AY, Jordan MI. On discriminative vs. generative classifiers: a comparison of logistic regression and naive bayes. In: Advances in neural information processing systems; 2002. p. 841–8.
45. Tunthanathip T, Sae-Heng S, Oearsakul T, Sakarunchai I, Kaewborisutsakul A, Taweesomboonyat C. Machine learning applications for the prediction of surgical site infection in neurological operations. Neurosurg Focus. 2019;47:E7. https://doi.org/10.3171/2019.5.FOCUS19241.
46. Rokach L, Maimon O. Clustering methods. In: Data mining and knowledge discovery handbook. New York, NY: Springer; 2005. p. 321–52.
47. Sneath PH, Sokal RR. Numerical taxonomy. The principles and practice of numerical classification. San Francisco, CA: W.H. Freeman; 1973.
48. MacQueen J. Some methods for classification and analysis of multivariate observations. In: Proceedings of the fifth Berkeley symposium on mathematical statistics and probability, Oakland, CA, USA, vol. 14; 1967. p. 281–97.
49. Dempster AP, Laird NM, Rubin DB. Maximum likelihood from incomplete data via the EM algorithm. J R Stat Soc Ser B Methodol. 1977;39:1–22.
50. Ester M, Kriegel H-P, Sander J, Xu X. A density-based algorithm for discovering clusters in large spatial databases with noise. In: Knowledge discovery and data mining, vol. 34; 1996. p. 226–31.
51. Schubert E, Sander J, Ester M, Kriegel HP, Xu X. DBSCAN revisited, revisited: why and how you should (still) use DBSCAN. ACM Trans Datab Syst. 2017;42:1–21.
52. Verhaak RG, Hoadley KA, Purdom E, Wang V, Qi Y, Wilkerson MD, Miller CR, Ding L, Golub T, Mesirov JP, Alexe G, Lawrence M, O'Kelly M, Tamayo P, Weir BA, Gabriel S, Winckler W, Gupta S, Jakkula L, Feiler HS, Hodgson JG, James CD, Sarkaria JN, Brennan C, Kahn A, Spellman PT, Wilson RK, Speed TP, Gray JW, Meyerson M, Getz G, Perou CM, Hayes DN, Cancer Genome Atlas Research N. Integrated genomic analysis identifies clinically relevant subtypes of glioblastoma characterized by abnormalities in PDGFRA, IDH1, EGFR, and NF1. Cancer Cell. 2010;17:98–110. https://doi.org/10.1016/j.ccr.2009.12.020.
53. Patel AP, Tirosh I, Trombetta JJ, Shalek AK, Gillespie SM, Wakimoto H, Cahill DP, Nahed BV, Curry WT, Martuza RL, Louis DN, Rozenblatt-Rosen O, Suva ML, Regev A, Bernstein BE. Single-cell RNA-seq highlights intratumoral heterogeneity in primary glioblastoma. Science (New York, NY). 2014;344:1396–401. https://doi.org/10.1126/science.1254257.
54. Wells WM, Grimson WEL, Kikinis R, Jolesz FA. Adaptive segmentation of MRI data. IEEE Trans Med Imaging. 1996;15:429–42.
55. Plant C, Teipel SJ, Oswald A, Bohm C, Meindl T, Mourao-Miranda J, Bokde AW, Hampel H, Ewers M. Automated detection of brain atrophy patterns based on MRI for the prediction of Alzheimer's disease. NeuroImage. 2010;50:162–74. https://doi.org/10.1016/j.neuroimage.2009.11.046.

Foundations of Bayesian Learning in Clinical Neuroscience

10

Gustav Burström, Erik Edström, and Adrian Elmi-Terander

10.1 Introduction

In part driven by the demands made by evidence-based medicine, recent years have seen an increased interest in the use of prediction models to forecast clinical outcomes within the fields of clinical neuroscience and neurosurgery [1–3]. Building upon the now common use of simple regression models, the field has moved towards the use of prediction models incorporating more advanced machine learning (ML) methods [4]. These methods have the potential to better integrate knowledge gained from large trials with patient-specific data than what has previously been possible, outperforming traditional statistical models for predicting patient outcomes [5–7]. However, with the increasing use of prediction models and improved availability of ML tools to clinicians, comes the responsibility of using them correctly. An understanding of key concepts and an awareness of analytical pitfalls is required for clinicians and researchers alike to avoid finding themselves unequipped to evaluate research based on ML methodologies [8].

Bayesian learning is a specific set of statistical and ML methods. Traditionally, it has consisted of a wide variety of classical statistical models for predicting outcomes based on known input variables. More recently, with the introduction of ML models working in conjunction with the traditional Bayesian statistical models, the field includes a number of different ML classifiers and prediction models. Bayesian belief networks, also called Bayesian networks (BNs) for short, are one group of ML tools that have been used in the field of neurosurgery. They enable visualization of the relationship between variables and provide the user some influence on how the prediction model is structured. A different form of Bayesian ML method is the naïve Bayes classifier, a supervised ML method that is similar in usage to other common ML classifiers such as random forests and support vector machines (SVMs).

In this chapter, we introduce Bayes theorem and predictive statistics and provide examples of its use in machine learning. The first section introduces the mathematics behind Bayesian learning, but an understanding of these mathematical concepts is not necessary in order to understand when and how to apply the models presented later in the text. To investigate predictors of neurosurgical outcomes, we introduce the use of machine learning-based Bayesian belief networks to structure and define associations between outcome predictors and final outcome. For issues related to the classification of neurosurgical problems or outcomes, where an understanding the underlying causes is less important, we focus on the naïve Bayes classifiers. The present work aims to orient researchers in Bayesian machine learning methods, and when and how to use them.

Previous presentations: No previous presentation.

G. Burström (✉) · E. Edström · A. Elmi-Terander
Department of Clinical Neuroscience, Karolinska Institutet, Stockholm, Sweden

Department of Neurosurgery, ME Neurokirurgi, Karolinska University Hospital, Stockholm, Sweden
e-mail: gustav.burstrom@ki.se

10.2 Bayes Theorem

To understand the foundations of Bayesian machine learning methods, a basic understanding of the underlying theory is of value. Bayes theorem, or Bayes rule, is one of the central rules of probability theory. It is used to calculate the probability of an event occurring given information about a conditional event, known as a conditional probability. For example, it can be used to calculate the probability of a patient having

V. E. Staartjes et al. (eds.), *Machine Learning in Clinical Neuroscience*, Acta Neurochirurgica Supplement 134,
https://doi.org/10.1007/978-3-030-85292-4_10

cancer, given that a medical test came out positive. The Bayes theorem is stated as:

$$P(A|B) = \frac{P(A) * P(B|A)}{P(B)}$$

In the above equation:

- *P*(*A*|*B*): Conditional probability of event *A* occurring, given event I
- *P*(*A*): Probability of event *A* occurring
- *P*(*B*): Probability of event *B* occurring
- *P*(*B*|*A*): Conditional probability of event *B* occurring, given event *A*

The Bayes theorem might seem far separated from the work as a clinician or neuroscientist. However, phrased in other terms, the equation is used in daily practice in a number of situations. As an example, consider a patient that has a positive finding on a CT scan and subsequently may, or may not, have glioblastoma. The probability of the patient having glioblastoma would equal the probability of having a positive finding among all patients with glioblastoma, divided by the probability of having a positive CT in the general population. Given this example, the above equation would be:

- *P*(*A*|*B*): Probability of patient having glioblastoma, given a finding on CT
- *P*(*A*): Incidence of glioblastoma in the population
- *P*(*B*|*A*): Probability of having a finding on CT given the presence of a glioblastoma, i.e. the sensitivity of the test
- *P*(*B*): Probability of having a finding on CT, in the population. *P*(*B*) can be calculated given that it is a sum of all true positives and all false positives, i.e. *P*(*B*) = sensitivity * prevalence + false positive rate * (1 − prevalence).

The above example includes one predictor variable (positive CT) for a binary classification (glioblastoma: yes/no). However, in real-world applications, there are usually more than one predictor variable and there can be many outcome variables. Due to the exponential growth in possible interdependencies with increased numbers of predictor and outcome variables, this creates both a computational load and an exponential demand for data to determine these interdependencies. This leads to a computational problem and a data problem when attempting to structure datasets with multiple predictors and classifications, unless certain assumptions (as in naïve Bayes classifiers) or stepwise methods are applied (as in Bayesian networks).

10.3 Bayesian Networks

A Bayesian network (BN) is a graphical model that describes the conditional probability between predictor variables and outcome variables (as depicted in Fig. 10.1). In order to structure complex problems, Bayesian learning methods typically employ the use of graphical representations of each predictor variable leading up to the outcome, or classification, variable. The dependencies between variables are visualized with arrows, as demonstrated in Fig. 10.1. Such a graph is called a directed acyclic graph (DAG). Each conditional probability is thereby separated into a specific place in the DAG, facilitating both interpretation and calculation of the resulting outcome prediction. However, when dealing with predictor and outcome variables with unknown relationships to each other, as is often the case when examining large datasets in neuroscience and neurosurgery, the structure of the BN is unknown. Finding a BN that describes reality as true to reality as possible is therefore a key step. Thus, ML methodology is well suited to incorporate into BNs, to find the optimal graphical representation and hence, a descriptive solution to prediction modelling.

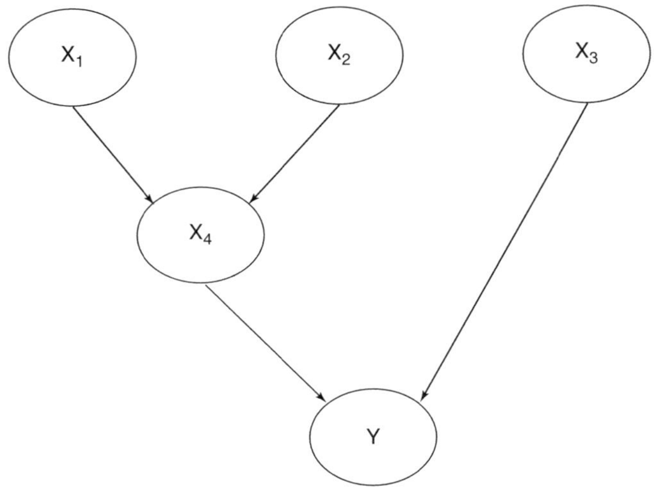

Fig. 10.1 A depiction of a Bayesian network structure with four input variables including interdependencies (X_1, X_2, X_3, and X_4) and one outcome variable (*Y*)

There are certain benefits of using BNs compared to other machine learning models. BNs structure problems in a sequential way, highlighting causalities and making interpretation possible. This is different from most other machine learning models such as random forests, neural networks or SVMs, which functions more like "black boxes" producing an output without revealing their inner workings. Given that the method is structured, it is also easier to exploit expert knowledge when building and interpreting BN models since spurious correlations can be identified and removed from models while already known correlations can be incorporated from the start.

In order to build a BN model, BN algorithms first try to learn the graphical structure of the Bayesian network and then estimate conditional probabilities (or more specifically, conditional probability distributions) given the learned BN structure. This two-step approach has the advantage that it considers one conditional probability function at a time, and it does not require modelling the global probability function a priori. The stepwise approach enables the method to be applicable to large datasets including multiple predictor and outcome variables that would otherwise pose a significant computational problem.

Structure learning algorithms used in Bayesian networks can be grouped in two categories, constraint-based algorithms and score-based algorithms. Constraint-based algorithms learn the network structure by identifying independences between variables with statistical tests, and linking nodes that are not found to be independent from each other [9, 10]. Score-based algorithms, on the other hand, develop a multitude of candidate BNs, assign scores to each candidate and then try to maximize it using a general-purpose heuristic search algorithm. These heuristic search algorithms use different techniques for solving the maximization problem faster than classical methods, and commonly used algorithms in for BNs are hill-climbing, simulated annealing, or tabu search [11–13].

A unique strength of Bayesian networks in the neurosurgical setting is that pre-existing knowledge can be used to define constraints to the algorithms. For example, a known relationship between O^6-methylguanine-DNA methyltransferase (MGMT) gene promoter methylation and temozolomide treatment on outcomes for glioblastoma patients can be pre-defined, so that a correlation exists as a precondition for the structure learning algorithm. Likewise, if the Bayesian network output exhibits nonsensical correlations, such a relationship can be inhibited as a precondition when running the algorithm again.

10.4 Naïve Bayes Classifiers

Naïve Bayes (NB) classifiers are a type of supervised machine learning algorithms that rely on a simplification of Bayes theorem. The simplification is to assume that all predictor variables are independent from each other (Fig. 10.2), hence the term "naïve." This enables calculation of conditional probabilities given reasonably small datasets. The reason for this simplification is that the Bayes theorem assumes that each input variable is (potentially) dependent upon all other variables, leading to increasing complexity in the calculation as the number of variables increases. If Bayes theorem was used, without the naïve simplification, to calculate the conditional probability of a certain outcome, one would need to calculate the interdependent conditional probabilities between all input variables. For every added input variable, the combinations to consider would increase exponentially. The computational cost would increase, and the input data required would become unmanageable for most situations.

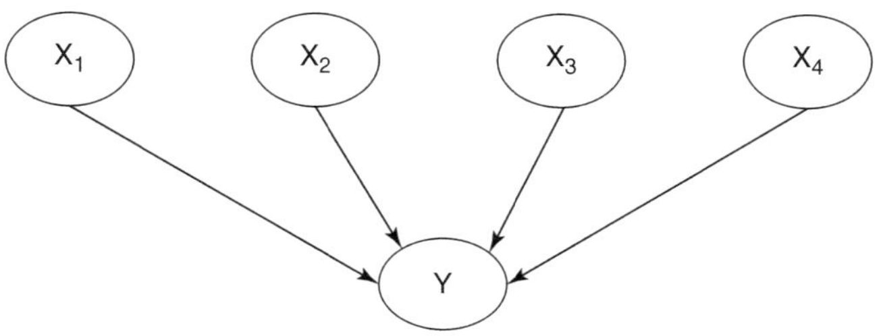

Fig. 10.2 A depiction of a Naïve Bayesian structure with four input fully independent variables (X_1, X_2, X_3, and X_4) and one outcome variable (Y)

Despite relying on a somewhat naïve simplification, NB classification can be used in a variety of classification problems in neurosurgical and neuroscientific settings with reliable results [3, 14–16]. When used in practice, NB classifiers are similar to other supervised ML algorithms such as random forests or SVMs. Data is first split into a training set and a test set. Typical methods can be used, such as a 2:1 split (2 training data for every 1 test data) or *n*-fold cross-validation [17]. After splitting the data, all independent variable data are normalized (i.e. feature scaling is performed) and the NB model is fitted to the training data (i.e. trained on the training data). Lastly, the NB model is evaluated by predicting classifications on the test data resulting in an estimation of sensitivity, specificity, and balanced accuracy for the model.

10.5 Discussion

Bayesian networks (BNs) and naïve Bayesian (NB) classification are two common machine learning methods relying on Bayesian statistics that can be used to create clinical prediction models and help clinicians and researchers to better understand how patient-specific circumstances can affect clinical outcomes. BNs are well suited for developing prediction models describing patient-specific risks in a structured matter, where known correlations can be incorporated in the models. NBs, on the other hand, offer a powerful tool for creating simple classification models with high efficacy. However, NBs and BNs only represent a fraction of available Bayesian methods that have been incorporated in machine learning models in some way or other, but these are beyond the scope of this introduction to Bayesian learning.

Although this text serves as an introduction to Bayesian learning, applying classification models without rigorous validation presents a risk, especially if deployed without fully understanding the implications. Bayesian statistics in general has a strength in that it includes prior probabilities, e.g. the frequency of a disease in the population being tested, when calculating the probability of an outcome. The importance of this step, often called "calibration" of a classification model, is not always apparent when deploying classification models in a neurosurgical context. Frequently, the sensitivity and specificity of a prediction model is reported but not necessarily the calibrated value that would say that "there is an *x%* chance of having the predicted outcome" [18]. This becomes even more important when employing prediction models outside of the population, or medical center, where they were developed, since the frequency of diseases or complications can vary significantly. Therefore, recalibration, or even retraining, of prediction models on the population in question may be necessary if the initial model was developed in a specific setting not generalizable to other centers [19]. Bayesian machine learning methods do not require this calibration step as part of building the classification models, however, but researchers working with Bayesian statistics should hopefully be primed to the importance of prior probabilities to calibrate their classification methods.

10.6 Conclusion

This introduction to Bayesian learning outlines Bayes theorem and the use of it in machine learning applications. Bayesian networks using machine learning methodology are particularly highlighted as a way to structure prediction modelling in a comprehensible way, while Naïve Bayes classifiers are outlined as powerful tools to create simple classification models with high efficacy in neurosurgical and neuroscientific settings.

Conflicts of Interest The authors declare that they have no conflict of interest.

References

1. Celtikci E. A systematic review on machine learning in neurosurgery: the future of decision-making in patient care. Turk Neurosurg. 2018;28:167–73.
2. Glaser JI, Benjamin AS, Farhoodi R, Kording KP. The roles of supervised machine learning in systems neuroscience. Prog Neurobiol. 2019;175:126–37.
3. Senders JT, Staples PC, Karhade AV, Zaki MM, Gormley WB, Broekman ML, Smith TR, Arnaout O. Machine learning and neurosurgical outcome prediction: a systematic review. World Neurosurg. 2018;109:476–486.e1.
4. Mijderwijk H-J, Steyerberg EW, Steiger H-J, Fischer I, Kamp MA. Fundamentals of clinical prediction modeling for the neurosurgeon. Neurosurgery. 2019;85:302–11.
5. Eftekhar B, Mohammad K, Ardebili HE, Ghodsi M, Ketabchi E. Comparison of artificial neural network and logistic regression models for prediction of mortality in head trauma based on initial clinical data. BMC Med Inform Decis Mak. 2005;5:1–8.
6. Ferragina A, de Los CG, Vazquez A, Cecchinato A, Bittante G. Bayesian regression models outperform partial least squares methods for predicting milk components and technological properties using infrared spectral data. J Dairy Sci. 2015;98:8133–51.
7. Singal AG, Mukherjee A, Elmunzer BJ, Higgins PD, Lok AS, Zhu J, Marrero JA, Waljee AK. Machine learning algorithms outperform conventional regression models in predicting development of hepatocellular carcinoma. Am J Gastroenterol. 2013;108:1723.
8. Kernbach JM, Staartjes VE. Machine learning-based clinical prediction modeling--a practical guide for clinicians. ArXiv. 2020:200615069.
9. Pearl J. Probabilistic reasoning in intelligent systems: networks of plausible inference. Amsterdam: Elsevier; 2014.
10. Verma T, Pearl J. Equivalence and synthesis of causal models. Los Angeles, CA: Computer Science Department, UCLA; 1991.
11. Daly R, Shen Q. Methods to accelerate the learning of Bayesian network structures. In: Proceedings of the 2007 UK Workshop on Computational Intelligence; 2007.
12. O'Gorman B, Babbush R, Perdomo-Ortiz A, Aspuru-Guzik A, Smelyanskiy V. Bayesian network structure learning using quantum annealing. Eur Phys J Spec Top. 2015;224:163–88.
13. Tsamardinos I, Brown LE, Aliferis CF. The max-min hill-climbing Bayesian network structure learning algorithm. Mach Learn. 2006;65:31–78.
14. Armañanzas R, Alonso-Nanclares L, DeFelipe-Oroquieta J, Kastanauskaite A, de Sola RG, DeFelipe J, Bielza C, Larrañaga P. Machine learning approach for the outcome prediction of temporal lobe epilepsy surgery. PLoS One. 2013;8:e62819.
15. Shamir RR, Dolber T, Noecker AM, Walter BL, McIntyre CC. Machine learning approach to optimizing combined stimulation and medication therapies for Parkinson's disease. Brain Stimul. 2015;8:1025–32.
16. Voglis S, van Niftrik CH, Staartjes VE, Brandi G, Tschopp O, Regli L, Serra C. Feasibility of machine learning based predictive modelling of postoperative hyponatremia after pituitary surgery. Pituitary. 2020;23:543–51.
17. Kohavi RA. Study of cross-validation and bootstrap for accuracy estimation and model selection. In: IJCAI, vol. 2; 1995. p. 1137–45.
18. Staartjes VE, Kernbach JM. Letter to the editor. Importance of calibration assessment in machine learning–based predictive analytics. J Neurosurg Spine. 2020;32:985–7.
19. Staartjes VE, Kernbach JM. Significance of external validation in clinical machine learning: let loose too early? Spine J. 2020;20:1159–60.

Introduction to Deep Learning in Clinical Neuroscience

11

Eddie de Dios, Muhaddisa Barat Ali, Irene Yu-Hua Gu, Tomás Gomez Vecchio, Chenjie Ge, and Asgeir S. Jakola

11.1 Introduction

The application of machine learning (ML) technology is rapidly increasing in the biomedical field and countless ML methods are already behind significant achievements in modern society. A few of these examples include speech, vision and face recognition, language processing, board games, and social network filtering, as well as applications in medical imaging, drug development, and bioinformatics. Deep learning (DL), a subtype of ML, has drawn much attention lately as it can be used to automatically extract *features* from input data, in order to detect, classify, or predict a certain *target variable*. DL can be *supervised* or *unsupervised*. In supervised learning, the algorithm is trained from *labeled* data in the training dataset, whereas in unsupervised learning, the algorithm is given *unlabeled* training data. The unsupervised learning methods thus attempt to find a structure within the dataset, in order to extract a meaningful output. DL is inspired by biological neural systems, consisting of deep layers for learning features and learning a classifier. While conventional ML methods use analytic models with human expert-defined hand-crafted features as input, DL methods are more attractive due to their plasticity for automatically learning features or building black box models from large datasets, e.g. predicting the overall survival in glioma, based on a model learned from large amounts of magnetic resonance image (MRI) data.

This section on DL will focus on several applications of DL techniques in the field of clinical neuroscience. In particular, DL has demonstrated remarkable performance in the area of computer vision, ranging from face recognition in smartphones to fracture detection in X-rays [1]. However, to perform well, DL methods need to be trained with a large amount of input data with a good coverage of data statistics, which is a challenge in a field such as neuroscience where the number of patients typically is rather small [2]. In addition, real-world clinical datasets frequently present missing or non-standardized data. These difficulties pose real challenges for the successful application of DL methods in clinical neuroscience.

This chapter describes several key issues encountered in DL-assisted clinical diagnosis of neurological diseases, where we specifically focus on MRI-based models for glioma, although the principles and methods can be useful in a range of applications in clinical neuroscience.

11.2 Materials and Methods: Useful DL Methods in Clinical Neuroscience

The DL field encompasses many conceptual aspects and a few of them will be described in this section. The core constituent of the "depth" of learning is normally regarded to be the number of "hidden layers" in the DL model. These hidden layers represent interneurons between the input and the output layers, and therefore not only the number of levels,

E. de Dios
Department of Neurosurgery, Sahlgrenska University Hospital, Gothenburg, Sweden

M. B. Ali · I. Y.-H. Gu · C. Ge
Department of Electrical Engineering, Chalmers University of Technology, Gothenburg, Sweden
e-mail: barat@chalmers.se; irenegu@chalmers.se

T. G. Vecchio
Department of Clinical Neuroscience, Institute of Neuroscience and Physiology, University of Gothenburg, Sahlgrenska Academy, Gothenburg, Sweden
e-mail: tomas.gomez.vecchio@gu.se

A. S. Jakola (✉)
Department of Neurosurgery, Sahlgrenska University Hospital, Gothenburg, Sweden

Department of Clinical Neuroscience, Institute of Neuroscience and Physiology, University of Gothenburg, Sahlgrenska Academy, Gothenburg, Sweden

Department of Neurosurgery, St. Olavs University Hospital HF, Trondheim, Norway
e-mail: jakola.asgeir@gu.se

V. E. Staartjes et al. (eds.), *Machine Learning in Clinical Neuroscience*, Acta Neurochirurgica Supplement 134,
https://doi.org/10.1007/978-3-030-85292-4_11

but also the "interconnectivity" of these layers for effectively learning meaningful representations through back and forth propagation and tuning of information, can be regarded as a measure of "depth." As an example, all the voxels from an MRI T1 contrast enhanced scan could represent the input layer with the goal of the output layer being to accurately predict the overall survival in glioma. The hidden layers will then be trained with training and validation sets for optimization in predicting the desired outcome with a high accuracy. How the hidden layers actually interact is not necessarily understandable for humans, but with enough data, the model can identify representations that are associated with a certain outcome.

Pre-processing of MRI Data

Pre-processing of MRI data is a crucial step, which may significantly impact the final performance (could be >10% or even more). The pipeline of pre-processing of MRI usually includes *cortical reconstruction*, *image size normalization*, and *intensity normalization* (Fig. 11.1). Cortical reconstruction includes a set of processing like image re-orientation, image registration to a reference image, skull and neck removal, and bias field correction. Some software, like the recon-all function in "FreeSurfer" [3] can handle the entire cortical reconstruction process, though a combination of other software packages like "FSL" [4], the "FLIRT FERIB" linear image registration tool, "BET" brain extraction tool, and "ANTs" [5] can also be used. The intensity normalization step scales image values in the range [0.0, 1.0]. Finally, software "MRIcron" can be used for visualizing and extracting MRI slices.

Segmentation of Region of Interest (ROI)

Segmentation of an *ROI* may serve as a mask/annotation to perform the desired task (e.g. molecular prediction). However, in some instances segmentation may also be the desired task [6]. Establishing tumor boundaries can provide important information in determining tumor burden and subtle tumor growth, and thus also to detect response or failure of therapies. The Brain Tumor Segmentation (BraTS) challenge [7] uses multi-institutional preoperative MRI scans and focuses on the segmentation of heterogenous brain tumors, specifically gliomas. The BraTS challenge top-ranked algorithms from 2017 to present 2020 are available on the BraTS algorithmic repository [7]. It is known that a fusion of these algorithms have a slight advantage over its single use [8]. We are also getting closer to much needed clinical usefulness in tumor segmentation. For instance, Kickingereder et al. used a DL technique called *U-Net*, for automated identification and segmentation of contrast-enhanced tumor and non-enhanced T2-signal abnormalities on MRI in a recent landmark study [9]. U-Net and its variants have been widely employed for MRI-based tumor segmentation, and other groups have also presented clinically relevant results [10, 11].

Deep Convolutional Neural Networks (CNNs)

There exist many introductory articles or websites that describe the basics of DL and in particular *CNNs* [12–14]. A deep CNN usually consists of many layers, with a typical architecture containing a repetition of *convolutional layers*, *nonlinear activation*, and *pooling layers* for feature learning, followed by several *fully connected* (FC) layers for classification. A convolutional layer computes the output of neurons from the input taken from small regions. The weights of neurons are learned from the supervised training. The size of *filter kernels* usually starts small and gradually increases with the layers. The nonlinear activation function is usually added to introduce nonlinearity, where a most commonly used function is "ReLU" (the rectified linear unit), which gives zero value output for any negative input x, i.e. $f(x) = max(0,x)$. Other nonlinear activation functions, e.g. "sigmoid," "tanh," and "softmax," can also be used. A pooling layer often achieves nonlinear down-sampling, e.g. a 2*2 *maxpool* outputs one maximum value from a 2*2 input. For the FC layers, multidimensional input is usually first converted into one-dimensional input by a *flatten layer*, then followed by two or three FC layers where all neurons are connected to each other. The number of layers is usually selected experimentally, as there is no general theory or guidelines on this. Some experimental guidelines for initially selecting the number of layers could be dependent on the dimension of input data (e.g. 2D or 3D data), and the size of the training dataset. One could then adjust the number of lay-

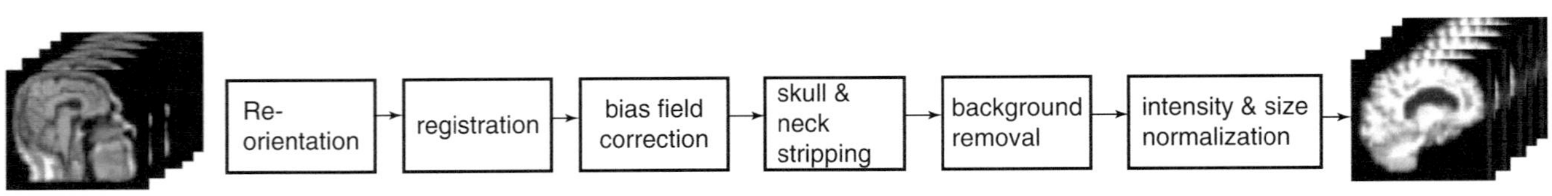

Fig. 11.1 Pre-processing pipeline for brain MR images

ers by examining the training and validation accuracy curves as a function of *epochs*, i.e. the number of passes of the entire training dataset that the algorithm has completed. Based on DL experience, if the accuracy from the training is much less than the desired value, more convolutional layers are probably needed. If the disparity of accuracy curves between the training and validation is large, it indicates that the CNN is overfitting, and one should consider either to reduce the number of layers or to increase the size of the training dataset. The number of layers in a CNN can vary significantly, e.g. the well-known VGG19 Net [15], GoogLeNet [16], and ResNet [17] consisted of 19, 22, and 152 layers, respectively. The outputs from convolutional layers for feature extraction result in feature maps, where the feature scale varies, from fine resolution in the first layer to the coarsest resolution in the last layer. One can then extract CNN feature maps for visualization. To evaluate the efficacy in feature learning from different DL methods, heatmap [18] is a useful tool that compares heatmaps from different methods and indicates which method is more effective. For human comprehension of these steps, several methods have been explored in an attempt to "look inside" a deep neural network, many of which have focused on visual interpretability. In the brain tumor segmentation context, for instance, the CNN model might have separate filters learning to detect normal brain tissue, followed by detecting brain edema, followed by detecting necrotic tissue, and so on, finally identifying the size of the active tumor component, contrast enhancing regions or other important predictive factors. However, one must also be aware that a CNN model is not necessarily possible to decode this way, as the network could spread information between its convolutional layers in entangled and non-interpretable forms for human conceptualization [19].

In essence, a CNN employs a set of nonlinear filters whose coefficients are learned from the training data through supervised learning. As demonstrated later, CNNs are found useful for learning features or MRI data representation.

Deep Autoencoders (AEs)

A deep *AE* consists of an *encoder* and a *decoder*, each containing many layers of neural networks. It is used for learning the compressed representation of data. The encoder/decoder coefficients are learned from the training data in an end-to-end manner that minimizes the reconstruction error under a selected criterion, either through supervised or unsupervised learning. One can choose different DL methods for realizing the encoder and decoder, e.g. by a CNN. In such a case, the encoder part of the *convolutional autoencoder* (CAE) is itself a CNN, though the size of the filter kernel usually decreases when the number of layers increases. A decoder is an exact reverse of the encoder. The code size from the encoder output is a choice from the designer, depending on how much details one wishes to keep in the learned data representation. After the training, only the encoder and its output are kept. As demonstrated later, AEs are useful DL tools for learning features or MRI data representation.

Generative Adversarial Networks (GANs)

A *GAN* is a DL method that is widely employed for distinguishing real and fake data, for preventing *adversarial attacks*, and also for generating synthetic data that is highly similar to the real ones. A GAN consists of two neural networks, a *generator* G and a *discriminator* D. They work together to produce highly realistic images or data through *adversarial learning*. D and G can be formed by CNNs. For G, the input is usually a random image or seed data z, and tries to generate an output image/data $G(z)$ as similar as the real one. A discriminator D tries to distinguish the real and fake image/data. The two networks D and G are trained sequentially in alternation until convergence, usually under the min-max criterion $\min_G \max_D V(D,G) = E_{x\sim p_{data(x)}}[\log D(x)] + E_{z\sim p_z(z)}[\log(1 - D(G(z)))]$. As demonstrated later, GANs are useful for effectively generating synthetic MRI data to increase the size of the training dataset, and for mapping MRI datasets presenting large variations.

When working with MRI datasets we often wish to use the complementary information provided by different sequences (e.g. T1, T1 contrast enhanced, T2, and FLAIR). Often the training dataset consists of data from a rather small number of patients, and missing sequences of MRI data in some patients can reduce the number of patients available for the training set even further. A so-called pairwise-GAN can be used to generate the missing MRI sequence based upon the already existing ones. A pair-wise GAN consists of two sets of GANs that are cross-linked between the two modalities, where the input of the second discriminator D_2 is connected to the output of the first generator G_1, whose input is the data from an existing modality (e.g. T2), and output is the synthetic data on the missing modality (e.g. T1). Similarly, G_1 and D_2 are also cross-linked.

Techniques to Effectively Combining Several Small Datasets

A common issue in datasets in clinical neuroscience is that they are usually small (i.e. collected from just a few hundred patients). This is undesirable for DL as it requires learning the statistics/representations from a large amount of data. To compensate for small single-institutional data, several small datasets from multiple institutions can be combined. However, directly combining these training datasets into a large one may not help to improve the generalization performance on the test data despite the steps of pre-processing mentioned above, since there may exist large variations between the obtained datasets. In the setting of MRI data, such differences may be due to different scanners and parameter settings.

To effectively merge such training datasets, *domain mapping* can be used. The essence of domain mapping [20] is to find a mapping function of each individual dataset onto a common dataset. This common dataset can be a newly created one or one of the existing datasets. After the mappings, these datasets may share more uniform properties. Domain mapping can be employed by the DL method *cycle-GAN*. A cycle-GAN is a technique for training unsupervised data mapping functions through the GAN architecture using unpaired collections of data from two different domains. Assuming there are two datasets *X* and *Y*, that one wishes to map onto a common dataset *Z*, let us first consider how to map *X* to *Z* by training a cycle-GAN. A cycle-GAN tries to minimize the *cycle consistency loss*, where its two GANs (i.e. GAN_{XZ_x}, GAN_{Z_xX}) are connected and trained together to minimize the loss. In a similar way, one can map the dataset *Y* onto *Z* by employing another cycle-GAN that learns its two GANs (i.e. GAN_{YZ_y}, GAN_{Z_yY}).

11.3 Results: DL-Assisted Diagnostics in Gliomas

Results of Tumor Segmentation Performed by DL Instead of Manual Outline

In the BraTS challenge 2012–2013 most of the individual DL-based segmentation methods did not outperform interrater agreement across expert clinicians, but the fusion of DL-based segmentation from top-ranked algorithms outperformed all individual methods and was comparable with the inter-rater agreement. The Dice score and Hausdorff distance of the fused segmentations consistently ranked first in both metrics [7]. In a recent publication segmentation with a U-Net architecture, consisting of an encoder and a decoder network interconnected with skip connections, was a significantly better surrogate endpoint than traditional image assessment using the central Response Assessment in Neuro-Oncology (RANO) criteria [21] for predicting overall survival in the European Organization for Research and Treatment of Cancer-26101 trial (EORTC-26101) test dataset, acquired from 38 institutions across Europe (hazard ratios DL 2.59 [95% CI 1.86–3.60] versus central RANO 2.07 [95% CI 1.46–2.92]; $p < 0.0001$) [9]. In this study, the median Dice coefficient was 0.89 (95% CI 0.86–0.90) and 0.93 (95% CI 0.92–0.94) for MRI contrast enhancing and non-enhancing tumors, respectively, in the Heidelberg test set of 239 MRI scans. For the EORTC-26101 trial test set, it was 0.91 (0.90–0.92) and 0.93 (0.92–0.94) for MRI contrast enhancing and non-enhancing tumors, respectively [9]. In the work of Yogananda et al. described subsequently for tumor classification, they included U-Net-based automatic segmentation in the process and achieved a whole tumor segmentation average Dice score of 0.80 ± 0.007 in T2 only [22], and 0.89 ± 0.006 when combining T1 contrast enhanced, T2, and FLAIR [23].

Prediction of Glioma Subtypes of New Patients with MRIs Only

Several glioma grading and molecular-subtype prediction methods have been developed with relatively good accuracy by using methods such as *3D Dense-Nets*, *residual neural networks (RNNs)*, CNNs, and CAEs. While some methods use automated segmentation [22–24], others rely on a more time-consuming manual segmentation. These prediction models have been tested in both institutional research datasets [20, 24–27] as well as open access datasets, including The Cancer Genome Atlas (TCGA), The Cancer Imaging Archive (TCIA), and the BraTS datasets. Some datasets contain both high-grade gliomas (HGG) and low-grade gliomas (LGG), while others rely exclusively on LGG [20, 24, 25, 27]. The datasets may also differ due to inter-institutional image variability [20]. Most DL implementations focus on predicting biomarkers such as IDH mutation and 1p/19q codeletion. Table 11.1 shows the results of some recent DL applications, including a brief description of their methods and results.

Results Following Expanding Training Data by DL

For DL tasks using MRI as source data, techniques to expand data by augmentation may include *flipping*, *rotation*, and *adding noise* [30]. However, as mentioned, pairwise GANs (red box in Fig. 11.2a) can be applied for generating missing sequences to avoid excluding patients, and for generating fake patient MRI data. The feature learning was performed by *3-stream 2D CNNs* (blue box in Fig. 11.2a) on the enlarged training dataset, containing real and GAN-generated sequences. After the training, the system is ready for tumor subtype prediction of new patients from their MRI scans. This system was tested for prediction of IDH mutation status where results from the enlarged training dataset improved the classification rate on the test set with 3–5% [28].

Table 11.1 Examples of MRI-based DL-assisted applications for prediction of glioma subtype (by type of classification and performance)

Authors	Methods	Significant findings	Comments
C. Yogananda [23]	3D Dense-UNet TCIA and TCGA datasets GBM and lower-grade glioma combined, $n = 214$	**Prediction of IDH mutation** Mean accuracy of 97.12% ± 0.09 on test set, 3 runs Sensitivity: 0.98 ± 0.02 Specificity: 0.97 ± 0.001 Whole tumor Dice score: 0.89 ± 0.006	Less pre-processing, similar results using one MRI sequence (T2) compared to multiple. The model includes automatic segmentation. Performance increased when using patients with quite dissimilar looking tumors (GBM and LGG included together). Strict data splitting according to patients into training and test. Each run was on the initial split for threefold cross validation.
Z. Li [24]	Convolutional neural network + support vector machine classifier Single institution dataset Lower-grade glioma only, $n = 118$	**Prediction of IDH mutation** Accuracy of 0.9118 on test set, single run Sensitivity: 0.9231 Specificity: 0.8750 Whole tumor Dice score: 0.77	DL used for feature extraction; ML support vector machine used as classifier The model includes automatic segmentation. Strict data splitting according to patients into training and test. Standard deviation was not reported.
C. Ge [28]	Multi-stream convolutional neural networks TCGA dataset GBM and lower-grade glioma combined, $n = 167$	**Prediction of IDH mutation** Mean accuracy of 88.82% ± 6.57 on test sets, 5 runs Sensitivity: 81,81% ± 11.13 Specificity: 92.17% ± 4.77	Strict data splitting according to patients into training and test sets. Each run was on re-split training and test sets.
K. Chang [26]	Residual convolutional neural network Multi-institutional research datasets and TCIA GBM and lower-grade glioma combined, $n = 496$	**Prediction of IDH mutation** Mean accuracy of 85.7% on test set, single run	Strict data splitting according to patients into training and test. Sensitivity, specificity, and standard deviation for MRI sequence network model were not reported.
S. Liang [29]	3D Dense-Net BraTS 2017 and TCGA datasets GBM and lower-grade glioma combined, $n = 167$	**Prediction of IDH mutation** Mean accuracy of 84.6% on validation set, 5 runs Sensitivity: 78.5% Specificity: 88.0%	No strict data splitting: Results based on fivefold cross-validation. Standard deviation was not reported.
Y. Matsui [27]	Residual neural networks Multimodal dataset, containing MRI, PET, CT, and clinical patient characteristics Lower-grade glioma only, $n = 217$	**Prediction of IDH mutation** Mean accuracy of 82.9	No strict data splitting: Results based on leave-one-out cross validation. The result was the average accuracy of the 217 models when predicting each set of training data. Sensitivity, specificity, and standard deviation were not reported.
M. Ali [20]	Multi-stream convolutional autoencoders Multi-institutional datasets Diffuse WHO grade 2 glioma only, $n = 161$	**Prediction of IDH mutation** Prediction of IDH mutation: Mean accuracy of 81.19% ± 3.70 on test sets, 5 runs Sensitivity: 93.33% ± 3.39 Specificity: not reported	Strict data splitting according to patients into training and test sets. Each run was on re-split training and test sets. Used rectangular bounding box of tumors (no segmentation).
Y. Matsui [27]	Residual networks. Multimodal dataset, containing MRI, PET, CT, and clinical patient characteristics Lower-grade glioma only, $n = 217$	**Prediction of 3-group molecular subtypes** Mean accuracy of 68.7%	No strict data splitting: Results based on leave-one-out cross validation. The result was the average accuracy of the 217 models when predicting each set of training data. Sensitivity, specificity, and standard deviation were not reported.

(continued)

Table 11.1 (continued)

Authors	Methods	Significant findings	Comments
C. Yogananda [22]	3D Dense-UNet. TCIA and TCGA datasets GBM and lower-grade glioma combined, $n = 368$	**Prediction of 1p/19q co-deletion** Mean accuracy of 93.46% ± 0.86 on test set, 3 runs Sensitivity: 0.90 ± 0.003 Specificity: 0.95 ± 0.01 Whole tumor Dice score: 0.80 ± 0.007	T2 images only. The model includes automatic segmentation. Results not reported in the strict LGG group Strict data splitting according to patients into training and test. Each run was on the initial split for threefold cross validation.
Z. Akkus [25]	Convolutional neural network. Single institution dataset Lower-grade glioma only $n = 159$	**Prediction of 1p/19q co-deletion** Accuracy of 87.7% on test set, single run. Sensitivity: 93.3% Specificity: 82.22%	No strict data splitting of patients into training and test. Standard deviation and AUC were not reported.
Y. Matsui [27]	Residual networks. Multimodal dataset, containing MRI, PET, CT, and clinical patient characteristics Lower-grade glioma only, $n = 217$	**Prediction of 1p/19q co-deletion** Mean accuracy of 75.1%	No strict data splitting: Results based on leave-one-out cross validation. The result was the average accuracy of the 217 models when predicting each set of training data. Sensitivity, specificity, and standard deviation were not reported.
M. Ali [20]	Multi-stream convolutional autoencoders Multi-institutional datasets Diffuse WHO grade 2 glioma only, $n = 161$	**Prediction of 1p/19q co-deletion** Mean accuracy of 74.81% ± 0.98 on test set, over 5 runs. Sensitivity: 75.93% ± 3.12 Specificity: not reported	Strict data splitting according to patients into training and test sets. Each run was on re-split training and test sets. Used rectangular bounding box of tumors (no segmentation).

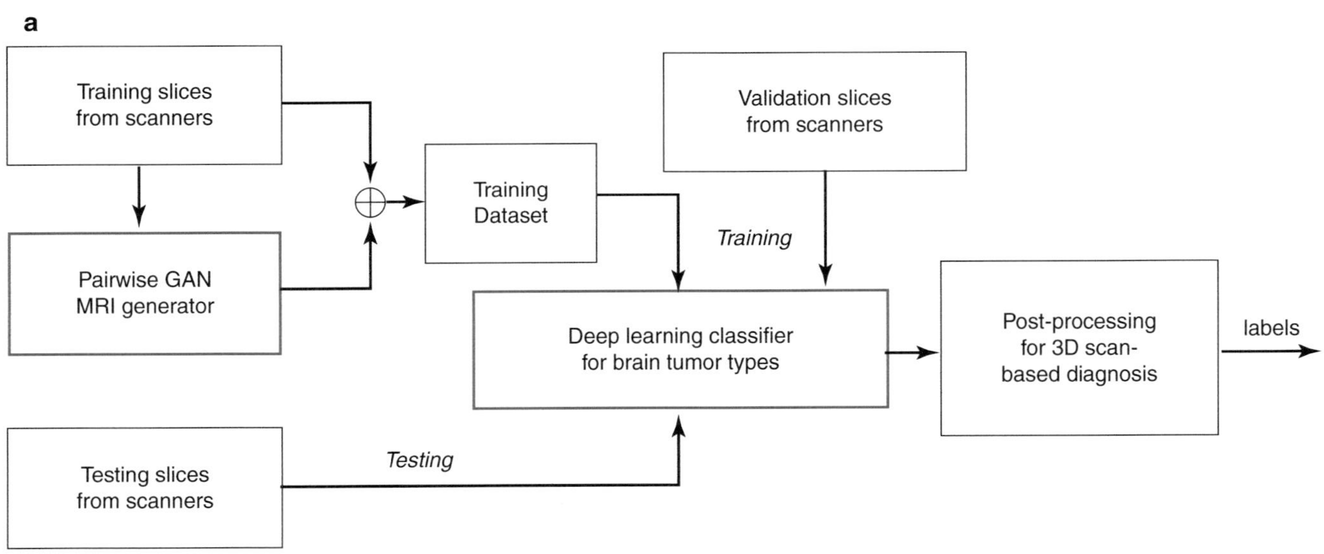

Fig. 11.2 A DL and classification scheme for brain tumor subtype prediction. (**a**) Pipeline of the scheme; (**b**) detailed architecture of the 3-stream 2D-CNNs in the blue box of (**a**)

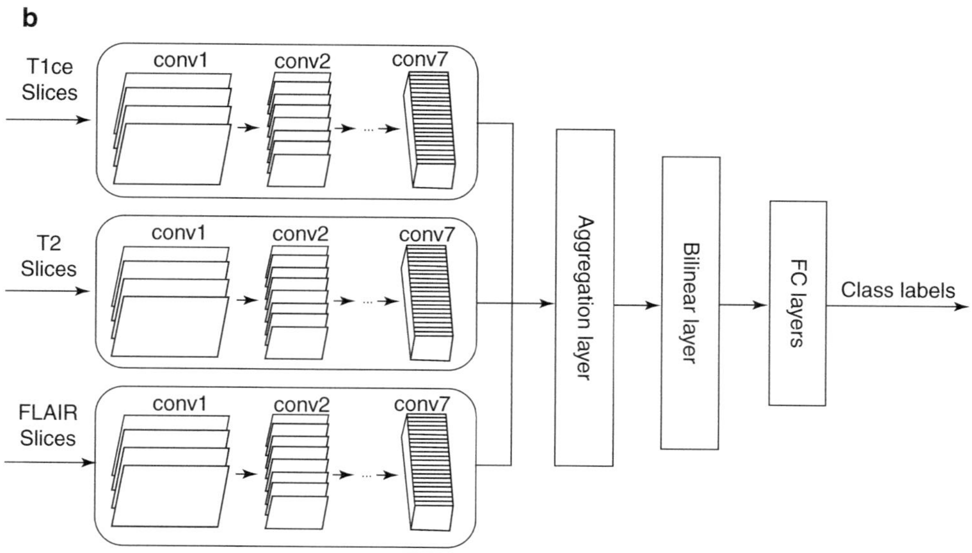

Fig. 11.2 (continued)

Results Following Fitting Data from Several Sources with Significant Variability

In the work of Ali et al. several DL techniques were employed (e.g. combining multi-institutional datasets by cycle-GAN domain adaptation, enlarging the training dataset by unpaired GANs, feature learning by CAEs and fusion) for predicting 1p/19q codeletion status. With the use of domain mapping the classification rate improved with 7.78% on the test set [20]. The pipeline of the system is shown in Fig. 11.3.

11.4 Discussion

Based on the results described in this chapter several DL techniques, including CNNs, CAEs, GANs, U-Nets, and others, are found to be promising tools for applications in neuroscience. On the more generic side, DL methods can expand the training data through data augmentation, either by generating fake patients (e.g. new MRI sets) or by replacing missing parts of a dataset (e.g. a missing T1 contrast enhanced sequence) to avoid excluding those patients. Also, if multi-institutional datasets with significant data variability exist, domain mapping or adaptation for combining training datasets can significantly improve the test results. Furthermore, although not strictly related to DL methods, we and others have experienced when analyzing brain tumors using MRI that (a) pre-processing is an important step that has a significant impact on performance, and (b) tumor segmentation before applying DL methods for learning tumor representation is needed, where again DL methods such as U-Net has been found effective.

Despite the success in the computer vision area, successfully applying DL methods in clinical neuroscience remains challenging, partly due to the lack of large datasets with annotated data, variations between datasets, and importantly, the current gaps between medical and engineering expertise requiring broad and close collaborations. Because of the relatively scarce data in clinical neuroscience [2], we have included aspects where DL-based methods can evade discarding data, in addition to boosting it. This generic DL use may assist more researchers to further explore areas in clinical neuroscience despite the rather small datasets. More specifically, examples in this chapter demonstrate that DL methods show potential applications for clinical neuroscience, especially for automatically learning features and representations of data if there exist medium/large annotated training datasets. Hybrid ML and DL can be combined when there exist clearly clinically related features. In cases of lack of expert knowledge, for example, associating features in MRIs with molecular subtypes of glioma, ML and DL show their strength in finding associated features that are notoriously difficult even for medical experts [31]. Another benefit of DL is that time-consuming tasks can be automated, like tumor segmentation, and this may ultimately pave the way for the much needed shift from qualitative or crude measures such as one- or two-diameter volumetric assessments [32].

Since DL methods are relatively new to most researchers within the field of clinical neuroscience, attention should be paid to several issues. First, whether training and testing datasets are partitioned according to patients. If they are not strictly separated, data correlation within each individual patient could give a false impression of the performance with high accuracy on the validation or test set, however, when

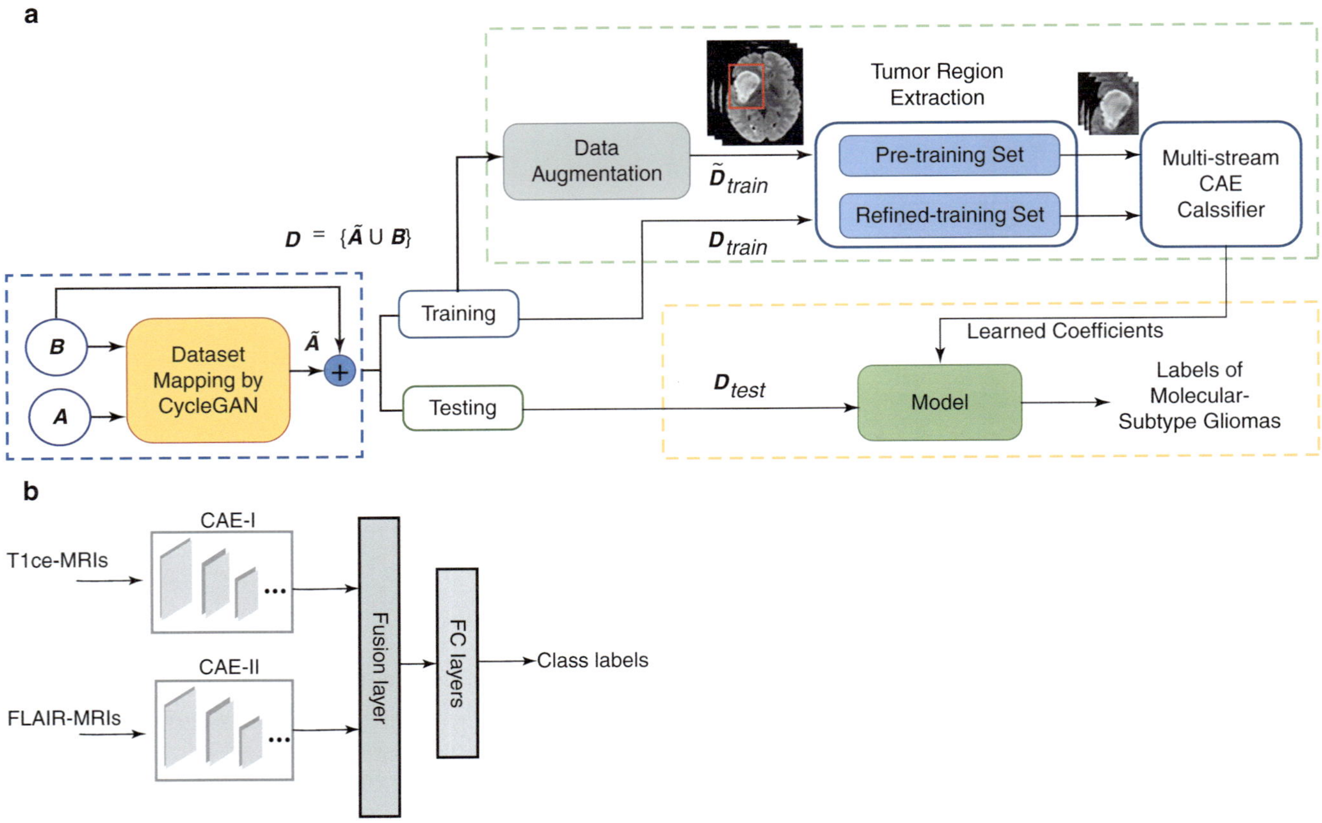

Fig. 11.3 A DL and classification scheme for predicting glioma subtypes where cycle-GAN is used for combining two small training datasets through domain mapping, and multi-stream CAEs and fusion are used for feature learning. (**a**) Pipeline of the scheme; (**b**) details of "multi-stream CAE classifier" in the blue box of (**a**)

testing data from unseen new patients is applied, the performance could drop significantly (sometimes a drop of 20% or more can be seen). Second, whether the performance is on the test set (if on validation set, the performance is usually significantly higher, as DL often uses an *early stopping* strategy in the training, hence validation performance is coupled with the training even though slightly lower). Third, the performance criteria on whether it is on average accuracy on two/multiple classes or using the Area under the ROC Curve (AUC), noting they are not directly comparable. Fourth, whether multiple tests are done on re-split test sets, as multiple times of random partition of training and test sets followed by re-training and re-testing processes give a better indication of the true test performance.

There are other obstacles in the implementation of novel prediction models by ML, and perhaps in particular when using DL. There already exist numerous prediction models where most are not in clinical use, and one could argue that a slight improvement achieved by an opaque method (i.e. "black box" prediction) is not likely to radically change clinical decision making [33, 34]. On the other hand, the benefit would be access to decision support systems that are not geographically constrained or restricted to certain centers of excellence. For this reason, improving the explainability of DL models has recently gained increased coverage in the scientific literature. For images, this is exemplified by a stepwise illustration of what parts of the image that are used by the algorithms into understandable concepts for humans, in order to tackle the mystifying "black box" effect [19]. Explaining the nuances of these highly complex models may positively affect the willingness of physicians to incorporate DL into their practices [35, 36]. Explainable models may also aid the researcher to identify the behavior of their networks on early stages of model development [37]. Furthermore, DL models are better equipped for tasks that are time-consuming or require rigorous attention to detail, such as detection of abnormalities or complex measurements on MRIs. As previously mentioned, a research group demonstrated that DL assessment of tumor response was significantly better in predicting overall survival than the RANO criteria [21], enabling an automated on-demand quantitative tumor response assessment in roughly 10 min [9]. Evidently, these findings require prospective validation before broad clinical implementation can be recommended, but this holds promise both for more efficient and accurate delivery of care in the future.

The use of DL for imaging data holds promise also outside the neuro-oncological field, which can be exemplified by the work of Chilamkurthy et al., where DL accurately identified abnormalities requiring urgent attention [38].

Their training set contained 313,318 head computed tomography (CT) scans, with a test set of 21,095 CT scans, achieving AUC scores between 0.90 and 0.96 for detecting different types of intracranial hemorrhage, demonstrating the potential for providing efficient care and rational allocation of human resources. Furthermore, in the epilepsy field, DL was applied to whole-brain presurgical structural connectomes from diffusion tensor imaging, thereby isolating abnormal individualized patterns, providing a highly accurate prediction of seizure outcomes after surgery [39].

Finally, outside the field of image analysis, DL has demonstrated encouraging results in several other areas of clinical neuroscience. A systematic review of DL-based electroencephalography (EEG) ascertained the exponential rise of DL-applications for EEG-processing in domains such as brain-computer interfacing, sleep, epilepsy, cognitive, and affective monitoring, with various DL architectures being used successfully, with CNNs, RNNs, and AEs being used most often [40]. Notably, a substantial proportion of medical data is tabular and for such data ML methods dominate, exemplified by *support vector machines* [41, 42]. Although still in the infancy it is possible for DL methods to transform tabular data to images and later classify images based upon conventional DL methods with apparent good results [43–45].

We acknowledge that these examples only constitute a minimal proportion of the large number of DL studies that have been published during the last few years in topics related to neuroscience. The increased interest in this field is assumed to reflect a need for clinical decision-making support systems, more efficient use of (limited) human resources, and that DL is believed to have a role in improving the management and outcome of patients. The examples provided in this chapter are only meant to serve as an introduction to this multidisciplinary and complex field, and it is beyond the scope of this chapter to give a complete overview of potential medical applications, or to provide in-depth technical data to allow readers to learn how to set up a functioning DL system.

11.5 Concluding Remarks

DL is a complex architecture of multiple sequential layers of learning algorithms, making its workings conceptually similar to the plasticity and the related learning capacity of the biological brain. For this reason, DL can be better than ML due to the more automatic and dynamic processing and learning of data that DL methods can offer. DL can also be better than the human brain due to its ability to handle much larger amounts of information and perform highly complex computations, without human errors or biases. However, for optimal performance DL requires large, pre-processed and integrated datasets, which pose practical challenges for its use in clinical neuroscience. Importantly, there is also a need for thorough external validation before it can be allowed to be implemented in a clinical support decision setting. Nevertheless, we believe that DL models have potential to be used effectively for data augmentation, segmentation, detection, classification, prediction, and prognostication, based on clinical, radiological, and several other diagnostic modalities, for a more rational, accurate, and time-efficient use of resources that could benefit clinical practice and improve patient outcome.

Acknowledgements This project was partly funded by research grant from the Swedish Research Council (2017-00944).

Conflict of Interests None declared.

References

1. Kim DH, MacKinnon T. Artificial intelligence in fracture detection: transfer learning from deep convolutional neural networks. Clin Radiol. 2018;73:439–45. https://doi.org/10.1016/j.crad.2017.11.015.
2. Button KS, Ioannidis JP, Mokrysz C, Nosek BA, Flint J, Robinson ES, Munafò MR. Power failure: why small sample size undermines the reliability of neuroscience. Nat Rev Neurosci. 2013;14:365–76. https://doi.org/10.1038/nrn3475.
3. Fischl B. FreeSurfer. NeuroImage. 2012;62:774–81.
4. Jenkinson M, Beckmann CF, Behrens TE, Woolrich MW, Smith SM. Fsl. NeuroImage. 2012;62:782–90. https://doi.org/10.1016/j.neuroimage.2011.09.015.
5. Avants BB, Tustison NJ, Song G, Cook PA, Klein A, Gee JC. A reproducible evaluation of ANTs similarity metric performance in brain image registration. NeuroImage. 2011;54:2033–44. https://doi.org/10.1016/j.neuroimage.2010.09.025.
6. Selbekk T, Jakola AS, Solheim O, Johansen TF, Lindseth F, Reinertsen I, Unsgård G. Ultrasound imaging in neurosurgery: approaches to minimize surgically induced image artefacts for improved resection control. Acta Neurochir. 2013;155:973–80.
7. Bakas S, Reyes M, Jakab A, Bauer S, Rempfler M, Crimi A, Shinohara RT, Berger C, Ha SM, Rozycki M. Identifying the best machine learning algorithms for brain tumor segmentation, progression assessment, and overall survival prediction in the BRATS challenge. arXiv preprint arXiv:181102629; 2018.
8. Kofler F, Berger C, Waldmannstetter D, Lipkova J, Ezhov I, Tetteh G, Kirschke J, Zimmer C, Wiestler B, Menze BH. BraTS toolkit: translating BraTS brain tumor segmentation algorithms into clinical and scientific practice. Front Neurosci. 2020;14:125.
9. Kickingereder P, Isensee F, Tursunova I, Petersen J, Neuberger U, Bonekamp D, Brugnara G, Schell M, Kessler T, Foltyn M, Harting I, Sahm F, Prager M, Nowosielski M, Wick A, Nolden M, Radbruch A, Debus J, Schlemmer HP, Heiland S, Platten M, von Deimling A, van den Bent MJ, Gorlia T, Wick W, Bendszus M, Maier-Hein KH. Automated quantitative tumour response assessment of MRI in neuro-oncology with artificial neural networks: a multicentre, retrospective study. Lancet Oncol. 2019;20:728–40. https://doi.org/10.1016/s1470-2045(19)30098-1.

10. Ronneberger O, Fischer P, Brox T. U-net: Convolutional networks for biomedical image segmentation. In: International conference on medical image computing and computer-assisted intervention. Berlin: Springer; 2015. p. 234–41.
11. Yogananda CGB, Shah BR, Vejdani-Jahromi M, Nalawade SS, Murugesan GK, Yu FF, Pinho MC, Wagner BC, Emblem KE, Bjørnerud A. A fully automated deep learning network for brain tumor segmentation. Tomography. 2020;6:186.
12. LeCun Y, Bengio Y, Hinton G. Deep learning. Nature. 2015;521:436–44. https://doi.org/10.1038/nature14539.
13. Saha S. A comprehensive guide to convolutional neural networks—the ELI5 way. Towards Data Science; 2018.
14. Wataya T, Nakanishi K, Suzuki Y, Kido S, Tomiyama N. Introduction to deep learning: minimum essence required to launch a research. Jpn J Radiol. 2020;38:907–21. https://doi.org/10.1007/s11604-020-00998-2.
15. Simonyan K, Zisserman A. Very deep convolutional networks for large-scale image recognition. arXiv preprint arXiv:14091556; 2014.
16. Szegedy C, Liu W, Jia Y, Sermanet P, Reed S, Anguelov D, Erhan D, Vanhoucke V, Rabinovich a going deeper with convolutions. In: Proceedings of the IEEE conference on computer vision and pattern recognition. 2015. p. 1–9.
17. He K, Zhang X, Ren S, Sun J. Deep residual learning for image recognition. In: Proceedings of the IEEE conference on computer vision and pattern recognition. 2016. p. 770–8.
18. Samek W, Binder A, Montavon G, Lapuschkin S, Muller KR. Evaluating the visualization of what a deep neural network has learned. IEEE Trans Neural Netw Learn Syst. 2017;28:2660–73. https://doi.org/10.1109/tnnls.2016.2599820.
19. Natekar P, Kori A, Krishnamurthi G. Demystifying brain tumor segmentation networks: interpretability and uncertainty analysis. Front Comput Neurosci. 2020;14:6.
20. Ali MB, Gu IY, Berger MS, Pallud J, Southwell D, Widhalm G, Roux A, Vecchio TG, Jakola AS. Domain mapping and deep learning from multiple MRI clinical datasets for prediction of molecular subtypes in low grade gliomas. Brain Sci. 2020;10(7):463. https://doi.org/10.3390/brainsci10070463.
21. van den Bent MJ, Wefel JS, Schiff D, Taphoorn MJ, Jaeckle K, Junck L, Armstrong T, Choucair A, Waldman AD, Gorlia T. Response assessment in neuro-oncology (a report of the RANO group): assessment of outcome in trials of diffuse low-grade gliomas. Lancet Oncol. 2011;12:583–93.
22. Yogananda CGB, Shah BR, Yu FF, Pinho MC, Nalawade SS, Murugesan GK, Wagner BC, Mickey B, Patel TR, Fei B, Madhuranthakam AJ, Maldjian JA. A novel fully automated MRI-based deep-learning method for classification of 1p/19q co-deletion status in brain gliomas. Neurooncol Adv. 2020;2:vdaa066. https://doi.org/10.1093/noajnl/vdaa066.
23. Bangalore Yogananda CG, Shah BR, Vejdani-Jahromi M, Nalawade SS, Murugesan GK, Yu FF, Pinho MC, Wagner BC, Mickey B, Patel TR, Fei B, Madhuranthakam AJ, Maldjian JA. A novel fully automated MRI-based deep-learning method for classification of IDH mutation status in brain gliomas. Neuro-Oncology. 2020;22:402–11. https://doi.org/10.1093/neuonc/noz199.
24. Li Z, Wang Y, Yu J, Guo Y, Cao W. Deep learning based radiomics (DLR) and its usage in noninvasive IDH1 prediction for low grade glioma. Sci Rep. 2017;7:5467. https://doi.org/10.1038/s41598-017-05848-2.
25. Akkus Z, Ali I, Sedlar J, Kline TL, Agrawal JP, Parney IF, Giannini C, Erickson BJ. Predicting 1p19q chromosomal deletion of low-grade gliomas from MR images using deep learning. arXiv preprint arXiv:161106939; 2016.
26. Chang K, Bai HX, Zhou H, Su C, Bi WL, Agbodza E, Kavouridis VK, Senders JT, Boaro A, Beers A, Zhang B, Capellini A, Liao W, Shen Q, Li X, Xiao B, Cryan J, Ramkissoon S, Ramkissoon L, Ligon K, Wen PY, Bindra RS, Woo J, Arnaout O, Gerstner ER, Zhang PJ, Rosen BR, Yang L, Huang RY, Kalpathy-Cramer J. Residual convolutional neural network for the determination of IDH status in low- and high-grade gliomas from MR imaging. Clin Cancer Res. 2018;24:1073–81. https://doi.org/10.1158/1078-0432.Ccr-17-2236.
27. Matsui Y, Maruyama T, Nitta M, Saito T, Tsuzuki S, Tamura M, Kusuda K, Fukuya Y, Asano H, Kawamata T, Masamune K, Muragaki Y. Prediction of lower-grade glioma molecular subtypes using deep learning. J Neuro-Oncol. 2020;146:321–7. https://doi.org/10.1007/s11060-019-03376-9.
28. Ge C, Gu IY-H, Jakola AS, Yang J. Enlarged training dataset by pairwise GANs for molecular-based brain tumor classification. IEEE Access. 2020;8:22560–70.
29. Liang S, Zhang R, Liang D, Song T, Ai T, Xia C, Xia L, Wang Y. Multimodal 3D DenseNet for IDH genotype prediction in gliomas. Genes (Basel). 2018;9:382. https://doi.org/10.3390/genes9080382.
30. Yordanova YN, Cochereau J, Duffau H, Herbet G. Combining resting state functional MRI with intraoperative cortical stimulation to map the mentalizing network. NeuroImage. 2019;186:628–36.
31. van der Voort SR, Incekara F, Wijnenga MM, Kapas G, Gardeniers M, Schouten JW, Starmans MP, Tewarie RN, Lycklama GJ, French PJ. Predicting the 1p/19q codeletion status of presumed low-grade glioma with an externally validated machine learning algorithm. Clin Cancer Res. 2019;25:7455–62.
32. Jakola AS, Reinertsen I. Radiological evaluation of low-grade glioma: time to embrace quantitative data? Acta Neurochir. 2019;161:577–8.
33. Chaudhari AS, Sandino CM, Cole EK, Larson DB, Gold GE, Vasanawala SS, Lungren MP, Hargreaves BA, Langlotz CP. Prospective deployment of deep learning in MRI: a framework for important considerations, challenges, and recommendations for best practices. J Magn Reson Imaging. 2020;54(2):357–71. https://doi.org/10.1002/jmri.27331.
34. Shah ND, Steyerberg EW, Kent DM. Big data and predictive analytics: recalibrating expectations. JAMA. 2018;320:27–8. https://doi.org/10.1001/jama.2018.5602.
35. Ibrahim A, Primakov S, Beuque M, Woodruff HC, Halilaj I, Wu G, Refaee T, Granzier R, Widaatalla Y, Hustinx R, Mottaghy FM, Lambin P. Radiomics for precision medicine: current challenges, future prospects, and the proposal of a new framework. Methods. 2021;188:20–9. https://doi.org/10.1016/j.ymeth.2020.05.022.
36. Wickstrom KK, OyvindMikalsen K, Kampffmeyer M, Revhaug A, Jenssen R. Uncertainty-aware deep ensembles for reliable and explainable predictions of clinical time series. IEEE J Biomed Health Inform. 2020. https://doi.org/10.1109/jbhi.2020.3042637.
37. Windisch P, Weber P, Fürweger C, Ehret F, Kufeld M, Zwahlen D, Muacevic A. Implementation of model explainability for a basic brain tumor detection using convolutional neural networks on MRI slices. Neuroradiology. 2020;62:1515–8. https://doi.org/10.1007/s00234-020-02465-1.
38. Chilamkurthy S, Ghosh R, Tanamala S, Biviji M, Campeau NG, Venugopal VK, Mahajan V, Rao P, Warier P. Deep learning algorithms for detection of critical findings in head CT scans: a retrospective study. Lancet. 2018;392:2388–96. https://doi.org/10.1016/s0140-6736(18)31645-3.
39. Gleichgerrcht E, Munsell B, Bhatia S, Vandergrift WA 3rd, Rorden C, McDonald C, Edwards J, Kuzniecky R, Bonilha L. Deep learning applied to whole-brain connectome to determine seizure control after epilepsy surgery. Epilepsia. 2018;59:1643–54. https://doi.org/10.1111/epi.14528.
40. Roy Y, Banville H, Albuquerque I, Gramfort A, Falk TH, Faubert J. Deep learning-based electroencephalography analysis: a systematic review. J Neural Eng. 2019;16:051001. https://doi.org/10.1088/1741-2552/ab260c.

41. Chen D, Liu S, Kingsbury P, Sohn S, Storlie CB, Habermann EB, Naessens JM, Larson DW, Liu H. Deep learning and alternative learning strategies for retrospective real-world clinical data. NPJ Digit Med. 2019;2:43. https://doi.org/10.1038/s41746-019-0122-0.
42. Munkhdalai T, Liu F, Yu H. Clinical relation extraction toward drug safety surveillance using electronic health record narratives: classical learning versus deep learning. JMIR Public Health Surveill. 2018;4:e29. https://doi.org/10.2196/publichealth.9361.
43. Buturovic L, Miljkovic D. A novel method for classification of tabular data using convolutional neural networks. BioRxiv; 2020.
44. López-García G, Jerez JM, Franco L, Veredas FJ. Transfer learning with convolutional neural networks for cancer survival prediction using gene-expression data. PLoS One. 2020;15:e0230536. https://doi.org/10.1371/journal.pone.0230536.
45. Sharma A, Vans E, Shigemizu D, Boroevich KA, Tsunoda T. DeepInsight: a methodology to transform a non-image data to an image for convolution neural network architecture. Sci Rep. 2019;9:11399. https://doi.org/10.1038/s41598-019-47765-6.

Machine Learning-Based Clustering Analysis: Foundational Concepts, Methods, and Applications

12

Miquel Serra-Burriel and Christopher Ames

12.1 Introduction

On a day-to-day basis, one after another, we make unconscious classifications around the things we perceive. From colors to personalities, we classify observations into groups. A recent hypothesis in neuroscience suggests that brains spontaneously learn statistical structure of images by extracting their properties such as geometry or illumination [1]. Clustering analysis is the branch of statistics that formally deals with this task, learning from patterns, and its formal development is relatively new in statistics compared to other branches.

Statistical learning can be broadly defined as supervised, unsupervised, or a combination of the previous two. While supervised learning aims at mapping inputs to pre-specified outputs, unsupervised learning aims at grouping objects so that elements in each group are more similar to each other than those in other groups. The advantage of this approach is that it does not require any assumptions regarding the underlying joint distribution of patterns, also unsupervised learning also does not require labelling, which is usually time- and cost-sensitive or entirely impossible for large, unstructured datasets.

There are a lot of types of clustering. However, the main thing that they share in common is the fact that they try to explain variance in the data with discrete partitions. Cluster analysis made its first public appearance in human anthropology by Driver and Kroeber in 1932 in their quantitative expression of cultural relationships [2]. They used a simple trait-count model of the populations of Polynesia, Plains Sun Dance, America Northwest Coast, and Peru to cluster them. Much has happened since, and the number of applications of such a simple principle is almost infinite. Marketing [3], genetics [4], politics [5], physics [6], ecology [7], and many more fields benefit from it. Most digital companies use it to segment their market and customer base according to their online preferences and behaviors.

How can we cluster? There are a lot of approaches to cluster observations, namely: connectivity-based clustering or hierarchical clustering, centroid-based clustering, and density-based clustering. We will go through each approach, with applications, review dimensionality reduction and two examples of papers that we find meaningful. The Supplementary Content 12.1 presents the R code to replicate our results and create your own, while following these examples.

Supplementary Information The online version contains supplementary material available at [https://doi.org/10.1007/978-3-030-85292-4_12].

M. Serra-Burriel (✉)
Epidemiology, Biostatistics and Prevention Institute, University of Zurich (UZH), Zurich, Switzerland
e-mail: miquel.serraburriel@uzh.ch

C. Ames
Department of Neurological Surgery, University of California San Francisco (UCSF), San Francisco, CA, USA
e-mail: Christopher.Ames@ucsf.edu

12.2 Connectivity-Based Clustering

Connectivity-based clustering is based on the idea of building a hierarchy of similar elements within a sample. It can be performed in two ways, bottom-up or agglomerative and top-down or divisive. The former begins with each observation being its own cluster and later pairing them recursively, the later starts with one cluster containing all observations and recursively splitting them into smaller clusters until each observation forms its own group. The results of clustering are usually presented in dendrograms, tree-shaped objects that represent the hierarchy of the clustering product.

To illustrate the basic functionality, let us begin with a toy example of hierarchical clustering with two dimensions or features of a population. We have a sample of 1000 individuals who were subject to two visual perception tasks, one of

V. E. Staartjes et al. (eds.), *Machine Learning in Clinical Neuroscience*, Acta Neurochirurgica Supplement 134,
https://doi.org/10.1007/978-3-030-85292-4_12

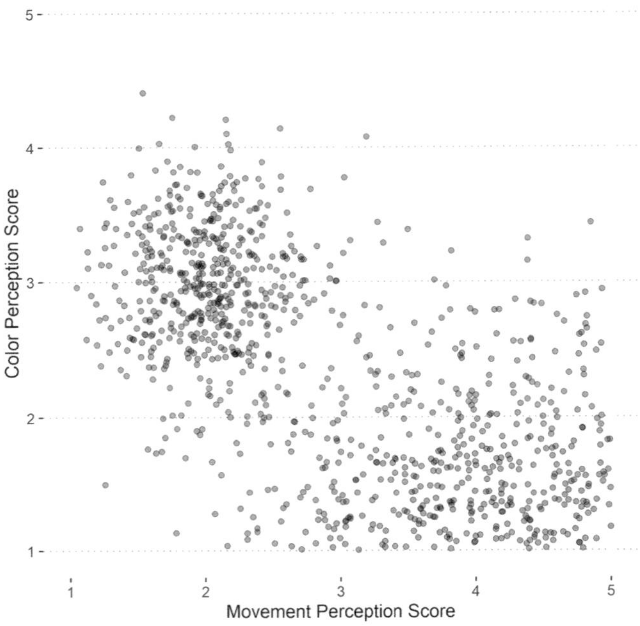

Fig. 12.1 Scatterplot of cognition performance

movement perception and another one of color perception. The scatterplot of the performance in both tasks is presented in Fig. 12.1.

Each dot presents an observation of our study, the x axis presents the score of the movement perception task and the y-axis presents the score of the color perception one. We want to create groups that are homogeneous within themselves and heterogenous across. The first step to clustering is to create a distance or dissimilarity matrix. This matrix contains the relative distance of each observation with respect to all other observations in the set. There are a lot of ways to create a distance matrix. The most widely used is the Euclidean distance (Eq. 12.1):

$$d(p,q) = \sqrt{\sum_{i=1}^{n} (p_i - q_i)^2} \tag{12.1}$$

where the distance between observations p and q is equal to the square root of the squared sum of differences in position of p and q for n dimensions. In our case, since we have 1000 observations, each Euclidean distance for participant i, with respect to participant j, takes form in the following way (Eq. 12.2):

$$d(i,j) = \sqrt{(\text{mps}_i - \text{mps}_j)^2 + (\text{cps}_i - \text{cps}_j)^2} \tag{12.2}$$

where mps is the movement perception score and cps is the color perception score. Figure 12.2 presents the matrix of distances as measured by different metrics.

The upper left panel of the figure presents the Euclidean distance, the upper right panel presents the maximum distance, the lower left the Manhattan distance, and the lower right panel presents the Canberra distance. It can be noted that irrespective of the distance measure, the overall structure of the matrix is fairly similar. Once the matrix has been constructed, two approaches are possible, the above-mentioned agglomerative (also called Agnes) and divisive (also called Diana) functions. In general terms, agglomerative methods are mainly used to find small clusters and divisive methods larger clusters. Let us use the Euclidean distance matrix from Fig. 12.2 to build a dendrogram for the bottom-up approach and split it into four clusters.

Figure 12.3 represents the resulting dendrogram. The x-axis presents each observation, while the y-axis connections present the pairs of observations and groups of observations. In the figure, the number of clusters is predefined to be 4. However, how can one determine the "natural" or optimal number of clusters in the sample? In our sample there are between 2 and 999 potential clusters. The hierarchy of the model aids us in distinguishing which subgroups stem from other bigger clusters recursively.

There are three main methods in determining the number of clusters: the elbow method [8], average silhouette method [9], and the gap statistic method [10].

The elbow method basically computes the resulting intra-cluster variation (also known as wss) for each of the potential cluster groupings. The location of the bend or "knee," meaning the inflexion point is usually chosen as the indicator of the appropriate number of clusters. The silhouette method computes a silhouette value that considers how close each observation is to its own cluster compared to the others and the value ranges from −1 to 1, with higher values indicating better clustering for each iteration on the number of clusters. The gap statistic method is similar to the silhouette method; however, it compares the resulting difference in intra-cluster variation from each clustering distribution with a random Monte Carlo simulated sample. Figure 12.4 presents the results on the optimal number of clustering by each of the described methods.

Independently, each method points toward two underlying clusters. We rebuild the previous dendrogram and plot clustered scatterplot of cognition performance groups (Fig. 12.5).

What are the advantages and disadvantages of hierarchical clustering?

Advantages:

- The clustering model has an imposed structural hierarchy, which tends to be more interpretable than other outputs.
- Its construction process is independent of the number of clusters, thus conserving some information that can be of value for the researcher.
- Their simplicity and transparency foster interpretation and reproducibility in external settings.

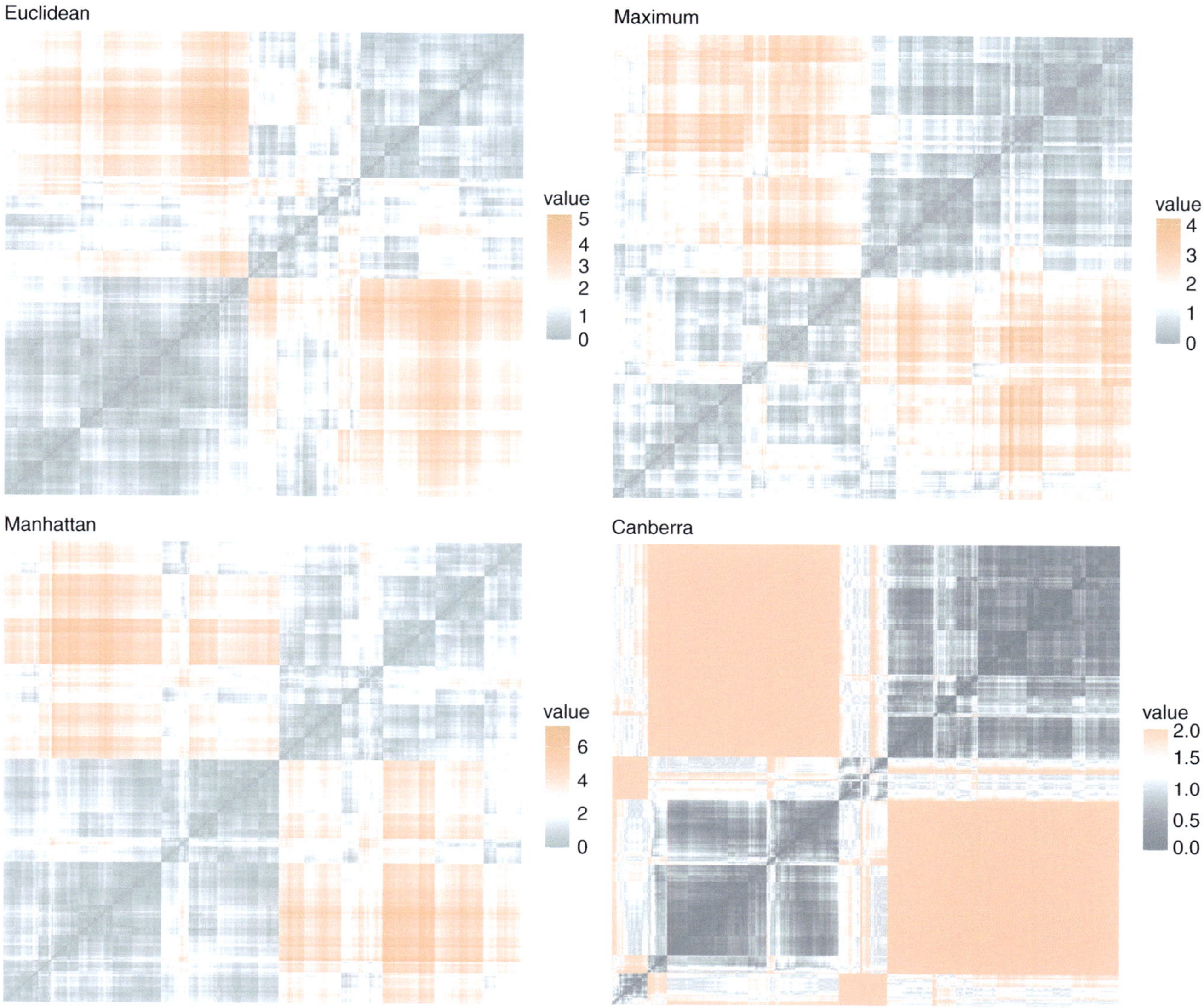

Fig. 12.2 Distance matrix according to different distance measures

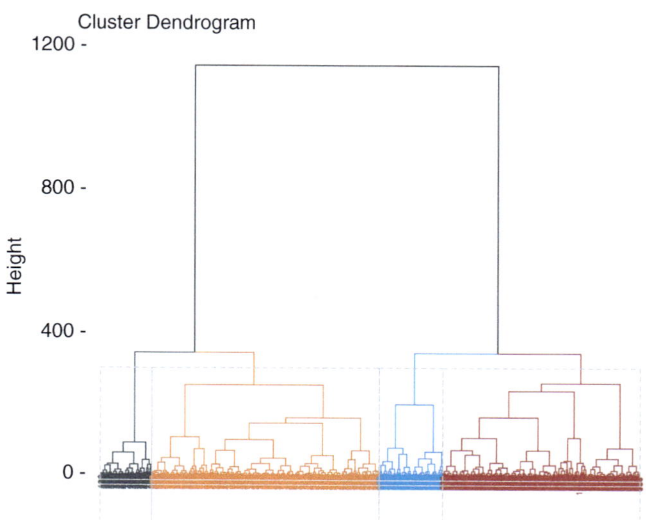

Fig. 12.3 Agnes Dendrogram built with Euclidean distance and four groups

Disadvantages:

- Given its static recursive approach, once a data point has been placed within a cluster, the model does not test for other potential combinations.
- It is more computationally demanding than other clustering algorithms.
- Its sensitivity to outliers requires caution in the preprocessing stage.
- Its results also depend on the metric used to compute the distance or dissimilarity matrix.

12.3 Centroid-Based Clustering

Instead of computing distance across observations and then recursively imposing a hierarchy over them, centroid-based clustering aims to partition observations into k groups in such a way that the sum of distances from points to the cen-

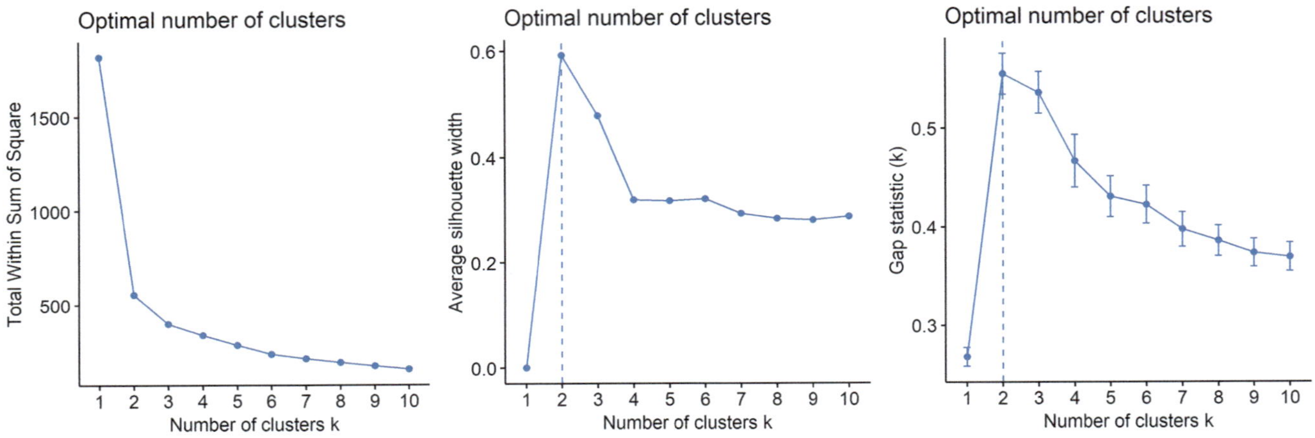

Fig. 12.4 Optimal number of clusters by method

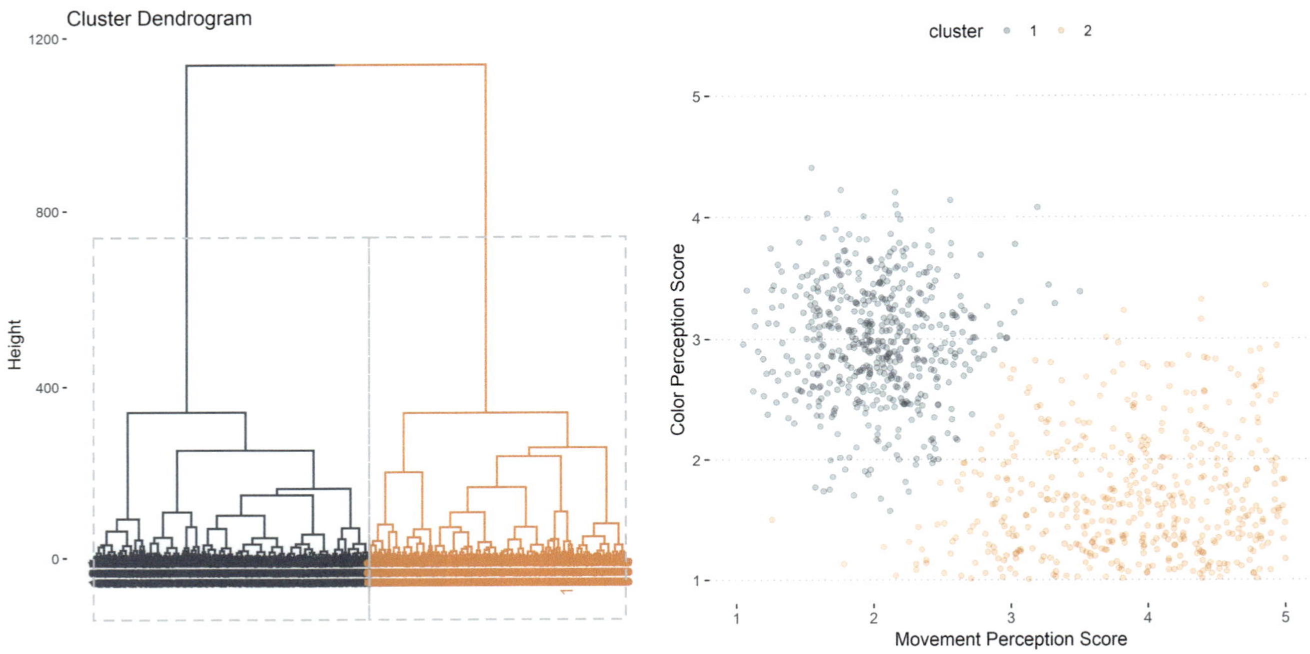

Fig. 12.5 Optimized Agnes Dendrogram Clustering built with Euclidean distances and scatterplot by cluster

troid of their respective clusters is minimized. A valid analogy would be to split a lot of identical pies into *k* pieces, not in even parts necessarily, and select the splitting pattern that is more satisfying. The history of this type of clustering started in the late 50s, with Hugo Steinhaus first in 1956 [11] and Stuart Lloyd in 1957 [12] as a technique for representing analog signals in a digital way. However, the algorithm was further refined by James MacQueen in 1967 [13] and the currently most used one was published in 1979 by Hartigan and Wong [14].

The algorithm has two steps, assignment, and update, preceded by an initialization method. The initialization can be done in two ways. Randomly choosing *k* (the same amount of desired clusters) observations and using them as the initial means or randomly assigning a cluster to each observation and using that cluster mean as the centroid. Then, with either method the assignment step follows. Each observation is assigned to the cluster that is nearer, measured with the Euclidean distance to the centroid as described in Eq. (12.1). Then, the update step follows by simply computing the centroid or mean again for the observations assigned to it. The process is repeated until the observations classified to each cluster do not change. Note that this process does not need to converge necessarily, and the general recommendation is to initialize the algorithm with several random starts, which sometimes prevents the algorithm from not converging.

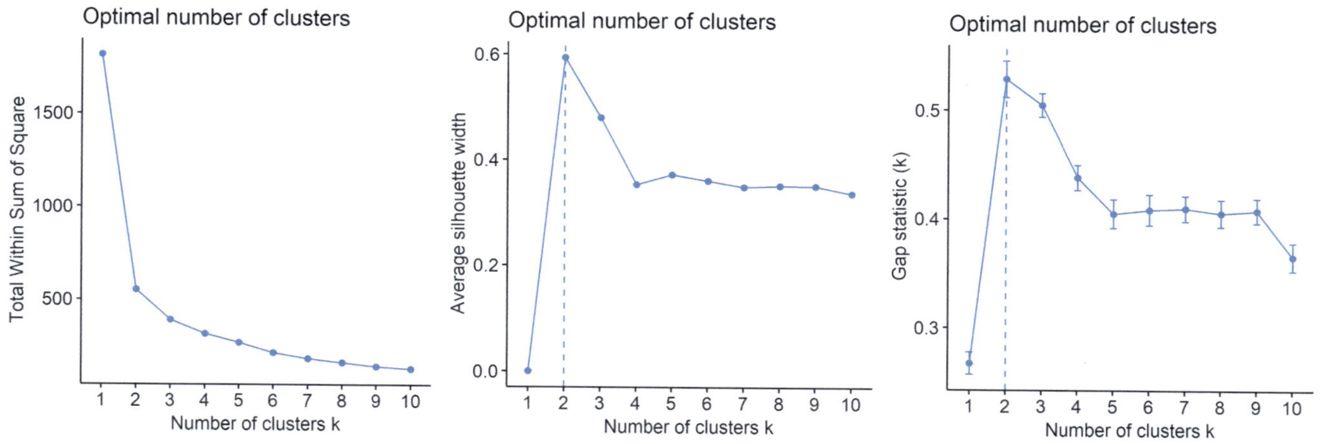

Fig. 12.6 *k*-means clustering partitions, from 2 to 7 clusters

Using the same dataset since the beginning of the chapter we perform a *k*-means clustering with the Hartigan–Wong algorithm, 5 random starts, and from 2 to 7 clusters. Figure 12.6 presents the results of the clustering.

To determine the optimal number of clusters, the same methods described before apply: the elbow method, the silhouette and the Gap method. Again, as with the hierarchical clustering approach the optimal amount is revealed to be two by all accounts. The results of both algorithms are strikingly similar. Figure 12.7 presents the results of the optimization process.

What are the advantages and disadvantages of centroid-based clustering?

Advantages:

- Simpler algorithm to implement.
- Computationally efficient.
- It has been shown to produce results with high external validity.
- Adapts and recognizes well clusters with distinct functional forms and relative sizes.

Disadvantages:

- It does not identify clusters with non-convex shapes.
- It has difficulties identifying clusters of different size.
- It is not completely suited to clustering exercises of high dimensionality, due to Euclidean distance causing the algorithm to converge almost immediately.

12.4 Density-Based Clustering

Compared to the previous two methods of clustering, density-based clustering does not impose a hierarchy or partitions the space. It rather choses clusters based on the defined areas higher statistical density than the rest. Different from before, all observations are not assigned a cluster, points outside the optimized clusters are considered to be noise.

The most used clustering method based on this principle is the density-based spatial clustering of applications with noise (DBSCAN) (Fig. 12.8). Developed in 1996 by Ester, Kriegel, Sander, and Xu, and it is a non-parametric algorithm [15]. The intuition of the algorithm is straightforward. The model uses what is called *minPts*, a threshold on the number of neighboring points, within a radius *e*. Points with more neighboring points than the threshold are considered as a core point, analogous to a centroid. The objective of the algorithm is then to find separated areas of high-density vs. areas of low density.

In abstract terms, the DBSCAN algorithm has three steps. Find the points within the *e* radius of every point, and identify core points with a number of observations above the threshold *minPts*. Then, the connected core points are merged, and finally points are assigned either to clusters or to noise.

What are the advantages and disadvantages of density-based clustering?

Advantages:

- It does not require a pre-specified or optimized number of clusters.
- It does recognize non-convex clusters, and even strange shapes such as circles within circles.
- Because density has a noise component, the method is robust with respect to eliminating outliers.
- It only requires two parameters which are independent of the order or functional forms of the underlying data-generating process.

Disadvantages:

- It does not cluster well data with different densities, meaning that if there are two clusters in the dataset, but

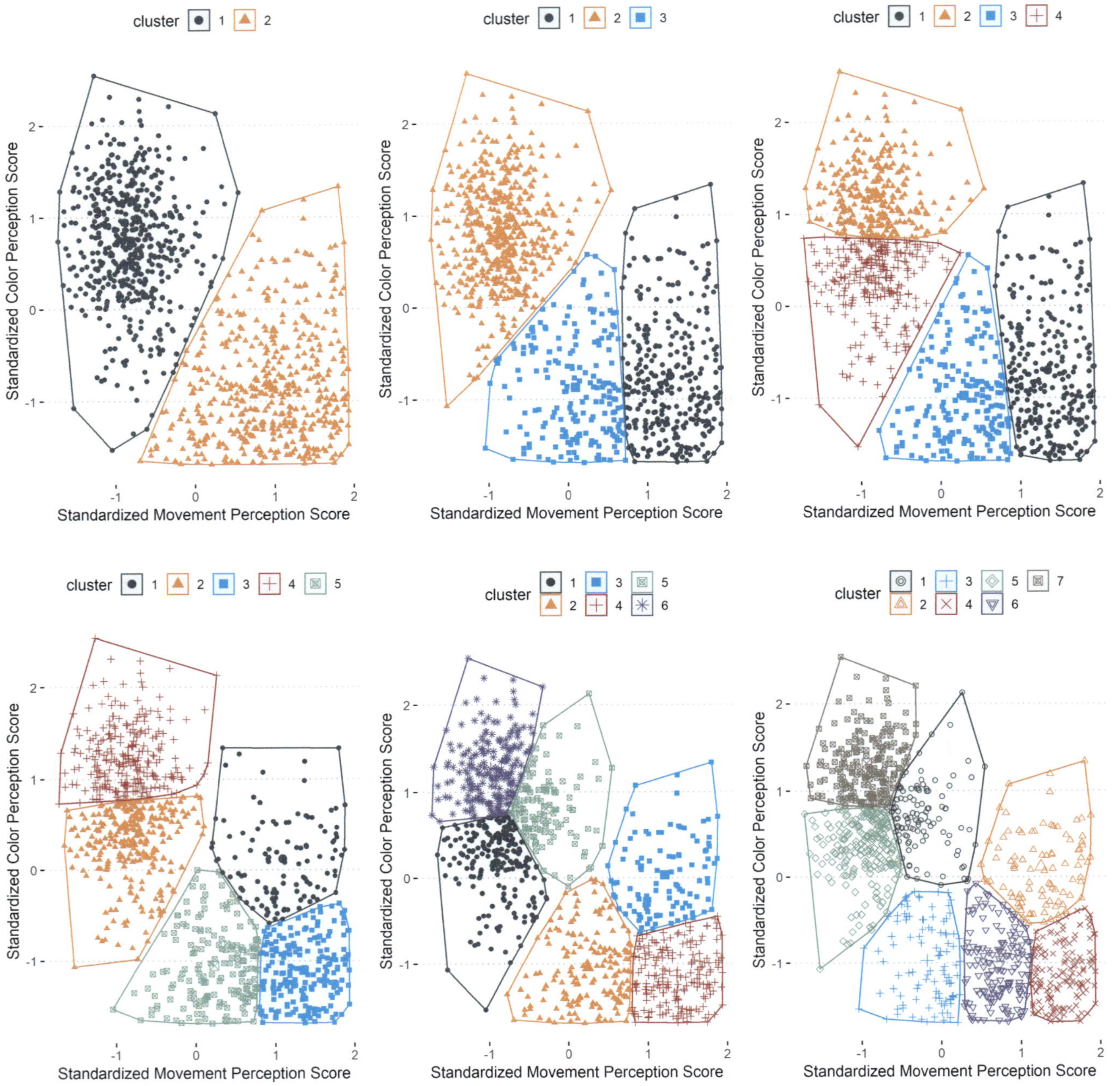

Fig. 12.7 Optimal number of clusters by method

one is highly dense and the other is not, density-based models will have difficulty recognizing them.

- Given some combinations of both parameters in the algorithm, irrelevant tiny clusters might appear.
- It requires the most user supervision of all the algorithms, as the results are highly unstable based on different combinations of parameters.

12.5 Dimensionality Reduction

Until now, all of our examples have been based on two dimensions, *x*- and *y*-axis values. However, in real-life scenarios, it is unlikely that setting investigated has only two. Most problems in clinical science appear within incredibly complex causal networks. Patients, their diseases, and realities are highly dimensional. We have highlighted that clustering algorithms tend to fail when the number of dimensions increases because distance-based metrics tend to be meaningless at high values. The response to this phenomena: to reduce dimensions of your data.

Dimension reduction is the task that transforms high dimensions of data to low dimensions while conserving the most important relations and features of the original. There is an almost infinity of ways to achieve such a purpose, from principal component analysis to uniform manifold approximation and projection algorithms. Let us demonstrate this with another toy example.

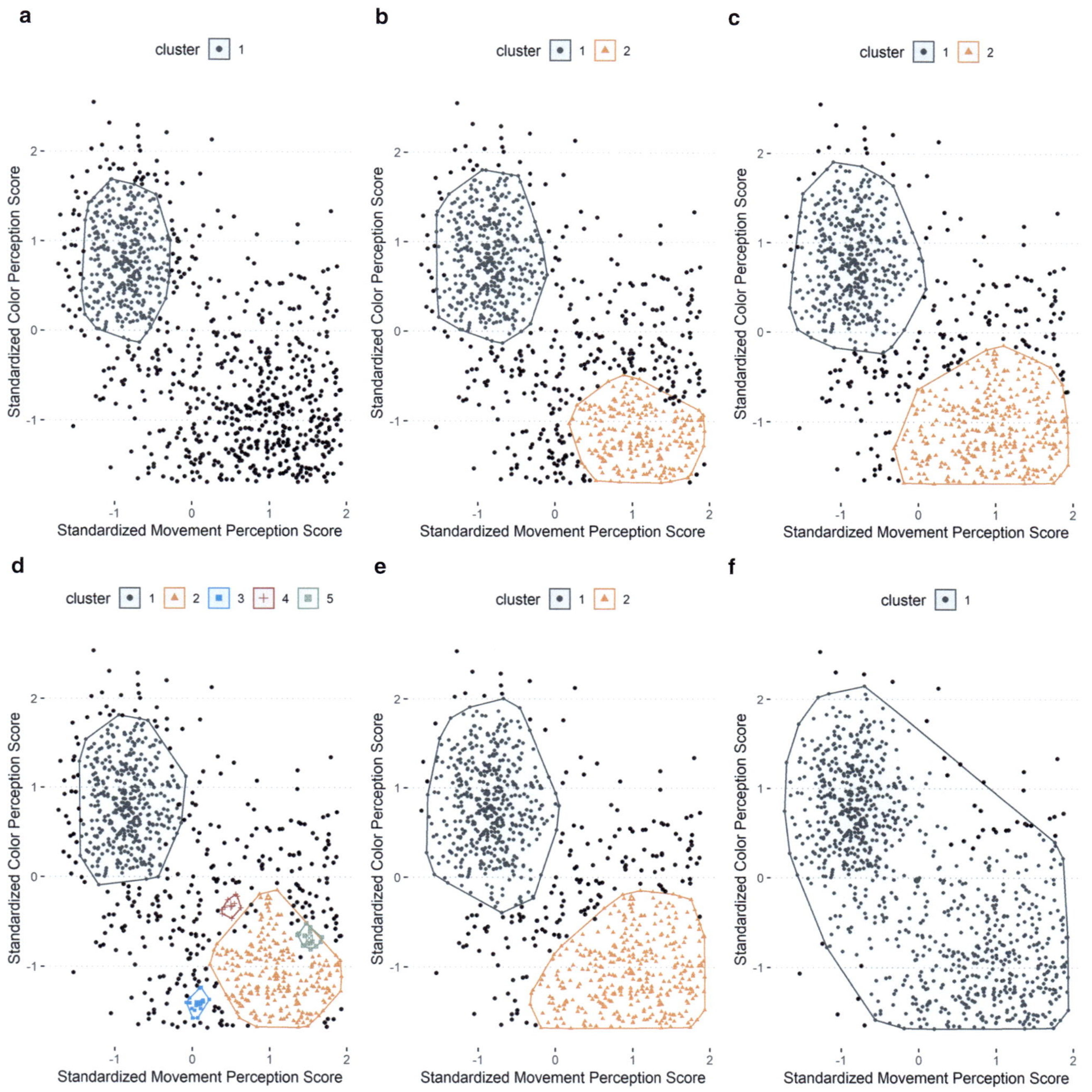

Fig. 12.8 DBSCAN clustering results with varying parameters. *Notes:* (**a**) $e = 0.25$, $minPts = 40$, (**b**) $e = 0.25$, $minPts = 30$, (**c**) $e = 0.25$, $minPts = 20$, (**d**) $e = 0.15$, $minPts = 10$, (**e**) $e = 0.30$, $minPts = 30$, (**f**) $e = 0.35$, $minPts = 30$

We have now performed six additional cognitive tasks on our imaginary sample, resulting in eight variables. However, we want to describe the sample with as little complexity as possible, let us say three components maximum. The first step is to compute the principal components of the dataset. To do so, the covariance matrix of the data has to be estimated, and the eigenvalues and eigenvectors are factored in to diagonalize the elements that form the variance of each respective dimensions. The proportion of explained variance that each eigenvector reflects is calculated by dividing the eigenvalue by the addition of each eigenvector. In our case, the first component explains 36% of the data variance, the second 20%, and the third around 12%. This means that by using the first three components we are resembling 68% of the original dataset, with of 3 out 8 dimensions, or 37.5% of the original data. Figure 12.9 shows the graphical presentation.

We cut the dimensions to three, and now we apply again the optimized hierarchical clustering algorithm of the

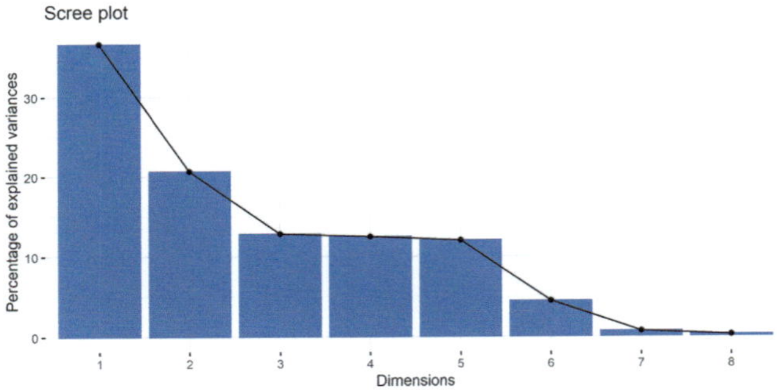

Fig. 12.9 Variance explained by each dimension

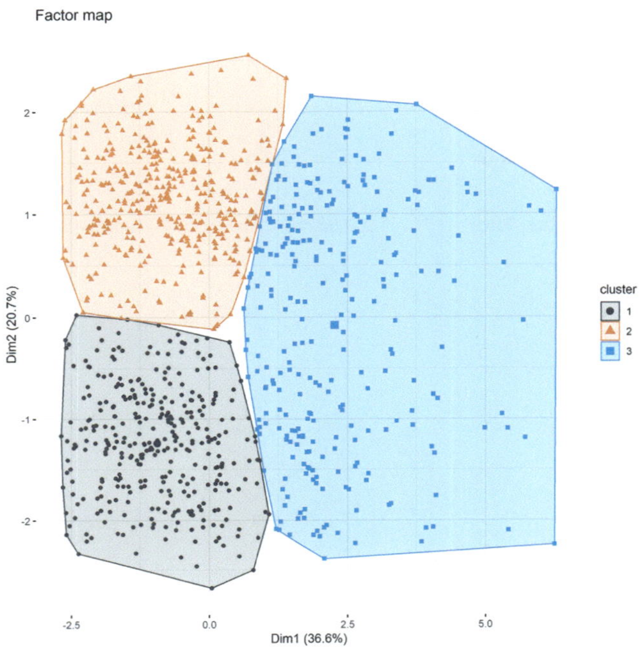

Fig. 12.10 Optimized hierarchical clusters of the simplified dataset

beginning of this chapter resulting in three clusters presented in Fig. 12.10.

12.6 Applications

Adult Spinal Deformity

We previously published one paper, in 2019 [16], using the methods described in this chapter. We did it in the adult spinal deformity (ASD) field. ASD, also known as scoliosis of the adult, is a highly heterogeneous and debilitating condition. Its defining feature is a physical deformation of the spine mainly measured in key angles of its shape. Up to that point, the available classifications of the disease were mainly based in X-ray measurements of the Spine, the Schwab [17] and Lenke [18] classifications. And, while it is true that the spine is a complex structure that entails a lot of features, to us, ignoring non-spine specific patient parameters seemed like an incomplete model of the disease process.

Using a combined data query from both the European Spine Study Group (ESSG) and the International Spine Study Group (ISSG) we set up to simply describe and characterize the potential latent patient clusters. Adding simple quality of life and demographic metrics, we performed a hierarchical clustering modelling to group similar patients from dissimilar ones. We found an optimal of three types of patients, we called them, young coronal patients, old first-timers, and old-revisions. The main descriptive characteristics of the groups were: young coronal patients typified by much younger patients with a coronal spinal deformity and little sagittal malalignment. Old first-timers were patients mostly in their late 50s or early 60s with a more severe deformity mostly related to the lumbar spine and with no previous spinal surgery. Finally, old revision patients were the oldest and the ones with the most severe malalignment, especially in the sagittal plane and who had undergone prior spinal surgery.

However, to us the task seemed incomplete, and on top of a patient-specific clustering exercise we also applied it to surgical techniques. The surgical treatment of scoliosis involves a wide variety of different techniques. The termination levels of fusions and placement of nerve decompressions and vertebral releases and osteotomies result in significant treatment heterogeneity. When we clustered the range of surgical treatments, we found four types of surgeries to be the main clusters.

Finally, by superimposing both the patient and surgery classification, we obtained a descriptive grid of patient and surgery heterogeneity. By doing so, we were able to look at what happened 2 years after surgery when patients within a same cluster where operated on by different surgical clusters. What we obtained was not only a descriptive result in terms of clusters, but also a simple prognostic model associating types of patients and surgeries to outcomes. We observed that, for instance, young coronal patients were the ones with the lowest functional and quality of life improvement, on average, while those young coronal patients receiving more aggressive surgeries were also experiencing higher levels of post-surgical complications. This allowed us to identify simple areas of improvement in terms of patient and surgical selection with a cost-benefit that might not justify more aggressive surgeries.

Sepsis

One of our favorite examples of a successful application of *k*-means clustering is an article by Seymour and coauthors published in 2019 in JAMA [19]. They developed and validated clinical phenotypes for sepsis and model the potential benefit and harm of treatments with data from an external randomized controlled trial.

Sepsis is highly heterogeneous condition defined by an unregulated immune response to an infection that leads to acute organ failure. Given the multidimensional array of clinical symptoms and biological features, the authors used a variety of variables that ranged from demographic, vital signs, markers of inflammation, to markers of organ dysfunction. Out of more than 50 potential candidate variables a total of 29 were selected and observations were clustered according to the consensus k-means clustering method. A total of four phenotypes, alpha, beta, gamma, and omega were found to be optimal using diverse measures of optimization. When looking at the outcomes at any time during hospitalization they found startling differences. The first phenotype, alpha, had only a 2% in-hospital mortality with only 25% of patients admitted to the ICU, while the last cluster or phenotype had a 32% in-hospital mortality and 85% ICU admissions rates. Compared to the standard classification of sepsis, the proposed "phenotypic" classification was fairly constant across the other scheme, highlighting that the human-proposed classification did not capture relevant variance.

The authors then, go a step further, analogous to the above-mentioned cost/benefit grid. They used external RCT data to estimate differential treatment effects across phenotypes. First, they assign the observations of three RCTs (ACCESS, PROWESS, and ProCESS) to each of their derived clusters. After, they vary the proportion of patients from each cluster in each trial to simulate scenarios and their causal effects. They find that out of the three interventions used in the RCTs, according to which phenotype they are applied, the effects varied remarkably: from total benefit to an extremely high likelihood of harm.

Common Pitfalls and Proposed Solutions

The three most common pitfalls in clustering research relate to (a) the use of high-dimensional data, (b) the lack of comparison of results across clustering methods, and (c) determining whether the results are meaningful. Geometry behaves irregularly in high-dimensional settings, hence measures of distance are rendered non-useful. Sparsity and the identification of relevant variables in the problem tend to be hidden under large numbers of irrelevant ones. We recommend to thoroughly inspect data in the pre-implementation stage and to make sure that each included feature has a potential meaningful implication. As we have discussed in this chapter, different methods can produce different results, hence judging one clustering configuration without comparing it to potential others can render the external validity of the results null. We recommend applying, at least, three different optimized algorithms to assess the robustness of the results. The determination of the usefulness of the results is perhaps the most crucial part, and where we researchers tend to use follow-up data or third-party linked results. It is imperative to pair any good clustering exercise with expert knowledge on the underlying data-generating process.

12.7 Conclusions

Any clustering task involves investigator-related choices, and many of them are critical to the validity of results, both internally and externally. In the present chapter we have introduced, with examples, a few of the most relevant unsupervised learning techniques for the practicing clinical neuroscience researcher. We have not extensively covered all potential algorithms or methods, as that would require a series of books in itself, but we have provided a few visual examples and applications that we hope successfully aid other researchers in the use of these tools. Moreover, the full capacities of data will only be achieved if everyone learns to pair the right research question with the appropriate tools. Clustering methods are the most important tool for data discovery and description, and its integration with both predictive and causal objectives is crucial to maximize its potential, as alone, it still is a descriptive method.

Our experience reveals that the advantages of using formal unsupervised learning algorithms are superior to standard supervised classification methods for the description of phenotypes or clusters. Not only that, but given their potential for heterogeneous treatment effects, they will be a cornerstone for trial design by selecting populations with expected effect sizes well below or above the mean.

In short, clustering is perhaps, more than other machine learning techniques, the most underused and underappreciated, and should be strongly considered in questioning scientific paradigms regarding classification of features.

For further reading we recommend the books by Trevor Hastie, Robert Tibshirani & Jerome Friedman. "The elements of statistical learning: data mining, inference, and prediction" Springer Science & Business Media, 2009, and M. Emre Celebi & Kemal Aydin. "Unsupervise learning algorithms" Berlin: Springer International Publishing, 2016.

Conflict of Interest Declaration Dr. Serra-Burriel reports receiving grant funding from the European Commission H2020 program and European Commission EiT Health program.

Dr. Ames reports receiving royalties from Stryker, Biomet Zimmer Spine, DePuy Synthes, NuVasive, Next Orthosurgical, K2M, and Medicrea; being a consultant to DePuy Synthes, Medtronic, Medicrea, and K2M; receiving research support from Titan Spine, DePuy Synthes, and ISSG; being on the editorial board of Operative Neurosurgery;

receiving grant funding from SRS; being on the executive committee of ISSG; and being a director of Global Spine Analytics.

None in relation to the present work.

References

1. Storrs KR, Fleming RW. Unsupervised learning predicts human perception and misperception of gloss. bioRxiv. 2020. https://doi.org/10.1101/2020.04.07.026120.
2. Driver HE, Kroeber AL. Quantitative expression of cultural relationships. Berkeley: University of California Press; 1932.
3. Sánchez-Hernández G, Chiclana F, Agell N, Aguado JC. Ranking and selection of unsupervised learning marketing segmentation. Knowl Based Syst. 2013;44:20–33.
4. Libbrecht MW, Noble WS. Machine learning applications in genetics and genomics. Nat Rev Genet. 2015;16:321–32. https://doi.org/10.1038/nrg3920.
5. Denny M, Spirling A. Text preprocessing for unsupervised learning: why it matters, when it misleads, and what to do about it. Polit Anal. 2017;26(2):168–89.
6. Wang L. Discovering phase transitions with unsupervised learning. Phys Rev B. 2016;94:195105.
7. Sonnewald M, Dutkiewicz S, Hill C, Forget G. Elucidating ecological complexity: unsupervised learning determines global marine eco-provinces. Sci Adv. 2020;6:eaay4740.
8. Syakur MA, Khotimah BK, Rochman EMS, Satoto BD. Integration K-means clustering method and elbow method for identification of the best customer profile cluster. In: IOP conference series: materials science and engineering. 2018.
9. Kodinariya TM, Makwana PR. Review on determining number of cluster in K-means clustering. Int J Adv Res Comput Sci Manag Stud. 2013;1:90–5.
10. Tibshirani R, Walther G, Hastie T. Estimating the number of clusters in a data set via the gap statistic. J R Stat Soc Ser B Stat Methodol. 2001;63:411–23.
11. Fichet B, Piccolo D, Verde R, Vichi M. Studies in classification, data analysis, and knowledge organization. In: Knowledge organization. 2011.
12. Lloyd S. Least squares quantization in PCM. IEEE Trans Inf Theory. 1982;28:129–37.
13. MacQueen J. Some methods for classification and analysis of multivariate observations. In: Proceedings of the fifth Berkeley symposium on mathematical statistics and probability, volume 1: statistics. Berkeley: University of California Press; 1967. p. 281–97. https://projecteuclid.org/euclid.bsmsp/1200512992.
14. Hartigan JA, Wong MA. Algorithm AS 136: a k-means clustering algorithm. J R Stat Soc Ser C (Appl Stat). 1979;28:100–8.
15. Ester M, Kriegel H-P, Sander J, Xu X. A density-based algorithm for discovering clusters in large spatial databases with noise. In: Kdd. 1996. p. 226–31.
16. Ames CP, Smith JS, Pellisé F, Kelly M, Alanay A, Acaroğlu E, et al. Artificial intelligence based hierarchical clustering of patient types and intervention categories in adult spinal deformity surgery: towards a new classification scheme that predicts quality and value. Spine (Phila Pa 1976). 2019;44:915–26.
17. Terran J, Schwab F, Shaffrey CI, Smith JS, Devos P, Ames CP, et al. The SRS-Schwab adult spinal deformity classification: assessment and clinical correlations based on a prospective operative and nonoperative cohort. Neurosurgery. 2013;73(4):559–68.
18. Lenke LG. The Lenke classification system of operative adolescent idiopathic scoliosis. Neurosurg Clin N Am. 2007;18(2):199–206.
19. Seymour CW, Kennedy JN, Wang S, Chang C-CH, Elliott CF, Xu Z, et al. Derivation, validation, and potential treatment implications of novel clinical phenotypes for sepsis. JAMA. 2019;321:2003–17. https://doi.org/10.1001/jama.2019.5791.

13 Deployment of Clinical Prediction Models: A Practical Guide to Nomograms and Online Calculators

Adrian E. Jimenez, James Feghali, Andrew T. Schilling, and Tej D. Azad

13.1 Introduction

Within the neurosurgical literature, there has been a proliferation of efforts to develop and validate clinical prediction models [1]. In addition to forecasting postoperative outcomes using traditional statistical regression techniques, predictive modeling efforts have also incorporated machine learning algorithms to automate tumor volumetric measurements, detect surgical complications within clinical texts, and explore a number of other novel applications [2–5].

Accompanying the burgeoning interest in neurosurgical predictive modeling has been important commentary aimed at delineating the best techniques for quantifying the accuracy and calibration of such models, an increased awareness of the strengths and limitations of various modeling strategies, and a renewed focus on the importance of external validation [1, 6–11]. Importantly, many neurosurgical predictive models have been made available to clinicians and patients through nomograms, web applications, and RStudio (Boston, MA) Shiny applications [4, 12, 13].

Here, we discuss deployment methods of predictive models and provide instructions on navigating model deployment using the R programming language for two common deployment modalities: nomograms and Shiny application calculators. The present work aims to make model deployment simple and intuitive in order to allow researchers to make their models more transparent and accessible, with the ultimate goal of facilitating the creation of tools that can aid clinicians in clinical decision making, thereby improving patient outcomes.

Supplementary Information The online version contains supplementary material available at [https://doi.org/10.1007/978-3-030-85292-4_13].

A. E. Jimenez · J. Feghali · A. T. Schilling · T. D. Azad (✉)
Department of Neurosurgery, Johns Hopkins University School of Medicine, Baltimore, MD, USA
e-mail: tazad1@jhmi.edu

The following tutorial requires both R programming language software (found at https://cran.r-project.org/) and RStudio (found at https://rstudio.com/products/rstudio/download/). Readers should also download the "Glioblastoma_Dataset.xlsx" and the "script_classification" files from the MICN lab website (https://micnlab.com/files/). After downloading the files, both should be saved within the same folder on your computer. The "script_classification" file should then be run within RStudio to load the glioblastoma dataset into the global environment, to load required R packages, and to train the predictive models that will be deployed into nomogram and calculator format in this chapter. Instructions for creating a Shinyapps account and linking the account to the version of RStudio installed on your computer are available at https://docs.rstudio.com/shinyapps.io/, specifically within Chap. 2. The required R packages necessary for constructing nomograms and building the online calculator are included within the relevant R code snippets displayed throughout the chapter, and the full R scripts containing the code used in this tutorial have been included as supplementary content (Supplementary Content 13.1 and 13.2).

13.2 Nomograms

Nomograms are visual representations of predictive models that allow for individualized risk-estimation based on a patient's unique demographic and clinical characteristics. Nomograms are used to calculate a patient-specific numeric score which is translated to a specific probability that the patient will experience the outcome of interest based on the underlying statistical model represented in the nomogram. Nomograms are simple and intuitive tools that may easily be incorporated into clinical workflows and used at the bedside for patient counseling. An important limitation of nomograms is that the required calculations may become overly time-consuming and therefore unfeasible in a clinical setting

V. E. Staartjes et al. (eds.), *Machine Learning in Clinical Neuroscience*, Acta Neurochirurgica Supplement 134,
https://doi.org/10.1007/978-3-030-85292-4_13

1. Obtain distribution summaries for variables within "train" dataset

```
library(rms)

train_dist <- datadist(train)
options(datadist='train_dist')
```

2. Define logistic regression model

```
lrfit_rms <- lrm(TwelveMonths ~.,data=train)
```

3. Construct and format nomogram

```
nom.lrfit_rms <- nomogram(lrfit_rms,fun=function(x)1/(1+exp(-x)),
                          lp=FALSE,
                          funlabel="Predicted Probability of 12-Month Postoperative Survival",
                          fun.at = c(0.01,0.25,0.95,0.99))
```

4. Plot nomogram

```
plot(nom.lrfit_rms)
```

Fig. 13.1 R code for constructing nomogram

as the number of prognostic factors that are considered increases, such as for models trained on very large datasets.

As shown in the R nomogram script (Fig. 13.1), the first step to creating a nomogram is to specify the distribution summaries for our predictor variables of interest using the "datadist()" rms function. This function determines metrics such as effect and plotting ranges, adjustment values, and overall ranges for predictor variables [14]. As specified within the MICN classification script, the following variables were selected for model-building using recursive feature elimination (RFE): age, hospital caseload, chemotherapy, comorbidity, *IDH* (isocitrate dehydrogenase) mutation status, KPS (Karnofsky Performance Score), sex, MGMT (O^6-alkylguanine DNA alkyltransferase)-methylation status, tumor midline localization, prior surgeries, radiotherapy dose, tumor size, and *TERT* (telomerase reverse transcriptase) promoter mutations. Age, hospital caseload, and KPS, radiotherapy dose, and tumor size were analyzed as continuous variables (specified using "as.numeric()"), while the remaining predictors were analyzed as categorial variables (specified using "as.factor()"). These variables are stored within the "train" dataset, and therefore the code within section 1 of Fig. 13.1 serves to both specify distribution summaries for these variables and to store these summaries using the "options()" function to streamline any future model-building that uses these predictors. Next, section 2 fits a logistic regression model predicting the probability of 12-month postoperative survival (binary outcome) following glioblastoma surgery using standard R formula syntax, and a nomogram object is generated and stored as "nom.lrfit_rms" within section 3. Within the "nomogram()" function, the "fun" argument transforms the logistic regression output of log-odds of 12-Month Postoperative Survival into the probability of 12-Month Postoperative Survival, allowing for a more intuitive clinical interpretation of the model's output. The "lp=FALSE" argument may be used to suppress the log-odds output from being displayed on the nomogram; "lp=TRUE" may be used to display both the log-odds output in addition to the predicted probability. "funlabel" is used to label the predicted probability on the nomogram, while the "fun.at" argument specifies the tick marks that are displayed on the predicted probability nomogram output. The final "nom.lrfit_rms" nomogram object may then be visualized using the "plot()" function as shown in section 4, with the final nomogram output displayed in Fig. 13.2.

13.3 Online Calculators

Shinyapps calculators are created using the Shiny R package and allow implementation of predictive models as online calculators that output predicted probabilities depending on user input. Predictive models are developed and serve as the functional backend of the calculator. A graphic user interface is generated to allow users to enter patient information. User interfaces may be customized using both the R programming language as well as HTML (Hypertext Markup Language), allowing for significant flexibility in how calculator results are presented. Calculators may be uploaded online with a Shinyapps account, allowing anyone with the calculator's web address to access the predictive model. While users may deploy up to 5 applications with a maximum of 25 h total use time with a free account, premium Shiny accounts and monthly payments are required to exceed these data caps.

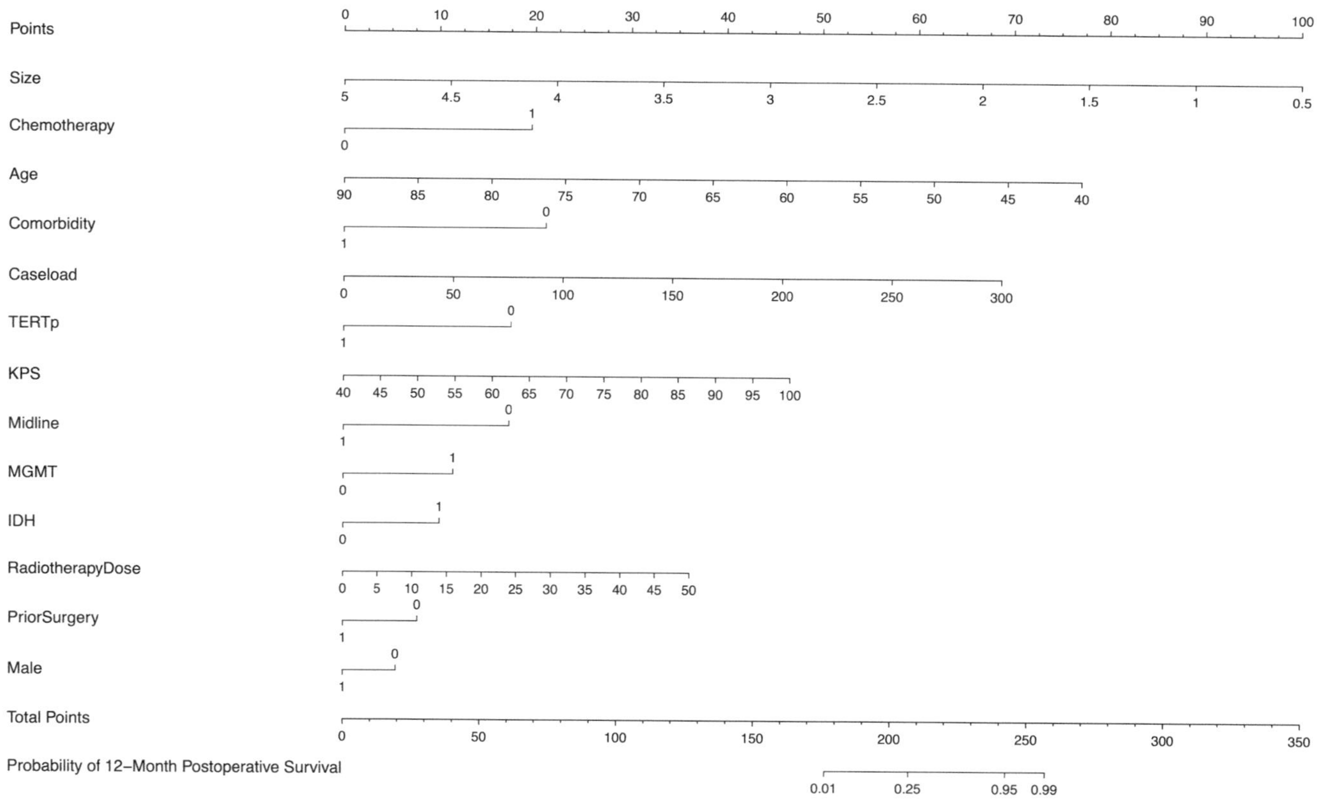

Fig. 13.2 Final nomogram

The R Shinyapps script (Figs. 13.3 and 13.4) contains code for specifying both the user interface and the server logic required to output predicted probabilities from a Caret model [15]. Importantly, any R script that will be used to create a Shiny application should have the file type "app.R," rather than the ".R" type utilized with normal R scripts. Prior to launching a Shiny application, a model generated using a separate R script must be saved as an individual file. This tutorial will use the stochastic gradient boosting machine (GBM) model that is trained after the MICN lab classification script is run within R studio. Once the "gbmfit" object appears in the global environment, the function "saveRDS()" may be used entered into the RStudio console to save the model under the file name "gbmfit":

```
> saveRDS(gbmfit, "gbmfit")
```

This file should then be saved into a dedicated folder alongside the app.R script file, as this folder will be uploaded to a Shiny server once the app.R calculator script is finalized.

Within the first part of the app.R calculator script (Fig. 13.3), running the code in section 0 will load the required packages or prompt installation if they have not yet been installed. Section 1 defines the code specifying the user interface (i.e. the components of the calculator that a user sees and is able to directly manipulate). Section 1.1, specifically the "titlePanel()" function, is used to label the calculator as a risk calculator for 12-month survival following glioblastoma surgery. The calculator sidebar, coded within section 1.2, is where users will enter the patient-specific predictive variables used to calculate an individualized predicted probability of 12-month survival. There are many ways to customize the sidebar (thereby affecting how users may enter information into the calculator), but the present worked example will only focus on three aspects of the sidebar sufficient for deploying the GBM model: "numericInput()," "selectInput()," and "helpText()." "numericInput()" is useful for specifying how users may enter continuous variables, such as age and hospital caseload. The "inputID" argument to the "numericInput()" function assigns an object name to the input that can be called later when reconstructing the predictive model, while the "label" argument displays a label on the user interface that can be used to specify what type of information should be inputted. Within "numericInput()," "min," and "max" designate the minimum and maximum value that a user may enter into the calculator, while "value" designates the numeric starting value utilized at calculator initialization. The "selectInput()" function, on the other hand, is useful for specifying how categorial variables are entered into the calculator. Within "selectInput()," "choices," and "list()" may be used to provide users with a

Fig. 13.3 R code for calculator user interface

0. Load required packages

```
library(shiny)
library(caret)
library(base64)
library(rsconnect)
library(readxl)
library(pROC)
library(gbm)
require(MASS)
library(ResourceSelection)
```

1. Define user interface for application

```
ui <- fluidPage(

  #1.1 Application title
  titlePanel("Risk Calculator for 12-Month Survival Following Glioblastoma Surgery"),

  #1.2 Sidebar with numeric and slider input
  sidebarLayout(
    sidebarPanel(
      numericInput(inputId = "age",
                   label = "Enter Patient Age",
                   min = 0,
                   max = 10000,
                   value = 50),
      numericInput(inputId = "caseload",
                   label = "Enter Caseload",
                   min = 0,
                   max = 10000,
                   value=100),
      selectInput(inputId = "chemotherapy",
                  label = "Select Patient Chemotherapy Status",
                  choices=
                    list(
                      "Received Chemotherapy"=1,
                      "Did Not Receive Chemotherapy"=0),
                  selected=1),
      selectInput(inputId = "comorbidity",
                  label = "Select Patient Comorbidity Status",
                  choices=
                    list(
                      "Yes"=1,
                      "No"=0),
                  selected=0),
      helpText("Comorbidity Status: Presence of any systemic comorbidity such as
               diabetes, coronary heart disease, chronic obstructive pulmonary disease, etc."),
      selectInput(inputId = "idh",
                  label = "Select IDH Status",
                  choices=
                    list(
                      "Mutated"=1,
                      "Wild-type"=0),
                  selected=1),
      numericInput(inputId = "kps",
                   label = "Enter KPS Score",
                   min = 1,
                   max = 100,
                   value = 100),
    selectInput(inputId = "sex",
                label = "Select Patient Sex",
                choices=
                  list(
                    "Male"=1,
                    "Female"=0),
                selected=1),
    selectInput(inputId = "mgmt",
                label = "Select MGMT Methylation Status",
                choices=
                  list(
                    "Methylated"=1,
                    "Not Methylated"=0),
                selected=1),
    selectInput(inputId = "midline",
                label = "Does Tumor Extend Into The Midline?",
                choices=
                  list(
                    "Yes"=1,
                    "No"=0),
                selected=0),
    selectInput(inputId = "prior_surgery",
                label = "Has The Patient Had Prior Surgery?",
                choices=
                  list(
                    "Yes"=1,
                    "No"=0),
                selected=0),
    numericInput(inputId = "radiotherapy_dose",
                 label = "Enter Radiotherapy Dose (in Gray)",
                 min = 1,
                 max = 10000,
                 value = 20),
    numericInput(inputId = "size",
                 label = "Enter Maximum Tumor Diameter (in cm)",
                 min = 1,
                 max = 10000,
                 value = 3),
    selectInput(inputId = "tert",
                label = "Select TERT Promoter Mutation Status",
                choices=
                  list(
                    "Mutated"=1,
                    "Not Mutated"=0),
                selected=1)),
    #1.3 Output probability of 12-Month Survival
    mainPanel(
      tabsetPanel(type="tabs",
                  tabPanel("Disclaimer",'The following calculator was developed using a simulated dataset and sho
uld only be
                           used for educational purposes to supplement the following publication:"Deployment of C
linical
                           Prediction Models: Nomograms and Online Calculators". Under no circumstances should th
is
                           calculator be used to provide medical advice.'),
                  tabPanel("Calculator Output",tableOutput("model_table")))
    )
  )
)
```

2. Define server logic required to output probability

```
server <- function(input, output) {

  #2.1 Load GBM model file
  gbmfit <- readRDS("gbmfit")

  #2.2 Define reactive output
  model_output <- reactive({

    #2.2.1 Specify type of output and formula for generating output
    data.frame(
      `Result` = c("Will Patient Be Alive 12 Months After Surgery?","Probability (%) of Survival Within 12 Months
of Surgery"),
      `Output` = c(as.character(predict.train(gbmfit,data.frame(Age=as.numeric(input$age),
                                              Caseload=as.numeric(input$caseload),
                                              Chemotherapy=as.factor(input$chemotherapy),
                                              Comorbidity=as.factor(input$comorbidity),
                                              IDH=as.factor(input$idh),
                                              KPS=as.numeric(input$kps),
                                              Male=as.factor(input$sex),
                                              MGMT=as.factor(input$mgmt),
                                              Midline=as.factor(input$midline),
                                              PriorSurgery=as.factor(input$prior_surgery),
                                              RadiotherapyDose=as.numeric(input$radiotherapy_dose),
                                              Size=as.numeric(input$size),TERTp=as.factor(input$tert)),
                              type="raw")),
                   (formatC(predict.train(gbmfit,data.frame(Age=as.numeric(input$age),
                                              Caseload=as.numeric(input$caseload),
                                              Chemotherapy=as.factor(input$chemotherapy),
                                              Comorbidity=as.factor(input$comorbidity),
                                              IDH=as.factor(input$idh),
                                              KPS=as.numeric(input$kps),
                                              Male=as.factor(input$sex),
                                              MGMT=as.factor(input$mgmt),
                                              Midline=as.factor(input$midline),
                                              PriorSurgery=as.factor(input$prior_surgery),
                                              RadiotherapyDose=as.numeric(input$radiotherapy_dose),
                                              Size=as.numeric(input$size),TERTp=as.factor(input$tert)),
                              type="prob")[,"yes"]*100))))

  })

  #2.3 Display output
  output$model_table <- renderTable(model_output())
}
```

3. Run the application

```
shinyApp(ui = ui, server = server)
```

Fig. 13.4 R code for calculator server logic

list of possible options, with each labeled option corresponding to a specific input that the model can use for prediction (i.e. selecting "Male" under "Select Patient Sex" will provide the model with a factor level of "1," while selecting "Female" would correspond to a factor level of "0"). Similar to the "value" option within "numericInput()," the "selected" option within "selectInput()" defines the factor level utilized for the default prediction at calculator initialization. Lastly, the "helpText()" option is useful for adding any additional instructions for user input, such as clarifying unintuitive clinical terms. In the present example, "helpText()" is used to more precisely define "comorbidity status" for the calculator user. In section 1.3, the "mainPanel()" function is used to customize the main panel of the calculator, defined as being comprised of two tabs via the "tabsetPanel()" function: a "Disclaimer" tab and a "Calculator Output" tab. The former is important for communicating important information to calculator users, such as the fact that this calculator is for educational use only and should not be utilized in clinical settings. The latter tab contains the actual numeric predictions generated by the statistical model. "tableOutput()" designates that the predictions generated by the GBM model (stored in the object "model_table") will be formatted within the "Calculator Output" tab as a table output element.

Section 2 of the app.R script contains the server function, which enters user input values into the GBM model and outputs the model's predicted probability of 12-month survival (Fig. 13.4). The code in section 2.1 loads our previously saved GBM Caret model using "readRDS()" and saves it as a Caret object labeled "gbmfit." Section 2.2 defines the model output as a *reactive* object, meaning that the predicted probability is automatically updated whenever input values are changed using the user interface. In this present example, this functionality allows calculator users to observe how changes in patient characteristics such as age, comorbidity status, and KPS affect 12-month survival probability in real time. Within the reactive function, and as detailed in section 2.2.1, an R data frame object is defined with a "Result" column to label what the model output signifies (i.e. the model's binary yes/no prediction of whether the patient will be alive 12 months after surgery as well as a predicted probability of 12-month postoperative survival) and an "Output" column of this data frame to contain the predicted yes/no output plus the numeric probability returned by the GBM model. Importantly, the "Output" column contains our "gbmfit" model object, a data frame (which contains our new data used for prediction) containing values extracted from our user interface inputs, and a "predict.train(object, newdata=, type=)" function to extract predictions using both the "gbmfit" model and the data frame containing the user interface inputs. Importantly, each entry within the data frame must be correctly specified as a continuous or categorical variable using "as.numeric()" and "as.factor()," respectively, and also must be saved using the same name as one of the predictor variables that the model was trained on. For example, "Age=as.numeric(input$age)" takes the user-specified patient age and saves it within the data frame as a value titled "Age," which may then be used by the GBM model to calculate the predicted probability of survival at 12 months of surgery. The "type=" argument within the "predict.train" function can be used to either specify that the output should be a yes/no prediction of 12-month postoperative survival (type="raw") or a predicted probability of 12-month postoperative survival (type="prob"). For the binary prediction, a default cutoff of 0.5 is used, with predicted probabilities ≥0.5 corresponding to an output of "yes" for 12-month postoperative survival and predicted probabilities of <0.5 corresponding to an output of "no." Furthermore, the argument for specifying a binary yes/no prediction is wrapped in an "as.character()" function to ensure that the output are the actual words "yes" or "no" rather than the integers "1" or "2," which is how R normally stores factor levels. When outputting predicted probabilities using the "type="prob" argument, the additional "[,"yes"]" argument is included so that only the predicted probability of the patient being alive is outputted. If "[,"no"]" was instead used, the predicted probability would instead correspond to patient mortality within 12 months of surgery. If neither is used, both probabilities are printed. Finally, the predicted probability output can be limited to two decimal places by using the function "formatC()."

The code within section 2.3 concludes the server logic segment of the app.R code by assigning the reactive object "model_output" to be displayed as a table on the main calculator panel, which was defined in section 1.3. Finally, the code under section 3 builds the shinyApp object by uniting the user interface and server logic components. Within R studio, Shiny applications can be directly uploaded to any shinyapps.io account. Detailed instructions on managing applications within a shinyapps.io account can be found at https://docs.rstudio.com/shinyapps.io/. A working example of the calculator developed in this chapter can be accessed using the following link: https://neurooncsurgery2.shinyapps.io/gbm_calculator/.

13.4 Other Methods of Deployment

Aside from nomograms and Shinyapps calculators, neurosurgical predictive models have also been deployed using native mobile applications (e.g. iOS and Android) and other web applications besides Shiny [12, 16]. Such alternatives may allow more nuanced customization of model deployment compared to the discrete set of functionalities available through Shinyapps. These modalities may also be a more cost-effective option compared to premium Shinyapps subscriptions depending on how much the applications will be accessed by users. Overall, the choice between deploying prediction models using nomograms, Shinyapps, or other custom web applications depends on technical website- and application-building knowledge, model accessibility, and personal preference.

13.5 Discussion

Nomograms and Shinyapps calculators are two common methods for deploying clinical prediction models and allowing users to better understand how patient-specific information affects the predicted probabilities of important clinical outcomes. Both tools may be created in R and have the potential to be easily incorporated into clinical workflows. Aside from these two methods, clinical prediction models may also be deployed into formats such as native mobile apps and other web applications. While the methodology detailed in the present chapter can be used to deploy predictive models trained on tabulated patient demographic and clinical data, the deployment of more complex models incorporating techniques such as radiographic image segmentation or conversion requires addition user interface and server capabilities beyond the scope of this tutorial.

Though the present chapter is focused on instructing researchers on how their predictive models may be deployed using nomograms or risk calculators, it is also important to consider the trade-offs involved with creating open-access prediction models. With the increasing use of prediction models and deployment methods allowing for open-access use of such models, clinicians and investigators have begun to express concerns over whether predictive models are being deployed preemptively in ways that may compromise patient safety [17–19]. Some researchers argue that deployment of predictive models into an open-access format may be potentially hazardous if rigorous external validation has not been performed or if all predictive performance metrics have not been reported [19]. Other investigators contend that deployment of predictive models, even with limited external validation, may serve as an educational aid by allowing readers to directly interact with the model via an accessible front-end (i.e. an online calculator) [18]. Regarding these concerns, if predictive models are employed prior to external validation, researchers should add disclaimers to their calculators specifying that the tool is not to be used in clinical settings and to direct users toward the peer-reviewed research articles which fully characterize the limitations of their training data or their statistical models. For example, a disclaimer might state that a model specifically trained on surgically-treated patients to predict postoperative outcomes should not be used to prognosticate outcomes for patients treated solely using medical therapy. The disclaimer might also clarify that the model deployed in an online calculator format is an artificial neural network (ANN), and that ANNs are prone to overfitting on their training datasets [20–22]. In this manner, researchers can allow readers to better understand their model while also avoiding preemptive clinical use that may compromise patient safety.

Overall, when deploying predictive models, it is important to thoroughly delineate the limitations of the model and to externally validate predictive performance metrics using novel datasets whenever possible. Establishing whether or not a predictive model was trained on data that is representative of a larger patient population can only be determined by assessing predictive performance on external datasets (e.g. patient data collected at a different medical center than where the model was created) and by quantifying metrics such as model calibration, discrimination, accuracy, sensitivity, and specificity [19, 23]. Such external validation is crucial for minimizing bias that results from single-center data such as surgeon caseloads, unique hospital workflows/protocols, and patient demographics specific to a particular geographic area [19]. These precautions are of paramount importance for establishing replicable scientific findings and for ensuring patient safety. By encouraging the responsible deployment of clinical predictions models though nomograms and online calculators may serve to further educate users about the utility of predictive analytics within neurosurgery and may also help streamline the implementation of predictive models into clinical and operative workflows.

13.6 Conclusion

The present chapter details step-by-step instructions on deploying clinical prediction models using nomograms and Shinyapps online calculators. When used appropriately, such tools may serve to improve understanding of predictive models and may also help streamline the implementation of such models into clinical and operative settings.

Acknowledgments None.

Disclosure of Funding None.

Financial Disclosure The authors received no financial support for the research, authorship, and/or publication of this article.

Conflict of Interest On behalf of all authors, the corresponding author states that there is no conflict of interest.

References

1. Mijderwijk HJ, Steyerberg EW, Steiger HJ, Fischer I, Kamp MA. Fundamentals of clinical prediction modeling for the neurosurgeon. Neurosurgery. 2019;85(3):302–11.
2. Chang K, Beers AL, Bai HX, et al. Automatic assessment of glioma burden: a deep learning algorithm for fully automated volumetric and bidimensional measurement. Neuro-Oncology. 2019;21(11):1412–22.
3. Karhade AV, Bongers MER, Groot OQ, et al. Natural language processing for automated detection of incidental durotomy. Spine J. 2020;20(5):695–700.
4. Khalafallah AM, Jimenez AE, Patel P, Huq S, Azmeh O, Mukherjee D. A novel online calculator predicting short-term postoperative outcomes in patients with metastatic brain tumors. J Neurooncol. 2020;149(3):429–36. https://doi.org/10.1007/s11060-020-03626-1.
5. Lubelski D, Ehresman J, Feghali J, Tanenbaum J, Bydon A, Theodore N, Witham T, Sciubba DM. Prediction calculator for nonroutine discharge and length of stay after spine surgery. Spine J. 2020;20(7):1154–8.
6. Azad TD, Ehresman J, Ahmed AK, Staartjes VE, Lubelski D, Stienen MN, Veeravagu A, Ratliff JK. Fostering reproducibility and generalizability in machine learning for clinical prediction modeling in spine surgery. Spine J. 2020; S1529-9430(20)31143-8. https://doi.org/10.1016/j.spinee.2020.10.006.
7. Kernbach J, Staartjes V. Machine learning-based clinical prediction modeling: a practical guide for clinicians. arXiv. 2020.

8. Muhlestein WE, Akagi DS, Davies JM, Chambless LB. Predicting inpatient length of stay after brain tumor surgery: developing machine learning ensembles to improve predictive performance. Neurosurgery. 2019;85(3):384–93.
9. Panesar SS, Kliot M, Parrish R, Fernandez-Miranda J, Cagle Y, Britz GW. Promises and perils of artificial intelligence in neurosurgery. Neurosurgery. 2020;87(1):33–44.
10. Steyerberg EW, Vergouwe Y. Towards better clinical prediction models: seven steps for development and an ABCD for validation. Eur Heart J. 2014;35(29):1925–31.
11. Van B, Mclernon DJ, Van Smeden M, Wynants L, Steyerberg EW, On behalf of Topic Group "Evaluating diagnostic tests and prediction models" of the STRATOS initiative. Calibration: the Achilles heel of predictive analytics. BMC Med. 2019;17:230.
12. Lubelski D, Alentado V, Nowacki AS, Shriver M, Abdullah KG, Steinmetz MP, Benzel EC, Mroz TE. Preoperative nomograms predict patient-specific cervical spine surgery clinical and quality of life outcomes. Neurosurgery. 2018;83(1):104–13.
13. Senders JT, Staples P, Mehrtash A, Cote DJ, Taphoorn MJB, Reardon DA, Gormley WB, Smith TR, Broekman ML, Arnaout O. An online calculator for the prediction of survival in glioblastoma patients using classical statistics and machine learning. Neurosurgery. 2020;86(2):E184–92.
14. Zhang Z, Kattan MW. Drawing nomograms with R: applications to categorical outcome and survival data. Ann Transl Med. 2017;5(10):211. https://doi.org/10.21037/atm.2017.04.01.
15. Kuhn M. Building predictive models in R using the caret package. J Stat Softw. 2008;28(5):1–26.
16. Veeravagu A, Li A, Swinney C, et al. Predicting complication risk in spine surgery: a prospective analysis of a novel risk assessment tool. J Neurosurg Spine. 2017;27(1):81–91.
17. D'Urso PI. Letter: an online calculator for the prediction of survival in glioblastoma patients using classical statistics and machine learning. Neurosurgery. 2020;87(2):E273–4.
18. Rajan PV, Karnuta JM, Haeberle HS, Spitzer AI, Schaffer JL, Ramkumar PN. Response to letter to the editor on "significance of external validation in clinical machine learning: let loose too early?". Spine J. 2020;20(7):1161–2.
19. Staartjes VE, Kernbach JM. Significance of external validation in clinical machine learning: let loose too early? Spine J. 2020;20(7):1159–60.
20. Karhade AV, Thio QCBS, Ogink PT, et al. Predicting 90-day and 1-year mortality in spinal metastatic disease: development and internal validation. Neurosurgery. 2019;85(4):E671–81.
21. Senders JT, Arnaout O, Karhade AV, Dasenbrock HH, Gormley WB, Broekman ML, Smith TR. Natural and artificial intelligence in neurosurgery: a systematic review. Neurosurgery. 2018;83(2):181–92.
22. Shah AA, Karhade AV, Bono CM, Harris MB, Nelson SB, Schwab JH. Development of a machine learning algorithm for prediction of failure of nonoperative management in spinal epidural abscess. Spine J. 2019;19(10):1657–65.
23. Staartjes VE, Schröder ML. Class imbalance in machine learning for neurosurgical outcome prediction: are our models valid? J Neurosurg Spine. 2018;29:611–2.

Updating Clinical Prediction Models: An Illustrative Case Study

14

Hendrik-Jan Mijderwijk, Stefan van Beek, and Daan Nieboer

14.1 Introduction

The performance of clinical prediction models may deteriorate over time as patient populations evolve over time. Application of a clinical prediction model to another setting, e.g. outpatient surgery vs. inpatient surgery, likely results in a different model performance. Such domain validation studies are especially suited for model updating due to the differences in case mix and event rate [1]. Model updating is an efficient method for the development of clinical prediction models and avoids the generation of multiple de novo prediction models [2, 3].

A range of updating methods are available for predictive analytic techniques. For prediction modeling with logistic regression analysis, updating methods include recalibration (adjusting intercept), model revision (adjusting the coefficient of the prognostic variables), and model extension (inclusion of new prognostic variables) [4, 5].

This paper provides a synopsis of these updating techniques. For illustration, we use data from two randomized controlled trials (RCTs) to illustrate this methodology with a case study.

H.-J. Mijderwijk (✉)
Department of Neurosurgery, Heinrich Heine University, Medical Faculty, Düsseldorf, Germany
e-mail: Hendrik-Jan.Mijderwijk@med.uni-duesseldorf.de

S. van Beek
Department of Anesthesiology, Erasmuc MC, University Medical Center, Rotterdam, The Netherlands

D. Nieboer
Department of Public Health, Erasmuc MC, University Medical Center Rotterdam, Rotterdam, The Netherlands

14.2 Methods

The case study uses data from two double-blinded placebo-controlled RCTs with a very similar methodological framework conducted at Erasmus MC [6, 7]. Therefore, some sections here are in line with previous publications reporting on these data. Both RCTs evaluated the effect (amongst others) of preoperative administered benzodiazepines on early (<24 h) postoperative anxiety. The studies were approved by the Medical Ethical Committee of Erasmus MC and by the Netherlands Central Committee on Research involving Human Subjects. Signed written informed consent was obtained from all patients.

Study Population and Design

Model Development Set

Between October 2010 and September 2011, 400 mixed patients undergoing minor surgery at the day-case surgery department of Erasmus MC were included. Inclusion criteria were as follows: all patients who were referred for ambulatory surgery and at least 18 years of age. Health care professionals, patients, and researchers were blinded to the treatment condition; however, nurses who were not involved directly in the care of these patients prepared the study medication according to the randomization table. Patients who consented to participate completed a set of online questionnaires when waiting for surgery (T0). Next, in the preoperative holding another nurse blinded to treatment condition injected the benzodiazepine by peripheral infusion before induction of anesthesia. The placebo group received an equal volume of 0.9% NaCl. After the surgical procedure, patients completed an online questionnaire before discharge (T1).

External Data Set for Domain Updating

Between July 2014 and September 2015, 192 mixed patients undergoing major surgery were recruited from the depart-

V. E. Staartjes et al. (eds.), *Machine Learning in Clinical Neuroscience*, Acta Neurochirurgica Supplement 134,
https://doi.org/10.1007/978-3-030-85292-4_14

ments of general surgery, gynecology, and urology at Erasmus MC. Inclusion criteria were the requirement for laparotomy, planned postoperative hospital stay for at least 3 days, and age at least 18 year. While waiting for surgery, patients completed the first set of questionnaires (T0). In the preoperative holding area, the independent recovery nurses prepared and administered the benzodiazepine prior to induction of anesthesia according to the group assignment document. The placebo group received an equal volume of 0.9% NaCl. Postoperative care was carried out according to the institution's *Enhanced Recovery after Surgery* protocol. After the surgical procedure, patients completed an online questionnaire on the first postoperative day (T1). The healthcare professionals who administered the questionnaires were blinded to the treatment allocation.

A modified flowchart from both studies is shown in Fig. 14.1.

Outcome Definition

Early postoperative anxiety was measured by the Dutch version of the State-Trait Anxiety Inventory (STAI) [8]. The STAI consists of 2 scales (State and Trait), each containing 20 items. We used the State scale (STAI-State) in this case study as outcome measure because this scale measures how the patient feels at the moment of completing the questionnaire [8]. We calculated the sum score by summing the scores on the items, theoretically ranging from 20 to 80. Greater scores indicate a greater level of anxiety. In line with on previous literature using normative data, we dichotomized patients into 2 groups: patients scoring <39 are considered having no anxiety and patients scoring ≥39 are considered having anxiety [9]. We note that ideally continuous variables should not be dichotomized to prevent loss of information.

Predictor Variables

To develop a simple prediction model, patient age and gender, in addition to preoperative anxiety (STAI-State) were considered. To illustrate updating with model extension, we added as predictor the STAI-Trait scale. In contrast to the State scale, the Trait scale measures how one generally feels [8]. Theoretically, the latter is not expected to be affected by a stressful situation like surgery.

Statistical Analysis

Binary logistic regression analysis was performed in the development set to develop the prediction model. Subsequently different model updating approaches were considered in the external data set and calibration and discrimination of the updated models were assessed in the external data set. Discrimination refers to the ability of a prediction model to discriminate between patients with and without the event of interest and is quantified using the *c*-statistic. The *c*-statistic ranges from 0.5 to 1, where 0.5 means that the prediction model is equivalent to a coin toss and 1 refers to perfect discrimination. Calibration refers to the agreement between predicted and observed outcome and was assessed visually using a calibration plot.

Updating Strategies

Reference Method

In this method, the original developed prediction model is applied, without any modifications, on the new external patient data set.

Recalibration Method

The recalibration method encompasses two options: intercept recalibration and logistic recalibration. In the former option, only the intercept of the model is adjusted to the new situation while keeping the relative effects of each predictor fixed. Technically this is done by fitting a logistic regression model using the linear predictor as an offset. In the latter option, all predictor effects are modified according to one common factor in addition to the intercept of the model. Technically this is performed by fitting a logistic regression

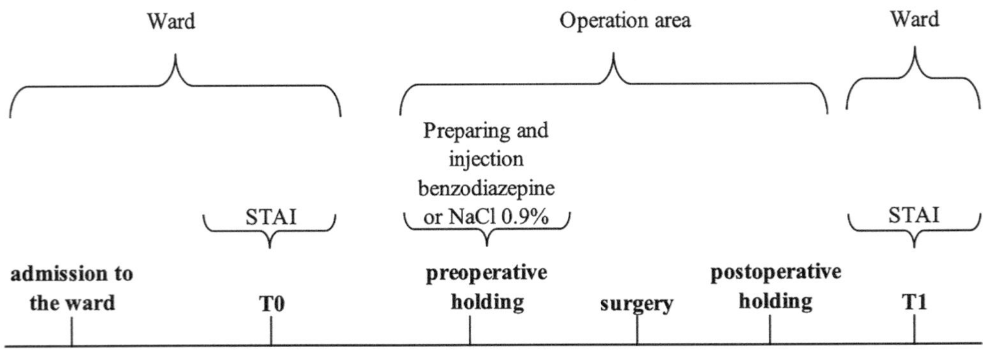

Fig. 14.1 Adapted time line of the RCTs. T0: baseline assessment on the day of surgery (self-reported questionnaire), T1: assessment <24 h postoperative (self-reported questionnaire), *STAI* Stait Trait Anxiety Inventory

model using the linear predictor of the developed model as the only predictor.

These relatively simple recalibration methods using logistic regression models are similar to "Platt scaling." More flexible approaches of recalibration can also be considered, such as allowing a non-linear transformation for the linear predictor in logistic recalibration. In machine learning, isotonic regression is also commonly applied besides Platt scaling, as the isotonic regression technique is nonparametric and can adjust for any—even non-linear—monotonic distortions. However, this is also the exact downfall of isotonic regression: The recalibration tends to be overfitted to the distortion in the training dataset, especially if sample sizes are relatively low and distortions are not entirely consistent among resamples of the training set—as is often the case in medical datasets. These more advanced recalibration techniques, however, require larger sample sizes to reduce the risk of overfitting and logistic recalibration may be preferred in clinical settings with limited data.

Model Revision

This approach updates all predictor estimates by re-estimating all regression coefficients. Consequently, the external data set should have a considerable amount of data corresponding to the data set used for model development.

Model Extension

Model extension is a powerful model updating method [4]. Here, the updated model provides new estimates on the initial parameters used for model development and for the new considered predictor(s).

Table 14.1 shows a summary of the updating strategies including rationale und caveats. Descriptive analysis and prediction modeling analysis were performed using R software version 3.5.2.

Table 14.1 Summary table of model updating methods

Updating method	Rationale	Caveats	How to perform?
Reference	No data needed.	No improvement in model performance.	–
Intercept updating	Simple updating method where only the model intercept is updated to reflect differences in baseline risk between settings. As only the model intercept is updated relative little data is required.	This approach does not improve discriminative ability or the calibration slope.	Fit a logistic regression model with the linear predictor of the original model as an offset.
Recalibration	Update the model intercept and additionally adjust all predictor effects by a common factor.	Does not improve discriminative ability.	Fit a logistic regression model using the linear predictor as the only covariate.
Model revision	Re-estimate all predictor effects and adjust baseline risk.	Requires extensive sample sizes comparable to model development and has relatively high risk of overfitting.	Fit a logistic regression model containing all individual predictors.
Recalibration + extension	Adjust the baseline risk and adjust individual predictor effects by a common factor and include extra predictor(s).	Simple adjustment method which may overestimate the added value of the new predictor based on performance of the original model.	Fit a logistic regression model using the linear predictor and new predictor(s) as covariates.
Revision + extension	Re-estimate the baseline risk all individual predictor effects and extend the model with new predictor(s).	Requires extensive sample size.	Fit a logistic regression model using all original predictors and new predictor(s) as covariates.

14.3 Results

The model development set contained 388 patients of which 60 (15%) showed early postoperative anxiety (Table 14.2). The external data set (i.e. domain updating set) contained 187 patients of which 49 (26%) showed postoperative anxiety. The patients in the development set were on average older and showed less preoperative state anxiety (Table 14.2).

The reference method as updating strategy reveals that the developed model underestimates the overall risk of postoperative anxiety in the external data set (Fig. 14.2). Regarding the recalibration method: updating the model intercept improved calibration while recalibration further improved the calibration. The more extensive model revision slightly improved the discriminative ability but showed a comparable calibration and discrimination to the recalibrated model (Table 14.3, Fig. 14.2). Extending the model with the new predictor (i.e. STAI-Trait) further improved the discriminative ability of the prediction model (Table 14.3). However, the simpler update method of recalibration and extension showed a similar performance to the more extensive model revision and extension (Table 14.3, Fig. 14.2).

14.4 Discussion

We discussed several approaches to update binary logistic regression models ranging from simple recalibration methods to model revision and extension. In this case study, we observed that updating methods improved the model performance in the external patient data set. Recalibration methods provided a model with similar model performance compared to model revision.

Model updating is a useful tool to develop more robust prediction models in the data at hand, however, from a clinical viewpoint it needs to be reasonable to apply the previously developed prediction model in the external update set. Relatively simple update methods such as intercept updating and recalibration assume there are only minor differences between the development and update populations, while more extensive model revision relaxes this assumption. However, a major drawback of model revision approaches is the large amount of data needed to reliably estimate the coefficients in the prediction model and limit the risk of overfitting. To further reduce the risk of overfitting shrinkage methods may be employed using a heuristic shrinkage factor [10].

Several methods of model updating have been shown; it can be challenging to select a priori the most appropriate update method for the data at hand [11]. A closed test procedure has been proposed to use a statistical test to compare several update methods simultaneously while controlling the significance level while performing multiple statistical tests. This approach aims to select the most appropriate update method in a data driven fashion, but requires sufficient data to ensure that the test has enough power to detect relevant differences [11]. In the present case study, the closed test method identified the intercept updating method as most appropriate update strategy.

It is recommended to update prediction models periodically because model performance deteriorates over time [12]. Calibration drift is a well-known phenomenon that jeopardizes the safe use of prediction models as it may induce flawed predictions. Reasons for this include, but are not limited to, variations in patient case mix, new clinical workflows and/or guidelines, or technical innovations. There is a need to detect calibration drift in an early stage to inform

Table 14.2 Patient descriptives of the used data sets

Variables	Model development set (n = 388)	External set for domain updating (n = 187)
Age (mean, SD)	37 (29–49)	59 (47–67)
Gender (n, %)	174 (45%)	70 (37%)
State anxiety (mean, SD)		
Preoperative	37 (32–44)	39 (33–45)
Early postoperative	30 (26–35)	32 (27–39)
Trait anxiety (mean, SD)	–	31 (26–36)
Early postoperative anxiety above 39 (n, %)	60 (15%)	49 (26%)

We analyzed the patients having no missing data. *SD* standard deviation

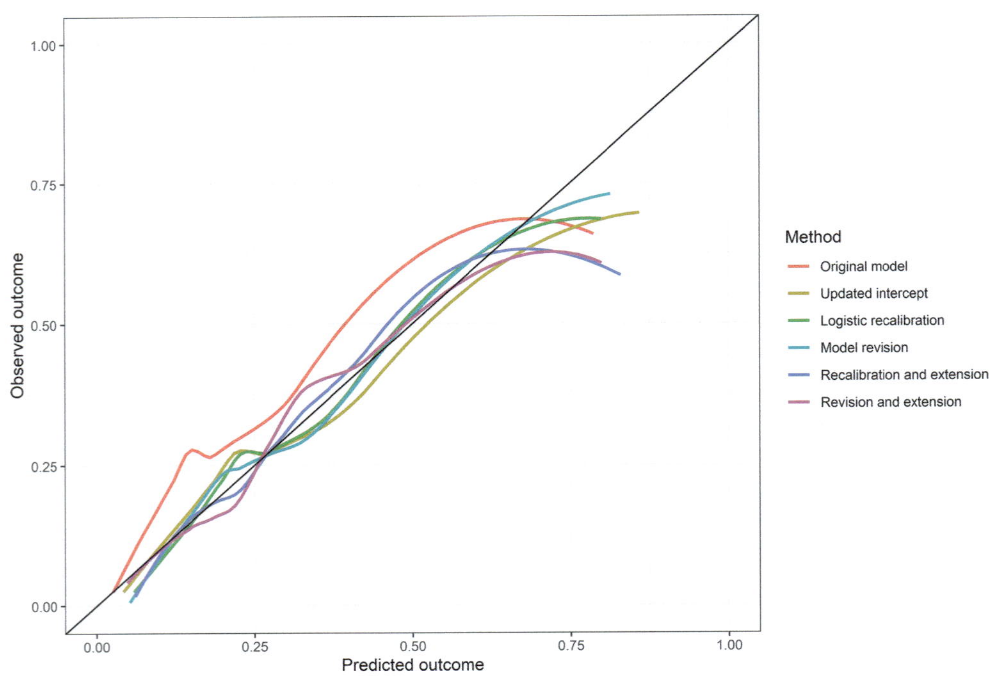

Fig. 14.2 Calibration plot for updated models in the external data set

Table 14.3 Parameter estimates of each of the updated models

Parameter	Update method					
	Original model	Update model intercept	Logistic recalibration	Model revision	Recalibration and extension	Model revision and extension
Intercept	−6.13	−5.63	−4.88	−3.95	−5.70	−4.03
Age (per decade)	0.06	0.06	0.05	−0.10	0.00	−0.01
Sex	0.36	0.36	0.30	0.14	0.24	0.06
Preopertive state anxiety	0.10	0.10	0.08	0.08	0.07	0.07
Preoperative trait anxiety	–	–	–	–	0.05	0.05
Apparent *c*-statistic	0.71	0.71	0.71	0.71	0.73	0.73

model updating. Recently, a detection system to continuously monitor calibration drift has been proposed [13].

The updating methods described here can be adapted to survival models and multinominal risk models, [14] and the recalibration methods may also be applied to more flexible machine learning techniques.

To conclude, model updating is an efficient technique and promising alternative to the de novo development of clinical prediction models [5].

Conflict of Interest On behalf of all authors, the corresponding author states that there is no conflict of interest.

References

1. Toll DB, Janssen KJM, Vergouwe Y, Moons KGM. Validation, updating and impact of clinical prediction rules: a review. J Clin Epidemiol. 2008;61:1085–94.
2. Janssen KJM, Moons KGM, Kalkman CJ, Grobbee DE, Vergouwe Y. Updating methods improved the performance of a clinical prediction model in new patients. J Clin Epidemiol. 2008;61:76–86.
3. Mijderwijk H-J, Steyerberg EW, Steiger H-J, Fischer I, Kamp MA. Fundamentals of clinical prediction modeling for the neurosurgeon. Neurosurgery. 2019;85:302–11.
4. Nieboer D, Vergouwe Y, Ankerst DP, Roobol MJ, Steyerberg EW. Improving prediction models with new markers: a comparison of updating strategies. BMC Med Res Methodol. 2016;16:128.
5. Steyerberg EW. Clinical prediction models: a practical approach to development, validation, and updating. Berlin: Springer International Publishing; 2019.
6. Mijderwijk H, van Beek S, Klimek M, Duivenvoorden HJ, Grüne F, Stolker RJ. Lorazepam does not improve the quality of recovery in day-case surgery patients. Eur J Anaesthesiol. 2013;30:743–51.
7. van Beek S, Kroon J, Rijs K, Mijderwijk H-J, Klimek M, Stolker RJ. The effect of midazolam as premedication on the quality of postoperative recovery after laparotomy: a randomized clinical trial. Can J Anesth. 2019;39:503–10.
8. van der Ploeg HM, Defares PB, Spielberger CD. Handleiding bij de Zelf Beoordelings Vragenlijst, een nederlandstalige bewerking van de Spielberger Stait-Trait Anxiety Inventory, STAI-DY. Lisse: Swets & Zeitlinger; 1980.
9. Mijderwijk H, Stolker RJ, Duivenvoorden HJ, Klimek M, Steyerberg EW. Clinical prediction model to identify vulnerable patients in ambulatory surgery: towards optimal medical decision-making. Can J Anaesth. 2016;63:1022–32.
10. Steyerberg EW, Borsboom GJJM, van Houwelingen HC, Eijkemans MJC, Habbema JDF. Validation and updating of predictive logistic regression models: a study on sample size and shrinkage. Stat Med. 2004;23:2567–86.
11. Vergouwe Y, Nieboer D, Oostenbrink R, Debray TPA, Murray GD, Kattan MW, Koffijberg H, Moons KGM, Steyerberg EW. A closed testing procedure to select an appropriate method for updating prediction models. Stat Med. 2016;36:4529–39.
12. te Velde ER, Nieboer D, Lintsen AM, Braat DDM, Eijkemans MJC, Habbema JDF, Vergouwe Y. Comparison of two models predicting IVF success; the effect of time trends on model performance. Hum Reprod. 2014;29:57–64.
13. Davis SE, Greevy RA Jr, Lasko TA, Walsh CG, Matheny ME. Detection of calibration drift in clinical prediction models to inform model updating. J Biomed Inform. 2020;112:103611–0.
14. van Calster B, Van Hoorde K, Vergouwe Y, Bobdiwala S, Condous G, Kirk E, Bourne T, Steyerberg EW. Validation and updating of risk models based on multinomial logistic regression. Diagn Progn Res. 2017;1:2.

15 Is My Clinical Prediction Model Clinically Useful? A Primer on Decision Curve Analysis

Hendrik-Jan Mijderwijk and Daan Nieboer

15.1 Introduction

The performance of clinical prediction models is commonly evaluated using performance measures that describe overall model performance or specific dimensions of model performance (e.g. calibration and discrimination). These performance measures, however, inadequately describe the potential impact of a prediction model on actual clinical practice. This impact, also called clinical usefulness, is a relevant metric by which to assess prediction models [1]. An increasingly popular method to assess the impact of a prediction model on medical decision making is a decision curve analysis [2]. Herein we aim to provide a short introduction of decision curve analysis for evaluating the clinical usefulness of clinical prediction models. We illustrate the interpretation of decision curves using a simulated dataset of glioblastoma patients.

15.2 Methodology

Imagine, a glioblastoma patient visits your outpatient clinic after post-operative radiochemotherapy. The routine follow-up MRI shows contrast enhancement in the radiated field. It is not possible to differentiate between glioblastoma progression or pseudoprogression. The patient will certainly ask the neurosurgeon what is best to do next. For didactic reasons, we consider two options: (1) intervening by doing a biopsy to obtain a histological diagnosis or (2) conservative treatment with clinical follow-up without biopsy. The threshold for the decision depends on the benefits and harms of either option. In this example the benefit consists of detecting a glioblastoma progression, while harms of performing a biopsy might be infection or bleeding.

Decision Curves

Figure 15.1 exemplifies the graphical summary of a decision curve analysis.

The *x*-axis shows the threshold probability. This represents the preference of the patient or the preference of the neurosurgeon, such as the minimum probability of glioblastoma progression at which the patient would undergo a biopsy, or the number of patients the neurosurgeon would be willing to biopsy to identify one patient with glioblastoma progression [3]. The link between the threshold probability and the harm-to-benefit ratio is the key component underpinning decision curve analysis. The odds of a particular threshold equals the harm-to-benefit ratio. Thus, if the neurosurgeon opts for a biopsy at a threshold probability of 20%, then the harm-to-benefit ratio is 1:4 (odds [20%] = 1/4) [4]. That means that the benefit of diagnosing glioblastoma progression is considered four times higher than the harm of a superfluous biopsy. In other words, the neurosurgeon accepts performing biopsies in five patients to correctly diagnose one patient with glioblastoma progression. Analogously, if the threshold probability is 10%, the harm-to-benefit ratio equals 1:9 and 10 biopsies are accepted to find one glioblastoma progression. Theoretically, the range of threshold probabilities can range from 0% to 100% but is often restricted to a range of clinically relevant thresholds which is dependent on the clinical context (Fig. 15.1, gray dotted lines). This would also reflect the variation in clinical practice where threshold probabilities may vary between neurosurgeons with an

Supplementary Information The online version contains supplementary material available at [https://doi.org/10.1007/978-3-030-85292-4_15].

H.-J. Mijderwijk (✉)
Department of Neurosurgery, Heinrich Heine University, Medical Faculty, Düsseldorf, Germany
e-mail: Hendrik-Jan.Mijderwijk@med.uni-duesseldorf.de

D. Nieboer
Department of Public Health, Erasmus MC, University Medical Center, Rotterdam, The Netherlands

V. E. Staartjes et al. (eds.), *Machine Learning in Clinical Neuroscience*, Acta Neurochirurgica Supplement 134,
https://doi.org/10.1007/978-3-030-85292-4_15

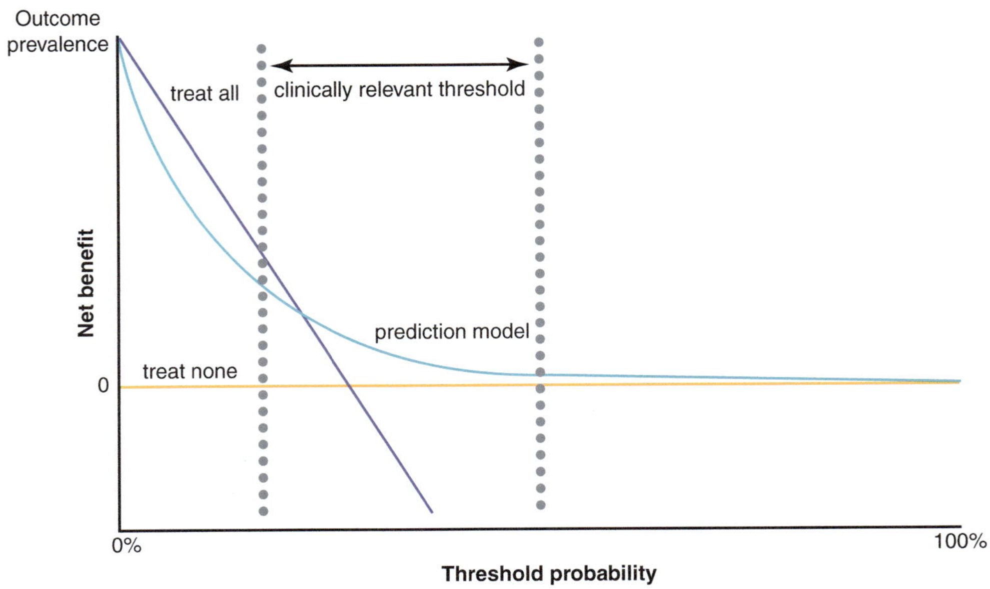

Fig. 15.1 Graphical summary of a hypothetical decision curve analysis

aggressive treatment strategy versus more conservative but can also vary between patients based on the comorbidities or anxiety level of a patient. It is imperative that the threshold probability is known before deploying a prediction model for medical decision making [5].

The *y*-axis shows the net benefit. This represents the difference in number of true positive classifications and false-positive classifications, weighted by the harm-to-benefit ratio [3, 6]. If a prediction model at a particular threshold probability has a net benefit of 0.05 higher compared to another strategy, then this means that a treatment strategy in which the prediction model is used for clinical decision making is equivalent to a strategy in which 5 extra true positive classifications per 100 patients are detected without obtaining extra false positives [3]. The net benefit can be negative and the maximum is equal to the prevalence of the outcome in the population (or event rate). The net benefit of using a prediction model is always compared to the default strategies of treating all patients and treating no patients, as these are often clinically reasonable strategies. In this example these strategies would be to biopsy all patients and to not perform a biopsy on the patients and monitor them.

The treat all line (Fig. 15.1, purple line) decreases with an increasing threshold probability. In a treat all strategy, the number of true positives and false positives is fixed, and only the weighting factor relating both changes. With an increasing probability threshold these harms are considered more important, i.e. one is willing to biopsy less patients to detect one progression.

The treat none line (Fig. 15.1, yellow line) has a net benefit of zero as nobody undergoes a biopsy and hence nobody experiences benefits or harms associated with the biopsy. The treat all line intersect the treat none line at the event rate.

The green line in Fig. 15.1 represents the net benefit of a hypothetical multivariable prediction model predicting glioblastoma progression. The prediction model is considered clinically useful if the net benefit of the prediction model is higher compared to the default strategies across the range of clinically relevant thresholds. Thus, the hypothetical prediction model depicted in Fig. 15.1 is of benefit for the majority of the clinical relevant thresholds. However, if there is a low threshold probability the net benefit of the prediction model is worse than the "treat all" strategy. In other words, the patient should be biopsied irrespective of the results provided by the prediction model.

Interventions Avoided

In many clinical examples the default strategies would be to perform an intervention in all patients. In the above mentioned hypothetical clinical example the default strategy of the neurosurgeons would be to perform a biopsy. In these scenarios the aim of a prediction model or would be to reduce the number of unnecessary biopsies. In this case the net benefit can also be transformed to the net number of interventions avoided. This is recommended if the default strategy would be to treat all patients. This would not change conclusions as to which the prediction model has the highest net benefit [5].

15.3 Example

To show an illustrative example of a decision curve analysis, we use the open-access files provided by the Machine Intelligence in Clinical Neuroscience (MICN) Lab (https://

mcinlab.com/files) from the Department of Neurosurgery and Clinical Neuroscience Center, University Hospital Zurich. This simulated dataset comprises 10,000 glioblastoma patients. Two multivariable clinical prediction models predicting 12-month mortality were developed. One model serves as a baseline model containing the predictors age, gender, Karnofsky performance score (KPS), and postoperative radiochemotherapy. We also developed an extended model containing the same predictors of the baseline model and additionally O^6-methylguanine-DNA methyltransferase promoter methylation (*MGMT*) status. The baseline model had a *c*-statistic equal to 0.73 while the extended model had a *c*-statistic of 0.74.

The decision curve analysis showed that both models had a higher net benefit compared to the default strategies in the range of thresholds of 20–80% (Fig. 15.2). This means that if the range of clinically relevant risk thresholds falls between 20% and 80%, then these results indicate that using the prediction models has a higher net benefit compared to the default strategies. The extended prediction model had higher net benefit compared to the base model. The R Code is provided in the supplementary material (Supplementary Material 15.1).

15.4 Final Comment

This paper provides a short introduction to decision curve analysis. This technique helps to identify models that may support medical decision making. Furthermore, it ranks competing clinical prediction models. To support a clinical prediction model for medical decision making, the model should outperform the default "treat all" and "treat none" strategies across the (whole) range of clinically relevant thresholds. If more than one model is analyzed, it is recommended to use the model that has the highest net benefit. However, if the superior model requires data that is associated with an increasing patient-risk or additional/expensive workload, clinicians may intuitively prefer the inferior model. It is possible to include harm associated with a clinical prediction model into a decision curve [2].

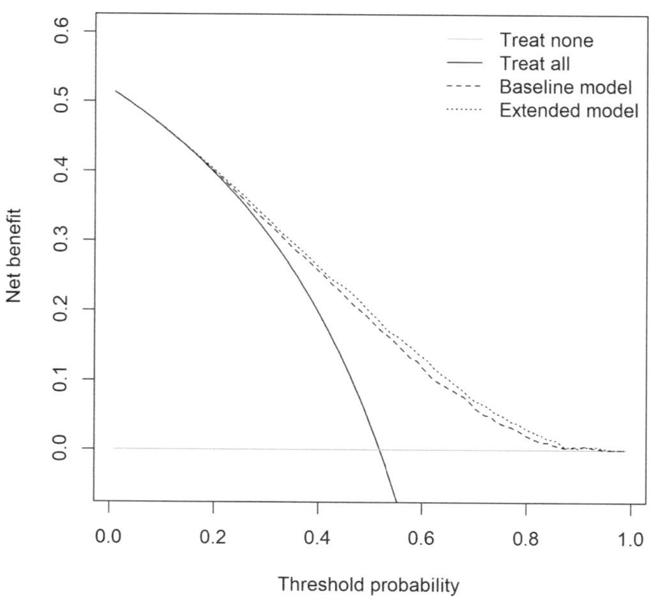

Fig. 15.2 Decision curves for the default strategies (i.e. treat none and treat all) and for the baseline model and extended model

Another decision analytic performance measure is the relative utility curve [7]. Relative utility curves are related to decision curve analysis [8]. In relative utility curves the net benefit of using a prediction model is related to the relevant baseline strategy (treat all/treat none) and to perfect classification.

Here we considered prediction models for a binary outcome measure for didactic reasons, but the decision curve analysis can be extended to survival data too [9]. Finally, we want to emphasize that decision curve analysis should not be used to identify an optimal risk threshold. This reverses threshold probability and risk provided by a prediction model. Before creating a decision curve, researchers should define a range of clinically relevant thresholds based on the relative harms and benefits of avoiding an intervention on a patient with the outcome versus unnecessarily performing an intervention on a patient who is disease free. Subsequently the net benefit of using a prediction model for decision making should be compared to the default strategies across the range of clinically relevant thresholds.

If used sensibly, a decision curve analysis is an elegant technique to assess the clinical usefulness of clinical prediction models. For the interested reader, more detailed information on decision curve analysis can be found elsewhere [2, 6, 9, 10].

Conflict of Interest On behalf of all authors, the corresponding author states that there is no conflict of interest.

References

1. Steyerberg EW, Vickers AJ, Cook NR, Gerds T, Gonen M, Obuchowski N, Pencina MJ, Kattan MW. Assessing the performance of prediction models: a framework for traditional and novel measures. Epidemiology. 2010;21:128–38.
2. Vickers AJ, Elkin EB. Decision curve analysis: a novel method for evaluating prediction models. Med Decis Mak. 2006;26:565–74.
3. Moons KGM, Altman DG, Reitsma JB, Ioannidis JPA, Macaskill P, Steyerberg EW, Vickers AJ, Ransohoff DF, Collins GS. Transparent reporting of a multivariable prediction model for individual prognosis or diagnosis (TRIPOD): explanation and elaboration. Ann Intern Med. 2015;162:W1–73.
4. van Calster B, Wynants L, Verbeek JFM, Verbakel JY, Christodoulou E, Vickers AJ, Roolbol MJ, Steyerberg EW. Reporting and inter-

preting decision curve analysis: a guide for investigators. Eur Urol. 2018;74:796–804.
5. Vickers AJ, van Calster B, Steyerberg EW. A simple, step-by-step guide to interpreting decision curve analysis. Diagn Progn Res. 2019;3:18.
6. Steyerberg EW. Clinical prediction models: a practical approach to development, validation, and updating. Berlin: Springer International Publishing; 2019.
7. Baker SG, Cook NR, Vickers A, Kramer BS. Using relative utility curves to evaluate risk prediction. J R Stat Soc Ser A Stat Soc. 2009;172:729–48.
8. van Calster B, Vickers AJ, Pencina MJ, Baker SG, Timmerman D, Steyerberg EW. Evaluation of markers and risk prediction models: overview of relationships between NRI and decision-analytic measures. Med Decis Mak. 2013;33:490–501.
9. Vickers AJ, Cronin AM, Elkin EB, Gonen M. Extensions to decision curve analysis, a novel method for evaluating diagnostic tests, prediction models and molecular markers. BMC Med Inform Decis Mak. 2008;8:1039–17.
10. Vickers AJ, van Calster B, Steyerberg EW. Net benefit approaches to the evaluation of prediction models, molecular markers, and diagnostic tests. BMJ. 2016;352:i6.

Part II

Neuroimaging

Introduction to Machine Learning in Neuroimaging

16

Julius M. Kernbach, Jonas Ort, Karlijn Hakvoort, Hans Clusmann, Georg Neuloh, and Daniel Delev

16.1 Introduction

In the last decade, the amount of biomedical data within the neuroscientific community has grown exponentially. The large amount of readily available information coining the age of "big data" comes in different types such as genomic data, gene expression, or multi-modal imaging data. Advances in scanning and imaging acquisition made it possible to accumulate rich, readily available, and high-resolution imaging data, including modalities such as magnetic resonance tomography (MRI), positron emission tomography, or electroencephalography. Consequently, the field of neuroimaging is projected to follow genetics as the next most data-rich biomedical specialty [1, 2]. The sheer increase in data complexity has led to efficient and sophisticated computational tools to analyze and interpret the large amount of granular data. Artificial intelligence (AI) and machine learning (ML) algorithms represent such computational tools. Although their presence in the literature has significantly increased during recent years, AI and ML are not novel. AI was first described in the 1950s and referred to computers that perform tasks typically requiring human intelligence [3, 4]. The overarching goal of AI is the emulation of natural intelligence, to not only learn but apply the gained knowledge and make elaborate decisions to solve complex problems mimicking human reasoning. ML, which represents a sub-methodology of AI, was described in the early 1950s and found its first medical applications in the 1960s. An ML algorithm inductively learns to automatically extract patterns from data to generate insight without being explicitly programmed [5]. This makes ML an attractive option to approximate and predict highly complex phenomena without pre-specifying an a priori theoretical model.

The gold-standard of functional magnetic resonance imaging (fMRI) analysis has been the standard mass-univariate analysis by modeling the brain response within an experimental paradigm as linear combinations of the applied experimental conditions [6, 7]. A statistical test has to be performed at each voxel to find regions associated with the condition, and different contrasts are applied over the succeeding conditions to reveal the underlying neural pattern to the corresponding cognitive function of interest. Recently, ML approaches, including multivariate pattern analysis, have been used to decode or predict *individual* brain states using neuroimaging data. Instead of using in-sample testing, the goodness of fit of the ML model is assessed by its predictive performance via cross-validation. ML-based studies have become successful in decoding brain states and enabled *personalized* clinical decisions by predicting disease phenotypes, course, or clinical outcome [8–10].

Julius M. Kernbach and Jonas Ort contributed equally.

J. M. Kernbach (✉) · J. Ort · K. Hakvoort · D. Delev
Neurosurgical Artificial Intelligence Laboratory Aachen (NAILA), RWTH Aachen University Hospital, Aachen, Germany

Department of Neurosurgery, Faculty of Medicine, RWTH Aachen University, Aachen, Germany
e-mail: jkernbach@ukaachen.de

H. Clusmann · G. Neuloh
Department of Neurosurgery, Faculty of Medicine, RWTH Aachen University, Aachen, Germany

16.2 Main Part

Neuroimaging techniques, including functional and resting-state magnetic resonance imaging (fMRI, rsMRI), are frequently applied to study brain function in vivo, aiming to find a mechanistic understanding of the nervous system. Neuroimaging data are complex, high dimensional, and come in a wide range of spatial and temporal resolu-

V. E. Staartjes et al. (eds.), *Machine Learning in Clinical Neuroscience*, Acta Neurochirurgica Supplement 134,
https://doi.org/10.1007/978-3-030-85292-4_16

tions; for these reasons, advanced analysis techniques are necessary to describe data derived from each imaging method. ML provides such opportunities. However, specific steps need to be executed before the data can be utilized by the ML algorithms. The necessary workflow includes image preprocessing, dimensionality reduction, and feature selection.

Image Preprocessing

Before feeding neuroimaging data into ML models, depending on the modality, standard preprocessing must be applied. For the modality of fMRI, a standard preprocessing pipeline includes motion correction, slice timing correction, co-registration, and normalization to a shared space, primarily the Montreal Neurologic Institute (MNI) template. Usually, signal cleaning is performed to remove non-informative trends and artifacts using detrending, normalization, or frequency filtering. Detrending removes a linear trend over the fMRI time-series due to the reasoning that the voxel intensity itself is non-informative, and the interest instead lies in the variation and correlation between voxels. Normalization remedies different scales and value ranges by setting the variance to one. Physiological or scanner-induced noise can be mitigated by low- or high-frequency filtering. There are various sources for code implementation, including the Python interface nipype [11], Matlab-based SPM [6], or FSL [12].

Dimensionality Reduction

Neuroimaging produces high-dimensional data with massively more features p than available samples n. In the case of fMRI, the number of features, that is, activation in each voxel, can quickly add up to $p = \sim 10^5$ features. However, in small sample settings, where $n \ll p$, statistical models and ML models alike tend to overfit. Based on the "curse of dimensionality," generalization to new data becomes increasingly difficult in $n < <p$ *situations*. To prevent the curse, the data's dimensionality has to be reduced to meaningful and concise information, finding a lower-dimensional representation of the given feature space [13, 14]. Therefore, neuroimaging data often requires the application of a dimensionality reduction step to decrease the complexity of the data before performing further analyses. Dimensionality reduction methods transform high-dimensional data into simpler representations while preserving most of the relevant information. Commonly applied methods include principal component analysis (PCA) or independent component analysis (ICA). For a detailed overview, see Chap. 8.

Feature Selection

Another possibility to reduce the complexity of neuroimaging data is the application of feature selection [15]. Different approaches can be used: (1) using domain knowledge, redundant features or features known to be of less importance for the investigated disorder can be removed. (2) Using feature engineering to construct new informative variables, e.g., by summarizing fMRI activation in a region of interest (ROIs) specific to the investigated neurological diseases. Furthermore, (3) numerous methods, including univariate and multivariate filter analyses, wrapper, and embedded methods, exist to select the most relevant features. In univariate analyses, every feature is examined on a single level and ranks individually. Although this approach is fast and robust, it misses dependencies between features, which can be assessed by multivariate analysis. While univariate and multivariate techniques identify the best set of features independently from model selection, wrapper methods and embedded methods combine model selection with a feature subset search. Embedded techniques for feature selection search for the optimal subset of features inside the classifier. This means that the search is performed in the combined space of feature subsets and hypotheses. Examples of wrapper selection approaches include greedy forward selection or backward elimination strategies (for more detail, see Chap. 7—Feature Selection).

fMRI Analyses: Supervised vs. Unsupervised

Supervised machine learning algorithms are trained using known targets, while unsupervised learning refers to algorithms, which learn on data with unknown targets. Once a target variable y is to be predicted, the problem becomes supervised. Depending on the type of the target variable, supervised learning can be divided into two subcategories. If the target variable is categorical, hence representing different classes (e.g., healthy versus disease), the problem is referred to as *classification*. If the target variable takes continuous values, the problem is referred to as *regression*. A popular example of supervised analysis in fMRI brain imaging is the *decoding/encoding* framework.

Decoding/Encoding Framework

Decoding refers to learning a model that predicts a target variable from the available brain imaging data (Fig. 16.1) and has become a powerful method in the neuroscientists' tool kit. The most famous example for decoding is the simplified experiment presented in Haxby et al. [17], which has been intensively studied and ultimately became the reference

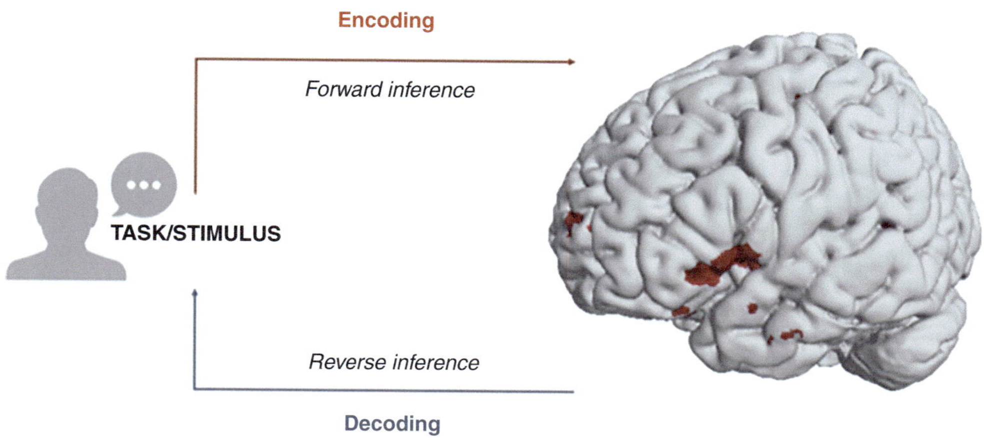

Fig. 16.1 Illustration of decoding and encoding in brain imaging using fMRI. Decoding refers to learning a model that predicts a target variable or stimulus from the available brain imaging data. Encoding describes the prediction of imaging data given an external variable or experimental stimulus [16]. Decoding applies reverse inference, e.g., drawing conclusions of behavioral processes from the neural process. In contrast, encoding applies forward inference, which is a statement on whether or not the neural signal is well explained by the stimulus

example for decoding [18, 19]. In the original work, participants are presented with eight different categories of visual stimuli. Given the recorded fMRI volumes, the goal is to decode and predict the category of the presented stimulus. The given inference of a decoding analysis tells us that if a certain pattern of brain activity is observed, we can deduce the underlying task or stimulus. Inversely to the encoding setting, such conclusions are often referred to as *reverse inference*. Hence, decoding answers questions of, e.g., "what is the underlying function of a neuronal subsystem?" while not probing the underlying task or cognitive process [20]. The applied predictive models can differ and are best chosen balancing modeling flexibility and regularization [21], including Bayesian models, Lasso- or ridge regression, support vector machines.

In contrast to decoding, *encoding* (Fig. 16.1) describes the prediction of imaging data given an external variable, such as experimental stimuli descriptors [16]. The applied type of inference in encoding is "forward inference." Based on the provided stimulus, we can conclude that the experimental task recruits certain brain regions. Specifically, the extent of variability captured by each voxel can be evaluated using techniques such as cross-validation and common metrics such as R^2 scores.

Clustering

The decoding/encoding framework is an example of supervised learning. In carefully designed fMRI experiments, a known target (e.g., a known behavioral or clinical stimulus) is used to investigate the underlying relation between brain and behavior. In contrast to task-related MRI, resting-state fMRI produces unlabeled data in the sense that the brain activity is recorded without specific task stimuli present. In ML, the analysis of unlabeled data is commonly known as unsupervised learning.

Cluster analysis is an unsupervised learning technique that can identify patterns in data and aggregate observations into groups without any previous knowledge of their target variable. The notion of similarity degree is essential to cluster analysis. The clustering results strongly depend on the adopted similarity measure. Even though a wide variety of clustering algorithms exists and many efforts have been allocated to solve the problems related to clustering, the main difficulty related to these methodologies concerns choosing the "optimal" number of clusters. However, this is an innately ill-posed question, as the optimal number of clusters depends on the complexity of the data and method used. Consequently, different indices have been introduced to approximate the optimal number of clusters, including the Davies–Bouldin, the Dunn, or the silhouette index [14]. In functional MRI, the similarity of neighboring voxels in regard to their connectivity can be used to form homogenous regions using cluster analysis [22]. Defining spatially distributed but functionally homogenous networks can be formulated as a problem of blind source separation. Typically, ICA is a common approach to recover these network structures [23].

16.3 Conclusion

Through technical advances, increased availability, and sophisticated analytical tools, the quality and quantity of neuroimaging data have risen exponentially in the last decades. This trend will likely continue and accelerate considering modern computational capacities. In this development, ML methods will rather act as catalysts than pure analytical armory. ML models will likely evolve into the dominating paradigm in neuroimaging analysis by observing, classifying, and clustering patterns beyond the scope of our human comprehension. However, any statistical or ML model is only an approximation to reality. To ensure that this approximation adds to the scientific signal—and not the noise—structured and standardized frameworks for data quality, preprocessing, dimensionality reduction, feature selection, and finally, the choice and tuning of the models are pivotal. Efforts towards such frameworks should become a priority to leverage ML's powerful technologies to their full benefit.

Acknowledgements

Funding J.M.K. and D.D. are supported by the Bundesministerium für Bildung und Forschung (BMBF COMPLS3-022).

Conflicts of Interest/Competing Interests None of the authors has any conflict of interest to disclose.

References

1. Editorial. Daunting data. Nature. 2016;539:467–8.
2. Smith SM, Nichols TE. Statistical challenges in "big data" human neuroimaging. Neuron. 2018;97(2):263–8. https://doi.org/10.1016/j.neuron.2017.12.018.
3. Rosenblatt F. The perceptron: a probabilistic model for information storage and organization in the brain. Psychol Rev. 1958;65(6):386–408. https://doi.org/10.1037/h0042519.
4. Turing AM. Computing machinery and intelligence. Mind. 1950;59:433–60.
5. Jordan MI, Mitchell TM. Machine learning: trends, perspectives, and prospects. Science (80-). 2015;349(6245):255–60. https://doi.org/10.1126/science.aaa8415.
6. Friston K. Statistical parametric mapping. Stat Parametr Mapp Anal Funct Brain Images. 2007; https://doi.org/10.1016/B978-012372560-8/50002-4.
7. Penny W, Friston K, Ashburner J, Kiebel S, Nichols T. Statistical parametric mapping: the analysis of functional brain images. Stat Parametr Mapp Anal Funct Brain Images. 2007; https://doi.org/10.1016/B978-0-12-372560-8.X5000-1.
8. Arbabshirani MR, Plis S, Sui J, Calhoun VD. Single subject prediction of brain disorders in neuroimaging: promises and pitfalls. NeuroImage. 2017;145(Pt B):137–65. https://doi.org/10.1016/j.neuroimage.2016.02.079.
9. Kernbach JM, Satterthwaite TD, Bassett DS, et al. Shared endophenotypes of default mode dysfunction in attention deficit/hyperactivity disorder and autism spectrum disorder. Transl Psychiatry. 2018;8(1):133. https://doi.org/10.1038/s41398-018-0179-6.
10. Mwangi B, Ebmeier KP, Matthews K, Douglas Steele J. Multicentre diagnostic classification of individual structural neuroimaging scans from patients with major depressive disorder. Brain. 2012;135(Pt 5):1508–21. https://doi.org/10.1093/brain/aws084.
11. Gorgolewski K, Burns CD, Madison C, Clark D, Halchenko YO, Waskom ML, Ghosh SS. Nipype: a flexible, lightweight and extensible neuroimaging data processing framework in python. Front Neuroinform. 2011;5:13. https://doi.org/10.3389/fninf.2011.00013.
12. Smith SM, Jenkinson M, Woolrich MW, et al. Advances in functional and structural MR image analysis and implementation as FSL. NeuroImage. 2004;23(Suppl 1):S208–19. https://doi.org/10.1016/j.neuroimage.2004.07.051.
13. Breiman L. Statistical modeling: the two cultures. Statist Sci. 2001;16(3):199–231.
14. Hastie T, Tibshirani R, Friedman JH. The elements of statistical learning: data mining, inference, and prediction. Berlin: Springer; 2009.
15. Mwangi B, Tian TS, Soares JC. A review of feature reduction techniques in neuroimaging. Neuroinformatics. 2014;12(2):229–44. https://doi.org/10.1007/s12021-013-9204-3.
16. Naselaris T, Kay KN, Nishimoto S, Gallant JL. Encoding and decoding in fMRI. NeuroImage. 2011;56(2):400–10. https://doi.org/10.1016/j.neuroimage.2010.07.073.
17. Haxby JV, Gobbini MI, Furey ML, Ishai A, Schouten JL, Pietrini P. Distributed and overlapping representations of faces and objects in ventral temporal cortex. Science (80-). 2001;293(5539):2425–30. https://doi.org/10.1126/science.1063736.
18. Hanke M, Halchenko YO, Sederberg PB, Hanson SJ, Haxby JV, Pollmann S. PyMVPA: a python toolbox for multivariate pattern analysis of fMRI data. Neuroinformatics. 2009;7(1):37–53. https://doi.org/10.1007/s12021-008-9041-y.
19. Hanson SJ, Matsuka T, Haxby JV. Combinatorial codes in ventral temporal lobe for object recognition: Haxby (2001) revisited: is there a "face" area? NeuroImage. 2004;23(1):156–66. https://doi.org/10.1016/j.neuroimage.2004.05.020.
20. Varoquaux G, Thirion B. How machine learning is shaping cognitive neuroimaging. Gigascience. 2014;3:28. https://doi.org/10.1186/2047-217X-3-28.
21. Poldrack RA, Huckins G, Varoquaux G. Establishment of best practices for evidence for prediction: a review. JAMA Psychiat. 2019;77(5):534–40. https://doi.org/10.1001/jamapsychiatry.2019.3671.
22. Thirion B, Flandin G, Pinel P, Roche A, Ciuciu P, Poline JB. Dealing with the shortcomings of spatial normalization: multi-subject parcellation of fMRI datasets. Hum Brain Mapp. 2006;27(8):678–93.
23. Beckmann CF, Smith SM. Probabilistic independent component analysis for functional magnetic resonance imaging. IEEE Trans Med Imaging. 2004;23(2):137–52. https://doi.org/10.1109/TMI.2003.822821.

17 Machine Learning Algorithms in Neuroimaging: An Overview

Vittorio Stumpo, Julius M. Kernbach, Christiaan H. B. van Niftrik, Martina Sebök, Jorn Fierstra, Luca Regli, Carlo Serra, and Victor E. Staartjes

17.1 Introduction

Machine learning (ML) and artificial intelligence (AI) applications in the field of neuroimaging have been rising in recent years, and their adoption is increasing worldwide [1]. Due to the availability of extensive amounts of data, their inherent complexity, and the potentially unlimited applications, neuroimaging is particularly attractive for ML, since virtually every step in clinical imaging spanning from image acquisition and processing to disease detection, diagnosis, and outcome prediction can be the target of ML algorithms [2–9].

Deep learning (DL) is a field of ML that can be defined as a set of algorithms enabling a computer to be fed with raw data and to then progressively discover—through multiple layers of representation—more complex and abstract patterns in large data sets [10–12]. The reports of DL algorithms in imaging tasks have been increasing, with applications in the context of several diseases of neurosurgical relevance including but not limited to brain tumors [7, 9, 13–15], aneurysms [16–18] and spinal diseases [19, 20]. In addition to anatomical imaging, ML-augmented histological diagnosis has been investigated [21]. Another field of ML in neuroimaging is radiomics. The workflow underlying DL applications for radiomics is often complex and may appear confusing for those unfamiliar with the field. Even so, reports combining both radiomic feature extraction and ML are increasing [22–24].

In the present chapter, we provide clinical practitioners, researchers, and medical students with the necessary foundations in a rapidly developing area of clinical neuroscience. We highlight the basic concepts underlying ML applications in neuroimaging, and discuss technical aspects of the most promising algorithms adopted into this field—with a specific focus on Convolutional Neural Networks (CNNs) and Generative Adversarial Networks (GANs) [25–27]. While in the recent past, segmentation and classification tasks have attracted the most interest, many other tasks exist [8, 28–31]. These tasks can be considered to some extent overlapping, even if the underlying algorithms may be different. While the vast potential of ML and AI can still be considered early in its development, a clearer categorization of tasks and reporting standardization would be valuable in favoring reproducibility and performance comparison of different studies. At present, this technology is still mainly confined to academic research centers and industry. Still, it is reasonable to expect that the near future will witness a variable integration of ML-based computer-aided tasks in patient management [32]. For this reason, reported applications from a practical standpoint are introduced in the last section of the chapter including image reconstruction and restoration, image synthesis and super-resolution, registration, segmentation, classification, and outcome prediction.

17.2 The Radiomic Workflow

Radiomics can be defined as the extraction of a significant number of features from medical images applying algorithms for data characterization. "Radiomic features" have the potential to highlight characteristics that are not identifiable by conventional image analysis. The underlying hypothesis is that these distinctive imaging characteristics

V. Stumpo · C. H. B. van Niftrik · M. Sebök · J. Fierstra · L. Regli
C. Serra · V. E. Staartjes (✉)
Machine Intelligence in Clinical Neuroscience (MICN) Lab, Department of Neurosurgery, Clinical Neuroscience Center, University Hospital Zurich, University of Zurich, Zurich, Switzerland
e-mail: victoregon.staartjes@usz.ch

J. M. Kernbach
Neurosurgical Artificial Intelligence Lab Aachen (NAILA), Department of Neurosurgery, RWTH University Hospital, Aachen, Germany

Department of Neurosurgery, Faculty of Medicine, RWTH Aachen University, Aachen, Germany

V. E. Staartjes et al. (eds.), *Machine Learning in Clinical Neuroscience*, Acta Neurochirurgica Supplement 134,
https://doi.org/10.1007/978-3-030-85292-4_17

invisible to the naked eye may provide additional relevant information to be exploited for enhanced image characterization, which can then in turn be applied for enhanced prognosis or prediction. Importantly, recent advances have moved the field from the use handcrafted characteristics such as shape-based (shape, size, surface information), first-order (mean, median ROI value—no spatial relations) and second-order features (inter-voxel relationships) towards data-driven and ML-based approaches, which can automatically perform feature extraction and classification [22, 33, 34].

In general, the radiomic pipeline [35] consists of a series of consecutive steps that may be summarized as following (Fig. 17.1):

1. Image Acquisition.
2. Processing.
3. Feature Selection/Dimensionality Reduction.
4. Downstream Analysis.

Image acquisition protocols depend on chosen imaging technique (ultrasound, X-ray, computed tomography (CT), magnetic resonance imaging (MRI), positron emission tomography (PET)). An important limitation with this respect is represented by intra- and inter-institutional differences in hardware, acquisition and imaging processing techniques, which—by definition—affect image quality, noise, and texture. For practical reasons, it has proven difficult to reach standardization of such heterogeneous equipment and acquisition pipeline, although increasingly pursued by means of international consortia and consensus statements [36]. Corrections during pre-processing may be necessary, with methods specific to the imaging modality of choice. For example, CT uses Hounsfield units which are absolute and anchored to the radiodensity of water, while MRI—due to differing voxel intensities—requires normalization relative to another structure.

Then, a region of interest (ROI) that has to be radiomically analyzed has to be defined through either manual or (semi-) automatic segmentation. Segmentation can be achieved in two-dimensional (2D) space or volume of interest (VOI) segmentation can be achieved in three-dimensional (3D) space. This process is required to identify the area where the radiomic features are to be calculated. This process can be either manual (the traditional gold-standard, even if affected by inter and intra-rater variability), semi-automatic or fully automatic (by means of ML, also affected by a series of pitfalls such as artifact and noise disturbances) [22, 36]. Once segmented images are obtained, additional processing steps may be necessary before feature extraction and analysis such as interpolation to isotropic voxel spacing, range re-segmentation and intensity outlier filtering (normalization), discretization.

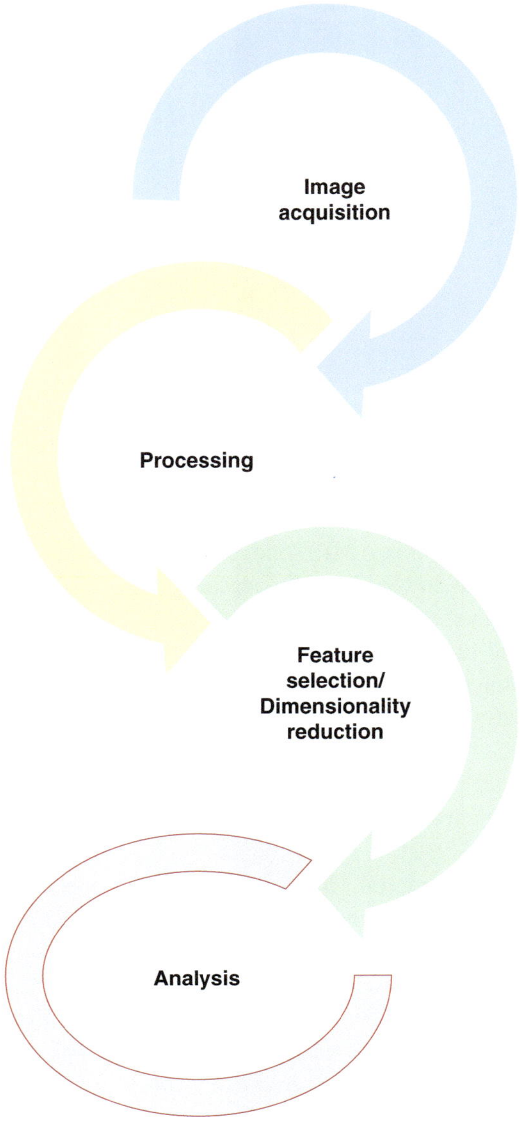

Fig. 17.1 Radiomic workflow. Schematic representation of the radiomic workflow is shown: image acquisition, processing, feature selection/dimension reduction, downstream analysis

For further details on this processing step please refer to van Timmeren et al. [35] Radiomic features to be extracted can be categorized into statistical —including histogram-based and texture-based—model-based, transformation-based, and shape-based [24]. The already introduced heterogeneity of the imaging modality—and therefore of their extracted features—have led to the recent introduction of recommendations, guidelines, definitions, and reference values for image features [37]. Interpretations of medical data remains to date largely in the hands of trained practitioners, with limitations due to inter-observer variability, complexity of the image, time constraints, and fatigue [5]. Conventional algorithms like Random Forest (RF), Support Vector Machine (SVM), Neural Networks (NN), *k*-Nearest Neighbor (KNN), and DL algorithms such as

Convolutional Neural Networks (CNN), Recurrent Neural Networks (RNN), and Generative Adversarial Networks (GANs) have been investigated to overcome these drawbacks [5, 38]. Among DL-based approaches for imaging applications, which led to the most astonishing results, CNNs and GANs have attracted considerable attention and will be introduced in the next section.

17.3 Introduction to Deep Learning Algorithms for Imaging

Convolutional Neural Networks (CNNs)

Architecture

CNNs have been applied to several tasks in radiological image processing (segmentation, classification, detection, et cetera) [25, 28]. CNN architecture is derived from the neurobiology of the visual cortex and is composed of neurons, each having a learnable weight and bias. The structure itself is made up of an input layer, multiple hidden layers (convolutional layers, pooling layers, fully connected layers, and various normalization layers), and one output layer (Fig. 17.2).

The next sections will detail the foundational concepts of these layers in more detail. As a brief summary, the convolutional layer is meant to merge two sets of information. On the other hand, the pooling layer reduces dimensionality by associating the output of neuron clusters in one layer with the single neuron. Fully connected layers connect every neuron in one layer to every neuron in another layer. Its primary purpose is to classify the input images into several classes, based on the training datasets [25]. To simplify, it can be stated that each new CNN layer learns filters—or kernels—of increasing complexity. In a commonly reported and straightforward example, the first layers learn basic feature detection filters such as edges, corners and similar. The middle layers can detect higher-order features, for example, eyes or ears in facial recognition tasks. The higher the layer, the more complex features are recognized, such as differences between faces, et cetera.

Convolution and Kernels

The convolution operation allows the network to detect the same feature in different regions of the image and for this reason, the convolutional layer can be considered the crucial building block of a CNN [39, 40]. In mathematics, convolution between two functions results in a third function expressing how the shape of one function is modified by another. In practice, this operation allows feature extraction by applying a kernel (or filter) to the input (or tensor), both numeric in nature. The product of each element of the kernel and input tensor is derived at each location and added to generate feature maps. The process is repeated through the application of different kernels resulting in an arbitrary number of feature maps, each representing different features of the input tensors. For this reason, different kernels are regarded as different feature extractors [41].

A single CNN layer detects only local features of the image, while multilayer CNNs allow increasing the perception field and synthesizing the features extracted at previous layers. Moreover, CNNs reduce the number of weights by sharing them between the network's neurons, which results in a considerable memory reduction.

Hyperparameter Optimization

CNNs aim to identify and "learn" the kernels that perform best for a chosen task based on a training dataset. Hyperparameter optimization of kernel size and number is crucial in defining the convolution operation. When visualizing the kernel as a matrix that moves over the input tensor, there are two other concepts that are relevant to be able to

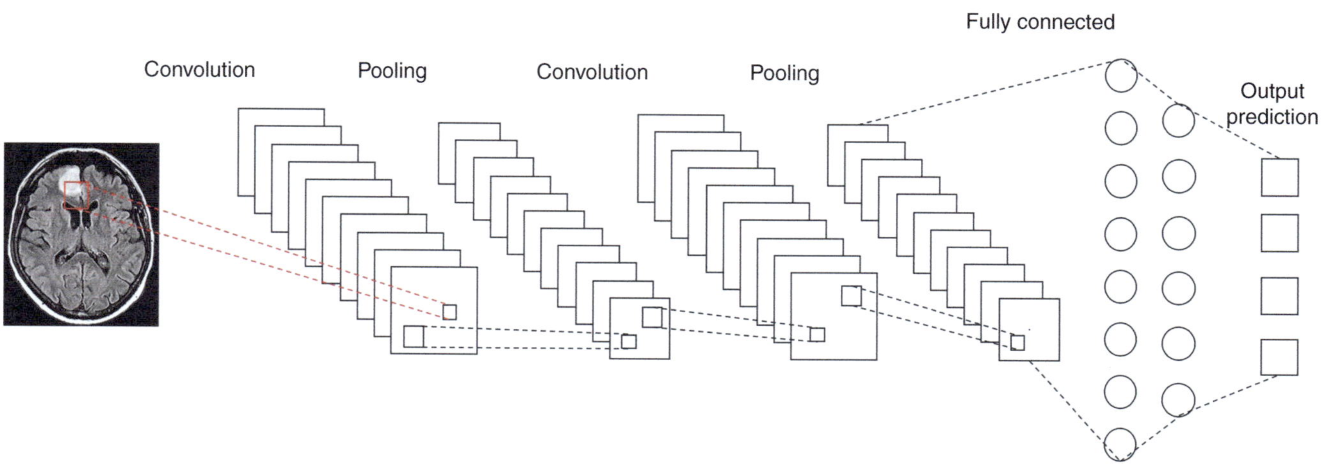

Fig. 17.2 CNN architecture. A simplified CNN architecture structure: input, convolutional, pooling, fully connected layer, and output are shown

grasp how a CNN processes imaging data: padding and stride.

Given that the convolution operation does not center the kernel to overlap the boundaries of the input data, this would result in reduction of the dimension of the output feature map, leaving out the very border of the image. For this reason, to solve the so-called border effect problem, padding is applied. This consists of adding rows and columns of data to the frame of the input tensor, most commonly zero-padding, i.e. columns and rows of zeros, allowing the kernel center to fit on the outermost element of the input, i.e. more space for the kernel to cover the image, and maintain in-plane dimension when the convolution operation is performed [41, 42].

Stride can instead be defined as the distance between two successive kernel positions. For a thorough overview of stride and padding, readers are encouraged to refer to Doumolin and Visin [43].

Of note, kernel values are learned during the training process in the convolution layer (parameter). In contrast, kernel size and number, padding, and stride require being set before training, and are then adjusted during hyperparameter tuning.

Another hyperparameter to be selected is the batch size, namely the number of samples that will be propagated through the network before "updating" its kernels. To explain this concept, we hypothesize to have 500 training samples and to set the batch size as 50. The algorithm will train the network based on the first 50 samples (1–50). Then, it will train using samples 51–100, and so on. A different concept is instead represented by the epoch, which is defined as the number of passes through the training data. Of course, batch size can take values between 1 and the number of samples in the training dataset, while the number of epochs can take any integer value ≥ 1 [44].

Activation Function and Backpropagation

Outputs of the convolutions, which are a linear function, are passed through an activation function. Activation functions allow learning more complex functional mappings between the different layers. Examples of activation functions are the binary step function, a simple linear activation function, or nonlinear functions such as sigmoid, hyperbolic tangent, or rectified linear unit (ReLU), and leaky ReLU [45]. A binary step function, where activation is single-threshold-based, does not support multi-value output (i.e. multiple categories as output). A linear function on the contrary, after receiving the input (modified by the weight of each neuron) produces an output signal that is proportional to its input. Although smooth nonlinear functions have been extensively used given their similarity with physiological neuronal behavior, ReLU is now more commonly used. In simple words these functions are equations determining the activation (or firing) of a neuron. Specifically, a ReLU will output the input directly in a linear way if it is positive—otherwise, it will output zero. A leaky ReLU will allow a small positive gradient when the input is negative, i.e. changing the slope to a minimum in these cases.

Two major drawbacks of linear activations are the following: they cannot use backpropagation, because the derivative of the function is a constant and is thus not related to the input, preventing weight adjustment. Also, the neural network would be constituted by one collapsed layer as the last function would still be linear, making the NN a linear regression model [46]. On the contrary, nonlinear activation functions allow the model to identify complex relationships among inputs and outputs—an essential feature for complex (or multi-dimensional) data analysis. In this case, backpropagation and multilayer representation is possible (allowing hidden layers to achieve higher abstraction levels on complex data).

Backpropagation

We have just introduced the important concept of backpropagation. When fitting a feed-forward neural network, backpropagation allows descending the gradient with respect to all the weights simultaneously. By chaining the gradients found using the "chain rule," backpropagation computes the gradient for any weight that is to be optimized—and consequently, can compute improvements with respect to the errors backwards towards the most upstream layer in the network [47, 48]. Due to its high efficiency, backpropagation is useful in many gradient descent methods for training multilayer networks, correcting weights to minimize loss. To better understand how this process works, we can describe that CNNs work in reverse. The gradient (updates to the weights) decreases closer to the input layer and increases towards the output layer as a result of backpropagation updating the weights from the final layer backwards towards the first. Minimization of error (loss) occurs at the final layer, where a higher level of abstraction is recognized and adjusted, tracing back through previous layers. Intuitively, starting from the input instead, a CNN can be described as progressively better at discriminating, e.g. an object that is to be identified, by stepping away from tiny details and looking instead at the "big picture" from a distance [40].

Optimization and Network Training

A loss (or cost) function computes the congruence between output predictions of the network through forward propagation and known ground truth labels. Loss functions are one of the hyperparameters to be determined according to the given task [41, 49]. The amount to which weights are updated during training is referred to as the step size or the "learning rate" [50]. This is an additional hyperparameter used in the training of neural networks, usually taking a small positive value.

A variety of algorithms can be applied for optimization of weights to reduce losses. These include gradient descent, stochastic gradient descent (SGD), mini-batch gradient descent, momentum, Nesterov-accelerated gradient, Adagrad, Adadelta, Adam, and RMSProp [51–55].

Gradient descent is a first-order optimization algorithm dependent on the first-order derivative of a loss function. It aims to compute in which direction weights should be modified so that the function can reach a minimum (Fig. 17.3a). The loss is transferred from one layer to another by means of backpropagation, as discussed before, and the model's parameters—or weights—are modified depending on the losses, so that loss itself can be minimized. Such optimization is performed after the gradient is calculated on the whole dataset. In addition to normal (batch) gradient descent, SGD and mini-batch descent are most commonly employed. SGD is particularly helpful to minimize the risk of reaching a local minimum (non-convex function) instead of the global minimum—one of the major drawbacks of normal gradient descent (Fig. 17.3b). In a commonly reported example, a normal gradient optimizes weights in a dataset with 1000 observations only after these are all analyzed (every epoch). In SGD, in contrast, the different data rows are analyzed individually, and thus model parameters are updated more often than in batch gradient descent. Of note, despite the higher fluctuations in updating weights, SGD requires significantly less time and less memory. In mini-batch gradient descent, model parameters are instead updated after every mini-batch (a certain subset of the training data). Normal batch gradient descent can be used for smoother curves. SGD can be used when the dataset is very large. In addition, batch gradient descent converges directly to minima, while SGD converges faster when datasets are very large.

The advantages and disadvantages of other optimization techniques are briefly discussed. Given the high variance in SGD, *momentum* was introduced—with the need for an additional hyperparameter, namely γ—to accelerate descent in the right directions, and to limit fluctuation to the wrong

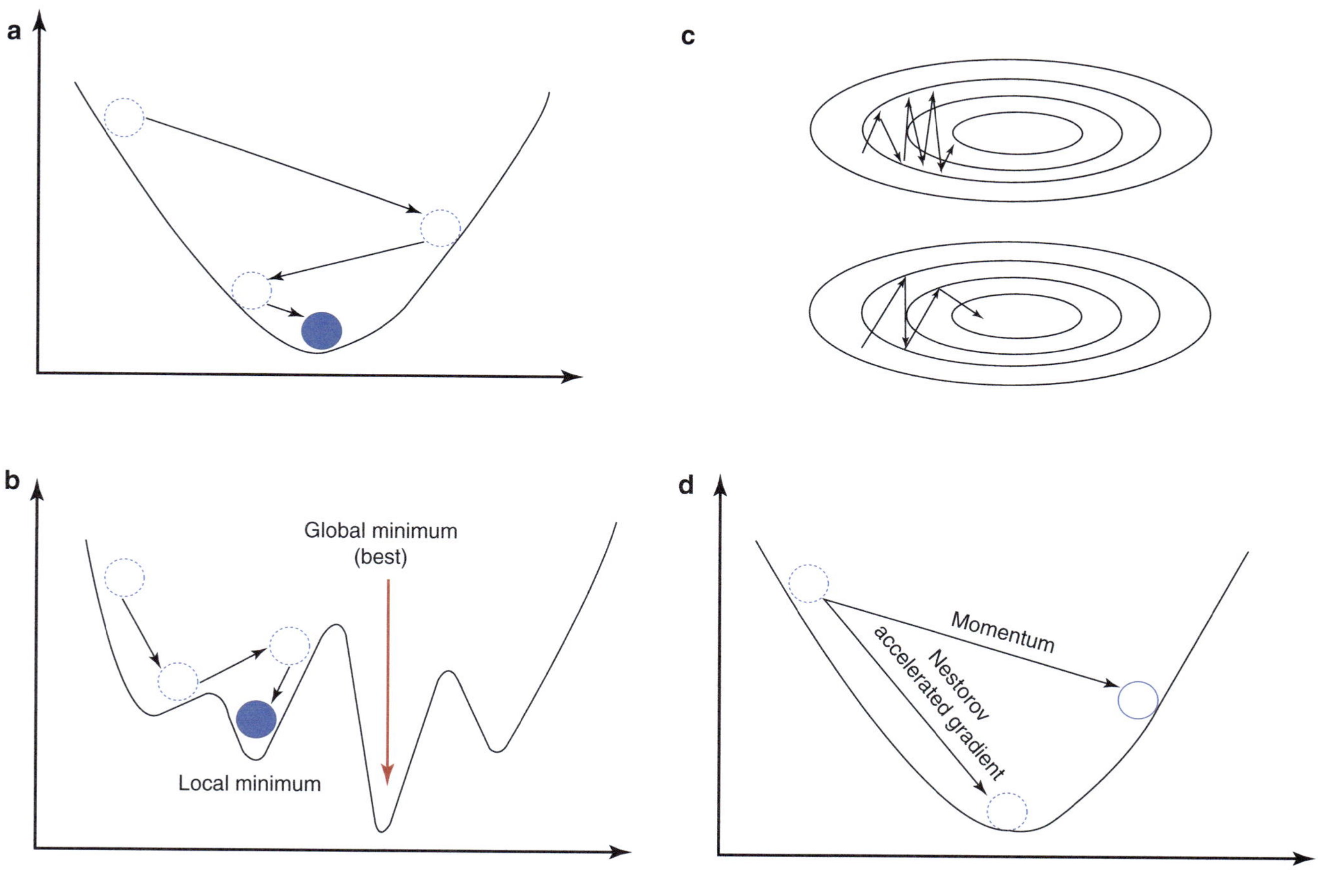

Fig. 17.3 Schematic representation of intuitions underlying: (**a**) gradient descent. Gradient descent is an optimization algorithm used to minimize a function by moving in the direction of steepest descent as defined by the negative of the gradient. In machine learning, it is used to update the parameters of the model; (**b**) stochastic gradient descent (SGD). While gradient descent risks to reach a local with respect to the global minimum, SGD fluctuations enable it to jump to new and potentially better local minima; (**c**) momentum. Momentum was introduced to limit the high fluctuations of SGD, allowing faster convergence in the right direction; (**d**) Nesterov-accelerated gradient (NAG). It can be used to modify a gradient descent-type method to improve its initial convergence

one (Fig. 17.3c) [56]. A too high momentum may miss a minimum and start to ascend again. To address this problem, Nesterov-Accelerated Gradient (NAG)—or *gradient descent with Nesterov momentum*—was introduced (Fig. 17.3d). The intuition of NAG consists in anticipating when the slope is going to decrease. To achieve this, previously calculated gradients are considered for the calculation of the momentum, instead of current gradients. This process guarantees that minima are not missed, but makes the operation slower when minima are close.

Differently from the previously discussed optimizers, where the learning rate is constant, both with respect to parameters and cycle, *Adagrad* changes the learning rate, making smaller updates for parameters associated with frequently occurring features, and larger updates for ones occurring less often. One advantage of such an approach is that the learning rate does not require manual tuning. Unfortunately, squared gradients are accumulated in the denominator, causing the learning rate to continuously decrease reaching infinitesimally small values. For this reason, *Adadelta* was introduced, in which the sum of gradients is recursively defined as a decaying average of all past squared gradients. A similar rationale was the basis for the development of the *RMSprop* optimizer. Lastly, *Adam* (Adaptive Moment Estimation), in addition to storing an exponentially decaying average of past squared gradients like Adadelta and RMSprop, is also characterized by an exponentially decaying average of past gradients, similar to momentum. Intuitively, when visualizing momentum as a ball slope, Adam can be described as a slower ball with friction, which thus prefers flat minima in the error surface. Still other optimizers have been developed (AdaMax, Nadam, AMSGrad), but their discussion is out of the scope of this chapter [51, 54].

Pooling, Fully Connected Layers, and Last Activation Function

Convolutional layers are limited to the fact that a precise position of the feature map is recorded and small changes in the position of the feature in the input image will determine rather different feature maps. Pooling layers perform a downsampling operation which decreases in-plane dimensionality of feature maps obtained in the convolution. This layer lacks learnable parameters, while still maintaining other hyperparameters previously described. The aim of the operation is to reduce the spatial size of the input while maintaining volume depths. This results in a decrease of the number of learnable parameters. The final objective of this step, as described above, is to make the representation resilient to minor translations of the input. This resilience means that if we translate the input by a small amount, the values of most of the pooled outputs do not change [41, 42].

There are different pooling operations, such as maximum pooling and average pooling [42]. Average pooling calculates an average for each patch of the feature map according to pre-specified criteria. Maximum pooling instead calculates the maximum value in each specified patch. The results are downsampled to the pooled feature maps that highlight the most present feature in the patch, but not the average presence of the feature in the case of average pooling. This has been found to work better in practice than average pooling for computer vision tasks like image classification (Fig. 17.4).

At the fully connected layer level, feature maps of the last convolution/pooling layer are said to be "flattened," i.e. converted into a one-dimensional vectors, in which every input is connected to every output by a learnable weight. The final fully connected layer typically has the same number of

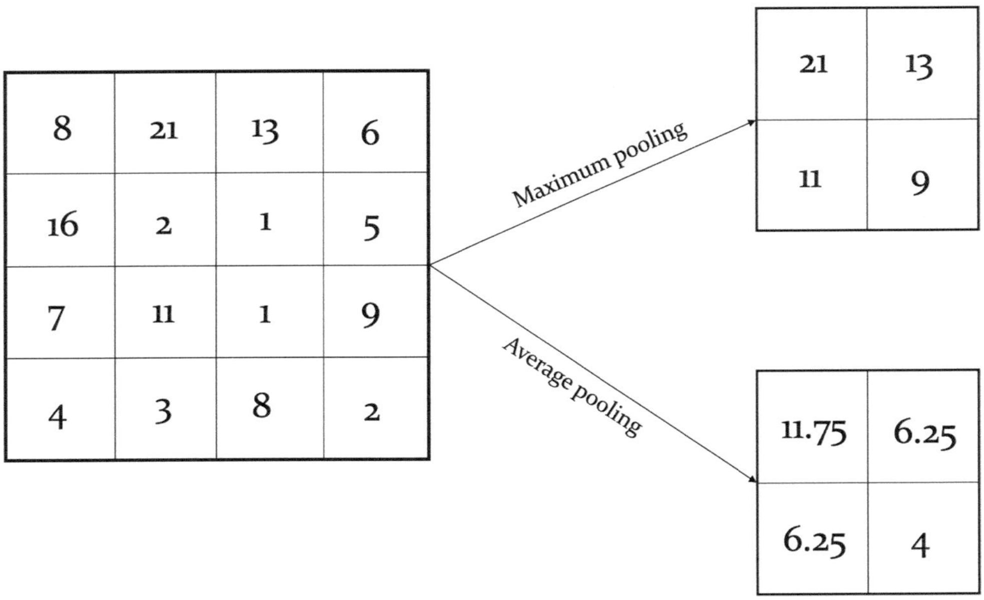

Fig. 17.4 Schematic representation of maximum and average pooling. Pooling reduced in-plane dimensionality of feature maps obtained in the convolution to make the representation become invariant to minor translations of the input (noise suppression). Average pooling calculates an average for each patch of the feature map according to pre-specified criteria. Maximum pooling, instead calculates the maximum value in each specified patch. Both approaches result in a downsampled feature map

output nodes as the number of output classes. Their function is essentially to compile the data extracted by previous layers to arrive at the final output [41].

The activation function applied to the last fully connected layer is different from the previous ones and is selected depending on the task of interest (linear, sigmoid, softmax). Also, the loss function is selected according to the last activation function implemented (mean square error, cross-entropy). As an example, for multiclass classification, a softmax function is chosen which normalizes output values from the last fully connected layer to target class probabilities, where each value ranges between 0 and 1 and all values sum to 1 [41, 57].

Overfitting and Dropout

When training a ML model, one of the most important problems is overfitting (Fig. 17.5a). This phenomenon occurs when an algorithm "learns" training data too closely, subsequently failing to generate accurate predictions on new samples. Data are usually split into training and validation set, and performance is tested on this unseen validation set to determine generalizability.

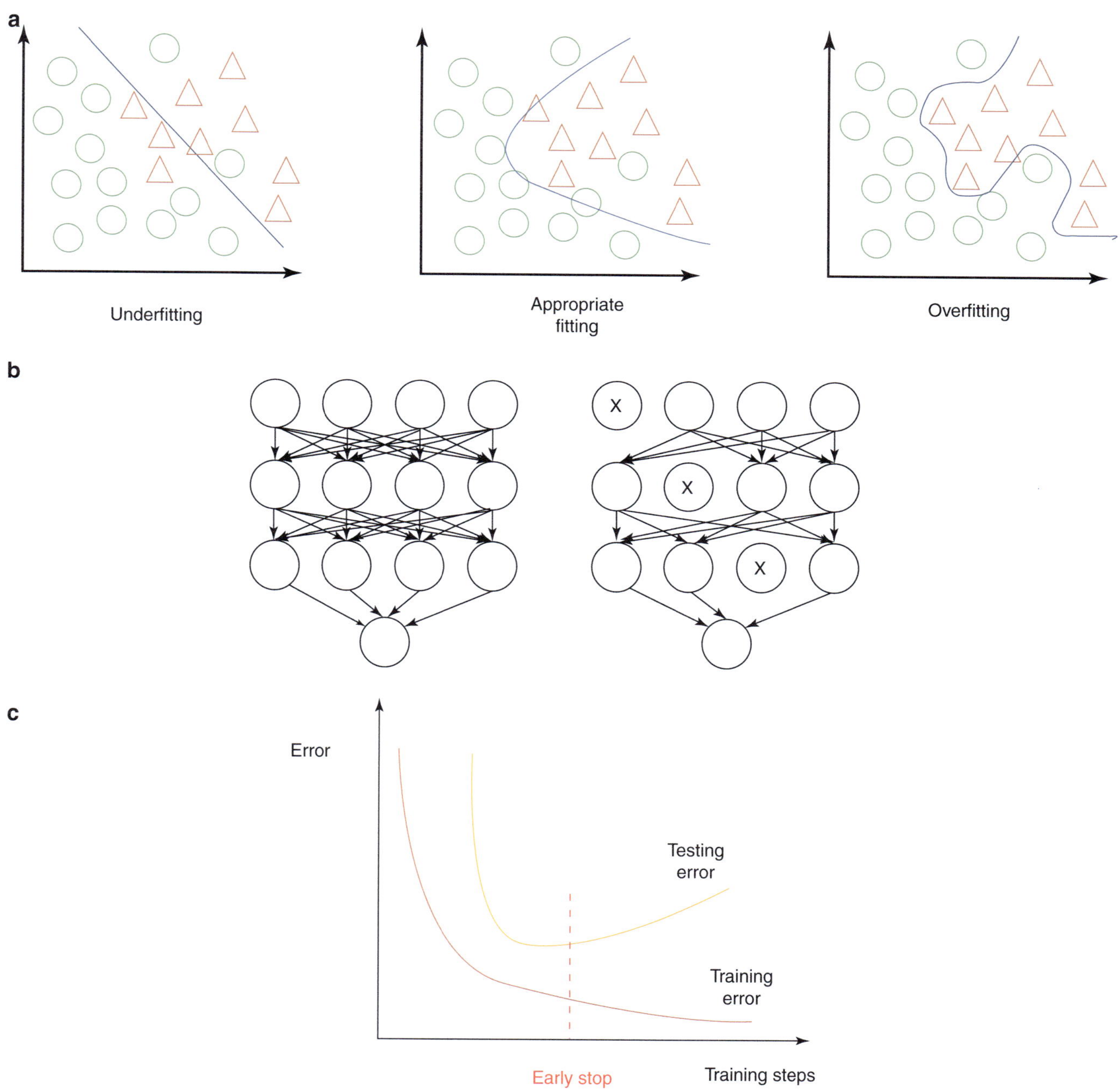

Fig. 17.5 Schematic representation of: (**a**) overfitting. In overfitting, algorithm training leads to a function that too closely fit a limited set of data, preventing generalizability on new unseen data; and selected regularization approaches, i.e. (**b**) dropout. Dropout allows to decrease complexity of the model by dropping a certain set of neurons chosen at random, forcing the network to rely on more robust feature for training; (**c**) early stopping. In early stopping, training stop as soon as the validation error reaches the minimum

Several strategies are available to help prevent overfitting, including increasing amounts of training data, data augmentation approaches, regularization (weight decay, dropout), batch normalization, early stopping, as well as reducing architectural complexity [41, 58]. Also, when a small training dataset is anticipated, novel approaches have focused on fine-tuning previously developed CNNs for adaptation to new applications in a process termed *transfer learning*, which is addressed in another paragraph below [14, 59, 60].

As stated, data augmentation may be required in the setting of limited sample availability. A variety of basic approaches have been used in the past, such as image flipping, rotation, scaling, cropping, translation, Gaussian noise, et cetera [61].

Regularization approaches to avoid overfitting include among others dropout and weight decay. The term "dropout" refers to dropping out units (hidden and visible) in a neural network. By dropping a unit out, we mean temporarily removing it from the network, along with all its incoming and outgoing connections. For this reason, this regularization technique can be described as a noise-adder to the hidden units. The choice of which units to drop at each iteration is random, and dropout probability is set as a hyperparameter [58, 62–64] (Fig. 17.5b).

Weight decay, reduces overfitting by penalizing the model's weights so that the weights take only small values. This is obtained by adding an additional error, proportional to the sum of weights (L1 norm) or squared magnitude (L2 norm) of the weight vector, to the error at each node. L2 regularization is most commonly used as it strongly penalizes peaky weight vectors and prefers diffuse weight vectors. Due to multiplicative interactions between weights and inputs this system encourages the network to distribute little use of more inputs rather than high selective use of less of them. L1 regularization is a less common alternative. Simply stated, neurons with L1 regularization use only a sparse subset of their most important inputs and ignore noisy features. A combination of L1 with L2 regularizations is the elastic net regularization [58, 65, 66].

Batch normalization consists of a supplemental layer which adaptively normalizes (centering and scaling) the input values of the following layer, mitigating the risk of overfitting, as well as improving gradient flow through the network, allowing higher learning rates, and reducing the dependence on initialization. This allows the use of increased learning rates, and may eliminate the need for dropout and results in reduction of the number of training epochs needed to train the network. For a more structured overview on batch normalization, we advise consulting Ioffe and Szegedy [67], and of a simplified overview by Brownlee [50].

Lastly, early stopping can be considered a form of cross-validation strategy in which a part of the training set is used as a validation set. When the performance on this retained validation set starts to deteriorate, training of the model is interrupted (Fig. 17.5c).

2D vs. 3D CNN

Past image segmentation research has focused on 2D images. For MRI, for example, the approach has been individual segmentation for each slice followed by post-processing to connect 2D segmented slices in a 3D volume. Of course, this approach is prone to inhomogeneity in the reconstruction of the 3D images and loss of anatomical information [68]. Recent reductions in computational costs and the advent of graphics processing units (GPUs) in ML have allowed application of CNNs to 3D medical images using 3D deep learning. The mathematical formulation of 3D CNNs is very similar to 2D CNNs, with an extra dimension added. Here, a 3D convolution is different from the 2D one as the kernel slides in three dimensions as opposed to two dimensions (Fig. 17.6). The implications are particularly relevant for medical imaging when a model is constructed using 3D images voxels, granting increased precision and spatial resolution, higher data reliability at the expense of increased model complexity and slower computation [68–70]. For further readings on 3D CNN use for medical imaging, consult Singh et al. and Despotovic et al. [68, 70]

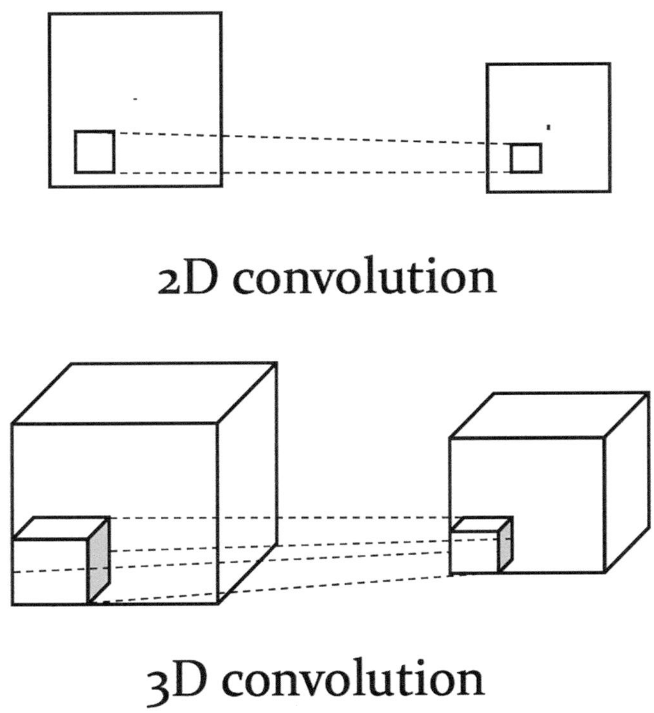

Fig. 17.6 Schematic representation of 2D versus 3D convolution. For imaging application, three-dimensional voxels increase spatial resolution and retain complex relationship for model training that would not be used otherwise

Transfer Learning

Recently the use of algorithms pre-trained for similar applications to be extended for other applications has proven valuable [60, 71]. This technique is named deep transfer learning (TL) and several reports in brain tumor research have been produced, for example, with CNNs [14, 59, 72, 73]. A pre-trained CNN has to be able to extract relevant features while maintaining irrelevant features and underlying noise. For a comprehensive overview of transfer learning, consult Zhuang et al. [71]

Available CNN Architectures

A variety of CNN architectures have been developed and are being extensively exploited in imaging applications: LeNet, AlexNet, GoogLeNet, ResNet, SENet, VGG16, VGG19 [74]. For a comprehensive overview of pre-trained CNN architectures we refer the readers to Khan et al. [75]

Generative Adversarial Networks

The basic function of GANs is to train a generator and discriminator in an adversarial way. Based on different requirements, either a stronger generator or a more sensitive discriminator is designed as the target goal [26, 76, 77]. These two models are typically implemented by neural networks such as CNNs. The generator tries to capture the distribution of true examples for new data example generation. The discriminator is usually a binary classifier, discriminating generated examples from the true examples as accurately as possible (Fig. 17.7). With improving generator performance, discriminator performance worsens. For this reason, GAN optimization is said to be a "minimax optimization problem." The optimization terminates at a saddle point (convergence) that is a minimum in terms of error with respect to the generator and a maximum in terms of error with respect to the discriminator [26]. Past the transitory convergent state, model training may continue with the discriminator providing only random feedback (50/50 or coin tossing), implying for the generator to train on meaningless feedback. This of course would result in decreased performance of the generator.

The contribution of GANs to medical imaging is therefore twofold. The generative part can help in exploring hidden structures in the training data leading to new image synthesis with valuable implications for addressing issues such as lack of data and privacy concerns. The discriminative part can be instead considered as a "learned prior" for normal images, so that it can be used as a regularizer or detector when presented with abnormal images [27].

Data Availability and Privacy

We have already mentioned how, to some extent, the "firepower" granted by DL techniques is difficult to implement

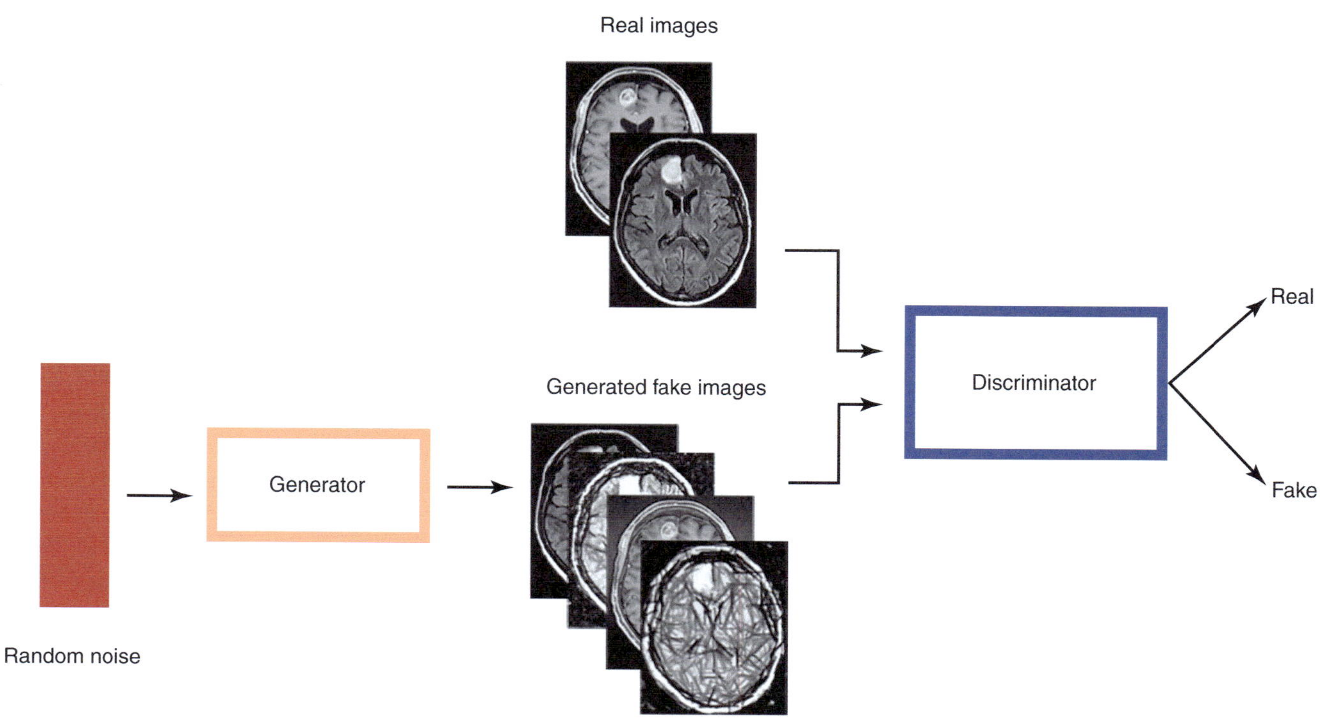

Fig. 17.7 GAN architecture. A simplified GAN is shown: generator and discriminator are trained in adversarial way. The discriminator attempts to distinguish generated examples from the true examples as accurately as possible

due to the poor availability of training data. Morever, the sensitive nature of patient medical information, data safety practices such as deidentification (anonymization and pseudo-anonymization) are crucial [78]. One solution to the lack of data availability has been proposed using ML approaches such as artificial image synthesis for data augmentation [79, 80]. Another option is federated learning, in which an algorithm is trained at various sites locally, without exchanging data—exchanging only the weights of the further trained model [81].

Deep Learning-Based Tasks in Imaging

The number of tasks that can be performed by DL in imaging is vast and intrinsically problem-oriented. A major distinction consists in supervised versus unsupervised machine learning approaches. In supervised learning, training data are given with known labels for which the correct outputs are already known, differently from unsupervised learning in which labels are not available, e.g. clustering [82]. Each of these methods carries its own advantages and disadvantages. Regardless of the approach, practical applications derive from widely appreciated clinical problems such as suboptimal image acquisition, time-consuming image analysis, and long learning curves for clinical experts or inter-observer variability in disease diagnosis and classification. In the next paragraphs, we aim to provide an overview of some clinical problems and the ML-based approaches that have been applied to tackle them. For descriptive purposes we identified the following tasks subgroups: image reconstruction and restoration, synthesis and super-resolution, registration, detection and classification, outcome prediction.

Image Reconstruction and Restoration

Image reconstruction refers to several scenarios where high-quality images are obtained from incomplete data or partial signal loss. The underlying issues are technique-dependent and can vary in different imaging modality for e.g. MRI, PET-CT, CT [33, 83]. Such problems are intimately connected to image restoration, whose aim is to improve the quality of suboptimal images acquired because of technical limitations or patient-related factors (e.g. respiration, discomfort, radiation doses). Other terminology to indicate issues of pertaining to image restoration are "denoising" and, more broadly, also artifact detection can be considered in this area. Few examples are here presented.

A study by Schramm et al. investigated anatomically-guided PET reconstruction aiming to improve bias-noise characteristics in brain PET imaging using a CNN. By applying a dedicated data augmentation during the training phase they showed encouraging results which could be generated in virtually real-time [84]. Yan et al. [85] trained a GAN algorithm to generate BOLD signals that were lost for technical reasons during fMRI. Intriguingly, reconstructed signals closely resembled the uncompromised signals and were coherent with each individual's functional brain organization. Kidoh et al. [86] have reported in five patients artificial noise addition to brain MRI, and training of a CNN to perform image reconstruction. The authors reported that their algorithm significantly reduced image noise while preserving image quality for brain MR images. CNNs have been most commonly reported for this task. Despite the preliminary encouraging results, recent reports point at instabilities in deep learning based methods raising concern on artifacts formation, failure to recover structural changes (from complete removal of details to more subtle distortions and blurring of the features) and others [87]. Additional applications are related to 3D reconstruction of anatomical regions. In spine surgery, DL can substitute manual segmentation and 3D reconstruction to aid surgical planning [88].

Image Synthesis and Super-Resolution

The applications of image synthesis are different and can be categorized in unconditional synthesis and cross-modality synthesis (image conversion), with the former meaning image generation from random noise without conditional information and the latter being instead referred to, for example, obtaining CT-like images from MRI or more in general to derive new parametric images or new tissue contrast [27, 89, 90].

This latter application has also been referred to as image super-resolution whose aim is to reconstruct a higher resolution image or image sequence from the observation of low-resolution images [91].

Especially for ML modeling, this allows training data to be augmented without recurring to traditional methods such as scaling, rotation, flipping, translation, and elastic deformation which do not account for variations resulting from different imaging protocols or sequences, not to mention variations in the size, shape, location, and appearance of specific pathology [27, 80]. Some examples of past studies are here discussed. Liu et al. [91] reported super-resolution reconstruction of experiments real datasets of MR brain images and demonstrated that multiscale fusion convolution network was able to recover detailed information from MR images outperforming traditional methods. A recent small preliminary study reported training of GANs to generate MRI T2w images from CT spine slices, obtaining far from optimal results [29]. The potential advantages of unconditional synthesis are related to overcoming privacy issues related to medical imaging use and the insufficient cases of patients positive for a given pathology [27, 79]. Generative Adversarial Networks (GANs) and Convolutional Neural Networks (CNNs) have been studied for this application.

Image Registration

Registration establishes anatomical correspondences between two images by mapping source and reference volume to the same coordinates [31, 92]. This task is required for intraoperative navigation, 3D reconstruction, multimodality image mappings, atlas construction, and arithmetic operations such as image averaging, subtraction, and correlation [31]. Implications are clear: Intraoperative neuronavigation requires mapping of a preoperative image onto an intraoperative image by registration. Another clinically relevant application in neuro-oncology is found in the context of rapid brain tumor growth, which requires longitudinal evaluation for disease evolution and for treatment results monitoring—both of which may greatly benefit from accurate registration to improve intra-individual imaging comparison [92]. Traditional methods can be summarized in deformable or elastic registration and linear registration or graph-based approaches [92].

Investigators have used a variety of approaches, with different degrees of manual interaction, to perform image registration. These approaches use either information obtained about the shape and topology of objects in the image or the presumed consistency in the intensity information from one slice to its immediate neighbor or from one brain or image set to another [31].

Despite the several strategies proposed, this task remains challenging due to the computational power needed, high-dimensional optimization, and task-dependent parameter tuning [93]. Recently, Fan et al. [93] reported the use of dual-supervised fully convolutional networks for image registration by predicting deformation from image appearance and showed promising registration accuracy and efficiency compared with the state-of-the-art methods. Estienne et al. [92] recently reported the introduction of DL-based framework to address segmentation and registration simultaneously.

Image Segmentation, Classification, and Outcome Prediction

Segmentation can be described as the process of partitioning an image into multiple non-overlapping regions that share similar attributes, enabling localization and quantification. Both supervised and unsupervised learning can play a role in segmentation tasks [12]. Segmentation from MR images is useful for diagnosis, growth prediction, and treatment planning. Its results are labels identifying each homogeneous region or a set of contours describing the region limits [68]. Of course, the higher the lesion complexity, the more problematic the segmentation. Well-defined lesions are easier to segment, while infiltrative, diffuse lesions are more daunting. Other obstacles to successful segmentation are represented by lesion variable shape, size, and location in addition to unstandardized voxel values in different modalities [28]. Segmentation applications have been reported for acute ischemic lesion segmentation [94], brain tumor (gliomas, meningiomas, metastases) [9, 15, 28, 79, 95–97], spine [19, 98], and aneurysms [4, 99] have been reported. Segmentation and classification are always intimately connected as segmentation implies a classification, while an imaging classifier implicitly segments an image. The segmentation results can be further used in several applications such as for analysis of anatomical structures, for the study of pathological regions, for surgical planning, et cetera [68]

The research area of disease detection, classification, and grading through machine learning based methods has also been referred as computer-aided diagnosis (CAD) [14]. A few examples are here discussed together with clinical implications. Deepak et al. [14] reported an automatic classification system designed for three brain tumor types (glioma, meningioma, and pituitary tumor) using a deep transfer learned CNN model for feature extraction from brain MRI images and classified using a SVM algorithm with high accuracy and AUC. CAD of a brain tumor can have a significant impact on clinical practice. For example, in the context of metastatic disease, early and accurate identification of brain metastases is crucial for optimal patient management. Given their small size, similarity to blood vessels and low technical contrast to background ratio, computer-assisted detection by means of DL algorithms can provide a valuable tool for early lesion identification [9]. Also, glioma recurrence can be difficult to identify at MRI due to post-treatment changes such as pseudo-progression and radiation necrosis and DL-based classification of these two lesions would be highly clinically relevant [13]. In the field of vascular neurosurgery, CNNs have proven useful in improving aneurysms detection at neuroimaging [100, 101]. Stemming from segmentation and classification tasks, outcome prediction – such as survival - has also been assessed preliminary by some studies [15, 102, 103].

17.4 Conclusions

The present chapter introduces ML applications in neuroimaging in a step-wise manner. The concept of radiomics has significantly increased expectations deriving from image analysis with respect to enhanced lesion diagnosis, characterization, segmentation, classification, outcome prediction, and prognosis evaluation. The computational power granted by ML—and DL in particular—has convincingly demonstrated preliminary potential to significantly impact patient management. CNNs and GANs, among other algorithms, constitute flexible tools to tackle multiple different ML tasks. Successful application in a variety of tasks spanning from image reconstruction and restoration, image synthesis and super-resolution, segmentation, classification, and outcome prediction have been introduced. Technical and ethical challenges posed by this technology are yet to be solved, with future research expected to improve upon the current limitations—Especially regarding explainable learning. Foundational knowledge of this field of ML by clinicians is required to safely guide the next medical revolution, truly introducing ML into neuroimaging.

References

1. Staartjes VE, Stumpo V, Kernbach JM, et al. Machine learning in neurosurgery: a global survey. Acta Neurochir. 2020;162(12):3081–91. https://doi.org/10.1007/s00701-020-04532-1.
2. Akeret K, Stumpo V, Staartjes VE, et al. Topographic brain tumor anatomy drives seizure risk and enables machine learning based prediction. NeuroImage Clin. 2020;28:102506.
3. Lubicz B, Levivier M, Francois O, Thoma P, Sadeghi N, Collignon L, Baleriaux D. Sixty-four-row multisection CT angiography for detection and evaluation of ruptured intracranial aneurysms: interobserver and intertechnique reproducibility. Am J Neuroradiol. 2007;28(10):1949–55.
4. Park A, Chute C, Rajpurkar P, et al. Deep learning–assisted diagnosis of cerebral aneurysms using the HeadXNet model. JAMA Netw Open. 2019;2(6):e195600.
5. Razzak MI, Naz S, Zaib A. Deep learning for medical image processing: overview, challenges and future. In: Dey N, Ashour A, Borra S, editors. Classification in BioApps. Lecture notes in computational vision and biomechanics, vol. 30. Cham: Springer; 2017.
6. Song J, Yin Y, Wang H, Chang Z, Liu Z, Cui L. A review of original articles published in the emerging field of radiomics. Eur J Radiol. 2020;127:108991.
7. Swinburne NC, Schefflein J, Sakai Y, Oermann EK, Titano JJ, Chen I, Tadayon S, Aggarwal A, Doshi A, Nael K. Machine learning for semiautomated classification of glioblastoma, brain metastasis and central nervous system lymphoma using magnetic resonance advanced imaging. Ann Transl Med. 2019; 7(11):232.
8. Zacharaki EI, Wang S, Chawla S, Soo Yoo D, Wolf R, Melhem ER, Davatzikos C. Classification of brain tumor type and grade using MRI texture and shape in a machine learning scheme. Magn Reson Med. 2009;62(6):1609–18.
9. Zhang M, Young GS, Chen H, Li J, Qin L, McFaline-Figueroa JR, Reardon DA, Cao X, Wu X, Xu X. Deep-learning detection of cancer metastases to the brain on MRI. J Magn Reson Imaging. 2020;52(4):1227–36.
10. Djuric U, Zadeh G, Aldape K, Diamandis P. Precision histology: how deep learning is poised to revitalize histomorphology for personalized cancer care. NPJ Precis Oncol. 2017;1(1):22.
11. LeCun Y, Bengio Y, Hinton G. Deep learning. Nature. 2015;521(7553):436–44.
12. Lundervold AS, Lundervold A. An overview of deep learning in medical imaging focusing on MRI. Z Med Phys. 2019;29(2):102–27.
13. Bacchi S, Zerner T, Dongas J, Asahina AT, Abou-Hamden A, Otto S, Oakden-Rayner L, Patel S. Deep learning in the detection of high-grade glioma recurrence using multiple MRI sequences: a pilot study. J Clin Neurosci. 2019;70:11–3.
14. Deepak S, Ameer PM. Brain tumor classification using deep CNN features via transfer learning. Comput Biol Med. 2019;111:103345.
15. Sun L, Zhang S, Chen H, Luo L. Brain tumor segmentation and survival prediction using multimodal MRI scans with deep learning. Front Neurosci. 2019;13:810.
16. Hainc N, Mannil M, Anagnostakou V, Alkadhi H, Blüthgen C, Wacht L, Bink A, Husain S, Kulcsár Z, Winklhofer S. Deep learning based detection of intracranial aneurysms on digital subtraction angiography: a feasibility study. Neuroradiol J. 2020;33(4):311–7.
17. Shi Z, Hu B, Schoepf UJ, Savage RH, Dargis DM, Pan CW, Li XL, Ni QQ, Lu GM, Zhang LJ. Artificial intelligence in the management of intracranial aneurysms: current status and future perspectives. Am J Neuroradiol. 2020;41(3):373–9.
18. Sichtermann T, Faron A, Sijben R, Teichert N, Freiherr J, Wiesmann M. Deep learning–based detection of intracranial aneurysms in 3D TOF-MRA. Am J Neuroradiol. 2019;40(1):25–32.
19. Huang J, Shen H, Wu J, Hu X, Zhu Z, Lv X, Liu Y, Wang Y. Spine explorer: a deep learning based fully automated program for efficient and reliable quantifications of the vertebrae and discs on sagittal lumbar spine MR images. Spine J. 2020;20(4):590–9.
20. Jamaludin A, Kadir T, Zisserman A. SpineNet: automated classification and evidence visualization in spinal MRIs. Med Image Anal. 2017;41:63–73.
21. Hollon TC, et al. Near real-time intraoperative brain tumor diagnosis using stimulated Raman histology and deep neural networks. Nat Med. 2020;26(1):52–8.
22. Avanzo M, Wei L, Stancanello J, Vallières M, Rao A, Morin O, Mattonen SA, El Naqa I. Machine and deep learning methods for radiomics. Med Phys. 2020;47(5):e185–202. https://doi.org/10.1002/mp.13678.
23. Lambin P, et al. Radiomics: the bridge between medical imaging and personalized medicine. Nat Rev Clin Oncol. 2017;14(12): 749–62.
24. Mayerhoefer ME, Materka A, Langs G, Häggström I, Szczypiński P, Gibbs P, Cook G. Introduction to Radiomics. J Nucl Med. 2020;61(4):488–95.
25. Dhillon A, Verma GK. Convolutional neural network: a review of models, methodologies and applications to object detection. Prog Artif Intell. 2020;9(2):85–112.
26. Gui J, Sun Z, Wen Y, Tao D, Ye J. A review on generative adversarial networks: algorithms, theory, and applications. arXiv:2001.06937 [cs, stat]. 2020.
27. Yi X, Walia E, Babyn P. Generative adversarial network in medical imaging: a review. Med Image Anal. 2019;58:101552.
28. Havaei M, Davy A, Warde-Farley D, Biard A, Courville A, Bengio Y, Pal C, Jodoin P-M, Larochelle H. Brain tumor segmentation with deep neural networks. Med Image Anal. 2017;35:18–31.
29. Lee JH, Han IH, Kim DH, Yu S, Lee IS, Song YS, Joo S, Jin C-B, Kim H. Spine computed tomography to magnetic resonance image synthesis using generative adversarial networks: a preliminary study. J Korean Neurosurg Soc. 2020;63(3):386–96.
30. Li Y, Sixou B, Peyrin F. A review of the deep learning methods for medical images super resolution problems. IRBM. 2020;42(2):120–33.
31. Toga AW, Thompson PM. The role of image registration in brain mapping. Image Vis Comput. 2001;19(1–2):3–24.
32. Topol EJ. High-performance medicine: the convergence of human and artificial intelligence. Nat Med. 2019;25(1):44–56.
33. Hammernik K, Knoll F. Machine learning for image reconstruction. Handbook of medical image computing and computer assisted intervention. Amsterdam: Elsevier; 2020. p. 25–64.
34. Rizzo S, Botta F, Raimondi S, Origgi D, Fanciullo C, Morganti AG, Bellomi M. Radiomics: the facts and the challenges of image analysis. Eur Radiol Exp. 2018;2(1):36.
35. van Timmeren JE, Cester D, Tanadini-Lang S, Alkadhi H, Baessler B. Radiomics in medical imaging—"how-to" guide and critical reflection. Insights Imaging. 2020;11(1):91.

36. Kocak B, Durmaz ES, Ates E, Kilickesmez O. Radiomics with artificial intelligence: a practical guide for beginners. Diagn Interv Radiol. 2019;25(6):485–95.
37. Zwanenburg A, Leger S, Vallières M, Löck S. Image biomarker standardisation initiative. Radiology. 2020;295(2):328–38.
38. Lambin P, Rios-Velazquez E, Leijenaar R, et al. Radiomics: extracting more information from medical images using advanced feature analysis. Eur J Cancer. 2012;48(4):441–6.
39. Brownlee J. How do convolutional layers work in deep learning neural networks? Machine Learning Mastery; 2019.
40. Convolutional neural networks—basics · machine learning notebook. https://mlnotebook.github.io/post/CNN1/. Accessed 27 Jan 2021.
41. Yamashita R, Nishio M, Do RKG, Togashi K. Convolutional neural networks: an overview and application in radiology. Insights Imaging. 2018;9(4):611–29.
42. Brownlee J. A gentle introduction to padding and stride for convolutional neural networks. Machine Learning Mastery; 2019.
43. Dumoulin V, Visin F. A guide to convolution arithmetic for deep learning. arXiv:1603.07285 [cs, stat]. 2018.
44. Brownlee J. Difference between a batch and an epoch in a neural network. Machine Learning Mastery; 2018.
45. Dutta-Roy T. Medical image analysis with deep learning—II. In: Medium. 2018. https://medium.com/@taposhdr/medical-image-analysis-with-deep-learning-ii-166532e964e6. Accessed 27 Jan 2021.
46. 7 types of activation functions in neural networks: how to choose? In: MissingLink.ai. https://missinglink.ai/guides/neural-network-concepts/7-types-neural-network-activation-functions-right/. Accessed 28 Jan 2021.
47. Agarwal M. Back propagation in convolutional neural networks—intuition and code. In: Medium. 2020. https://becominghuman.ai/back-propagation-in-convolutional-neural-networks-intuition-and-code-714ef1c38199. Accessed 27 Jan 2021.
48. Backpropagation - Wikipedia. Accessed 26 Sep 2021. https://en.wikipedia.org/wiki/Backpropagation.
49. Brownlee J. Loss and loss functions for training deep learning neural networks. Machine Learning Mastery; 2019.
50. Brownlee J. How to configure the learning rate when training deep learning neural networks. Machine Learning Mastery; 2019.
51. Doshi S. Various optimization algorithms for training neural network. In: Medium. 2020. https://towardsdatascience.com/optimizers-for-training-neural-network-59450d71caf6. Accessed 27 Jan 2021
52. Peixeiro M. The 3 best optimization methods in neural networks. In: Medium. 2020. https://towardsdatascience.com/the-3-best-optimization-methods-in-neural-networks-40879c887873. Accessed 27 Jan 2021.
53. Smolyakov V. Neural network optimization algorithms. In: Medium. 2018. https://towardsdatascience.com/neural-network-optimization-algorithms-1a44c282f61d. Accessed 27 Jan 2021.
54. Soydaner D. A comparison of optimization algorithms for deep learning. Int J Patt Recogn Artif Intell. 2020;34(13):2052013.
55. MLTut. What Is Stochastic Gradient Descent- A Super Easy Complete Guide! 2020. https://www.mltut.com/stochastic-gradient-descent-a-super-easy-complete-guide/.
56. Bushaev V. Stochastic gradient descent with momentum. In: Medium. 2017. https://towardsdatascience.com/stochastic-gradient-descent-with-momentum-a84097641a5d. Accessed 28 Jan 2021.
57. Deep learning: which loss and activation functions should I use? | By Stacey Ronaghan | towards data science. https://towardsdatascience.com/deep-learning-which-loss-and-activation-functions-should-i-use-ac02f1c56aa8. Accessed 28 Jan 2021.
58. Analytics Vidhya. Regularization Techniques | Regularization In Deep Learning. 2018. https://www.analyticsvidhya.com/blog/2018/04/fundamentals-deep-learning-regularization-techniques/.
59. Ahmed KB, Hall LO, Goldgof DB, Liu R, Gatenby RA. Fine-tuning convolutional deep features for MRI based brain tumor classification. In: Armato SG, Petrick NA, editors. Orlando, Florida, United States. 2017. p 101342E.
60. Tajbakhsh N, Shin JY, Gurudu SR, Hurst RT, Kendall CB, Gotway MB, Liang J. Convolutional neural networks for medical image analysis: full training or fine tuning? IEEE Trans Med Imaging. 2016;35(5):1299–312.
61. Data Augmentation | How to Use Deep Learning When You Have Limited Data. Accessed 26 Sep 2021. https://nanonets.com/blog/data-augmentation-how-to-use-deep-learning-when-you-have-limited-data-part-2/.
62. Hinton GE, Srivastava N, Krizhevsky A, Sutskever I, Salakhutdinov RR. Improving neural networks by preventing co-adaptation of feature detectors. arXiv:1207.0580 [cs]. 2012.
63. Srivastava N, Hinton G, Krizhevsky A, Sutskever I, Salakhutdinov R. Dropout: a simple way to prevent neural networks from overfitting. J Mach Learn Res. 2014;15(1):1929–58.
64. Wu H, Gu X. Towards dropout training for convolutional neural networks. Neural Netw. 2015;71:1–10.
65. Murugan P, Durairaj S. Regularization and optimization strategies in deep convolutional neural network. arXiv:1712.04711 [cs]. 2017.
66. Nagpal A. L1 and L2 regularization methods. In: Medium. 2017. https://towardsdatascience.com/l1-and-l2-regularization-methods-ce25e7fc831c. Accessed 28 Jan 2021.
67. Ioffe S, Szegedy C. Batch normalization: accelerating deep network training by reducing internal covariate shift. arXiv:1502.03167 [cs]. 2015.
68. Despotović I, Goossens B, Philips W. MRI segmentation of the human brain: challenges, methods, and applications. Comput Math Methods Med. 2015;2015:1–23.
69. Ji S, Xu W, Yang M, Yu K. 3D convolutional neural networks for human action recognition. IEEE Trans Pattern Anal Mach Intell. 2013;35(1):221–31.
70. Singh SP, Wang L, Gupta S, Goli H, Padmanabhan P, Gulyás B. 3D deep learning on medical images: a review. arXiv:2004.00218 [cs, eess, q-bio]. 2020.
71. Zhuang F, Qi Z, Duan K, Xi D, Zhu Y, Zhu H, Xiong H, He Q. A comprehensive survey on transfer Learning. arXiv:1911.02685 [cs, stat]. 2020.
72. Mehrotra R, Ansari MA, Agrawal R, Anand RS. A transfer learning approach for AI-based classification of brain tumors. Mach Learn Appl. 2020;2:100003.
73. Liu R, Hall LO, Goldgof DB, Zhou M, Gatenby RA, Ahmed KB. Exploring deep features from brain tumor magnetic resonance images via transfer learning. In: 2016 international joint conference on neural networks (IJCNN). IEEE, Vancouver, BC, Canada, 2016. p. 235–42.
74. Chelghoum R. Transfer learning using convolutional neural network architectures for brain tumor classification from MRI images.
75. Khan A, Sohail A, Zahoora U, Qureshi AS. A survey of the recent architectures of deep convolutional neural networks. Artif Intell Rev. 2020;53(8):5455–516.
76. Goodfellow IJ, Pouget-Abadie J, Mirza M, Xu B, Warde-Farley D, Ozair S, Courville A, Bengio Y Generative adversarial networks. arXiv:1406.2661 [cs, stat]. 2014.

77. Lan L, You L, Zhang Z, Fan Z, Zhao W, Zeng N, Chen Y, Zhou X. Generative adversarial networks and its applications in biomedical informatics. Front Public Health. 2020;8:164.
78. Montagnon E, Cerny M, Cadrin-Chênevert A, Hamilton V, Derennes T, Ilinca A, Vandenbroucke-Menu F, Turcotte S, Kadoury S, Tang A. Deep learning workflow in radiology: a primer. Insights Imaging. 2020;11(1):22.
79. Mok TCW, Chung ACS. Learning data augmentation for brain tumor segmentation with coarse-to-fine generative adversarial networks. arXiv:180511291 [cs]. 2019; 11383:70–80.
80. Nalepa J, Marcinkiewicz M, Kawulok M. Data augmentation for brain-tumor segmentation: a review. Front Comput Neurosci. 2019;13:83.
81. Yang Q, Liu Y, Chen T, Tong Y. Federated machine Learning: concept and applications. arXiv:1902.04885 [cs]. 2019.
82. Kotsiantis S, Zaharakis I, Pintelas P, et al. Supervised machine learning: a review of classification techniques. Emerging Artificial Intelligence Applications in Computer Engineering. 2007;160(1):3–24.
83. Zhang H, Dong B. A review on deep learning in medical image reconstruction. arXiv:1906.10643 [physics]. 2019.
84. Schramm G, Rigie D, Vahle T, Rezaei A, Van Laere K, Shepherd T, Nuyts J, Boada F. Approximating anatomically-guided PET reconstruction in image space using a convolutional neural network. NeuroImage. 2021;224:117399.
85. Yan Y, Dahmani L, Ren J, et al. Reconstructing lost BOLD signal in individual participants using deep machine learning. Nat Commun. 2020;11(1):5046.
86. Kidoh M, Shinoda K, Kitajima M, Isogawa K, Nambu M, Uetani H, Morita K, Nakaura T, Yamashita Y, Yamashita Y. Deep learning based noise reduction for brain MR imaging: tests on phantoms and healthy volunteers. Magn Reson Med Sci. 2020; 19(3):195–206.
87. Antun V, Renna F, Poon C, Adcock B, Hansen AC. On instabilities of deep learning in image reconstruction and the potential costs of AI. Proc Natl Acad Sci U S A. 2020;117(48):30088–95.
88. Fan G, Liu H, Wu Z, Li Y, Feng C, Wang D, Luo J, Wells WM, He S. Deep learning–based automatic segmentation of lumbosacral nerves on CT for spinal intervention: a translational study. Am J Neuroradiol. 2019;40(6):1074–81.
89. Nie D, Cao X, Gao Y, Wang L, Shen D. Estimating CT image from MRI data using 3D fully convolutional networks. In: Deep learning and data labeling for medical applications—1st international workshop, LABELS 2016, and 2nd international workshop, DLMIA 2016 held in conjunction with MICCAI 2016, proceedings. 2016. https://doi.org/10.1007/978-3-319-46976-8_18.
90. Staartjes VE, Seevinck PR, Vandertop WP, van Stralen M, Schröder ML. Magnetic resonance imaging–based synthetic computed tomography of the lumbar spine for surgical planning: a clinical proof-of-concept. Neurosurg Focus. 2021;50(1):E13.
91. Liu C, Wu X, Yu X, Tang Y, Zhang J, Zhou J. Fusing multi-scale information in convolution network for MR image super-resolution reconstruction. Biomed Eng Online. 2018;17(1):114.
92. Estienne T, Lerousseau M, Vakalopoulou M, et al. Deep learning-based concurrent brain registration and tumor segmentation. Front Comput Neurosci. 2020;14:15.
93. Fan J, Cao X, Yap P-T, Shen D. BIRNet: brain image registration using dual-supervised fully convolutional networks. Med Image Anal. 2019;54:193–206.
94. Chen L, Bentley P, Rueckert D. Fully automatic acute ischemic lesion segmentation in DWI using convolutional neural networks. NeuroImage Clin. 2017;15:633–43.
95. Bennai MT, Guessoum Z, Mazouzi S, Cormier S, Mezghiche M. A stochastic multi-agent approach for medical-image segmentation: application to tumor segmentation in brain MR images. Artif Intell Med. 2020;110:101980.
96. Laukamp KR, Thiele F, Shakirin G, Zopfs D, Faymonville A, Timmer M, Maintz D, Perkuhn M, Borggrefe J. Fully automated detection and segmentation of meningiomas using deep learning on routine multiparametric MRI. Eur Radiol. 2019;29(1):124–32.
97. Zhou T, Canu S, Ruan S. Fusion based on attention mechanism and context constraint for multi-modal brain tumor segmentation. Comput Med Imaging Graph. 2020;86:101811.
98. Fan G, Liu H, Wang D, et al. Deep learning-based lumbosacral reconstruction for difficulty prediction of percutaneous endoscopic transforaminal discectomy at L5/S1 level: a retrospective cohort study. Int J Surg. 2020;82:162–9.
99. Shahzad R, Pennig L, Goertz L, Thiele F, Kabbasch C, Schlamann M, Krischek B, Maintz D, Perkuhn M, Borggrefe J. Fully automated detection and segmentation of intracranial aneurysms in subarachnoid hemorrhage on CTA using deep learning. Sci Rep. 2020;10(1):21799.
100. Duan H, Huang Y, Liu L, Dai H, Chen L, Zhou L. Automatic detection on intracranial aneurysm from digital subtraction angiography with cascade convolutional neural networks. Biomed Eng Online. 2019;18(1):110.
101. Nakao T, Hanaoka S, Nomura Y, Sato I, Nemoto M, Miki S, Maeda E, Yoshikawa T, Hayashi N, Abe O. Deep neural network-based computer-assisted detection of cerebral aneurysms in MR angiography. J Magn Reson Imaging. 2018;47(4):948–53.
102. Bhandari A, Koppen J, Agzarian M. Convolutional neural networks for brain tumour segmentation. Insights Imaging. 2020;11(1):77.
103. Lao J, Chen Y, Li Z-C, Li Q, Zhang J, Liu J, Zhai G. A deep Learning-based radiomics model for prediction of survival in glioblastoma multiforme. Sci Rep. 2017;7(1):10353.

Machine Learning-Based Radiomics in Neuro-Oncology

18

Felix Ehret, David Kaul, Hans Clusmann, Daniel Delev, and Julius M. Kernbach

18.1 Introduction

With synergistic advances in the development of novel learning algorithms and the increasing availability of low-cost computation, artificial intelligence (AI) has conquered various fields in modern biomedical research. AI is commonly understood as the ambition to enable computers to behave in a human-like nature to solve a broad array of tasks. Machine learning (ML), which falls under the umbrella term of AI, can be understood as a technique that enables algorithms to learn inductively from data without being explicitly programmed and make predictions about new data. Deep learning (DL) is a subsequent branch of AI and ML, based on multilayered neural networks, which are well-suited to discover intricate patterns in high-dimensional data [1, 2]. Especially in data-rich disciplines, such as biomedical imaging or genetics, DL- or AI-based research has the potential to improve diagnostic and therapeutic methods in medicine. At the forefront of neuro-oncology and AI-research, the field of radiomics has emerged using non-invasive assessments of quantitative radiological biomarkers mined from complex imaging characteristics across various imaging modalities, such as magnetic resonance imaging (MRI) or positron emission tomography (PET), that are beyond human perception [3, 4]. The objective of this review is to provide an overview of common applications of ML- and DL-based radiomics in primary and secondary brain tumors and their implications for future research in the field.

F. Ehret
Berlin Institute of Health at Charité – Universitätsmedizin Berlin, Berlin, Germany

Charité – Universitätsmedizin Berlin, Corporate Member of Freie Universität Berlin and Humboldt-Universität zu Berlin, Department of Radiation Oncology, Berlin, Germany

European Cyberknife Center Munich, Munich, Germany

D. Kaul
Charité – Universitätsmedizin Berlin, Corporate Member of Freie Universität Berlin and Humboldt-Universität zu Berlin, Department of Radiation Oncology, Berlin, Germany

German Cancer Consortium (DKTK), Partner Site Berlin, German Cancer Research Center (DKFZ), Heidelberg, Germany

H. Clusmann
Department of Neurosurgery, Faculty of Medicine, RWTH Aachen University, Aachen, Germany

D. Delev · J. M. Kernbach (✉)
Department of Neurosurgery, Faculty of Medicine, RWTH Aachen University, Aachen, Germany

Neurosurgical Artificial Intelligence Laboratory Aachen (NAILA), RWTH Aachen University Hospital, Aachen, Germany
e-mail: jkernbach@ukaachen.de

18.2 Methodological Foundations

The term "radiomics" usually comprises processes and methods to extract quantitative variables from available imaging data [3, 4]. These values and features are usually beyond human perception and cannot be adequately utilized during clinical routine [3, 4]. Thus, a significant amount of obtained data and information are not incorporated into the reading of images. The overachieving objective of radiomics is to make full use of the obtained (quantitative) imaging data in a reproducible, ideally user-independent way to advance diagnostic testing and outcome prediction [3–6]. Radiomics can be subdivided into a supervised feature-based and a DL-based approach. Both analytical streams require various preprocessing steps, including intensity normalization, spatial resampling and smoothing, noise reduction, and de-confounding of scanner- and movement-introduced noise [5, 7].

In feature-based radiomics, mathematically pre-defined characteristics of varying complexity, ranging from shape features, including diameter, volume, or sphericity, and distributional features, including mean, median, entropy, skewness, and other histogram-based characteristics to complex textural features of contrast, energy, homogeneity and intensity, and higher-order features mined by computational

V. E. Staartjes et al. (eds.), *Machine Learning in Clinical Neuroscience*, Acta Neurochirurgica Supplement 134,
https://doi.org/10.1007/978-3-030-85292-4_18

transformations or filters are extracted and computationally selected [7]. These variables, known as agnostic features, usually include Haralick and Laws textures, wavelets, Laplacian transforms, Minowski functionals, and fractional dimensions [3]. These features complement the semantic annotations of radiologists. Semantic annotations are mostly used to describe imaging findings in a qualitative way [3, 4]. Such terms may refer to the tumor size, shape, location, vascularity, spiculation, necrosis, and lepidics and large efforts are being made to standardize the usage of these terms to avoid heterogeneity among imaging readings [3]. Before feature extraction, the respective regions of interest (ROI) must be identified manually, semi-automatically, or automatically. This process bears the risk of a user-dependent selection of ROI, potentially limiting the reproducibility of the obtained features and subsequent study results. Once a standardized approach of ROI selection is developed and applied, feature extraction can be realized. Today, several software options are available to extract features from imaging data, including many open-source tools [8–12]. As the amount of extracted features may be in the hundreds and, thus, often larger than the actual size of the study cohort, it is required to perform some form of feature selection to avoid model overfitting [3]. Feature selection commonly includes the elimination of features that highly correlate with each other or those that do not correlate with the study endpoint [3, 7, 13]. In general, feature selection is divided into supervised and unsupervised methodologies and is described in detail elsewhere [7]. After the features have been selected, they can be used for the model generation to assess the respective research question.

In contrast, DL-based radiomics can automatically extract relevant granular features at different levels of abstraction using complex network architectures with multiple hierarchical layers, including convolutional layer designs [7, 14]. Thus, a manual or semi-automatic segmentation of the ROI is not necessary. The network layers are identifying and extracting the relevant features without prior input. However, this approach demands larger datasets compared to the classic feature-based radiomics approach and, thus, may have a limited applicability in neuro-oncology [7]. Both approaches, feature- and DL-based radiomics have been successfully applied in various cancer imaging studies showing promising results for future implementation in daily clinical routine [6]. Radiomics can be an effective way to leverage imaging data to improve patient care, risk stratification, and treatment planning [4, 6]. Current challenges, especially in the field of neuro-oncology, comprise the lack of methodological standardization in regard to image acquisition, feature extraction and selection, availability of multicenter datasets and, therefore, reproducibility [4, 6, 13].

18.3 Recent Implications for Neuro-Oncology

DL-based radiomics have recently made remarkable progress along with advances in biomedical imaging, most notable in central nervous system (CNS) neoplasms. Gliomas are the most common primary brain tumors. Pathologic grading is made according to the WHO classification and ranges from grade I to IV. Grade IV gliomas, including glioblastomas (GB), have an extremely poor prognosis and dismal overall survival [15, 16]. As secondary brain tumors, cerebral metastases pose another considerable neurooncological challenge. A third of all patients with solid tumors will eventually develop brain metastases (BM), with often subsequent clinical deficits and need for treatment [17, 18]. In total, approximately 170,000 patients are annually diagnosed with cerebral metastases in the USA alone [19–21]. Clinical diagnostics and treatment monitoring for both metastatic and primary brain tumors routinely include MRI studies, and thus generate large imaging datasets containing data from the initial diagnosis to follow-up imaging. ML and DL are well-suited and increasingly used for radiomic analysis in primary and secondary brain tumors leading to numerous high-quality studies and literature reviews [22–25]. As lesion delineation is explicitly required before any radiomic analysis, we also include DL-based studies for tumor identification and segmentation in our review. Common applications include outcome prediction (e.g. survival, local control), discrimination between primary and secondary tumors, as well as between progression and pseudo-progression, and molecular phenotyping, envisioned in the field of radiogenomics. The results of respective studies and analyses are depicted herein.

18.4 Automated Tumor Segmentation

Accurate lesion segmentation of both primary and secondary brain tumors is essential for radiomic analyses. A variety of methodological approaches have been proposed so far, ranging from manual delineation to semi-automated methods and user-independent DL methods. Manual or semi-automated segmentation performed by experienced neuroradiologists and clinicians is often time-consuming and subject to a high rate of inter-rater variability [26, 27]. Ideally, fully-automated segmentations should reliably detect a tumor or peritumoral areas as regions of interest on standard imaging data and accurately contour them to mitigate user variability. Various studies have since explored ML- or DL-based automated segmentation in primary and secondary brain tumors [28–34]. Advances in automated segmentation tools have been facilitated by the release of large public databases such as The Cancer Imaging Archive (TCIA) and further accelerated by the annual Multimodal Brain Tumor Image Segmentation Benchmark (BraTS) challenge, which provided a well-accepted platform for the development and critical evaluation of novel algorithms [35–37]. With high reported performances, DL-based methods have since surpassed the more traditional segmentation approaches [37].

Among other highly competitive DL methods, convolutional neural networks (CNNs) gained popularity based on their tremendous success in complex image analysis [1]. By maintaining local topological relationships between layers, CNNs are well-suited to perform highly complex image recognition tasks by leveraging and preserving local image relations and low-level abstraction. With their success in the ImageNet Challenge, CNNs are now considered the benchmark in many fields, including image segmentation and radiomics [32, 38–41]. For instance, the DeepMedic 3D-CNN was successfully applied to multimodal MRI data for the segmentation of brain metastases and glioma [40]. The applied network structure achieved a fair model performance, with a promising DICE similarity coefficient of 0.79 [40]. By adding an additional sub-path with larger convolutional filters, the tweaked DeepMedic network used by Liu and colleagues to contour metastases, with a dedicated focus on metastases with less than 1.5 cc, achieved a mean DICE of 0.67 [32]. Different model architectures, such as the inception module-based GoogLeNet, were previously applied to detect and segment brain metastases [33, 42]. Results were grouped by the number of brain metastases (1–3, 4–10, >10 lesions per patient) in a cohort of 156 patients, with the network achieving overall DICE scores of 0.76, 0.83, and 0.78, respectively [33]. Curated by the BraTs Challenge, an increased number of the state-of-the-art segmentation algorithms specifically for low- and high-grade glioma was proposed. Successful model architectures included 2D-convolutions, as well as fully-connected multi-scale CNNs with 3D-convolutions [28, 43–45]. Based on the in 2015 introduced U-Net Structure, the segmentation performance of the complete tumor, core, and enhancing area, successively increased, reaching promising DICE scores in the BraTs 2017 competition of 0.89, 0.79 and 0.73, respectively [46, 47]. Building upon U-Net, the encoder–decoder architectures were subsequently modified with the addition of residual connections, densely connected layers, second decoder implementations, or different loss functions, e.g. DICE or focal loss [14, 48–53]. The winning approach of the 2020 challenge implemented an ensemble-based “no new net” U-Net (nnU-Net) architecture achieving highest DICE scores of 0.88, 0.85, and 0.82 for the whole tumor, tumor core, and enhancing tumor, respectively [36].

18.5 Molecular Phenotyping and Radiogenomics

Radiomics has advanced our understanding of neuro-oncology by seeking associations between the imaging domain and other disciplines, and hence evolved into a vital part of multi-omics. Perhaps most intriguing is the combination of radiomic image analyses with genetic or mutational expression patterns, which—depending on the source—has been coined the field of radiogenomics [54, 55]. Given the high clinical relevance of molecular biomarkers and the potential of providing non-invasive in vivo characterizations of molecular heterogeneity, radiogenomics has since advanced diagnostics and treatment stratification of patients with primary and secondary brain tumors [56].

In glioma radiogenomics, the non-invasive prediction of molecular markers includes clinically relevant targets such as the isocitrate dehydrogenase (IDH) genotype, the O^6-methylguanine-DNA methyltransferase (MGMT) promoter methylation status, or the 1p19q codeletion. Based on the TCIA dataset, Lu and colleagues successfully applied a three-level ML-framework based upon support vector machines to predict IDH genotype and 1p19q-status from MRI data achieving accuracies of 88.9–91.7% and 80%, respectively [57]. Chang et al. applied CNNs to conventional MRI of 259 patients with glioma yielding classification accuracies of 94% for IDH mutation status, 92% for 1p19q codeletion, and 83% for MGMT promoter methylation [58]. DL-implementations such as multimodal 3D-DenseNet architectures reached comparable classification accuracy regarding IDH mutation status of 84.6% in The Cancer Genome Atlas (TCGA) data set [59]. While most studies focus on conventional MRI data, other sequences, including texture analysis of diffusion tensor imaging or different imaging modalities such as *O*-(2-[^{18}F] fluoroethyl)-L-tyrosine (FET)-PET have been investigated [60–64]. For instance, Lohmann and colleagues predicted the IDH genotype with an evaluated accuracy of 86% in a tenfold cross-validated logistic regression model in 86 glioma patients based on combined FET-PET/MRI radiomic parameters [62].

Molecular subtypes and mutation status of secondary brain tumors are equally crucial given the recent developments in the field of targeted therapies. While lung cancer often bears a dismal prognosis, several molecular targets have been identified in the last years, which fostered the development of targeted drugs to exploit altered cellular pathways [65, 66]. One target of particular interest is the epidermal growth factor receptor (EGFR). It has been shown that patients with respective mutations show improved survival after treatment with EGFR-associated tyrosine kinase inhibitors [65–67]. Ahn et al. extracted radiomic features from T1 contrast-enhanced MRI scans of 61 lung cancer patients with 210 BM to predict the EGFR mutation status [68]. Twenty-nine patients in the study cohort had a confirmed EGFR mutation and six cases of SCLC were included, the rest were NSCLC patients [68]. Notably, mutation status was obtained by lung biopsy samples, not by examination of the BM tissue. The authors tested four different classification systems with a random forest algorithm demonstrating the best overall performance (Area under the curve (AUC) 0.86) [68]. Another recent study by Park et al. followed a similar approach but limited their sampling to NSCLC patients and acquisition of the EGFR mutation status from BM tissue as well as from the primary lung tumor [69]. Twenty-three out of 28 samples were EGFR-mutant tumors [69]. Preoperative imaging sequences included T1 contrast-enhanced and diffusion tensor images (DTI). The best-performing algorithm (linear discriminant algorithm) with the five best-performing imaging features achieved an AUC of 0.73 [69]. The EGFR mutation discordance rate between the primary lung lesion and the BM was 12% [69]. Like the EGFR mutation in lung cancer, proto-oncogene B-Raf (BRAF) expression in malignant melanoma can be specifically addressed by targeted therapies, with subsequent improvements in overall survival [70]. Shofty et al. utilized imaging radiomics to predict the BRAF mutation status based on MRI data [71]. The study cohort comprised 25 BRAF positive and 29 negative BM from 53 patients [71]. With the implementation of an support vector machine (SVM), an AUC of 0.78 was achieved [71].

18.6 Prediction of Clinical Outcome

For both primary and secondary brain tumors, the prediction of clinical outcome in current practice is mainly based on clinical parameters, including functional impairment, age, tumor grade and histology, as well as the molecular fingerprint [72, 73]. Notably, radiomic features are currently not adopted in prognostic models regarding primary or secondary brain tumors. Simple feature-based parameters, such as tumor enhancing volume or maximal diameter, were shown to be predictive beyond clinical models, yet, more complex DL-based features may facilitate the prediction of outcome for both metastatic brain tumors as well as glioma even further [74, 75].

Recent radiomic models were proposed to predict overall survival (OS) in glioblastoma in a supervised as well as unsupervised fashion [76–80]. SVM based on features extracted from traditional and advanced MRI sequences predicting survival (stratified into a low-, medium-, and high-risk group) with an accuracy approaching 80% identified volume, angiogenesis, peritumoral infiltration, cell density, and distance to the ventricular system as most predictive features. Combining a supervised principal component analysis on 12,190 features yielding eleven radiomic variables combined with clinical data resulted in a fair performance of OS prediction (*C*-index of 0.696), surpassing the performance of the radiomic and clinical subset alone [78, 80]. A fully-automated DL-model applied by Li and colleagues based on multiparametric radiomic signatures achieved even better performance, with a *C*-index of 0.705, and stratified patients into a low- and high-risk group [76] . Using CNN-based transfer learning, Lao and colleagues combined clinical risk factors with six-deep-feature phenotypes based on least absolute shrinkage and selection operator (LASSO) Cox regressions achieving prediction of overall survival (*C*-index 0.739) [77]. In an unsupervised fashion, Rathore et al. identified rim-enhancing, irregular, and solid as three latent imaging phenotypes using *K*-means clustering, which showed differential clinical outcomes and corresponded to different expression levels of molecular characteristics [79].

ML- and DL-based radiomics may be a suitable tool for enhanced prediction of OS and local failure in secondary brain tumors as well. Studies have shown that various imaging features, including the associated perilesional edema, the presence of a necrotic core, and the degree of contrast enhancement, may influence local failure or even survival [81–83]. Cha et al. were the first to assess whether a CT-trained neural network can predict the treatment response after stereotactic radiosurgery [84]. The authors trained ten CNNs on 110 BM CT scans [84]. Responses were classified as “responders” (complete and partial response per RECIST 1.1) and “non-responders” (stable and progressive disease per RECIST 1.1) [84, 85]. The AUC of the ensemble networks ranged between 0.76 and 0.85 [84]. A more recent study by Mouraviev et al. showed that the addition of radiomics features of T1 contrast-enhanced and T2 fluid-attenuated inversion recovery (FLAIR) imaging data to a set of clinical, dosimetric, and structural radiographic features improves local response prediction after stereotactic radiosurgery [86]. In contrast to the previously described study, the RANO-BM criteria were applied [87]. While the non-radiomic features achieved an AUC of 0.66, the addition of the top twelve radiomic features improved the performance to an AUC of 0.79 [86]. In another study, 133 BM from 100 patients were analyzed to extract the top five radiomic features for response prediction after hypo-fractionated stereotactic radiation therapy [88]. The optimal radiomic feature composition achieved an AUC of 0.79 for the overall local failure prediction and 0.80 as well as 0.81 for the 6-month and 12-month local-failure prediction, respectively [88].

18.7 Discriminating Radiation Necrosis from Tumor Progression and Primary from Secondary Brain Lesions

With the general availability of radiosurgery and multimodal treatments of brain tumors in combination with radiotherapy, the incidence of radiation necrosis is rising and may be apparent in up to 26% of patients after treatment [89, 90]. This underlines the necessity for reliable and fast discrimination between radiation necrosis and tumor progression, given their often indistinguishable appearance on conventional MRI and CT scans [91]. The current gold standard for diagnosing a radiation injury or necrosis is the pathological examination of the suspicious brain area. However, even after biopsy, a risk for misdiagnosis may be present as lesions can be heterogeneous [92]. As the pathophysiological processes of a radiation injury and tumor growth substantially differ, differences may be hidden within the imaging data that cannot be perceived by the radiologist's eye. Thus, the application of radiomics to this persistent clinical problem may improve clinical decision making. So far, radiomic analyses on this matter have focused on plain MRI data but also investigated emerging functional imaging methods like the FET-PET [93–97]. An early feasibility study from Tiwari et al. investigated a set of radiomic features from T1 contrast-enhanced, T2 weighted, and T2 FLAIR MRI data of 43 patients to discriminate radiation injury from tumor progression [93]. The performance of the top five most discriminating features on each MRI sequence was tested against two senior neuroradiologist [93]. For the 15 test cases, the established SVM identified twelve cases correctly, whereas the neuroradiologists were correct in seven and eight cases, respectively [93]. A comparable approach was applied by Hettal et al., extracting radiomics features from T1 contrast-enhanced imaging to achieve an AUC of 0.83 [96]. Moreover, the prediction accuracy for radiation necrosis and tumor progression were 75% and 91%, respectively [96]. Peng et al. investigated 82 lesions of 66 patients who had received stereotactic radiosurgery with radiomics [94]. Again, T1 contrast-enhanced imaging and T2 FLAIR imaging were analyzed. With an optimized IsoSVM, an overall AUC of 0.81 was obtained, showing a sensitivity and specificity of 65% and 86%, respectively [94]. In contrast, the reviewing senior neuroradiologist was able to classify 73% of cases, with a high sensitivity of 97% and low specificity of 19% [94]. As for the plain MRI studies, Zhang et al. have chosen a slightly different approach as they implemented radiomic features from two different time points to investigate potential changes and robustness in radiomic features over time (so-called delta radiomics) [97]. In this study, 87 patients with pathologically confirmed radiation necrosis or tumor progression after GammaKnife-based radiosurgery were included [97]. With five delta radiomic features, an algorithm with an AUC of 0.73 was obtained [97]. Given these results, future studies implementing delta radiomics may help to identify more robust radiomic features that can improve future algorithms. This objective may also be reached by implementing functional imaging modalities like FET-PET, which is gaining more and more attention in neuro-oncology. In a recent study from Lohmann et al., 52 patients with pathologically confirmed recurrent brain metastasis (21 patients) and radiation injury (31 patients) were investigated by means of contrast-enhanced MRI and additional FET-PET data [98]. Radiomic features were extracted for both imaging modalities, and respective prediction models were created. While no independent test cohort was available, cross-validation with different numbers of subsamples was utilized [98]. The best results were obtained when MRI and FET-PET features were combined, as the AUC improved by 0.05–0.11 up to 0.86, depending on the validation method [98]. The highest achieved AUC during validation for the models using only contrast-enhanced MRI and FET-PET data were 0.77 and 0.79, respectively [98].

Not only in regard to subsequent medical treatment, the discrimination between primary and secondary brain lesions is of utmost importance for further patient management. This is especially relevant for the differentiation between a single BM and GB. So far, several studies have investigated the usefulness of ML and radiomics for this task [99–105]. Bae et al. applied seven traditional ML classifiers and multi-input deep neural networks on a cohort of 248 patients [102]. The deep neural network outperformed the best-performing traditional ML model, achieving an AUC 0.95 (vs. an AUC of 0.89), indicating the potential of DL for such a task [102]. Other authors tackling the same neurooncological challenge applied classic methods like SVM, random forest, naïve Bayes, ensemble classifiers, linear discriminant analysis, and *k*-nearest neighbor, achieving AUCs ranging from 0.80 to 0.98 [99, 101, 103, 104]. Swinburne et al. also included another important entity into their radiomic study: CNS lymphoma [105]. The trained multiclass model achieved an overall maximum accuracy of 0.69 in a small cohort of 26 patients [105]. The exclusive differentiation between CNS lymphoma and GB was investigated by Chen et al., applying three classifiers based on various radiomic features on a cohort of 138 patients, obtaining excellent AUCs ranging from 0.95 to 0.97 [106].

18.8 Conclusions

Medicine has evolved into an increasingly data-centered discipline. In this context, AI and ML are promising methods to analyze multi-dimensional data. Along with the steep rise in the development and advancements of AI, the field of radiomics has gained popularity across various aspects of neuro-oncology. Due to its inherent ability to intricately mine patterns beyond human perception, radiomics is placed at the crossroad between radiology and precision medicine. The retrieved information or imaging phenotypes may have far-reaching potential to revolutionize the diagnosis, patient stratification, treatment selection and monitoring. Despite the remarkable progress towards personalized medicine, analytical and practical challenges remain.

Overall, the published studies have shown promising results. However, due to the manifold of analytical knobs and choices, small sample sizes, and lacking external validation, they rarely remain comparable (Table 18.1). This is

Table 18.1 Selected summary of published ML studies in neuro-oncology

Author	Year	Sample size	Objective	Imaging modality (sequences)	Overall performance
Detection and automatized segmentation					
Charron et al. [40]	2018	182 patients with BM	Detection/segmentation	MRI (T1, T1 w/ CE, T2 FLAIR)	Sensitivity: 98% FPC: 7.2 DICE: 0.79
Liu et al. [32]	2017	490 patients with BM	Segmentation	MRI (T1 w/ CE)	DICE: 0.67 AUC: 0.98
Grøvik et al. [33]	2020	156 patients with BM	Detection/segmentation	MRI (T1 CUBE, T1 w/ CE CUBE, T1 BRAVO, T2 FLAIR)	AUC: 0.98 DICE: 0.79 Overall FPC: 8.2 FPC lesion ≤10 mm^3: 3.4
Zhou et al. [34]	2020	266 patients	Detection	MRI (T1 w/ CE)	Sensitivity: 81% PPV: 36% BM ≥6 mm: Sensitivity: 98% PPV: 36% BM <3 mm: Sensitivity: 15% PPV: 100%
Havaei et al. [43]	2017	BRATS 2013	Segmentation	MRI (T1, T1 w/ CE, T2, FLAIR)	DICE 0.88 (whole tumor), 0.79 (core), 0.73 (enhancing)
McKinley et al. [50]	2019	BRATS 2018	Segmentation	MRI (T1, T1 w/ CE, T2, FLAIR)	DICE 0.88 (whole tumor), 0.79 (core), 0.73 (enhancing)
Myronenko et al. [51]	2018	BRATS 2018	Segmentation	MRI (T1, T1 w/ CE, T2, FLAIR)	DICE 0.82 (whole tumor), 0.86 (core), 0.82 (enhancing)
Jiang et al. [48]	2019	BRATS 2019	Segmentation	MRI (T1, T1 w/ CE, T2, FLAIR)	DICE 0.88 (whole tumor), 0.83 (core), 0.83 (enhancing)
Isensee et al. [36]	2020	BRATS 2020	Segmentation	MRI (T1, T1 w/ CE, T2, FLAIR)	DICE 0.88 (whole tumor), 0.85 (core), 0.82 (enhancing)
Predicting treatment responses and survival					
Cha et al. [84]	2018	110 BM	Treatment response	CT w/ CE	AUC range for ensemble models: 0.76–0.85
Mouraviev et al. [86]	2020	408 BM in 87 patients	Treatment response	MRI (T1 w/ CE, T2 FLAIR)	AUC w/o RM: 0.66 AUC w/ RM: 0.79
Karami et al. [88]	2019	133 BM in 100 patients	Treatment response	MRI (T1 w/ CE, T2 FLAIR)	AUC w/ top five features: 0.79 AUC best performance: 0.82
Bhatia et al. [107]	2019	196 BM in 88 patients w/ MM	PFS and OS	MRI (T1 w/ CE)	LoG was significantly associated with OS in multivariate analysis ($p = 0.003$)
Macyszyn et al. [80]	2015	105 patients with GB	OS	MRI (T1, T1 w/ CE, T2, FLAIR, DTI)	Accuracy 0.82 (6 month), 0.83 (18 month)
Kickingereder et al. [78]	2016	119 patients with GB	PFS and OS	MRI (T1 w/ CE, FLAIR)	*C*-index 0.696, 0.637
Lao et al. [77]	2017	112 patients with GB	OS	MRI (T1, T1 w/ CE, T2, FLAIR)	*C*-index 0.739
Li et al. [76]	2017	92 patients with GB	OS	MRI (T1, T1 w/ CE, T2, FLAIR)	*C*-index 0.705

Discriminating radiation necrosis from tumor progression					
Tiwari et al. [93]	2016	58 patients	Discrimination	MRI (T1 w/ CE, T2, T2 FLAIR)	AUC RN: 0.79 AUC TR: 0.75
Hettal et al. [96]	2020	20 patients	Discrimination	MRI (T1 w/ CE)	AUC: 0.83 Prediction accuracy RN: 75% Prediction accuracy TR: 91%
Zhang et al. [97]	2018	87 patients	Discrimination	MRI (T1 w/ CE, T2, T2 FLAIR)	AUC: 0.73 Prediction accuracy RN: 0.58 Prediction accuracy TR: 0.78
Lohmann et al. [98]	2018	52 patients	Discrimination	MRI (T1 w/ CE), FET-PET	AUC: 0.96 Sensitivity: 0.85 Specificity: 0.96
Peng et al. [94]	2018	66 patients with 82 BM	Discrimination	MRI (T1 w/ CE, T2 FLAIR)	AUC: 0.81 Sensitivity: 0.65 Specificity: 0.86
Radiogenomics and molecular phenotyping					
Kniep et al. [108]	2019	189 patients	Subtype characterization (primary cancer)	MRI (T1, T1 w/ CE, T2 FLAIR)	AUC BC: 0.78 AUC MM: 0.82 AUC GI: 0.68 AUC SCLC: 0.76 AUC NSCLC: 0.64
Ahn et al. [68]	2020	61 patients with 210 BM	Subtype characterization (EGFR status NSCLC/SCLC)	MRI (T1 w/ CE)	AUC: 0.86 AUC BM >10 mm: 0.78 AUC BM ≤10 mm: 0.89
Park et al. [69]	2020	51 patients with 99 BM	Subtype characterization (EGFR status NSCLC)	MRI (T1 w/ CE, DTI)	AUC: 0.73
Shofty et al. [71]	2020	53 patients with 54 BM	Subtype characterization (BRAF status MM)	MRI (T1 w/ CE)	AUC: 0.78
Zhang et al. [109]	2020	144 patients with 302 BM	Subtype characterization (NSCLC: AD vs. SCC)	CT w/ CE	AUC: 0.82
Li et al. [110]	2018	193 patients with GB	MGMT methylation	MRI (T1w, T1c, T2w, FLAIR)	AUC: 0.88
Wei et al. [111]	2018	105 patients with WHO II–IV glioma	MGMT methylation	MRI (T1c, FLAIR, ADC)	AUC: 0.902
Drabycz et al. [112]	2010	103 patients with GB	MGMT methylation	MRI (T1w, T1c, T2w, FLAIR)	AUC: 0.71
Lu et al. [57]	2018	214 with LGG and GB	IDH, 1p/19q	MRI (T1w, T2w, FLAIR, ADC, DWI)	AUC: 0.88–0.91
Chang. et al. [58]	2018	259 with LGG and GB	IDH, 1p/19q, MGMT methylation	MRI (T1w, T1c, T2w, FLAIR)	Accuracy 0.94, 0.92, 0.83
Liang et al. [59]	2018	167 with LGG and GB	IDH, WHO-grade	MRI (T1w, T1c, T2w, FLAIR)	AUC: 85.7, 91.4%
Lohman et al. [62]	2018	84 WHO grade II–IV	IDH	FET-PET, PET/MRI	Accuracy 0.93
Verger et al. [63]	2018	90 patients with WHO II–IV glioma	IDH, 1p/19q	FET-PET	Accuracy 0.81
Vettermann et al. [64]	2019	341 patients	IDH	FET-PET	AUC: 0.87
Zhao et al. [61]	2019	52 patients	IDH	DTI	AUC: 0.72–0.93

(continued)

Table 18.1 (continued)

Author	Year	Sample size	Objective	Imaging modality (sequences)	Overall performance
Discriminating single BM, CNS lymphoma and GB					
Artzi et al. [104]	2019	439 patients (212 w/ GB, 227 w/ BM)	Discrimination (GB and BC, lung cancer, other BM)	MRI (T1 w/ CE)	AUC GB: 0.98 AUC BC: 0.81 AUC lung cancer: 0.83 AUC other BM: 0.57
Dong et al. [99]	2020	120 patients (60 GB and 60 BM)	Discrimination (GB and BM)	MRI (T1, T1 w/ CE, T2)	Accuracy: 0.56–0.64 Sensitivity: 0.39–0.78 Specificity: 0.50–0.89
Ortiz-Ramón et al. [100]	2020	100 patients (50 GB and 50 BM)	Discrimination (GB and BM)	MRI (T1)	AUC: 0.89 Sensitivity: 0.82 Specificity: 0.80
Qian et al. [101]	2019	412 patients (242 GB and 170 BM)	Discrimination (GB and BM)	MRI (T1 w/ CE, T2)	AUC: 0.90 Sensitivity: 0.79 Specificity: 0.87
Bae et al. [102]	2020	248 patients (159 GB and 89 BM)	Discrimination (GB and BM)	MRI (T1 w/ CE, T2)	AUC: 0.95 Sensitivity: 0.90 Specificity: 0.88
Chen et al. [103]	2019	134 patients (76 GB and 58 BM)	Discrimination (GB and BM)	MRI (T1 w/ CE)	AUC: 0.80 Sensitivity: 0.69 Specificity: 0.86
Swinburne et al. [105]	2019	26 patients (9 GB, 8 CNS lymphoma, 9 BM)	Discrimination (GB, CNS lymphoma and BM)	MRI (T1 w/ CE, T2 FLAIR, DWI, DCE, DSC, perfusion maps)	Overall accuracy: 0.69 AUC GB: 0.72 AUC BM: 0.83 AUC CNS lymphoma: 0.76 Accuracy GB/BM: 0.83 Accuracy BM/CNS lymphoma: 0.82 Accuracy CNS lymphoma/GB: 0.64
Chen et al. [106]	2020	138 patients (76 GB and 62 CNS lymphoma)	Discrimination (GB and CNS lymphoma)	MRI (T1, T1 w/ CE, T2, T2 FLAIR)	AUC: 0.97

BM brain metastasis, *DL* deep learning, *RM* radiomics, *NN* neural network, *FPC* false positive cases, *AUC* area under the curve, *DICE* dice similarity coefficient, *PPV* positive predictive value, *PFS* progression-free survival, *OS* overall survival, *LoG* Laplacian of Gaussian edge feature, *RN* radiation necrosis, *TR* tumor recurrence, *LGG* low grade glioma, *GB* glioblastoma, *MM* malignant melanoma, *GI* gastrointestinal cancer, *SCLC* small cell lung cancer, *NSCLC* non-small cell lung cancer, *AD* adenocarcinoma, *SCC* squamous cell carcinoma, *CNS* central nervous system, *CE* contrast-enhanced, *DTI* diffusion tensor imaging, *w/* with, *w/o* without, *DCE* dynamic contrast enhanced, *DWI* diffusion weighted imaging, *DSC* dynamic susceptibility contrast

particularly critical for insatiable data-hungry DL methods, which often require an extensive sample size beyond the applied patient cohort. Accordingly, simulation studies suggest to scale the minimum sample size to the problem and the applied method at hand [113, 114]. As many studies frame their objective as classification problems, for instance, MGMT promoter methylation versus non-methylated, imbalances between classes can cause additional bias and lead to poor generalizability [115]. Additionally, there is a paramount need for standardized image acquisition in radiomic analysis. Multiple studies addressed the impact of varying acquisition parameters, including sequence variations, image reconstruction, and scanner specifications, as well as the influence of different spatial resolutions and differences regarding 2D versus 3D analysis [116–120]. Various software implementations were introduced to unify the analytical workflow. For instance, the BraTS Toolkit offers a joint approach from Digital Imaging and Communications in Medicine (DICOM) to brain tumor segmentation. Furthermore, multiple open-source tools were introduced to allay inhibiting factors for successful implementation into clinical routine [9, 10, 121]. Despite their current limitations, the swift translation of ML- and DL-based radiomics into clinical practice will potentially provide a significant benefit to diagnostics and treatment monitoring in primary and secondary brain tumors. However, future multicenter studies will be essential to validate the robustness and generalizability of the respective methods.

Acknowledgements FE is participant in the BIH Charité Junior Clinician Scientist Program funded by the Charité – Universitätsmedizin Berlin and Berlin Institute of Health at Charité (BIH).

Funding JMK and DD are supported by the Bundesministerium für Bildung und Forschung (BMBF COMPLS3-022).

Conflicts of Interest/Competing Interests None of the authors has any conflict of interest to disclose.

DK received travel grants from Accuray and has served as an advisory board member for Novocure, no conflicts of interest with regard to the current work exist.

References

1. LeCun Y, Bengio Y, Hinton G. Deep learning. Nature. 2015;521(7553):436–44. https://doi.org/10.1038/nature14539.
2. Goodfellow I, Bengio Y, Courville A, Bengio Y. Deep learning, vol. 1. Cambridge: MIT Press; 2016.
3. Gillies RJ, Kinahan PE, Hricak H. Radiomics: images are more than pictures, they are data. Radiology. 2016;278(2):563–77. https://doi.org/10.1148/radiol.2015151169.
4. Aerts HJ. The potential of radiomic-based phenotyping in precision medicine: a review. JAMA Oncol. 2016;2(12):1636–42. https://doi.org/10.1001/jamaoncol.2016.2631.
5. Kumar V, Gu Y, Basu S, Berglund A, Eschrich SA, Schabath MB, Forster K, Aerts HJWL, Dekker A, Fenstermacher D, et al. Radiomics: the process and the challenges. Magn Reson Imaging. 2012;30(9):1234–48. https://doi.org/10.1016/j.mri.2012.06.010.
6. Bi WL, Hosny A, Schabath MB, Giger ML, Birkbak NJ, Mehrtash A, Allison T, Arnaout O, Abbosh C, Dunn IF, et al. Artificial intelligence in cancer imaging: clinical challenges and applications. CA Cancer J Clin. 2019;69(2):127–57. https://doi.org/10.3322/caac.21552.
7. Lohmann P, Galldiks N, Kocher M, Heinzel A, Filss CP, Stegmayr C, Mottaghy FM, Fink GR, Jon Shah N, Langen KJ. Radiomics in neuro-oncology: basics, workflow, and applications. Methods. 2021;188:112–21. https://doi.org/10.1016/j.ymeth.2020.06.003.
8. Szczypiński PM, Strzelecki M, Materka A, Klepaczko A. MaZda—a software package for image texture analysis. Comput Methods Programs Biomed. 2009;94(1):66–76. https://doi.org/10.1016/j.cmpb.2008.08.005.
9. Nioche C, Orlhac F, Boughdad S, Reuzé S, Goya-Outi J, Robert C, Pellot-Barakat C, Soussan M, Frouin F, Buvat I. LIFEx: a freeware for radiomic feature calculation in multimodality imaging to accelerate advances in the characterization of tumor heterogeneity. Cancer Res. 2018;78(16):4786–9. https://doi.org/10.1158/0008-5472.Can-18-0125.
10. van Griethuysen JJM, Fedorov A, Parmar C, Hosny A, Aucoin N, Narayan V, Beets-Tan RGH, Fillion-Robin JC, Pieper S, Aerts H. Computational radiomics system to decode the radiographic phenotype. Cancer Res. 2017;77(21):e104–7. https://doi.org/10.1158/0008-5472.Can-17-0339.
11. Zhang L, Fried DV, Fave XJ, Hunter LA, Yang J, Court LE. IBEX: an open infrastructure software platform to facilitate collaborative work in radiomics. Med Phys. 2015;42(3):1341–53. https://doi.org/10.1118/1.4908210.
12. Fedorov A, Beichel R, Kalpathy-Cramer J, Finet J, Fillion-Robin JC, Pujol S, Bauer C, Jennings D, Fennessy F, Sonka M, et al. 3D Slicer as an image computing platform for the Quantitative Imaging Network. Magn Reson Imaging. 2012;30(9):1323–41. https://doi.org/10.1016/j.mri.2012.05.001.
13. Yip SS, Aerts HJ. Applications and limitations of radiomics. Phys Med Biol. 2016;61(13):R150–66. https://doi.org/10.1088/0031-9155/61/13/r150.
14. He K, Zhang X, Ren S, Sun J. Deep residual learning for image recognition. In: 2016 IEEE conference on computer vision and pattern recognition (CVPR). 2016.
15. Surawicz TS, McCarthy BJ, Kupelian V, Jukich PJ, Bruner JM, Davis FG. Descriptive epidemiology of primary brain and CNS tumors: results from the Central Brain Tumor Registry of the United States, 1990-1994. Neuro Oncol. 1999;1(1):14–25. https://doi.org/10.1093/neuonc/1.1.14.
16. Ostrom QT, Cioffi G, Gittleman H, Patil N, Waite K, Kruchko C, Barnholtz-Sloan JS. CBTRUS statistical report: primary brain and other central nervous system tumors diagnosed in the United States in 2012-2016. Neuro Oncol. 2019;21(Suppl 5):v1–v100. https://doi.org/10.1093/neuonc/noz150.
17. Patchell RA. The management of brain metastases. Cancer Treat Rev. 2003;29(6):533–40. https://doi.org/10.1016/s0305-7372(03)00105-1.
18. Posner JB. Management of brain metastases. Rev Neurol (Paris). 1992;148(6–7):477–87.
19. Ellis TL, Neal MT, Chan MD. The role of surgery, radiosurgery and whole brain radiation therapy in the management of patients with metastatic brain tumors. Int J Surg Oncol. 2012;2012:952345. https://doi.org/10.1155/2012/952345.
20. Gavrilovic IT, Posner JB. Brain metastases: epidemiology and pathophysiology. J Neurooncol. 2005;75(1):5–14. https://doi.org/10.1007/s11060-004-8093-6.

21. Brem S, Panattil JG. An era of rapid advancement: diagnosis and treatment of metastatic brain cancer. Neurosurgery. 2005;57(5 Suppl):S5–9; discusssion S1-4. https://doi.org/10.1093/neurosurgery/57.suppl_5.s4-5.
22. Rudie JD, Rauschecker AM, Bryan RN, Davatzikos C, Mohan S. Emerging applications of artificial intelligence in neuro-oncology. Radiology. 2019;290(3):607–18. https://doi.org/10.1148/radiol.2018181928.
23. Zhou M, Scott J, Chaudhury B, Hall L, Goldgof D, Yeom KW, Iv M, Ou Y, Kalpathy-Cramer J, Napel S, et al. Radiomics in brain tumor: image assessment, quantitative feature descriptors, and machine-learning approaches. Am J Neuroradiol. 2018;39(2):208–16. https://doi.org/10.3174/ajnr.A5391.
24. Chaddad A, Kucharczyk MJ, Daniel P, Sabri S, Jean-Claude BJ, Niazi T, Abdulkarim B. Radiomics in glioblastoma: current status and challenges facing clinical implementation. Front Oncol. 2019;9:374. https://doi.org/10.3389/fonc.2019.00374.
25. Narang S, Lehrer M, Yang D, Lee J, Rao A. Radiomics in glioblastoma: current status, challenges and potential opportunities. Transl Cancer Res. 2016;5(4):383–97.
26. Odland A, Server A, Saxhaug C, Breivik B, Groote R, Vardal J, Larsson C, Bjørnerud A. Volumetric glioma quantification: comparison of manual and semi-automatic tumor segmentation for the quantification of tumor growth. Acta Radiol. 2015;56(11):1396–403. https://doi.org/10.1177/0284185114554822.
27. Joe BN, Fukui MB, Meltzer CC, Huang QS, Day RS, Greer PJ, Bozik ME. Brain tumor volume measurement: comparison of manual and semiautomated methods. Radiology. 1999;212(3):811–6. https://doi.org/10.1148/radiology.212.3.r99se22811.
28. Kamnitsas K, Ledig C, Newcombe VF, Simpson JP, Kane AD, Menon DK, Rueckert D, Glocker B. Efficient multi-scale 3D CNN with fully connected CRF for accurate brain lesion segmentation. Med Image Anal. 2017;36:61–78.
29. Bakas S, Zeng K, Sotiras A, Rathore S, Akbari H, Gaonkar B, Rozycki M, Pati S, Davatzikos C. GLISTRboost: combining multimodal MRI segmentation, registration, and biophysical tumor growth modeling with gradient boosting machines for glioma segmentation. Brainlesion: glioma, multiple sclerosis, stroke and traumatic brain injuries. BrainLes (Workshop). 2016;9556:144–55. https://doi.org/10.1007/978-3-319-30858-6_1.
30. Gooya A, Pohl KM, Bilello M, Cirillo L, Biros G, Melhem ER, Davatzikos C. GLISTR: glioma image segmentation and registration. IEEE Trans Med Imaging. 2012;31(10):1941–54. https://doi.org/10.1109/TMI.2012.2210558.
31. Pérez U, Arana E, Moratal D. Brain metastases detection algorithms in magnetic resonance imaging. IEEE Latin Am Trans. 2016;14(3):1109–14. https://doi.org/10.1109/TLA.2016.7459586.
32. Liu Y, Stojadinovic S, Hrycushko B, Wardak Z, Lau S, Lu W, Yan Y, Jiang SB, Zhen X, Timmerman R, et al. A deep convolutional neural network-based automatic delineation strategy for multiple brain metastases stereotactic radiosurgery. PLoS One. 2017;12(10):e0185844. https://doi.org/10.1371/journal.pone.0185844.
33. Grøvik E, Yi D, Iv M, Tong E, Rubin D, Zaharchuk G. Deep learning enables automatic detection and segmentation of brain metastases on multisequence MRI. J Magn Reson Imaging. 2020;51(1):175–82. https://doi.org/10.1002/jmri.26766.
34. Zhou Z, Sanders JW, Johnson JM, Gule-Monroe MK, Chen MM, Briere TM, Wang Y, Son JB, Pagel MD, Li J, et al. Computer-aided detection of brain metastases in T1-weighted MRI for stereotactic radiosurgery using deep learning single-shot detectors. Radiology. 2020;295(2):407–15. https://doi.org/10.1148/radiol.2020191479.
35. Clark K, Vendt B, Smith K, Freymann J, Kirby J, Koppel P, Moore S, Phillips S, Maffitt D, Pringle M, et al. The cancer imaging archive (TCIA): maintaining and operating a public information repository. J Digital imaging. 2013;26(6):1045–57. https://doi.org/10.1007/s10278-013-9622-7.
36. Isensee F, Jaeger PF, Full PM, Vollmuth P, Maier-Hein KH. nnU-Net for brain tumor segmentation. arXiv preprint arXiv:2011.00848. 2020.
37. Ghaffari M, Sowmya A, Oliver R. Automated brain tumor segmentation using multimodal brain scans: a survey based on models submitted to the BraTS 2012-2018 challenges. IEEE Rev Biomed Eng. 2020;13:156–68. https://doi.org/10.1109/rbme.2019.2946868.
38. Deng J, Dong W, Socher R, Li L, Li K, Fei-Fei L. ImageNet: a large-scale hierarchical image database. In: 2009 IEEE conference on computer vision and pattern recognition. 2009. p. 248–55.
39. Krizhevsky A, Sutskever I, Hinton GE. ImageNet classification with deep convolutional neural networks. In: CACM. 2017.
40. Charron O, Lallement A, Jarnet D, Noblet V, Clavier JB, Meyer P. Automatic detection and segmentation of brain metastases on multimodal MR images with a deep convolutional neural network. Comput Biol Med. 2018;95:43–54. https://doi.org/10.1016/j.compbiomed.2018.02.004.
41. López-Zorrilla A, de Velasco-Vázquez M, Serradilla-Casado O, Roa-Barco L, Graña M, Chyzhyk D, Price CC. Brain white matter lesion segmentation with 2D/3D CNN. Cham: Springer International Publishing; 2017.
42. Szegedy C, Wei L, Yangqing J, Sermanet P, Reed S, Anguelov D, Erhan D, Vanhoucke V, Rabinovich A. Going deeper with convolutions. In: 2015 IEEE conference on computer vision and pattern recognition (CVPR). 2015.
43. Havaei M, Davy A, Warde-Farley D, Biard A, Courville A, Bengio Y, Pal C, Jodoin PM, Larochelle H. Brain tumor segmentation with Deep Neural Networks. Med Image Anal. 2017;35:18–31. https://doi.org/10.1016/j.media.2016.05.004.
44. Pereira S, Pinto A, Alves V, Silva CA. Brain tumor segmentation using convolutional neural networks in MRI images. IEEE Trans Med Imaging. 2016;35(5):1240–51. https://doi.org/10.1109/tmi.2016.2538465.
45. Urban, G., Bendszus M, Hamprecht F, Kleesiek J. Multi-modal brain tumor segmentation using deep convolutional neuralnetworks. In: MICCAI multimodal brain tumor segmentation challenge (BraTS) 2014. 2014. p. 31–5.
46. Ronneberger O, Fischer P, Brox T. U-Net: convolutional networks for biomedical image segmentation. Cham: Springer International Publishing; 2015.
47. Isensee F, Kickingereder P, Wick W, Bendszus M, Maier-Hein KH. Brain tumor segmentation and radiomics survival prediction: contribution to the BRATS 2017 challenge. Cham: Springer International Publishing; 2018.
48. Jiang Z, Ding C, Liu M, Tao D. Two-stage cascaded U-net: 1st place solution to BraTS challenge 2019 segmentation task. In: Brainlesion: glioma, multiple sclerosis, stroke and traumatic brain injuries. Cham: Springer International Publishing; 2020.
49. Gao H, Zhuang L, van der Maaten L, Weinberger K. Densely connected convolutional networks. arXiv preprint arXiv:1608.06993. 2018.
50. McKinley R, Meier R, Wiest R. Ensembles of densely-connected CNNs with label-uncertainty for brain tumor segmentation. In: BrainLes@MICCAI. 2018.
51. Myronenko A. 3D MRI brain tumor segmentation using autoencoder regularization. In: BrainLes@MICCAI. 2018.
52. Lin T-Y, Goyal P, Girshick RB, He K, Dollár P. Focal loss for dense object detection. In: 2017 IEEE international conference on computer vision (ICCV). 2017. p. 2999–3007.
53. Drozdzal M, Vorontsov E, Chartrand G, Kadoury S, Pal C. The importance of skip connections in biomedical image segmentation. In: Deep learning and data labeling for medical applications. Cham: Springer; 2016. p. 179–87.

54. Beig N, Patel J, Prasanna P, Hill V, Gupta A, Correa R, Bera K, Singh S, Partovi S, Varadan V, et al. Radiogenomic analysis of hypoxia pathway is predictive of overall survival in glioblastoma. Sci Rep. 2018;8(1):7. https://doi.org/10.1038/s41598-017-18310-0.
55. Ellingson BM. Radiogenomics and imaging phenotypes in glioblastoma: novel observations and correlation with molecular characteristics. Curr Neurol Neurosci Rep. 2015;15(1):506. https://doi.org/10.1007/s11910-014-0506-0.
56. Louis DN, Perry A, Reifenberger G, von Deimling A, Figarella-Branger D, Cavenee WK, Ohgaki H, Wiestler OD, Kleihues P, Ellison DW. The 2016 World Health Organization classification of tumors of the central nervous system: a summary. Acta Neuropathol. 2016;131(6):803–20. https://doi.org/10.1007/s00401-016-1545-1.
57. Lu CF, Hsu FT, Hsieh KL, Kao YJ, Cheng SJ, Hsu JB, Tsai PH, Chen RJ, Huang CC, Yen Y, et al. Machine learning-based radiomics for molecular subtyping of gliomas. Clin Cancer Res. 2018;24(18):4429–36. https://doi.org/10.1158/1078-0432.Ccr-17-3445.
58. Chang P, Grinband J, Weinberg BD, Bardis M, Khy M, Cadena G, Su MY, Cha S, Filippi CG, Bota D, et al. Deep-learning convolutional neural networks accurately classify genetic mutations in gliomas. Am J Neuroradiol. 2018;39(7):1201–7. https://doi.org/10.3174/ajnr.A5667.
59. Liang S, Zhang R, Liang D, Song T, Ai T, Xia C, Xia L, Wang Y. Multimodal 3D DenseNet for IDH genotype prediction in gliomas. Genes (Basel). 2018;9(8):382. https://doi.org/10.3390/genes9080382.
60. Eichinger P, Alberts E, Delbridge C, Trebeschi S, Valentinitsch A, Bette S, Huber T, Gempt J, Meyer B, Schlegel J, et al. Diffusion tensor image features predict IDH genotype in newly diagnosed WHO grade II/III gliomas. Sci Rep. 2017;7(1):13396. https://doi.org/10.1038/s41598-017-13679-4.
61. Zhao J, Wang YL, Li XB, Hu MS, Li ZH, Song YK, Wang JY, Tian YS, Liu DW, Yan X, et al. Comparative analysis of the diffusion kurtosis imaging and diffusion tensor imaging in grading gliomas, predicting tumour cell proliferation and IDH-1 gene mutation status. J Neurooncol. 2019;141(1):195–203. https://doi.org/10.1007/s11060-018-03025-7.
62. Lohmann P, Lerche C, Bauer EK, Steger J, Stoffels G, Blau T, Dunkl V, Kocher M, Viswanathan S, Filss CP, et al. Predicting IDH genotype in gliomas using FET PET radiomics. Sci Rep. 2018;8(1):13328. https://doi.org/10.1038/s41598-018-31806-7.
63. Verger A, Stoffels G, Bauer EK, Lohmann P, Blau T, Fink GR, Neumaier B, Shah NJ, Langen K-J, Galldiks N. Static and dynamic 18F–FET PET for the characterization of gliomas defined by IDH and 1p/19q status. Eur J Nucl Med Mol Imaging. 2018;45(3):443–51. https://doi.org/10.1007/s00259-017-3846-6.
64. Vettermann F, Suchorska B, Unterrainer M, Nelwan D, Forbrig R, Ruf V, Wenter V, Kreth F-W, Herms J, Bartenstein P, et al. Non-invasive prediction of IDH-wildtype genotype in gliomas using dynamic 18F-FET PET. Eur J Nucl Med Mol Imaging. 2019;46(12):2581–9. https://doi.org/10.1007/s00259-019-04477-3.
65. Lynch TJ, Bell DW, Sordella R, Gurubhagavatula S, Okimoto RA, Brannigan BW, Harris PL, Haserlat SM, Supko JG, Haluska FG, et al. Activating mutations in the epidermal growth factor receptor underlying responsiveness of non–small-cell lung cancer to gefitinib. N Engl J Med. 2004;350(21):2129–39. https://doi.org/10.1056/NEJMoa040938.
66. Johnson ML, Sima CS, Chaft J, Paik PK, Pao W, Kris MG, Ladanyi M, Riely GJ. Association of KRAS and EGFR mutations with survival in patients with advanced lung adenocarcinomas. Cancer. 2013;119(2):356–62. https://doi.org/10.1002/cncr.27730.
67. Novello S, Barlesi F, Califano R, Cufer T, Ekman S, Levra MG, Kerr K, Popat S, Reck M, Senan S, et al. Metastatic non-small-cell lung cancer: ESMO Clinical Practice Guidelines for diagnosis, treatment and follow-up. Ann Oncol. 2016;27:v1–v27. https://doi.org/10.1093/annonc/mdw326.
68. Ahn SJ, Kwon H, Yang JJ, Park M, Cha YJ, Suh SH, Lee JM. Contrast-enhanced T1-weighted image radiomics of brain metastases may predict EGFR mutation status in primary lung cancer. Sci Rep. 2020;10(1):8905. https://doi.org/10.1038/s41598-020-65470-7.
69. Park YW, An C, Lee J, Han K, Choi D, Ahn SS, Kim H, Ahn SJ, Chang JH, Kim SH, et al. Diffusion tensor and postcontrast T1-weighted imaging radiomics to differentiate the epidermal growth factor receptor mutation status of brain metastases from non-small cell lung cancer. Neuroradiology. 2021;63(3):343–52. https://doi.org/10.1007/s00234-020-02529-2.
70. Luke JJ, Flaherty KT, Ribas A, Long GV. Targeted agents and immunotherapies: optimizing outcomes in melanoma. Nat Rev Clin Oncol. 2017;14(8):463–82. https://doi.org/10.1038/nrclinonc.2017.43.
71. Shofty B, Artzi M, Shtrozberg S, Fanizzi C, DiMeco F, Haim O, Peleg Hason S, Ram Z, Bashat DB, Grossman R. Virtual biopsy using MRI radiomics for prediction of BRAF status in melanoma brain metastasis. Sci Rep. 2020;10(1):6623. https://doi.org/10.1038/s41598-020-63821-y.
72. Curran WJ Jr, Scott CB, Horton J, Nelson JS, Weinstein AS, Fischbach AJ, Chang CH, Rotman M, Asbell SO, Krisch RE, et al. Recursive partitioning analysis of prognostic factors in three Radiation Therapy Oncology Group malignant glioma trials. J Natl Cancer Inst. 1993;85(9):704–10. https://doi.org/10.1093/jnci/85.9.704.
73. Stelzer KJ. Epidemiology and prognosis of brain metastases. Surg Neurol Int. 2013;4(Suppl 4):S192–202. https://doi.org/10.4103/2152-7806.111296.
74. Zinn PO, Sathyan P, Mahajan B, Bruyere J, Hegi M, Majumder S, Colen RR. A novel volume-age-KPS (VAK) glioblastoma classification identifies a prognostic cognate microRNA-gene signature. PLoS One. 2012;7(8):e41522. https://doi.org/10.1371/journal.pone.0041522.
75. Gutman DA, Cooper LA, Hwang SN, Holder CA, Gao J, Aurora TD, Dunn WD Jr, Scarpace L, Mikkelsen T, Jain R, et al. MR imaging predictors of molecular profile and survival: multi-institutional study of the TCGA glioblastoma data set. Radiology. 2013;267(2):560–9. https://doi.org/10.1148/radiol.13120118.
76. Li Q, Bai H, Chen Y, Sun Q, Liu L, Zhou S, Wang G, Liang C, Li Z-C. A fully-automatic multiparametric radiomics model: towards reproducible and prognostic imaging signature for prediction of overall survival in glioblastoma multiforme. Sci Rep. 2017;7:14331. https://doi.org/10.1038/s41598-017-14753-7.
77. Lao J, Chen Y, Li ZC, Li Q, Zhang J, Liu J, Zhai G. A deep learning-based radiomics model for prediction of survival in glioblastoma multiforme. Sci Rep. 2017;7(1):10353. https://doi.org/10.1038/s41598-017-10649-8.
78. Kickingereder P, Burth S, Wick A, Götz M, Eidel O, Schlemmer HP, Maier-Hein KH, Wick W, Bendszus M, Radbruch A, et al. Radiomic profiling of glioblastoma: identifying an imaging predictor of patient survival with improved performance over established clinical and radiologic risk models. Radiology. 2016;280(3):880–9. https://doi.org/10.1148/radiol.2016160845.
79. Rathore S, Akbari H, Rozycki M, Abdullah KG, Nasrallah MP, Binder ZA, Davuluri RV, Lustig RA, Dahmane N, Bilello M, et al. Radiomic MRI signature reveals three distinct subtypes of glioblastoma with different clinical and molecular characteristics, offering prognostic value beyond IDH1. Sci Rep. 2018;8(1):5087. https://doi.org/10.1038/s41598-018-22739-2.

80. Macyszyn L, Akbari H, Pisapia JM, Da X, Attiah M, Pigrish V, Bi Y, Pal S, Davuluri RV, Roccograndi L, et al. Imaging patterns predict patient survival and molecular subtype in glioblastoma via machine learning techniques. Neuro Oncol. 2016;18(3):417–25. https://doi.org/10.1093/neuonc/nov127.
81. Della Seta M, Collettini F, Chapiro J, Angelidis A, Engeling F, Hamm B, Kaul D. A 3D quantitative imaging biomarker in pre-treatment MRI predicts overall survival after stereotactic radiation therapy of patients with a singular brain metastasis. Acta Radiol. 2019;60(11):1496–503. https://doi.org/10.1177/0284185119831692.
82. Tini P, Nardone V, Pastina P, Battaglia G, Vinciguerra C, Carfagno T, Rubino G, Carbone SF, Sebaste L, Cerase A, et al. Perilesional edema in brain metastasis from non-small cell lung cancer (NSCLC) as predictor of response to radiosurgery (SRS). Neurol Sci. 2017;38(6):975–82. https://doi.org/10.1007/s10072-017-2876-y.
83. Kocher M, Voges J, Treuer H, Sturm V, Müller R-P. Reduced response rate of necrotic brain metastases to radiosurgery. In: Kondziolka D, editor. Radiosurgery 1999. Basel: Karger; 2000. p. 240–6.
84. Cha YJ, Jang WI, Kim MS, Yoo HJ, Paik EK, Jeong HK, Youn SM. Prediction of response to stereotactic radiosurgery for brain metastases using convolutional neural networks. Anticancer Res. 2018;38(9):5437–45. https://doi.org/10.21873/anticanres.12875.
85. Eisenhauer EA, Therasse P, Bogaerts J, Schwartz LH, Sargent D, Ford R, Dancey J, Arbuck S, Gwyther S, Mooney M, et al. New response evaluation criteria in solid tumours: revised RECIST guideline (version 1.1). Eur J Cancer. 2009;45(2):228–47. https://doi.org/10.1016/j.ejca.2008.10.026.
86. Mouraviev A, Detsky J, Sahgal A, Ruschin M, Lee YK, Karam I, Heyn C, Stanisz GJ, Martel AL. Use of radiomics for the prediction of local control of brain metastases after stereotactic radiosurgery. Neuro Oncol. 2020;22(6):797–805. https://doi.org/10.1093/neuonc/noaa007.
87. Lin NU, Lee EQ, Aoyama H, Barani IJ, Barboriak DP, Baumert BG, Bendszus M, Brown PD, Camidge DR, Chang SM, et al. Response assessment criteria for brain metastases: proposal from the RANO group. Lancet Oncol. 2015;16(6):e270–8. https://doi.org/10.1016/s1470-2045(15)70057-4.
88. Karami E, Soliman H, Ruschin M, Sahgal A, Myrehaug S, Tseng CL, Czarnota GJ, Jabehdar-Maralani P, Chugh B, Lau A, et al. Quantitative MRI biomarkers of stereotactic radiotherapy outcome in brain metastasis. Sci Rep. 2019;9(1):19830. https://doi.org/10.1038/s41598-019-56185-5.
89. Chao ST, Ahluwalia MS, Barnett GH, Stevens GH, Murphy ES, Stockham AL, Shiue K, Suh JH. Challenges with the diagnosis and treatment of cerebral radiation necrosis. Int J Radiat Oncol Biol Phys. 2013;87(3):449–57. https://doi.org/10.1016/j.ijrobp.2013.05.015.
90. Kohutek ZA, Yamada Y, Chan TA, Brennan CW, Tabar V, Gutin PH, Jonathan Yang T, Rosenblum MK, Ballangrud Å, Young RJ, et al. Long-term risk of radionecrosis and imaging changes after stereotactic radiosurgery for brain metastases. J Neurooncol. 2015;125(1):149–56. https://doi.org/10.1007/s11060-015-1881-3.
91. Furuse M, Nonoguchi N, Yamada K, Shiga T, Combes J-D, Ikeda N, Kawabata S, Kuroiwa T, Miyatake S-I. Radiological diagnosis of brain radiation necrosis after cranial irradiation for brain tumor: a systematic review. Radiation Oncol (London, England). 2019;14(1):28. https://doi.org/10.1186/s13014-019-1228-x.
92. Ehrenfeld CE, Maschke M, Dörfler A, Reinhardt V, Koeppen S. Is stereotactic biopsy a reliable method to differentiate tumor from radiation necrosis? Clin Neuropathol. 2002;21(1):9–12.
93. Tiwari P, Prasanna P, Wolansky L, Pinho M, Cohen M, Nayate AP, Gupta A, Singh G, Hatanpaa KJ, Sloan A, et al. Computer-extracted texture features to distinguish cerebral radionecrosis from recurrent brain tumors on multiparametric MRI: a feasibility study. Am J Neuroradiol. 2016;37(12):2231–6. https://doi.org/10.3174/ajnr.A4931.
94. Peng L, Parekh V, Huang P, Lin DD, Sheikh K, Baker B, Kirschbaum T, Silvestri F, Son J, Robinson A, et al. Distinguishing true progression from radionecrosis after stereotactic radiation therapy for brain metastases with machine learning and radiomics. Int J Radiat Oncol Biol Phys. 2018;102(4):1236–43. https://doi.org/10.1016/j.ijrobp.2018.05.041.
95. Lohmann P, Stoffels G, Ceccon G, Rapp M, Sabel M, Filss CP, Kamp MA, Stegmayr C, Neumaier B, Shah NJ, et al. Radiation injury vs. recurrent brain metastasis: combining textural feature radiomics analysis and standard parameters may increase (18)F-FET PET accuracy without dynamic scans. Eur Radiol. 2017;27(7):2916–27. https://doi.org/10.1007/s00330-016-4638-2.
96. Hettal L, Stefani A, Salleron J, Courrech F, Behm-Ansmant I, Constans JM, Gauchotte G, Vogin G. Radiomics method for the differential diagnosis of radionecrosis versus progression after fractionated stereotactic body radiotherapy for brain oligometastasis. Radiat Res. 2020;193(5):471–80. https://doi.org/10.1667/rr15517.1.
97. Zhang Z, Yang J, Ho A, Jiang W, Logan J, Wang X, Brown PD, McGovern SL, Guha-Thakurta N, Ferguson SD, et al. A predictive model for distinguishing radiation necrosis from tumour progression after gamma knife radiosurgery based on radiomic features from MR images. Eur Radiol. 2018;28(6):2255–63. https://doi.org/10.1007/s00330-017-5154-8.
98. Lohmann P, Kocher M, Ceccon G, Bauer EK, Stoffels G, Viswanathan S, Ruge MI, Neumaier B, Shah NJ, Fink GR, et al. Combined FET PET/MRI radiomics differentiates radiation injury from recurrent brain metastasis. Neuroimage Clin. 2018;20:537–42. https://doi.org/10.1016/j.nicl.2018.08.024.
99. Dong F, Li Q, Jiang B, Zhu X, Zeng Q, Huang P, Chen S, Zhang M. Differentiation of supratentorial single brain metastasis and glioblastoma by using peri-enhancing oedema region-derived radiomic features and multiple classifiers. Eur Radiol. 2020;30(5):3015–22. https://doi.org/10.1007/s00330-019-06460-w.
100. Ortiz-Ramón R, Ruiz-España S, Mollá-Olmos E, Moratal D. Glioblastomas and brain metastases differentiation following an MRI texture analysis-based radiomics approach. Phys Med. 2020;76:44–54. https://doi.org/10.1016/j.ejmp.2020.06.016.
101. Qian Z, Li Y, Wang Y, Li L, Li R, Wang K, Li S, Tang K, Zhang C, Fan X, et al. Differentiation of glioblastoma from solitary brain metastases using radiomic machine-learning classifiers. Cancer Lett. 2019;451:128–35. https://doi.org/10.1016/j.canlet.2019.02.054.
102. Bae S, An C, Ahn SS, Kim H, Han K, Kim SW, Park JE, Kim HS, Lee SK. Robust performance of deep learning for distinguishing glioblastoma from single brain metastasis using radiomic features: model development and validation. Sci Rep. 2020;10(1):12110. https://doi.org/10.1038/s41598-020-68980-6.
103. Chen C, Ou X, Wang J, Guo W, Ma X. Radiomics-based machine learning in differentiation between glioblastoma and metastatic brain tumors. Front Oncol. 2019;9:806. https://doi.org/10.3389/fonc.2019.00806.
104. Artzi M, Bressler I, Ben Bashat D. Differentiation between glioblastoma, brain metastasis and subtypes using radiomics analysis. J Magn Reson Imaging. 2019;50(2):519–28. https://doi.org/10.1002/jmri.26643.
105. Swinburne NC, Schefflein J, Sakai Y, Oermann EK, Titano JJ, Chen I, Tadayon S, Aggarwal A, Doshi A, Nael K. Machine learning for semi-automated classification of glioblastoma, brain metastasis and central nervous system lymphoma using magnetic resonance advanced imaging. Ann Transl Med. 2019;7(11):232. https://doi.org/10.21037/atm.2018.08.05.

106. Chen C, Zheng A, Ou X, Wang J, Ma X. Comparison of radiomics-based machine-learning classifiers in diagnosis of glioblastoma from primary central nervous system lymphoma. Front Oncol. 2020;10:1151. https://doi.org/10.3389/fonc.2020.01151.
107. Bhatia A, Birger M, Veeraraghavan H, Um H, Tixier F, McKenney AS, Cugliari M, Caviasco A, Bialczak A, Malani R, et al. MRI radiomic features are associated with survival in melanoma brain metastases treated with immune checkpoint inhibitors. Neuro Oncol. 2019;21(12):1578–86. https://doi.org/10.1093/neuonc/noz141.
108. Kniep HC, Madesta F, Schneider T, Hanning U, Schönfeld MH, Schön G, Fiehler J, Gauer T, Werner R, Gellissen S. Radiomics of brain MRI: utility in prediction of metastatic tumor type. Radiology. 2019;290(2):479–87. https://doi.org/10.1148/radiol.2018180946.
109. Zhang J, Jin J, Ai Y, Zhu K, Xiao C, Xie C, Jin X. Differentiating the pathological subtypes of primary lung cancer for patients with brain metastases based on radiomics features from brain CT images. Eur Radiol. 2021;31(2):1022–8. https://doi.org/10.1007/s00330-020-07183-z.
110. Li ZC, Bai H, Sun Q, Li Q, Liu L, Zou Y, Chen Y, Liang C, Zheng H. Multiregional radiomics features from multiparametric MRI for prediction of MGMT methylation status in glioblastoma multiforme: a multicentre study. Eur Radiol. 2018;28(9):3640–50. https://doi.org/10.1007/s00330-017-5302-1.
111. Wei J, Yang G, Hao X, Gu D, Tan Y, Wang X, Dong D, Zhang S, Wang L, Zhang H, et al. A multi-sequence and habitat-based MRI radiomics signature for preoperative prediction of MGMT promoter methylation in astrocytomas with prognostic implication. Eur Radiol. 2019;29(2):877–88. https://doi.org/10.1007/s00330-018-5575-z.
112. Drabycz S, Roldán G, de Robles P, Adler D, McIntyre JB, Magliocco AM, Cairncross JG, Mitchell JR. An analysis of image texture, tumor location, and MGMT promoter methylation in glioblastoma using magnetic resonance imaging. Neuroimage. 2010;49(2):1398–405. https://doi.org/10.1016/j.neuroimage.2009.09.049.
113. Chan HP, Sahiner B, Wagner RF, Petrick N. Classifier design for computer-aided diagnosis: effects of finite sample size on the mean performance of classical and neural network classifiers. Med Phys. 1999;26(12):2654–68. https://doi.org/10.1118/1.598805.
114. Way TW, Sahiner B, Hadjiiski LM, Chan HP. Effect of finite sample size on feature selection and classification: a simulation study. Med Phys. 2010;37(2):907–20. https://doi.org/10.1118/1.3284974.
115. Mazurowski MA, Habas PA, Zurada JM, Lo JY, Baker JA, Tourassi GD. Training neural network classifiers for medical decision making: the effects of imbalanced datasets on classification performance. Neural Netw. 2008;21(2–3):427–36. https://doi.org/10.1016/j.neunet.2007.12.031.
116. Ford J, Dogan N, Young L, Yang F. Quantitative radiomics: impact of pulse sequence parameter selection on MRI-based textural features of the brain. Contrast Media Mol Imaging. 2018;2018:1729071. https://doi.org/10.1155/2018/1729071.
117. Yang F, Dogan N, Stoyanova R, Ford JC. Evaluation of radiomic texture feature error due to MRI acquisition and reconstruction: a simulation study utilizing ground truth. Phys Med. 2018;50:26–36. https://doi.org/10.1016/j.ejmp.2018.05.017.
118. Mayerhoefer ME, Szomolanyi P, Jirak D, Materka A, Trattnig S. Effects of MRI acquisition parameter variations and protocol heterogeneity on the results of texture analysis and pattern discrimination: an application-oriented study. Med Phys. 2009;36(4):1236–43. https://doi.org/10.1118/1.3081408.
119. Waugh SA, Lerski RA, Bidaut L, Thompson AM. The influence of field strength and different clinical breast MRI protocols on the outcome of texture analysis using foam phantoms. Med Phys. 2011;38(9):5058–66. https://doi.org/10.1118/1.3622605.
120. Hainc N, Stippich C, Stieltjes B, Leu S, Bink A. Experimental texture analysis in glioblastoma: a methodological study. Invest Radiol. 2017;52(6):367–73. https://doi.org/10.1097/rli.0000000000000354.
121. Kofler F, Berger C, Waldmannstetter D, Lipkova J, Ezhov I, Tetteh G, Kirschke J, Zimmer C, Wiestler B, Menze BH. BraTS toolkit: translating BraTS brain tumor segmentation algorithms into clinical and scientific practice. Front Neurosci. 2020;14:125. https://doi.org/10.3389/fnins.2020.00125.

19 Foundations of Brain Image Segmentation: Pearls and Pitfalls in Segmenting Intracranial Blood on Computed Tomography Images

Antonios Thanellas, Heikki Peura, Jenni Wennervirta, and Miikka Korja

19.1 Introduction

Among the medical emergencies that have a devastating impact, especially if left undiagnosed or misdiagnosed, are intracranial haemorrhages. In subarachnoid haemorrhage (SAH), which is usually of a spontaneous nature, blood bursts through a damaged intracranial vessel and accumulates widely in the subarachnoid space. In contrast, in epidural (EDH) and subdural haemorrhages (SDH), which are most often caused by head traumas, blood accumulation happens in much more restricted spaces. Because of the ever-growing number of diagnostic head computer tomography (CT) scans, which seem to retain their position as the first-line modality in busy emergency units, these critical brain haemorrhages may sometimes be missed. Given the global and increasing trend of a shortage of radiologists, the likelihood of misdiagnoses in emergency imaging is rising. For these reasons, machine learning (ML) models are required for head CT scans and not only for magnetic resonance (MR) images, which are rarely performed in an emergency setting. To develop supervised ML models, which are often preferred over the unsupervised models (that require much more extensive training material), a high-quality set of segmented lesions is needed to train the models.

Despite ML methods in the field of radiology enjoy an increased popularity with a seemingly unmatched performance, relatively few ML models have been put into use in radiology departments worldwide. This may be linked to the fact that in the clinical setting the performance of developed ML models is often inferior to the performance described in the product descriptions. Superior results of ML models can only be achieved by a sequence of successful decisions, ranging from the selection of a proper model and relevant features to the appropriate hyperparameters and representative datasets. Any mistake in this chain will inevitably propagate and reflect upon the final performance level. In this sense, preparing the training material to represent a wide variety of clinical cases is not a trivial undertaking. Furthermore, choosing the most appropriate segmentation strategy for a lesion of interest, adopting an adequate granularity depth in segmentation, and selecting a proper software that will assist experts in the creation of the training sets are other important decisions to be made. In the current book chapter, we discuss these topics and explain why high-quality segmentations should be a priority in developing ML models for radiology. Moreover, we provide practical advice on how to fasten the segmentation step and choose the proper software.

19.2 Segmentation: What, Why, and How

During a standard labelling process a binary value (0 or 1) is assigned to the imaging series, every slice in the series, or every true positive voxel in a single slice. Such binary classification divides imaging series, slices, or voxels into a foreground (only the lesion) and background (anything but the lesion), which are the key components in training ML models. A distinct difference between annotations and segmentations is that the former operates at a fuzzy and binary level in identifying the region of interest, while the latter accurately delineates the target lesion at the voxel level. Annotations do not aim at a voxel-level accuracy and can be done, for example, in the form of bounding boxes [1, 2]. Segmentations, by contrast, aim at maximizing the labelling precision since their scope is at the voxel level [3]. A flowchart showing the segmentation design rationale is presented in Fig. 19.1, and

A. Thanellas
Department of Information Management, Helsinki University Hospital, Helsinki, Finland
e-mail: antonios.thanellas@hus.fi

H. Peura · J. Wennervirta · M. Korja (✉)
Department of Neurosurgery, Helsinki University Hospital and University of Helsinki, Helsinki, Finland
e-mail: Miikka.Korja@hus.fi

V. E. Staartjes et al. (eds.), *Machine Learning in Clinical Neuroscience*, Acta Neurochirurgica Supplement 134,
https://doi.org/10.1007/978-3-030-85292-4_19

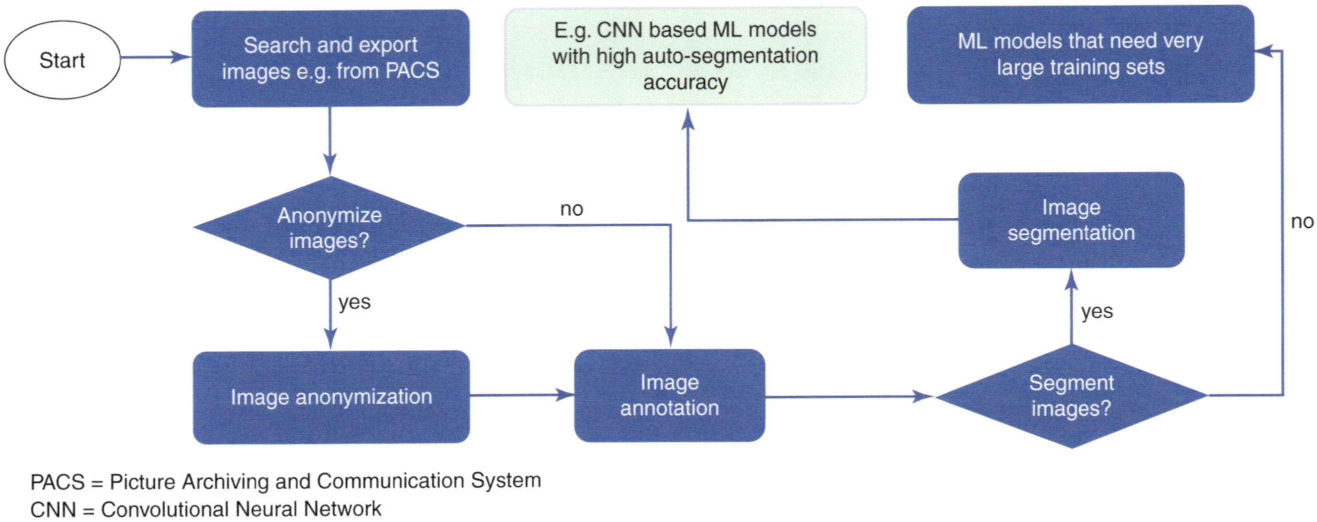

Fig. 19.1 Segmentation design rationale

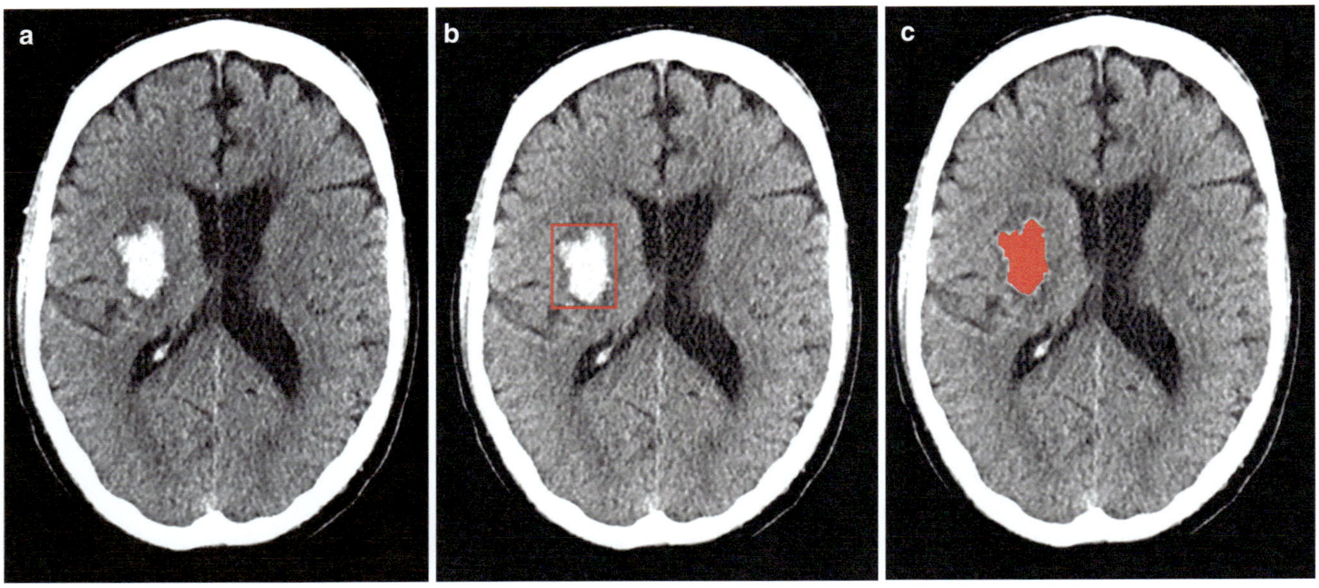

Fig. 19.2 (**a**) A single slice of a non-contrast head CT scan with intracerebral haemorrhage. (**b**) An example of a box annotation where the lesion is surrounded with a square box. This bounding box is binary (it either exists or not in a given slice) and it marks multiple voxels (all voxels covered by the edges of the rectangle). (**c**) An example of a segmentation where the lesion is delineated as accurately as possible

the differences between a box annotation and segmentation are illustrated in Fig. 19.2.

Every slice out of the stack of slices that comprises the 3D CT volume consists of pixel elements. Each slice is spaced a certain distance from its preceding and successive slices. This distance gives the slice a particular depth, which is a third dimension. Therefore, instead of talking about pixels we are talking about "volume pixels," which are better known as voxels. If only one structure or lesion is to be segmented, which is the most common case, then all voxels are labelled with the same categorical value (typically 1), while the rest of the scan's voxels get the background value (typically 0). In a less common case, where more than one structure or lesion is going to be segmented (multi-label segmentation), structures' voxels will get a unique categorical value (e.g. 1, 2, 3, etc.), while the rest will get the same background value of 0. In all of these cases, segmentation leads to a new image layer, which is called an image mask. The image mask has exactly the same dimensions as the original image layer, but its voxels contain categorical values instead of intensity units. In daily clinical CT imaging, a CT scanner generates an attenuation profile of the X-ray beams, and this profile is expressed as tissue attenuation coefficient maps. These maps, in turn, are converted into the intensity units, i.e. Hounsfield units [4], so that they are relative to a reference quantity. This reference quantity is the water at room temperature, and different tissues can be compared with this reference quantity based on their Hounsfield units.

The necessity for voxel-level accuracy in the segmentation process makes the task much more laborious than that of an annotation. The time required to complete an accurate segmentation of, for example, blood in a head CT scan of one patient can be hours. Still, we prefer segmentations over annotations. The inherent characteristic of segmentations to localize the areas of interest at the maximum precision results in a high-quality training material, which in turn leads to a ML model accuracy [5] that can be only achieved with much larger annotated image sets [6].

Assessing reliably the quality of any segmentation, regardless of whether it is produced by an algorithm or an expert, has been studied extensively [7]. Knowing that a trained expert can create variable results while segmenting the same structure twice (intra-rater variability), or that there can be considerable variation between one expert's results and those of others (inter-rater variability), reveals the complexity of the task. The methodologies employed to address agreement among experts' segmentations range from majority voting rules [8] to expert agreement measures [9], label fusion [10, 11], and hybrid methods that combine different principles [12]. Similarly, comparing segmentations made by algorithms with those prepared by experts requires various metrics. Among the ones most used are volumetry (i.e. total volume in cubic millimetres), volumetric overlap estimates (i.e. Dice and Jaccard coefficients [13, 14]) and boundary differences (i.e. Hausdorff [15] distance). Combining the various metrics that quantify different aspects of the segmentation's quality into one final score has also been addressed in the literature [16].

19.3 Multi-label Segmentation

A multi-label segmentation often appears as a single image mask with every structure's or lesion's voxels having their specific categorical value (e.g. 1, 2, 3, etc., with the value 0 often reserved for the background). A multi-label segmentation can also exist in the form of multiple binary image masks or a mask that stores voxel values in multiple 3D arrays. An example of a multi-label segmentation is illustrated in Fig. 19.3a.

A multi-label segmentation requires that every structure or pathology gets all of its voxels labelled, as discussed earlier, which translates into an increased time of completing the segmentation. As an example, in a binary label segmentation, all blood clusters will be given the same categorical value, i.e. will be segmented equally, regardless of the bleeding subtype. In contrast to the binary label segmentation, a multi-label segmentation enables us to give every blood cluster a specific categorical value, depending on whether the blood represents EDH, SDH, SAH, intraventricular (IVH), or intraparenchymal haemorrhage (ICH) (Fig. 19.3c). The need to differentiate various types of bleedings, e.g. multi-

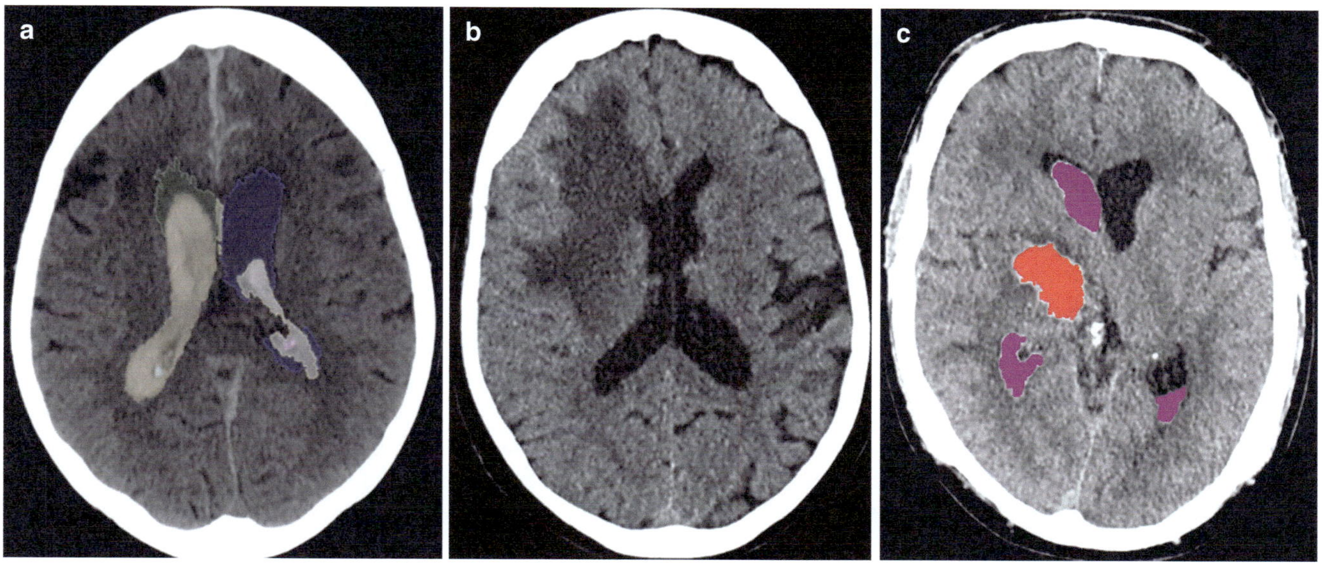

Fig. 19.3 A single slice of a non-contrast head CT scan with (**a**) multi-label segmentation. The right ventricle is segmented in green, the IVH inside this ventricle in brown, and its calcified choroid plexuses in turquoise. In a similar fashion, the left ventricle is segmented in blue, its IVH in yellow, and the calcification in pink. This compartmentalization allows for individual metrics for each region of interest. (**b**) A glioblastoma in the right hemisphere is hypodense with ill-defined borders. (**c**) Multi-label segmentation. The IVH of the lateral ventricles is segmented in magenta and the intracerebral haemorrhage of the right basal ganglia in red

label the head CT images with intracranial haemorrhages, becomes crucial when, for example, the aim of training convolution neural networks is to develop a comprehensive clinical solution for an emergency setting.

19.4 Segmentation of Blood Detected in Head CT Scans

One of the most challenging segmentation tasks is a diffuse intracranial bleeding, such as SAH, which is scattered around the brain. The segmentation burden in such cases is proportional to the amount of blood and its dispersion inside the subarachnoid space. Other obstacles complicating the segmentation task arise from the various stages of haematoma evolution. In an intracranial haemorrhage, the initial hyperdense (acute) presentation of the blood (i.e. haematoma) in a non-contrast CT scan (NCCT) will first evolve to an isodense (subacute) and then to a hypodense (chronic) stage. Unless the delay from symptom onset to imaging has been controlled, the dataset may include cases with, for instance, acute and chronic haematomas with highly varying Hounsfield units. An algorithm that primarily detects, for example, subacute bleedings may not serve the purpose for which it was meant. Depending on the application's objectives, segmentations on stringently selected images inevitably lead to more specific ML models, which often is the desired end goal. Therefore, a careful consideration of the study's aims, options, and limitations should be dealt with beforehand. Simply put, if your aim is to create a ML solution for acute intracranial haemorrhages your dataset should consist of acute cases. When segmenting intracranial blood detected in a head CT scan, it must be stressed that reaching a 100% voxel accuracy in the segmentation process is a virtually impossible goal. There will always be some ambiguous voxel clusters about which even experienced neuroradiologists disagree (whether they represent blood or not). Therefore, this also means that there will never be a ML algorithm that has a 100% voxel accuracy relative to a gold standard, which represents expert segmentation of intracranial blood. In this sense, a voxel-level performance reporting of an algorithm is merely of academic interest, and the slice level (how many of the slices are rated/diagnosed correctly) reporting should be the rule for clinical algorithms.

19.5 Confounders in Segmenting Blood

The complexity of a structure (or lesion) determines, to a large extent, the time that will be spent on segmentation. A vascular tree segmentation, for example, can be prohibitively time consuming, without any form of automatic or semi-automatic assistance [17]. An accurate segmentation of the finer branches of the tree might even become impossible not only because of the image noise interference at such a small scale but also because it can be very difficult to follow all of the tiny branches, especially if using 2D projections. In a similar fashion, structures with unclear borders create uncertainties during the demarcation, which can lead to further challenges. For example, gliomas that are surrounded by oedema have unclear margins in NCCT scans [18], thus falling into this category (Fig. 19.3b). The dynamic intensity range of soft tissues in NCCT is quite restrictive [19]. As a result, soft tissues tend to map into very similar intensity ranges, leading to low contrast and ill-defined borders. A smooth reconstruction filter, typically used with multi-planar reformat (MPR) images emphasizing soft tissues, will reduce the innate granular noise of NCCT at the expense of its spatial accuracy. This means that the higher the smoothing, the lower the noise and the poorer the tissue borders. In addition to these challenges, numerous other factors may confound segmentations.

Calcifications are a common radiological finding that can be attributed to physiological or pathological aetiologies. Calcifications are observed in different sites of the parenchyma, dura, and leptomeninges [20]. For example, calcified choroid plexuses (Fig. 19.4c) have in their periphery intensities that overlap with those of intracranial blood. Therefore, an accurate segmentation of, for instance, blood in the cisterns and ventricles is sometimes challenging.

Normal vasculature can become a source of confounding when segmenting intracranial blood. Normal vascularization around the cavernous sinus (Fig. 19.4b) has often intensity ranges that resemble acute blood. In the case of subarachnoid haemorrhage, once again, the presence of blood in the carotid or chiasmatic cistern may complicate the delineation of the borders that separate the blood from the normal vasculature. Similar phenomena can be present around other major brain sinuses (Fig. 19.4c).

Secondary pathologies, such as oedemas, herniations, and mass effects (Fig. 19.4e), also complicate the segmentation task. They are often responsible for large deformations, therefore disrupting the natural anatomy and increasing the delineation difficulty. Moreover, as the anatomy is deformed, segmented lesions or structures are not in their usual locations, making it more difficult for a convolutional neural network to learn the spatial presentation of a classified lesion.

Previous intracranial interventions, such as microneurosurgical clippings or endovascular coilings of aneurysms, introduce streak image artefacts, which vary markedly depending on the materials used. Serious metallic artefacts have the potential not only to substantially hinder the seg-

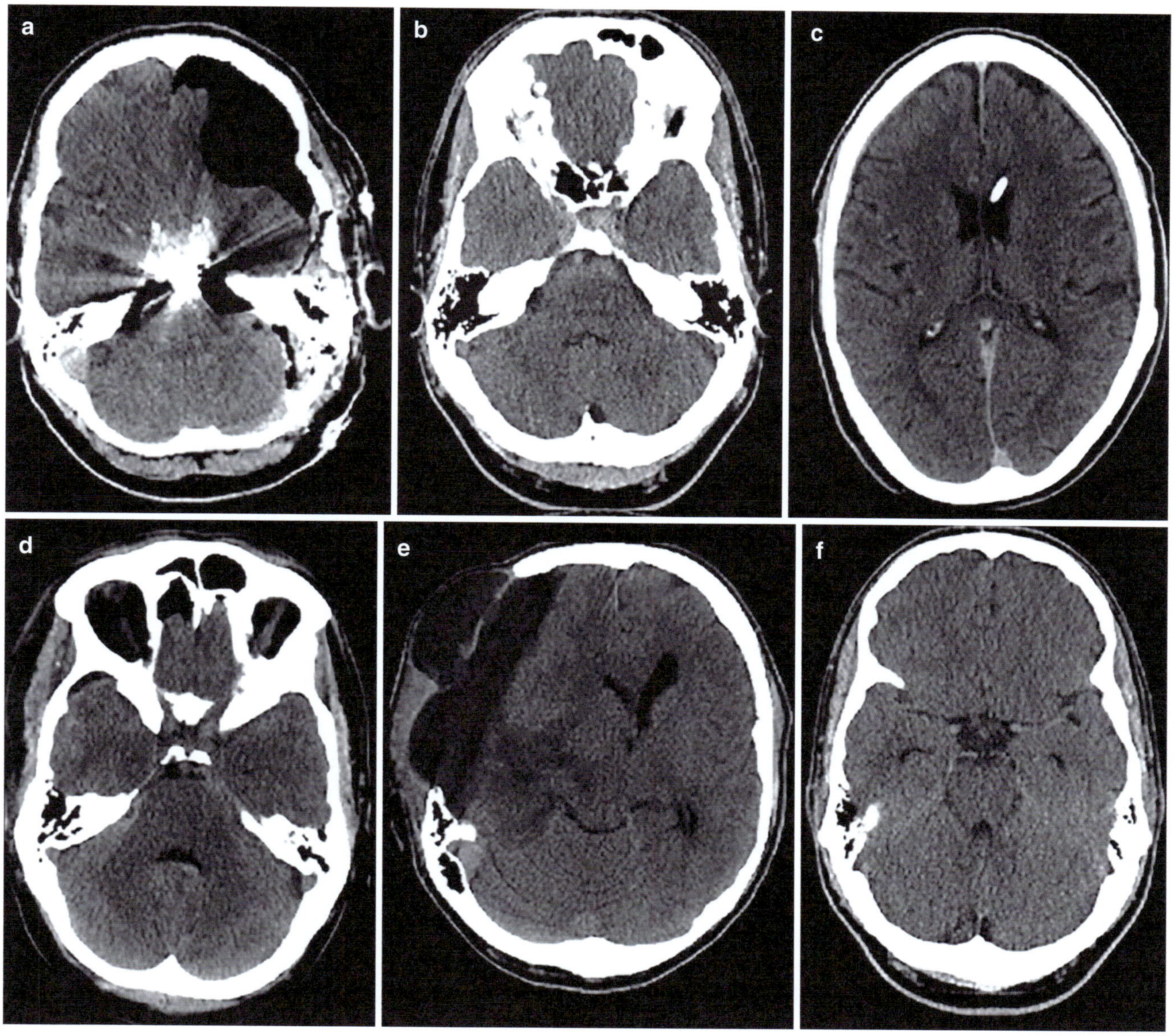

Fig. 19.4 A single slice of a non-contrast head CT scan with (**a**) aneurysm clips that introduce very strong streak artefacts, (**b**) a normal vasculature of the cavernous sinus and the sella turcica (can be confused with acute blood), (**c**) a ventricular catheter may cause a few artefacts and the calcification of the choroid plexuses of the lateral ventricles can be confused with acute blood, (**d**) a pneumocephalus in the frontal and middle fossae, (**e**) an extra-axial cerebrospinal fluid collection and a subfalcine herniation, and (**f**) hyperattenuated (calcified) left and right middle cerebral arteries

mentation process but also to make it impossible (Fig. 19.4a). Similarly to aneurysm clips and coils, ventricular shunts (Fig. 19.4c) or ventriculostomies may cause artefacts that sometimes complicate the blood segmentations. These very same artefacts are a true challenge for a real-world ML solution, which is developed to assist on-call radiologists to detect intracranial blood in various case scenarios. Therefore, these confounding cases must be included in the datasets used to train convolutional neural networks.

19.6 Selecting a Segmentation Software

Selecting the appropriate segmentation software is an important step. Finding a fully integrated and functioning-as-designed software is not a straightforward process. Functionalities should be carefully examined to determine the extent to which they fulfil the needs and objectives of an institution's research group. Commercial demos of the software's capabilities can give an excellent impression, but an exciting demo does not always guarantee an exciting software. Therefore, the segmentation software selection process, particularly in the case of a commercial solution, should include a proper trial period. Among the appealing characteristics of open-source solutions is that they have no trial periods, and they most often come at much lower costs than their commercial counterparts. One downside with many open-source segmentation programmes is that they are targeted to somewhat smaller sized research-oriented groups with some prior knowledge of similar open-source solutions. The learning curve for some of them can be quite long particularly if the user has no previous experience with a similar software. Therefore, even though these open-source segmentation programmes are excellent tools for many users, they are often less intuitive and user-friendly for clinicians. If a segmentation task requires a major input from clinicians, it is perhaps wise to test various commercial segmentation programmes and choose more than one to meet varying end-user requirements. As a rule of thumb, clinicians prefer a simple user interface. At the same time, one should bear in mind that simplicity versus functionality is not always a good trade-off. Another aspect that should be carefully considered is the software's maturity, which can be estimated based on the time passed since its initial release, its development rate with new releases, and its number of active users. Using an immature software that falls behind in functionality might very well mean spending time as its involuntary beta tester. On a more practical level, a segmentation software needs to have proper tools that will help the user to carry out different segmentation tasks. These tools include a colour palette to do multi-label segmentations, adjustable opacities for each label when overlapping segmentations should be visualized simultaneously, 3D-rendering of the images and their overlaid segmentations for a better perspective, semi-automatic or fully automatic routines to complete segmentations, and an option to choose proper settings of the window width and window level. Of the open-source solutions that offer semi- or fully automatic segmentation tools, the ITK-Snap [21] and 3DSlicer [22] with a history of more than a decade of development are among the most established ones. In brief, selecting a user-friendly and sufficiently versatile segmentation software is key to efficiently segmenting a high-quality dataset for ML training.

19.7 Practical Segmentation Tips

As stated earlier in this chapter, image segmentation is a crucial step in achieving high-accuracy ML models. If segmentation is done with high accuracy, less than 100 CT volumes per lesion type will in most cases be sufficient to create a clinically reliable ML model that can detect certain haemorrhage types. Since there are multiple intracranial haemorrhage types, the required workload of clinical experts to segment the training dataset for the ML training can still be extensive.

A high-quality image dataset that will be used to train the ML model should contain diverse images that cover a real-world spectrum of cases encountered in hospital. In addition to different intracranial haemorrhage types, the image set should contain, for instance, pre- and postoperative images. Perhaps the best way to start with segmentations is to focus on simple but clinically meaningful entities. Of the intracranial bleeding types, ICH is among the easiest ones to segment, whereas SAH is probably the most demanding. People doing the segmentations should have medical experience, skills, and time for the task. Therefore, we recommend that a neurosurgeon or neuroradiologist at least verifies the accuracy of every segmentation. Preferably, a neurosurgeon or neuroradiologist will segment the training datasets. A ground truth segmentation can be derived from the segmentations of multiple experts using fusion labelling, which is available as an open-source solution in, among others, the ITK-Snap (using c3d staple) [21].

Before starting the segmentation work, it should be considered whether the ML training is going to be performed in collaboration with non-medical personnel. Such collaboration can in fact save a lot of time and money. If, for example, companies are involved in the algorithm development process, then anonymization of the images may become a necessity, as it is crucial that all patient data are handled with caution and according to national data privacy laws and legislation during the whole process. If data anonymization needs to be done, a conversion from the Digital Imaging and Communications in Medicine (DICOM) file format to the Neuroimaging Informatics Technology Initiative (NIfTI) format is perhaps the easiest way to ensure anonymization. However, unnecessary conversions between image file formats, such as, e.g. DICOM or NIfTI, should be avoided along with image data pre-processing to minimize data loss, which may negatively affect the algorithm's final accuracy.

When segmenting blood from CT scans, a useful tip to increase the segmentation accuracy and reduce the time spent is to create an additional mask using a Hounsfield unit-based approach. This additional mask, which should enclose all areas except the blood, permits an easier inspection of the actual borders of the bleeding and can guide the user through the segmentation process. Hounsfield unit-based masking is an available functionality in most segmentation software.

Last, it should be decided at the beginning whether the aim is to create individual ML algorithms for each haemorrhage type or to create one that handles all types. If more than one intracranial haemorrhage type is to be tackled with a single ML algorithm, the multi-label segmentation technique is, in our opinion, preferred. If the aim is to create individual algorithms, then the binary approach is perhaps the way to start. For the reader interested in understanding the fundamentals of image segmentation and processing, the book by Gonzalez et al. [23] reviews these concepts and methodologies, while keeping the mathematical complexity at a reasonable level. A book by Ranscharet et al. [24] offers a more general overview of these topics and focuses on the use of artificial intelligence in the field of medical imaging without going into programming detail.

19.8 Conclusions

The ultimate goal of any ML method in radiology is to accurately pinpoint every abnormal voxel on an image stack and provide a structured report that describes the findings and makes a list of useful and understandable metrics that support the findings report. In practice, a realistic goal in developing clinically useful algorithms for intracranial haemorrhages is to achieve 100% accuracy at the slice level, not the voxel level. Such solution would be sufficiently accurate to be deployed in emergency room settings. To achieve this goal, regions of interest should often be segmented by clinical experts. The segmentation step, indeed, is the most crucial step in developing clinically useful and reliable ML algorithms. The capabilities and potential of ML methods to accurately locate regions of interest on radiological images depend almost entirely on the quality and diversity of segmented images. A carefully designed and executed game plan that has considered all options, from selecting the most appropriate software to choosing the most suitable segmentation strategy, can be decisive regarding both the project's completion time and the algorithm's performance.

Conflict of Interest The authors have no conflicts of interest to declare.

References

1. Lempitsky V, Kohli P, Rother C, Sharp T. Image segmentation with a bounding box prior. In: 2009 IEEE 12th international conference on computer vision. 2009. p. 277–84.
2. Rajchl M, Lee MC, Oktay O, Kamnitsas K, Passerat-Palmbach J, Bai W, Damodaram M, Rutherford MA, Hajnal JV, Kainz B, Rueckert D. Deepcut: object segmentation from bounding box annotations using convolutional neural networks. IEEE Trans Med Imaging. 2016;36(2):674–83.
3. Veeraraghavan H. MO-A-207B-01: radiomics: segmentation & feature extraction techniques. Med Phys. 2016;43:3694.
4. Hounsfield GN. Computed medical imaging. Nobel lecture, December 8, 1979. J Comput Assist Tomogr. 1980;4(5):665.
5. Grewal M, Srivastava MM, Kumar P, Varadarajan S. Radnet: radiologist level accuracy using deep learning for hemorrhage detection in CT scans. In: 2018 IEEE 15th international symposium on biomedical imaging. 2018. p. 281–4.
6. Lee H, Yune S, Mansouri M, Kim M, Tajmir SH, Guerrier CE, Ebert SA, Pomerantz SR, Romero JM, Kamalian S, Gonzalez RG. An explainable deep-learning algorithm for the detection of acute intracranial haemorrhage from small datasets. Nat Biomed Eng. 2019;3(3):173.
7. Zhang YJ. A survey on evaluation methods for image segmentation. Pattern Recogn. 1996;29(8):1335–46.
8. Warfield S, Dengler J, Zaers J, Guttmann CR, Wells WM, Ettinger GJ, Hiller J, Kikinis R. Automatic identification of gray matter structures from MRI to improve the segmentation of white matter lesions. J Image Guided Surg. 1995;1(6):326–38.
9. Zijdenbos AP, Dawant BM, Margolin RA, Palmer AC. Morphometric analysis of white matter lesions in MR images: method and validation. IEEE Trans Med Imaging. 1994;13(4):716–24.
10. Gerig G, Jomier M, Chakos M. Valmet: a new validation tool for assessing and improving 3D object segmentation. In: International conference on medical image computing and computer-assisted intervention. Berlin: Springer; 2001. p. 516–23.
11. Warfield SK, Zou KH, Wells WM. Simultaneous truth and performance level estimation (STAPLE): an algorithm for the validation of image segmentation. IEEE Trans Med Imaging. 2004;23(7):903–21.
12. Mahapatra D. Semi-supervised learning and graph cuts for consensus based medical image segmentation. Pattern Recogn. 2017;63:700–9.
13. Dice LR. Measures of the amount of ecologic association between species. Ecology. 1945;26(3):297–302.
14. Jaccard P. The distribution of the flora in the alpine zone. 1. New Phytol. 1912;11(2):37–50.
15. Huttenlocher DP, Klanderman GA, Rucklidge WJ. Comparing images using the Hausdorff distance. IEEE Trans Pattern Anal Mach Intell. 1993;15(9):850–63.
16. Heimann T, Van Ginneken B, Styner MA, Arzhaeva Y, Aurich V, Bauer C, Beck A, Becker C, Beichel R, Bekes G, Bello F. Comparison and evaluation of methods for liver segmentation from CT datasets. IEEE Trans Med Imaging. 2009;28(8):1251–65.
17. Livne M, Rieger J, Aydin OU, Taha AA, Akay EM, Kossen T, Sobesky J, Kelleher JD, Hildebrand K, Frey D, Madai VI. A U-Net deep learning framework for high performance vessel segmentation in patients with cerebrovascular disease. Front Neurosci. 2019;13:97.
18. Alexiou GA, Tsiouris S, Voulgaris S, Kyritsis AP, Fotopoulos AD. Glioblastoma multiforme imaging: the role of nuclear medicine. Curr Radiopharm. 2012;5(4):308–13.
19. Rorden C, Bonilha L, Fridriksson J, Bender B, Karnath HO. Age-specific CT and MRI templates for spatial normalization. Neuroimage. 2012;61(4):957–65.
20. Saade C, Najem E, Asmar K, Salman R, El Achkar B, Naffaa L. Intracranial calcifications on CT: an updated review. J Radiol Case Rep. 2019;13(8):1.
21. Yushkevich PA, Gao Y, Gerig G. ITK-SNAP: an interactive tool for semi-automatic segmentation of multi-modality biomedical images. In: 2016 38th annual international conference of the IEEE engineering in medicine and biology society (EMBC). 2016. p. 3342–5.
22. Pieper S, Halle M, Kikinis R. 3D slicer. In: 2004 2nd IEEE international symposium on biomedical imaging: nano to macro (IEEE Cat No. 04EX821). 2004. p. 632–5.
23. Gonzalez R. Digital image processing fourth edition. Global ed. New York: Pearson; 2018.
24. Ranscharet ER, Morozov S, Algra PR. Artificial intelligence in medical imaging, opportunities, applications and risks. Berlin: Springer; 2019.

Applying Convolutional Neural Networks to Neuroimaging Classification Tasks: A Practical Guide in Python

20

Moumin A. K. Mohamed, Alexander Alamri, Brandon Smith, and Christopher Uff

20.1 Introduction

The utilisation of machine learning in medical imaging is an area of growing interest. It is widely believed that it has the capacity to reform the way we interact with medical imaging [1]. Imaging in clinical practice is used to screen, diagnose, monitor, stage and prognosticate illnesses, and machine learning has been implemented in each of these aspects [1, 2]. Usually, the process of generating a machine learning application is conducted outside the treating medical team/hospital, which creates numerous regulatory and confidentiality challenges that could vary between institutes and countries [3]. As treating clinicians, the access to such data, although difficult, is significantly simpler. In this chapter we aim to give a practical guide for interested clinicians with some programming experience on how to work with medical imaging data in the context of neurotrauma. This will be done using open source software tools and can be applied to any type of medical imaging. Throughout this practical explanation, the authors assume that the reader has basic knowledge and understanding of the Python programming language and associated libraries such as matplotlib and Keras [1, 2].

When a patient sustains a traumatic brain injury (TBI), an emergency computed tomography (CT) scan is indicated in the vast majority of patients with severe and moderate head injuries, and in some patients with mild TBI [4, 5]. This type of imaging is key to determine the type and reversibility of the injury, and to guide management plans for the patient. Multiple attempts have been made to automate the detection of abnormalities on CT scans in TBI [6–8]; the algorithms were able to successfully identify the type and location of intracranial pathologies. Two- or three-dimensional analyses of the scans have been utilised with satisfying results [9]. Following the acute phase of TBI, the focus of imaging is shifted to assess the delayed sequelae of TBI, for instance vascular and venous injuries. Although there are some publications depicting the utilisation of machine learning in vascular imaging in other contexts, no literature exists in the context of intracranial vascular imaging in TBI, and thus this may become an area of future interest. Further down the timeline of TBI, magnetic resonance imaging (MRI) is used to visualise injuries not visible on the CT scan, or for prognostication [10]. For example, the authors are working on a model to interpret susceptibility weighted imaging for prognostication. Single Photon Emission CT (SPECT) and positron emission tomography (PET) scans may also be utilised in the context of TBI to visualise lesions, estimate cerebral blood flow, and prognostication [10]. In this chapter the authors will explain the structure of medical imaging files, how to obtain the images from said files, and how to implement them in a two-dimensional convolutional neural network (CNN).

M. A. K. Mohamed (✉) · A. Alamri (✉) · C. Uff
Department of Neurosurgery, Royal London Hospital, London, UK

The London Neuro-Machine Learning Institute, Barts Health NHS Trust, London, UK

B. Smith
The London Neuro-Machine Learning Institute, Barts Health NHS Trust, London, UK

20.2 Digital Imaging and Communications in Medicine (DICOM)

Developed in 1993 by The American College of Radiology (ACR) and the National Electrical Manufacturers Association (NEMA), the Digital Imaging and Communications in Medicine (DICOM) file protocol has become the beating heart of the modern medical imaging industry [11]. It has been updated multiple times since its launch, and the DICOM protocol has been used to standardise the storage and communication of patient data, imaging and therapeutic information [11, 12]. Maintained by NEMA, the DICOM standard is freely available online (https://www.dicomstandard.org/), and is recognised by the International Organization for

V. E. Staartjes et al. (eds.), *Machine Learning in Clinical Neuroscience*, Acta Neurochirurgica Supplement 134,
https://doi.org/10.1007/978-3-030-85292-4_20

Standardization (ISO) as ISO 12052:2017. Describing the detailed structure of the DICOM file system is outside the scope of this chapter, nevertheless, in order to understand how to extract and pre-process medical imaging we need a basic understanding of it.

When stored offline, all DICOM data have a dictionary file named DICOMDIR, the absence of this file indicates a non-DICOM protocol of storage [13–15]. The DICOMDIR file is arranged in a hierarchical structure, storing data into four principal DICOM tables: patient, study, series, and image illustrated in Fig. 20.1. Accessing a specific study is a multistep process; first you will need to select the patient, then the study, the series, and finally the images.

To read and view the DICOM images, we used Pydicom [16] and Matplotlib [17] libraries on an Anaconda installation of Python (Python Software Foundation. Python Language Reference, version 3.7.9. Available at http://www.python.org). We use a Jupyter Notebook as the text editor, and to visualise the code and the images.

20.3 Practical Steps

Before you can start any step in this practical guide, you need to import essential libraries as shown in Fig. 20.2. You also want to ensure that your graphs can be visualised by running *%matplotlib inline*. Following this, you need to obtain the path to the DICOMDIR file directory. The code below refers to where our DICOMDIR file exists in relation to the Jupyter notebook that is concurrently running, Fig. 20.3.

Once you have opened the DICOMDIR file, you need to identify and select the patient record, the study and the series of interest, Fig. 20.4. To list them in between each step you can run a *for* loop for patient records, studies and all series. By listing *all_series*, you can visualise and select the targeted series by standard Python indexing. Once you have identified the series you are interested in, you need to extract the list of locations for the files storing the series, Fig. 20.5.

Now that you have the desired list of paths, several steps must be performed before it is possible to visualise the images. First, the paths must be converted to string format using the *str* Python function, adding the directory relative to the notebook, as mentioned above, to the beginning of the path. Next, obtain the image dimensions and spacing and store them into a single array as per the code in Fig. 20.6. You can read more about this code on the Pydicom website (https://pydicom.github.io/). To view each image with its index in the scan, you will have to iterate though the *ArrayDicom* pre-built array in the for loop, and use *pyplot* to view it, as shown in Fig. 20.7.

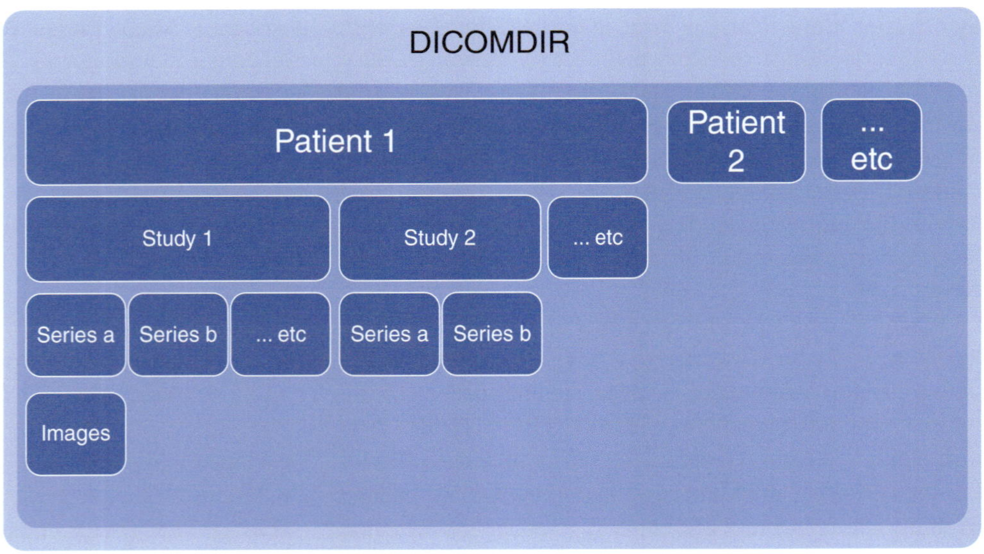

Fig. 20.1 Illustrates the structure of the standard DICOMDIR file

```
In [1]:
import numpy as np
import matplotlib
import pydicom
from pydicom import dcmread
from pydicom.data import get_testdata_file
import os
from pathlib import Path
%matplotlib inline
```

Fig. 20.2 Start by importing essential libraries

Fig. 20.3 Locate, import and read the DICOMDIR file and print its directory

```
In [2]:
directory='6'
# fetch the path to the DICOM dictionary and files
path = get_testdata_file('{}\\DICOMDIR'.format(directory))
ds = dcmread('{}/DICOMDIR'.format(directory))
root_dir = Path(ds.filename).resolve().parent
print(f'Root directory: {root_dir}\n')
```

```
Root directory: C:\Users\      \Desktop\code\extraction\6
```

Fig. 20.4 Selecting the targeted patient, study and series

```
In [3]:
#To list the patients in the record
ds.patient_records

# to select the only patient in this record
for patient in ds.patient_records:
    patient

# Find all the STUDY records for the patient
studies = [ii for ii in patient.children if ii.DirectoryRecordType == "STUDY"]

# Select the only study in this patient record
for study in studies:
    study

# Find all the SERIES records in the study
all_series = [ii for ii in study.children if ii.DirectoryRecordType == "SERIES"]
```

```
#Choose the target series
selected_series=all_series[7] # 7 is the index of the target series in the all_series list
```

```

# Find all the IMAGE records in the series
images = [ii for ii in selected_series.children if ii.DirectoryRecordType == "IMAGE"]

plural = ('', 's')[len(images) > 1]

descr = getattr(selected_series, "SeriesDescription", "(no value available)")

print(f"{'  ' * 2}SERIES: SeriesNumber={selected_series.SeriesNumber}, "
    f"Modality={selected_series.Modality}, SeriesDescription={descr} - "
    f"{len(images)} SOP Instance{plural}")
# Get the absolute file path to each instance
#   Each IMAGE contains a relative file path to the root directory
elems = [ii["ReferencedFileID"] for ii in images]
# Make sure the relative file path is always a list of str
paths = [[ee.value] if ee.VM == 1 else ee.value for ee in elems]
paths = [Path(*p) for p in paths]

# List the instance file paths
for p in paths:
    print(f"{'  ' * 3}IMAGE: Path={os.fspath(p)}")
```

Fig. 20.5 Select the targeted series, locate images and read paths

20.4 Image Preprocessing

Now that the DICOM images are organised into arrays and you are able to view them, a decision must be made whether the images will be viewed in two or three dimensions. In this chapter, we describe the two-dimensional image process. Once the images are identified, they need to be labelled based on target features. This can be done by appending the image and its label to separate empty lists using *listname.append(the image), listname.append(thelable)*. The author prefers to create a tuple with the image and its label at this stage because tuples are immutable [18]. Each image is stored using the *pickle* module in python [18, 19]. Only when aggregating all the data to a single file is the tuple broken into

```
# Get ref file
RefDs = pydicom.filereader.dcmread(str(complete_path[0]))

# Load dimensions based on the number of rows, columns, and slices (along the Z axis)
ConstPixelDims = (int(RefDs.Rows), int(RefDs.Columns), len(complete_path))

# Load spacing values (in mm)
ConstPixelSpacing = (float(RefDs.PixelSpacing[0]), float(RefDs.PixelSpacing[1]), float(RefDs.SliceThickness))
```

```
# The array is sized based on 'ConstPixelDims'
ArrayDicom = np.zeros(ConstPixelDims , dtype=RefDs.pixel_array.dtype)

# loop through all the DICOM files
for filenameDCM in complete_path:
    # read the file
    ds = pydicom.read_file((filenameDCM))
    # store the raw image data
    ArrayDicom[:, :, complete_path.index(filenameDCM)] = ds.pixel_array
```

Fig. 20.6 Obtain image dimensions and creating a single array for 3-dimensional series (like CT scans)

Fig. 20.7 The code shows you how to view the images from the array built in the previous step

```
for s in range(ArrayDicom.shape[2]):
    matplotlib.pyplot.figure(dpi=250)
    matplotlib.pyplot.axes().set_aspect('equal', 'datalim')
    matplotlib.pyplot.set_cmap(matplotlib.pyplot.gray())
    matplotlib.pyplot.pcolormesh(np.flipud(ArrayDicom[:, :, s]))
    matplotlib.pyplot.show()
    print(s)
```

Fig. 20.8 Resize all images into a uniform size using OpenCV

```
# Resize all images into a single size
img_size=640
for x in range(len(X)):
    X[x]=cv2.resize(X[x],(img_size,img_size))

X = np.array(X).reshape(-1, img_size, img_size,1)
```

its forming elements. For the purpose of simplicity and standardisation, all the images should be added to a list named X, and all the targets in a list named Y. Unifying the size of all images is part of the good coding practice in machine learning [20–22]. This can be done using the OpenCV 2 resize function [23, 24]; the OpenCV 2 library has been imported as cv2, Fig. 20.8.

Now that we have images (X) and labels (Y), you will need to create a holdout group and split the rest of the data into training and testing, using the Scikit-learn train-test split function [25]. There are no specific guidelines for the ratio used in splitting the data into holdout, train and test subsets, however a 20:60:20 ratio is generally accepted. This can be achieved by using train-test split function twice (the first time to generate the hold out group, the second time to generate train and test data). Alternatively, an 80:20 split followed by K fold splitting of the training data is a reasonable approach, like shown below. You will eventually integrate a CNN into a stratified K fold cross validation process with adjusted class weights, Fig. 20.10 [25]. In order to do so, the required libraries need to be imported. Subsequently, class weights will need to be calculated, and the Keras data generator will need to be setup, illustrated in Figs. 20.9 and 20.10.

It is possible to now use custom performance assessment functions to return values for the true positive, true negative, false positive and false negative. In addition to this, you will be able to calculate a precision score, accuracy score, F1 score and compute the area under the receiver operating characteristic curve (ROC AUC), Fig. 20.11. Finally, the K fold cross validation code structure is detailed in Fig. 20.12. The CNN part has been omitted at this stage, and will be discussed separately in the following segment.

```python
# Importing essential libraries
import numpy as np
import pandas as pd
import matplotlib.pyplot as plt
%matplotlib inline
import seaborn as sns
import sklearn
import imblearn
import itertools
import os as os
import pickle
import random
import cv2
import time
import PIL
from PIL import Image
import tensorflow as tf
import keras

import tensorflow.keras.backend as K
from keras.optimizers import Adam, SGD, RMSprop,Adagrad,Adadelta,Adamax,Nadam
from keras.metrics import categorical_crossentropy
from keras.preprocessing.image import ImageDataGenerator
from keras.layers.normalization import BatchNormalization
from keras.layers.convolutional import *
from keras.models import Sequential
from keras.layers import Dense, Dropout, Activation, Flatten, Conv2D, MaxPooling2D
from keras.callbacks import TensorBoard
from keras.layers import LeakyReLU
from keras.callbacks import ModelCheckpoint
from keras.utils import multi_gpu_model
from keras.callbacks import EarlyStopping
from keras.regularizers import l1, l2

from sklearn.metrics import confusion_matrix, recall_score, classification_report,\
                            roc_auc_score, roc_curve, precision_score,accuracy_score,f1_score
from sklearn.model_selection import train_test_split
from sklearn.model_selection import KFold, StratifiedKFold
from IPython.display import display
```

Fig. 20.9 Importing libraries and functions important for CNN development and for K fold process

Fig. 20.10 Top: calculating the weights of the different classes. Bottom: data augmentation generator setup

```python
# Calculate and assign class weights to a dictionary:
class_weights = sklearn.utils.class_weight.compute_class_weight('balanced',
                                                                np.unique(y),
                                                                y)
class_weight={}
class_weight[0]=class_weights[0]
class_weight[1]=class_weights[1]
```

```python
# Preparing the data augumentation generator specifications:
datagen = ImageDataGenerator(
    featurewise_center=True,
    featurewise_std_normalization=True,
    rotation_range=20,
    width_shift_range=0.2,
    height_shift_range=0.2,
    horizontal_flip=True,
    rescale=1/255
    )
```

Fig. 20.11 Customised performance assessment metrics

```
# Independent performance functions
def perf_measure(y_actual, y_hat, ypredic_per):
    TP = 0
    FP = 0
    TN = 0
    FN = 0


    for i in range(len(y_hat)):
        if y_actual[i]==y_hat[i]==1:
            TP += 1
        if y_hat[i]==1 and y_actual[i]!=y_hat[i]:
            FP += 1
        if y_actual[i]==y_hat[i]==0:
            TN += 1
        if y_hat[i]==0 and y_actual[i]!=y_hat[i]:
            FN += 1

    precision = precision_score(y_actual, y_hat)
    recall = recall_score(y_actual, y_hat)
    accuracy = accuracy_score(y_actual, y_hat)
    f1 = f1_score(y_actual, y_hat)
    auc_keras=roc_auc_score(y_actual,ypredic_per)

    return(TP, FP, TN, FN,precision,recall,accuracy,f1,auc_keras )

```

20.5 Convolutional Neural Network (CNN) Building and Assessment

Building a CNN is not overly onerous, however optimising the structure of the network to achieve tangible results whilst avoiding under or overfitting can be a time-consuming exercise. There are multiple well-known architectures of CNN reported in the literature, and the reader may wish to refer to the bibliography for further detail [26–30]. In this practical example we will use a modified AlexNet [26] architecture. Classically, AlexNet is composed of five convolutional layers and three densely connected layers. In this example there will be three convolutional layers, two densely connected layers and a single outcome layer.

In building a CNN model, start with a two (or three) dimensional image, and apply a small filter (2–3 pixels * 2–3 pixels) to all areas of the image (Fig. 20.13). This will be followed by an activation function—in this case, we will use the rectified linear unit (*relu*) activation function [31]. The outcomes will be summarised by a pooling function; in this use case we employ a maximum pooling function, which has been reported to outperform other pooling functions [32]. For the purpose of this exercise we repeated this convolution step two more times and added a 30% neuron drop out to these layers. The outcome of these layers will be a two-dimensional array, and before it is possible to connect it to a dense neural network it must be converted to a one-dimensional array by using a *Flatten* layer. The dense connected layers will also have a *relu* activation function and a 0.3 neuron drop out. Finally, a single output layer with a sigmoid activation function will generate the prediction. In the code above, we chose Adaptive Moment Estimation (Adam) as an optimisation function with modified parameters and binary cross entropy as a loss function. We also utilised the *early stopping* function to optimise the training time, and restore the best performing model.

Before incorporating this model into the K fold cross validation code structure, it is imperative to experiment and test the model on the data, and modify the model's depth, layer's density (number of neurons), the structure of the model, deferent activation and optimisation functions. Learning about different functions used in similar classification problems is useful in identifying the best option, however, trial and error is also an accepted method. The model needs to be assessed using standard classification metrics, area under the curve (AUC) and different cross validation methods, such as the prementioned K fold cross validation. Lastly, the final predictions will be calculated by averaging the predictions of the different models in the K fold process. The code is published in more detail with accompanying example data on a GitHub repository (https://github.com/Mouminakm/DICOM-Machine-Learning.git).

```
# Prepare the 5 fold cross validation function specification:
skf = StratifiedKFold(n_splits = 5, random_state = 7, shuffle = True)
# This table will contain the performance of each fold of the cross validation
final_table=pd.DataFrame(columns=['TP', 'FP', 'TN', 'FN','precision','recall','accuracy','f1'])
# The directory where the models are going to be saved
save_dir = '/saved_models/'
# fold counter
fold_var = 1


for train_index, val_index in skf.split(X,Y):
    K.clear_session()
    #Trainig and validation assigniment
    trainingX=X[train_index]
    trainingY=Y[train_index]

    valX=X[val_index]
    valY=Y[val_index]

    K.clear_session()
    # Creating the model, this wil be explained in the next step

    model = Sequential()
    '''Model structure '''

    opt=keras.optimizers.Adam(lr=0.00003, beta_1=0.9, beta_2=0.999, amsgrad=False, decay=1e-6)


    #compile the model

    model.compile(loss='binary_crossentropy',
                  optimizer=opt,
                  metrics=['val_loss'])
    #callback
    es = EarlyStopping(monitor='val_loss', mode='min', verbose=1, patience=100,restore_best_weights=True )

    # train the K fold with data augmentation generator
    model.fit(datagen.flow(trainingX,trainingY, batch_size=5),callbacks=[es],\
             class_weight=class_weight,verbose=0,epochs=1500 ,validation_data=(valX,valY))

    # Predict on the out of boot (validation)
    result = model.evaluate(valX,valY)
    results = dict(zip(model.metrics_names,result))
    ypredic_per=model.predict(valX)

    yvalpred=model.predict_classes(valX)
    print(perf_measure(valY,yvalpred,ypredic_per))
    pd.concat([final_table,perf_measure(valY,yvalpred,ypredic_per)], axis=0)

    model.save(save_dir+str(fold_var)+".h5")




    print( 'model {} accuracy is {} and the loss is {}'.format(fold_var,results['accuracy'], results['loss']))
    K.clear_session()
    fold_var += 1
```

Fig. 20.12 Illustration of the stratified K fold code

```
# Creating the convolutional neural network model this structure is simpler/modified model from AlexNet architecture
model = Sequential()
# The input shape needs to be the unified shape of the images in the training data.
model.add(Conv2D(60, (3, 3),input_shape= trainingX.shape[1:],kernel_regularizer=l2(l=0.1)  ))
model.add(Activation('relu'))
model.add(MaxPooling2D(pool_size=(2, 2)))

model.add(Conv2D(60, (2,2),kernel_regularizer=l2(l=0.1)))
model.add(Activation('relu'))
model.add(MaxPooling2D(pool_size=(2, 2)))
model.add(Dropout(0.3))

model.add(Conv2D(60, (3, 3),kernel_regularizer=l2(l=0.1)))
model.add(Activation('relu'))
model.add(MaxPooling2D(pool_size=(2, 2)))
model.add(Dropout(0.3))


model.add(Flatten())


model.add(Dense(64, activation='relu', activity_regularizer=l1(0.001)))
model.add(Dropout(0.3))

model.add(Dense(32, activation='relu',activity_regularizer=l1(0.001)))
model.add(Dropout(0.3))

model.add(Dense(1))
model.add(Activation('sigmoid'))
```

Fig. 20.13 CNN model structure and specification

References

1. Langlotz CP, et al. A roadmap for foundational research on artificial intelligence in medical imaging: from the 2018 NIH/RSNA/ACR/The Academy Workshop. Radiology. 2019;291(3):781–91.
2. Erickson BJ, Korfiatis P, Akkus Z, Kline TL. Machine learning for medical imaging. Radiographics. 2017;37(2):505–15.
3. Willemink MJ, et al. Preparing medical imaging data for machine learning. Radiology. 2020;295(1):4–15.
4. Saboori M, Ahmadi J, Farajzadegan Z. Indications for brain CT scan in patients with minor head injury. Clin Neurol Neurosurg. 2007;109(5):399–405.
5. Smits M, et al. External validation of the Canadian CT Head Rule and the New Orleans Criteria for CT scanning in patients with minor head injury. JAMA. 2005;294(12):1519–25.
6. Chilamkurthy S, et al. Deep learning algorithms for detection of critical findings in head CT scans: a retrospective study. Lancet. 2018;392(10162):2388–96.
7. Chilamkurthy S, et al. Development and validation of deep learning algorithms for detection of critical findings in head CT scans. 2018. arXiv preprint arXiv:1803.05854.
8. Keshavamurthy KN, et al. Machine learning algorithm for automatic detection of CT-identifiable hyperdense lesions associated with traumatic brain injury. Med Imaging 2017 Comput Diagn. 2017;10134(1):101342G. https://doi.org/10.1117/12.2254227.
9. Gong T, et al. Classification of CT brain images of head trauma. Lect Notes Comput Sci (including Subser Lect Notes Artif Intell Lect Notes Bioinformatics). 2007;4774 LNBI:401–8. https://doi.org/10.1007/978-3-540-75286-8_38.
10. Lee B, Newberg A. Neuroimaging in traumatic brain imaging. NeuroRx. 2005;2(2):372–83.
11. Mustra M, Delac K, Grgic M. Overview of the DICOM standard. In: 2008 50th International Symposium ELMAR, vol. 1; 2008. p. 39–44.
12. Mildenberger P, Eichelberg M, Martin E. Introduction to the DICOM standard. Eur Radiol. 2002;12(4):920–7.
13. Gibaud B. The DICOM standard: a brief overview. In: Molecular imaging: computer reconstruction and practice. New York: Springer; 2008. p. 229–38.
14. Huang J, Ling A, Summers RM, Yao J. Integration of PACS and CAD systems using DICOMDIR and open-source tools. In: Medical imaging 2013: advanced PACS-based imaging informatics and therapeutic applications, vol. 8674; 2013. p. 86740V.
15. Villegas R, Montilla G, Villegas H. A software tool for reading DICOM directory files. Int J Healthcare Inf Syst Informatics. 2007;2(1):54–70.
16. Mason D, et al. pydicom/pydicom: pydicom 2.1.1; 2020. https://doi.org/10.5281/ZENODO.4248192.
17. Caswell TA, et al. matplotlib/matplotlib: REL: v3.3.1; 2020. https://doi.org/10.5281/ZENODO.3984190.
18. Beazley DM. Python essential reference. Boston: Addison-Wesley Professional; 2009.
19. Dalcin LD, Paz RR, Kler PA, Cosimo A. Parallel distributed computing using Python. Adv Water Resour. 2011;34(9):1124–39.
20. Wang H, Li S, Song L, Cui L. A novel convolutional neural network based fault recognition method via image fusion of multi-vibration-signals. Comput Ind. 2019;105:182–90.
21. Howard AG. Some improvements on deep convolutional neural network based image classification. arXiv Prepr. arXiv1312.5402; 2013.
22. Jifara W, Jiang F, Rho S, Cheng M, Liu S. Medical image denoising using convolutional neural network: a residual learning approach. J Supercomput. 2019;75(2):704–18.
23. Bradski G. The OpenCV library. Dr Dobbs J Softw Tools. 2000;120:122–5.
24. Howse J, Joshi P, Beyeler M. Opencv: computer vision projects with python. Birmingham: Packt Publishing Ltd; 2016.
25. Pedregosa F, et al. Scikit-learn: machine learning in {P}ython. J Mach Learn Res. 2011;12:2825–30.

26. Krizhevsky A, Sutskever I, Hinton GE. Imagenet classification with deep convolutional neural networks. In: Advances in neural information processing systems; 2012. p. 1097–105.
27. Zeiler MD, Fergus R. Visualizing and understanding convolutional networks. In: European conference on computer vision; 2014. p. 818–33.
28. Simonyan K, Zisserman A. Very deep convolutional networks for large-scale image recognition. arXiv Prepr. arXiv1409.1556; 2014.
29. Szegedy C, et al. Going deeper with convolutions. In: Proceedings of the IEEE conference on computer vision and pattern recognition; 2015. p. 1–9.
30. He K, Zhang X, Ren S, Sun J. Deep residual learning for image recognition. In: Proceedings of the IEEE conference on computer vision and pattern recognition; 2016. p. 770–8.
31. Hara K, Saito D, Shouno H. Analysis of function of rectified linear unit used in deep learning. In: 2015 International Joint Conference on Neural Networks (IJCNN); 2015. p. 1–8.
32. Scherer D, Müller A, Behnke S. Evaluation of pooling operations in convolutional architectures for object recognition. In: International conference on artificial neural networks; 2010. p. 92–101.

Foundations of Lesion Detection Using Machine Learning in Clinical Neuroimaging

21

Manoj Mannil, Nicolin Hainc, Risto Grkovski, and Sebastian Winklhofer

21.1 Introduction

Radiology has made great advances since X-rays were first used to detect broken bones and bullet fragments at the turn of the nineteenth century. But even with the plethora of computing power driving today's machine learning (ML) algorithms one aspect has remained constant over the years: the endeavor to detect lesions, to differentiate normal from abnormal, and to single out and define abnormalities within organs or amongst organs within a population. Lesion detection is central to the radiological process and precedes all further processes which include but are not limited to segmentation, characterization, quantification, longitudinal disease assessment, prognosis, and prediction of treatment response. For purposes of lesion detection, four distinct categories exist: lesions that are clearly detectable by the human reader, lesions that are incidentally found, lesions where the human reader benefits from assisted lesion detection, and lesions that are yet to be discovered through ML.

Brain tumors, intracranial hemorrhage, and stroke are examples of lesions that a human reader will detect with a high sensitivity. The premise is simple: we know exactly what we are looking for and will scrutinize images until satisfied, either by detecting a lesion or deeming the study unremarkable. With certain lesions, ML-based lesion detection may not necessarily aid the human reader with the study they are presently reading, but can help improve patient outcome in other manners, for example by highlighting scans with critical/acute findings waiting to be read in the list. In other clinical settings, such as follow-up studies of multiple sclerosis patients, ML-based detection will aid the human reader to discover new lesions, especially in patients with a tediously high lesion burden. Furthermore, ML-based lesion detection can help decrease inter-reader variability when lesion detection has direct implications for patient management, e.g., through automated ASPECT scoring in acute stroke [1].

The second category of lesion encompasses incidental findings. Brain aneurysms, for example, will be detected by a human reader with a high sensitivity given an MR angiography. However, for routine follow up of brain tumors and multiple sclerosis, a dedicated MR angiography is not routinely performed and the focus of the human reader is elsewhere. Here, a system assessing for relevant incidental findings running in the background could provide additional value in patient care.

The third category of lesion includes cases where human readers need help with visual perception, i.e., the lesion in question lingers near the threshold of a human reader's ability to correctly detect it. We know exactly what we are looking for but we may not always be able to detect the lesion. Focal cortical dysplasia type 1 is an example of this. Here, we scrutinize the entire cortex, searching for a tiny area of gray-white blurring or relative cortical signal alteration, but these findings may not always be apparent. Work is constantly being done to improve sequences and thus detection

M. Mannil
Clinic of Radiology, University Hospital Münster, Münster, Germany
e-mail: manoj.mannil@ukmuenster.de

N. Hainc
Department of Medical Imaging, Division of Neuroradiology, Toronto Western Hospital, University Health Network, Toronto, ON, Canada

Department of Neuroradiology, Clinical Neuroscience Center, University Hospital Zürich, University of Zurich, Zurich, Switzerland
e-mail: Nicolin.Hainc@usz.ch

R. Grkovski
Department of Neuroradiology, Clinical Neuroscience Center, University Hospital Zürich, University of Zurich, Zurich, Switzerland

Department of Radiology, University Medical Center Maribor, Maribor, Slovenia

S. Winklhofer (✉)
Department of Neuroradiology, Clinical Neuroscience Center, University Hospital Zürich, University of Zurich, Zurich, Switzerland
e-mail: Sebastian.winklhofer@usz.ch

V. E. Staartjes et al. (eds.), *Machine Learning in Clinical Neuroscience*, Acta Neurochirurgica Supplement 134,
https://doi.org/10.1007/978-3-030-85292-4_21

[2] but help in the form of statistical pixel-value based ML lesion detection would be a welcome addition. The same can be said for dementia, where detection of a mildly atrophied cortex remains a challenge through visual assessment alone. Tiny aneurysms also fall into this category.

The fourth category of lesion involves syndromes for which an imaging biomarker has yet to be discovered, if at all. In schizophrenia, imaging has always played a secondary, exclusionary role, performed to rule out physical or structural causes, while diagnosis is made based on clinical assessment of behavior, emotional expression, psychotic symptoms, etc. Recently, ML techniques have been applied to resting state functional MRI describing an 87% accuracy in differentiating drug-native schizophrenia patients from healthy controls [3]. In other words, the capability to detect schizophrenia based on imaging has now been presented to human readers through machine learning. It is conceivable that ML will one day be able to detect lesions in other clinical syndromes for which an established imaging biomarker does not yet exist, ultimately challenging our notion of normal by highlighting areas on imaging studies we have not yet attributed importance to.

21.2 Technical Considerations

The field of radiomics involves the extraction of predefined features such as shape, intensity, and texture from a segmented (tumor) volume of interest [4]. Texture analysis (TA) is commonly used for quantitative medical image analysis and computer-aided classification [5, 6]. The texture features are derived from different groups, i.e., Histogram, Gradient distortion, Gray-Level-Co-Occurrence-Matrix (GLCM), Gray-Level-Dependency-Matrix (GLDM), Gray-Level-Run-Length-Matrix (GLRM), Gray-Level-Size-Zone-Matrix (GLZM), Neighboring-Gray-Tone-Difference-Matrix (NGTM), and Gray-Level-Dependence-Matrix (GLDM). These groups can be divided into several levels. Histogram analysis for example takes into account the mere frequency distribution of pixel intensities within a given region-of-interest and is therefore considered a first order TA feature. GLCM is considered a higher level feature, as it takes into account the spatial co-occurrence of certain pixel intensities as well. These predefined TA features allow for transparency when one considers to develop a generalizable algorithm for the purpose of lesion detection. The computed TA features are generally used as input to several machine learning algorithms to predict the abnormalities of interest. The resulting algorithms are graded according to their sensitivity, specificity, F1 score and the area-under-the-curve in receiver-operating-characteristics (ROC-AUC). In case the training data sets are either of insufficient size or include unnecessary features, the results will not be reproducible on an independent data set. To avoid this so called *overfitting* problem, it is important to perform dimension reduction (e.g., reproducibility, redundancy, information criterion) and split of data into training, testing and independent validation data sets.

In contrast to Texture analysis with custom-engineered features, deep learning allows for automatic feature extraction from imaging inputs. Multilayer artificial neural networks for instance are roughly comparable to biologic neural systems. For this purpose, weighted connections between neurons/ nodes are iteratively adjusted based on example pairs of inputs and target outputs. Back-propagation is used as a corrective measure through the network architecture. For computer vision tasks, convolutional neural networks (CNNs) have proven to be effective. Recently, several clinical applications of CNNs have been proposed and studied in radiology for classification, detection, and segmentation tasks [7].

Deep learning architecture based on CNNs consist of multiple layers. This network can represent a hierarchy of features that are of an increasingly complex composition of low-level input features, thereby modeling higher levels of abstractions (e.g., shape, edges, texture, contrast) from the input data. Predictions from a sample image require the sequential activation of each node of each layer, starting from the input layer up to the output layer, a process called forward propagation. In the setting of a classification task, the activation of the output layer is typically submitted to a function, e.g., a normalized "squashing" function that maps a vector of real values to a probability distribution. Therefore, this softmax function converts raw activation signals from the output layer to target class probabilities [7].

Training of a deep learning network is performed by repeatedly adjusting these parameters, which consist of the weights and biases of each node. Starting from a random initial configuration, the parameters are then adjusted via an optimization algorithm [7].

For the purpose of lesion detection, deep learning can be used in various ways. Recently, a novel method called "masked R-CNN" has been proposed. It allows for parallel evaluation of region proposal (attention), object detection (classification), and instance segmentation. In short, it is a combination of object detection within bounding boxes around each instance of a class and subsequent semantic segmentation within each of the bounding boxes.

Initially, a preconfigured distribution of bounding boxes at various shapes and resolutions is tested for the presence of a potential abnormality. Next, the highest ranking bounding boxes are identified and used to generate region proposals, therefore focusing algorithm attention on specific regions within the medical image. These composite region proposals are pruned using e.g., non-maximum suppression and are then used as input into a classifier to determine the presence or absence of a pathology [8]. In the case of a positive detection, a final segmentation branch of the network is used to generate binary masks (Fig. 21.1). The efficiency of a mask R-CNN architecture arises from a common backbone network that generates a shared set of image features for the various parallel detection, classification, and segmentation tasks [8].

To assess the quality of Radiomics studies for lesion detection, a Radiomics Quality Score (RQS) has been recently proposed [9]. The RQS consists of 16 parameters ranging from image protocol standards to calibration statistics. The resulting score positively correlates with the quality and reliability of the presented results (Table 21.1).

21.3 Clinical Applications

Introduction to Clinical Applications

Neuroimaging is frequently vital to rule out or to detect abnormalities of the central nervous system for the diagnosis and clinical management of patients with neurological conditions. Precise detection, characterization and interpretation of any changes are required for a quick and accurate assessment, in order to decrease the burden of the condition and prevent permanent functional impairment [10]. Machine learning and deep learning technology may be better suited for certain tasks in comparison to humans, such as detection and classification of abnormalities. Furthermore, it may be helpful for extracting patterns and features from images, which include automatic identification, notation, segmenta-

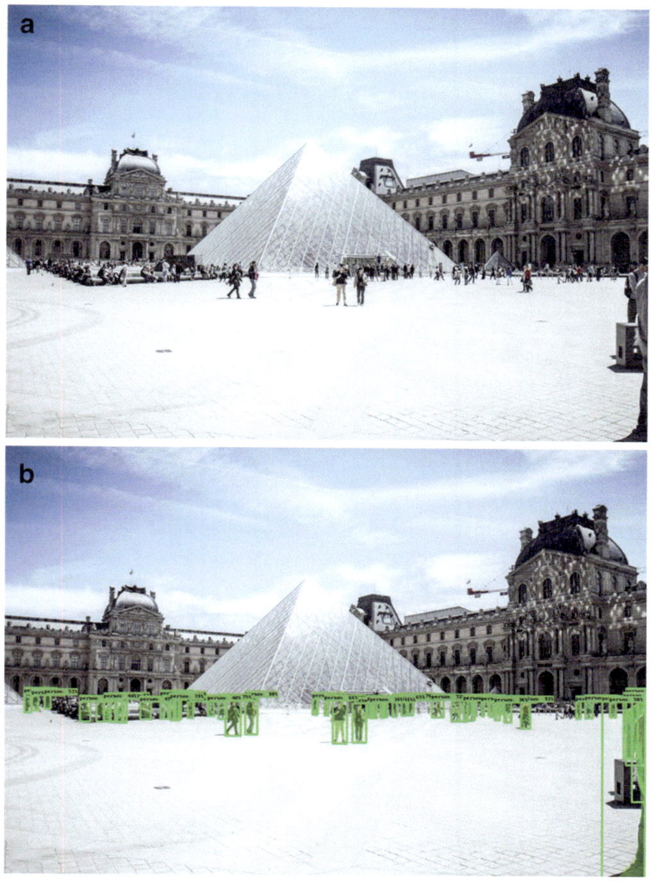

Fig. 21.1 Sample detection of people using a masked R-CNN: (**a**) Source image (Stacy Wyss/Realistic Shots), (**b**) Application of masked R-CNN to identify people within the image by use of COCO index mapping and Tensorflow deep learning architecture

Table 21.1 Radiomics Quality Score (modified from [9])

RQS criteria		Points
1	Image protocol quality—well-documented image protocols and/or usage of public image protocols allow reproducibility/replicability	+1 (if protocols are well-documented) +1 (if public protocol is used)
2	Multiple segmentations—possible actions are: segmentation by different physicians/algorithms/software, perturbing segmentations by (random) noise, segmentation at different breathing cycles. Analysis of feature robustness to segmentation variabilities	+1
3	Phantom study on all scanners—Detection of inter-scanner differences and vendor-dependent features. Analysis of feature robustness to these sources of variability.	+1
4	Imaging at multiple time points—collect images of individuals at additional time points. Analyze feature robustness to temporal variabilities	+1
5	Feature reduction or adjustment for multiple testing—decreases the risk of overfitting. Overfitting is inevitable if the number of features exceeds the number of samples	−3 (if neither measure is implemented) +3 (if either measure is implemented)
6	Multivariable analysis with non radiomics features—is expected to provide a more holistic model	+1
7	Detect and discuss biological correlates—demonstration of phenotypic differences.	+1
8	Cutoff analyses—determine risk groups by either the median, a previously published cutoff or report a continuous risk variable	+1
9	Discrimination statistics—report discrimination statistics (for example, C-statistic, ROC curve, AUC) and their statistical significance (for example, *p*-values, confidence intervals). One can also apply resampling method (for example, bootstrapping, cross-validation)	+1 (if a discrimination statistic and its statistical significance are reported) +1 (if a resampling method technique is also applied)

(continued)

Table 21.1 (continued)

RQS criteria		Points
10	Calibration statistics—report calibration statistics and their statistical significance (for example, *P*-values, confidence intervals). One can also apply resampling method	+1 (if a calibration statistic and its statistical significance are reported) +1 (if a resampling method technique is also applied)
11	Prospective study registered in a trial database—provides the highest level of evidence supporting the clinical validity and usefulness of the radiomics biomarker	+7 (for prospective validation of a radiomics signature in an appropriate trial)
12	Validation—the validation is performed without retraining and without adaptation of the cutoff value, provides crucial information with regard to credible clinical performance	−5 (if validation is missing) +2 (if validation is based on a dataset from the same institute) +3 (if validation is based on a dataset from another institute) +4 (if validation is based on two datasets from two distinct institutes) +4 (if the study validates a previously published signature) +5 (if validation is based on three or more datasets from distinct institutes) *Datasets should be of comparable size and should have at least 10 events per model feature
13	Comparison to "gold standard"—assess the extent to which the model agrees with/is superior to the current "gold standard" method	+2
14	Potential clinical utility—report on the current and potential application of the model in a clinical setting	+2
15	Cost-effectiveness analysis—report on the cost-effectiveness of the clinical application	+1
16	Open science and data—make code and data publicly available. Open science facilitates knowledge transfer and reproducibility of the study	+1 (if scans are open source) +1 (if region-of-interest segmentations are open source) +1 (if code is open source) +1 (if radiomics features are calculated on a set of representative ROIs and the calculated features and representative ROIs are open source)

Total points 36 (100%)

tion and delineation or outlining of the potentially abnormal changes (stroke, hemorrhage, tumors, and other structural abnormalities). Such applications are not only important for initial diagnosis, but in follow up imaging as well, i.e., for monitoring of any morphological or functional changes of the abnormalities [11, 12].

These same principles can be applied to normal changes. However, radiologists should be involved in setting up (sometimes subjective) threshold values of normal and abnormal findings and should take the lead role in determining the benefit of such applications to provide clinical value in everyday workflow [13, 14].

21.4 Stroke

In stroke and especially in ischemic stroke, time is an utmost important factor for successful recovery, thus a rapid and accurate diagnosis is crucial for optimal treatment and decrease in permanent disability in these patients. The protocol of appropriate assessment and triage of these patients, however, relies on a number of steps, which include collaboration among different clinical professions such as radiologists and neurologists. This process may absorb valuable time and the subspecialized infrastructure may not be fully accessible to all patients in need. Therefore, an automated support of image evaluation would be desirable to optimize the stroke detection step [15, 16].

Different imaging modalities are used when diagnosing stroke, but even these might sometimes not be enough for a successful identification of abnormalities by an imaging specialist. Computer-aided diagnosis (CAD) and machine learning algorithms, which have gained a lot of popularity in other fields of medicine, could provide additional image information in a shorter amount of time [11, 17, 18].

ASPECTS

The Alberta Stroke Program Early CT Score is a 10-point quantitative topographic CT scan score in patients with middle cerebral artery stroke to determine appropriate management [19].

This scoring is a challenging methodology to standardize [20], however currently there are a number of commercially available applications (software platforms), which provide a ML algorithm for automated ASPECTS assessment: Brainomix e-ASPECTS (Oxford, UK), Siemens Frontier (Erlangen, Germany), iSchemaView ASPECTS (Menlo Park, California, USA), and others that are in use or in development [16, 21, 22]. Both Nagel et al. [23] and Herweh [24] have shown a non-inferior performance of e-ASPECTS to the clinical experts. In patients with preexisting neurostructural changes the performance was somewhat inferior [25]. In a recent study [26], a recurrent residual convolutional neural network (RRCNN) for ASPECTS classification using diffusion-weighted imaging (DWI) achieved better performance than pre-trained convolutional neural networks (CNNs), such as VGG16, Inception V3, and a 3D convolutional neural network (3DCNN). Maegerlein et al. [27] showed RAPID ASPECTS (iSchemaView) software of having higher consensus correlation in comparison to two neuroimaging specialists. An advantage of RRCNN is that of the residual unit, which aids the deep architecture learning and feature accumulation with recurrent residual convolutional layers ensuring better feature representation for segmentation tasks [28].

Large Vessel Occlusion (LVO)

For large vessel occlusion (LVO) detection, CNNs might be the most suitable method applied to computed tomography (CT) and CT angiography images [16]. A U-Net based model created by You et al., which used clinical and imaging data for hyperdense middle cerebral artery (MCA) sign detection, showed a 68% sensitivity and 61% specificity [29]. Amukotuwa et al. achieved 95% sensitivity and 79% specificity [30] and Chatterjee et al. a 82% sensitivity and 94% specificity in a study with 650 patients [31]. Olive-Gadea et al. [32] tested Methinks LVO software in 1453 patients with non-contrast CT scans and achieved 83% sensitivity and 71% specificity. In a recent study, Stib et al. achieved an AUC of 0.89, a sensitivity of 100% and a specificity of 77%, by utilizing CNN in multiphase CT examinations with delayed phases [33].

Identification of Infarct Core and Tissue at Risk/Penumbra

In ischemic brain tissue, two main types of changes are observed: the core (irreversible) and the penumbra or tissue at risk (reversible). The detection of these changes is difficult to train on automated algorithms, as the reference values do not depend solely on imaging values. Training is mostly done by manual delineation [16]. Applications using a threshold lesion detection method can show a high variability of lesion volumes due to individually chosen different cutoff values [34–36]. One such algorithm, RAPID [37], achieved 100% sensitivity and 93% specificity for detecting a mismatch on perfusion images on patients from the DEFUSE trial [38]. A CNN based technique for segmentation of acute ischemic changes based on diffusion-weighted magnetic resonance imaging (MRI) images, by including two separate CNNs (DeconvNets (EDD Net) and a multi-scale convolutional label evaluation net (MUSCLE Net)), achieved a mean accuracy of the Dice coefficient of 0.67 (range 0–1) [39]. Lee et al. [40] showed a ML algorithm outperforming imaging experts in detecting diffusion-weighted imaging—fluid-attenuated inversion recovery (DWI-FLAIR) mismatch for the identification of patients with acute ischemic stroke within 4.5 h window for thrombolysis therapy in a study of 355 patients.

Hemorrhagic Transformation

Recently, CNN-based methods have also been utilized for detection of hemorrhagic transformation after reperfusion therapy [41] in patients with acute ischemic stroke, with one study showing comparable results to that of a radiological SEDAN score, with improved performance after including clinical data from NIHSS [42].

Intracranial Hemorrhage

The detection of an intracranial hemorrhage is usually done using computed tomography or magnetic resonance imaging. In particular, the detailed diagnosis is done by examining non-contrast CT images [13] and standard MRI sequences as well as dedicated susceptibility weighted imaging (SWI) sequences for the detection of microbleeds [43]. Detection based on CNN transfer-learning technology has shown promising results, with the advantage of being able to execute it on a small number of testing data [12]. For instance, Chang et al. demonstrated the high performance of masked R-CNNs fully automated, deep learning architecture to accurately detect and quantify intraparenchymal, epidural, subdural, and subarachnoidal hemorrhage on non-contrast CT examinations of the head [8]. However, the goal of such tasks should not only be to quantify, but also to qualify the imaging data in order to help in triage, re-prioritize, and modify workflow in order to improve assessment of critical cases and decrease the time from diagnosis to treatment. Qualification and standardization of data may be somewhat difficult, as it needs to be objectivized into which findings are important or urgent and which are expected in which patient group (e.g., microhemorrhages in stroke, postoperative hemorrhages). There are many factors that need to be taken into account for such decision making, which complicates automatic assessment or worklist prioritization, thus clinical experience still plays a key role [10, 13]. The Radiological Society of North America (RSNA) 2019 Brain CT Hemorrhage Challenge involved a publicly available

874,035-image, multi-institutional, and multinational brain hemorrhage CT dataset, composed of annotations of the five hemorrhage subtypes (subarachnoid, intraventricular, subdural, epidural, and intraparenchymal hemorrhage), in order to encourage machine learning development in this field [44]. The winners showed the potential of AI to improve the efficiency and quality of care in radiology with high complexness.

21.5 Multiple Sclerosis

The manual assessment of MRI images regarding multiple sclerosis (MS) lesions may be a time consuming process. The main task of machine learning in multiple sclerosis is lesion detection and classification, for which different imaging modalities can be used [45]. Shui-Hua Wang et al. developed a 14-Layer convolutional neural network with batch normalization, dropout, and stochastic pooling for MS detection on MRI images from 64 subjects, which were validated by MS imaging experts. They achieved an impressive 99% sensitivity, 99% specificity, and 99% accuracy [46]. Zurita et al. [47] developed an algorithm to confidently identify multiple sclerosis patients from healthy subjects by using support vector machine classifications of functional and diffusion MRI data. Ion-Mărgineanu et al. [48] used magnetic resonance spectroscopy (MRS) data from 87 patents together with clinical data for differentiating between relapsing-remitting, primary and secondary progressive forms of MS. Yoo et al. [49] used 3D image patches of myelin maps and corresponding T1-weighted MR images to distinguish between multiple sclerosis patients and healthy controls. Narayana et al.'s [50] algorithm predicted lesion enhancement in multiple sclerosis from unenhanced multiparametric MRI images with good accuracy. With this information, it might be possible to avoid the use of contrast agents. Duong [51] and Gessert [52] both constructed a CNN based method for lesion segmentation using FLAIR images, achieving a median Dice score of 0.79 and a true positive rate of 74% respectively.

21.6 Neuro-Oncology

The large variety of neurooncological imaging appearances frequently remains a challenge for the human reader. Brain tumor detection and segmentation of numerous features is important for clinical management [12, 45]. New applications can be tested using the publicly available The Brain Tumor Image Segmentation dataset of images of manually segmented brain tumors [53]. Since then, there has been an explosion of machine learning software available for tumor classification and segmentation [12, 45, 54]. Different approaches have been used, examples of most recent studies include: a transfer-learning approach based on a Convolutional Neural Network (CCN) for better classification of five multiclass tumor datasets compared to six different ML models [55], a fully automated 3D-Dense-UNets deep learning method for accurate segmentation of low grade and high grade gliomas from Brain Tumor Segmentation Challenge 2019 [56], radiomics including imaging data [57], successful automated brain tumor segmentation on FLAIR images from Brain Tumor Segmentation Challenge 2019, namely gliomas [58], using CNNs for detecting glioma heterogeneity [59], an outlier detecting framework using one-class support vector machine to extract features from post-contrast T1-weighted and FLAIR images [60] and classification of brain tumors based on IDH Status and 1p/19q-codeletion [61, 62] (Fig. 21.2). Methods based on CNN (such as 3D U-Net) can also be utilized for detection and segmentation of brain metastases from multimodal MR images [63–65] or different types of head and neck tumors from MRI, CT and fluorodeoxyglucose positron emission tomography (FDG PET) imaging modalities [45, 66], such as parotid gland tumors [67], nasopharyngeal carcinoma [68] and superficial laryngopharyngeal cancer [69].

21.7 Epilepsy

ML techniques can be beneficial in detection, localization and segmentation of potentially abnormal morphologic epileptogenic areas [10, 70]. A variety of potential clinical applications are described in the literature, mostly based on CNN technology, for example: CNN based on transfer learning using diffusion kurtosis images (DKI) for foci detection on segmented hippocampus images [70], a combination of electroencephalography (EEG) in functional magnetic resonance imaging (rs-fMRI) for separating preictal (pre-seizure) from non-preictal states [71], automatic segmentation of hippocampus with combination of a deep belief network (DBN) and the lattice Boltzmann (LB) method [72] and a newly developed method of iterative local linear mapping (ILLM) for hippocampus segmentation on both 1.5 and 3T MR images achieving similar mean Dice coefficients 0.89 and 0.88 respectively [73].

21.8 Aneurysms

Intracranial aneurysms are not uncommon. The majority of them will be asymptomatic, however a rupture of an aneurysm might result in severe morbidity or mortality. Their prevalence in general population consist of roughly 3% [74] (in the population with connective tissue disease even more than 10% [75]), around 85% out of which account for non-traumatic subarachnoid hemorrhages [76]. Thus detection

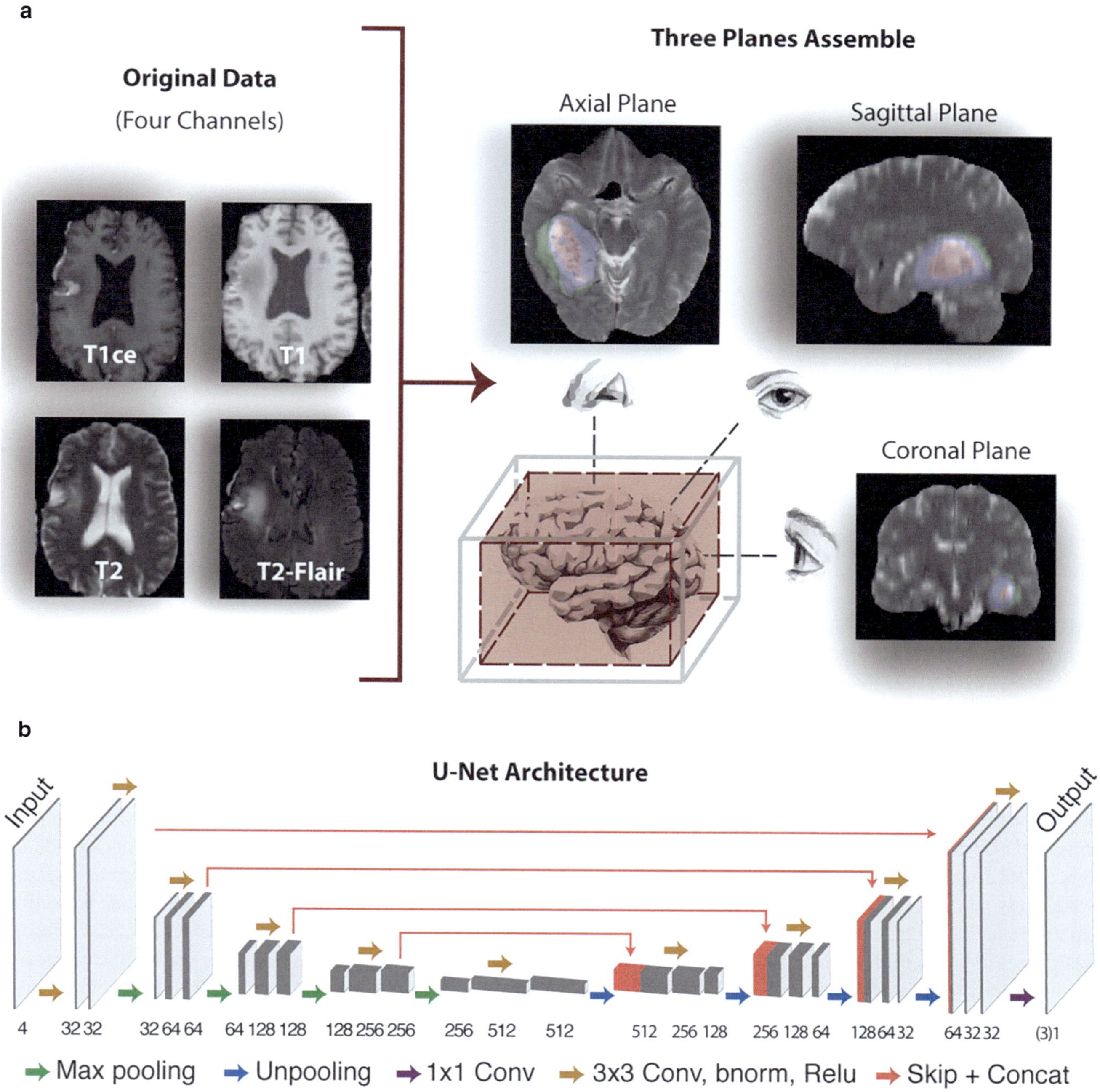

Fig. 21.2 Example of a U-Net Architecture for automated glioma segmentation of multimodal magnetic resonance imaging scans. Two-dimensional axial, sagittal, and coronal planes were generated from 3D multimodal T1ce, T1, T2 and T2-FLAIR images (**a**), which were used as an input into the U-Net Architecture (**b**) to segmentate areas of the whole tumor, tumor core, and enhancing tumor. (Adapted with reprint permission from Wu S, Li H, et al. Three-Plane-assembled Deep Learning Segmentation of Gliomas. Radiology: Artificial Intelligence Vol. 2 No. 2, 2020. Published online March 11, 2020. https://doi.org/10.1148/ryai.2020190011. © Radiological Society of North America [54])

and segmentation of unruptured aneurysms is also a relevant field to explore in ML [45]. Existing deep learning algorithms, mainly CNN based, can utilize images from 3D time-of-flight (TOF) MR angiography [77–79], 2D images from digital subtraction angiography (DSA) [80, 81] or computed tomographic angiography (CTA) [82] (Fig. 21.3). All showed impressive results and could greatly aid the diagnostic physician.

21.9 Neurodegeneration and Others

Detection and differentiation of dementia types from image data sets may sometimes prove challenging. As such, effective AI tools might assist in giving a correct diagnosis [10], with development being facilitated in recent years due to a number of publicly available databases [83]. As a result, a

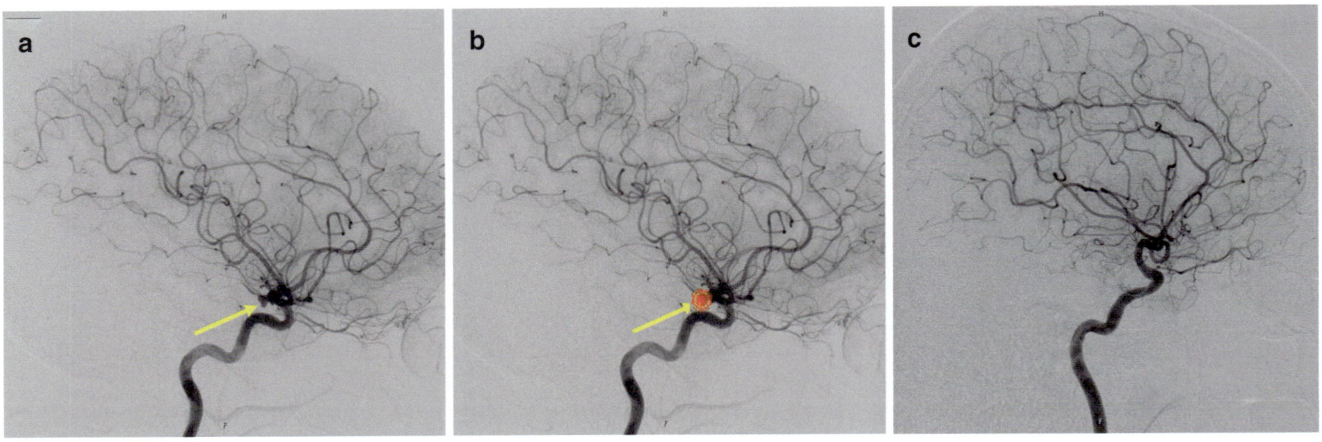

Fig. 21.3 Deep learning based detection of intracranial aneurysms on digital subtraction angiography (DSA) images [81]. (**a**, **b**) Demonstrate the case of a patient with an incidental aneurysm (yellow arrow in **a**) of the posterior communicating artery. (**b**) is the same image with the correctly detected and localized aneurysm by using a deep learning algorithm with machine learning (arrow indicates the correct labeling). (**c**) Demonstrates the case of another patient without an aneurysm. The deep learning algorithm correctly classified this case as a DSA image without an aneurysm

variety of machine learning applications with promising results have been developed, which include combinations of CNN, RNN, and other techniques for differentiating of Alzheimer's disease (AD) and mild cognitive impairment (MCI) from MR images [84–88] or from positron emission tomography (PET) with fluorodeoxyglucose (FDG) data [89, 90], separating symptomatic Alzheimer's Disease from depression [91], multiclass differentiation of neurodegenerative diseases (such as Alzheimer's disease, frontotemporal lobe degeneration, Dementia with Lewy bodies and vascular dementia) [92] and detection of heterogeneity in such conditions by utilizing imaging data with other biomarkers [93].

Kalmady et al. demonstrated the capability to detect schizophrenia based on imaging through machine learning. This diagnosis is used to be made on the basis of clinical parameters, and imaging has been used at most to exclude a structural cause for the symptoms. Using resting state functional MRI, the authors described an 87% accuracy in differentiating drug-native schizophrenia patients from healthy controls [3].

21.10 Conclusion

A number of machine learning algorithms focusing on lesion detection have been developed in recent years. They may either support or extend imaging tasks and an increasing number of applications are currently under development. Emphasis has been put on AI algorithms to assist (neuro-) radiologists and other clinicians in managing the growing everyday workflow by improving diagnostic accuracy and automation of time consuming repetitive clinical tasks. Selected established and proven applications have already found their way into daily clinical routine, and many other highly interesting and promising projects are currently under development.

However, despite the high and rapidly growing number of AI related applications in medical imaging, regular and widespread usage of such AI technology in clinical practice is not yet established. There are many important aspects which have to be considered for the implementation of AI applications in the clinical routine. Some of them are complex and have to be thoroughly and critically considered from various facets. Next to the technical requirements, these points include the need for standardization, evidence based research, assessing legal responsibility in case of adverse events, data protection, economic and ethical aspects, valid guidelines, as well as the confidence and trust in the technique by healthcare professionals, patients and other stakeholders. In addition, some human factors, such as emotional intelligence, communication skills in difficult situations or a mindful and critical thinking might not be fully reproducible by AI.

Future efforts have to focus on these aspects. Thus, it is important that the different disciplines from a variety of backgrounds including clinicians, radiologists, vendors, startups, and venture capitalist work closely together to achieve this demanding task, which will yield to the future of medical imaging.

References

1. Gupta AC, Schaefer PW, Chaudhry ZA, Leslie-Mazwi TM, Chandra RV, González RG, Hirsch JA, Yoo AJ. Interobserver reliability of baseline noncontrast CT Alberta Stroke Program Early CT Score for intra-arterial stroke treatment selection. AJNR Am J Neuroradiol. 2012;33:1046–9. https://doi.org/10.3174/ajnr.A2942.

2. Middlebrooks EH, Lin C, Westerhold E, Okromelidze L, Vibhute P, Grewal SS, Gupta V. Improved detection of focal cortical dysplasia using a novel 3D imaging sequence: Edge-Enhancing Gradient Echo (3D-EDGE) MRI. Neuroimage Clin. 2020;28:102449. https://doi.org/10.1016/j.nicl.2020.102449.
3. Kalmady SV, Greiner R, Agrawal R, Shivakumar V, Narayanaswamy JC, Brown MRG, Greenshaw AJ, Dursun SM, Venkatasubramanian G. Towards artificial intelligence in mental health by improving schizophrenia prediction with multiple brain parcellation ensemble-learning. NPJ Schizophr. 2019;5:2. https://doi.org/10.1038/s41537-018-0070-8.
4. Gillies RJ, Kinahan PE, Hricak H. Radiomics: images are more than pictures, they are data. Radiology. 2016;278:563–77. https://doi.org/10.1148/radiol.2015151169.
5. Bhandari AP, Liong R, Koppen J, Murthy SV, Lasocki A. Noninvasive determination of. AJNR Am J Neuroradiol. 2020; https://doi.org/10.3174/ajnr.A6875.
6. Summers RM. Texture analysis in radiology: does the emperor have no clothes? Abdom Radiol (NY). 2017;42:342–5. https://doi.org/10.1007/s00261-016-0950-1.
7. Chartrand G, Cheng PM, Vorontsov E, Drozdzal M, Turcotte S, Pal CJ, Kadoury S, Tang A. Deep learning: a primer for radiologists. Radiographics. 2017;37:2113–31. https://doi.org/10.1148/rg.2017170077.
8. Chang PD, Kuoy E, Grinband J, Weinberg BD, Thompson M, Homo R, Chen J, Abcede H, Shafie M, Sugrue L, Filippi CG, Su MY, Yu W, Hess C, Chow D. Hybrid 3D/2D convolutional neural network for hemorrhage evaluation on head CT. AJNR Am J Neuroradiol. 2018;39:1609–16. https://doi.org/10.3174/ajnr.A5742.
9. Lambin P, Leijenaar RTH, Deist TM, Peerlings J, de Jong EEC, van Timmeren J, Sanduleanu S, Larue RTHM, Even AJG, Jochems A, van Wijk Y, Woodruff H, van Soest J, Lustberg T, Roelofs E, van Elmpt W, Dekker A, Mottaghy FM, Wildberger JE, Walsh S. Radiomics: the bridge between medical imaging and personalized medicine. Nat Rev Clin Oncol. 2017;14:749–62. https://doi.org/10.1038/nrclinonc.2017.141.
10. Duong MT, Rauschecker AM, Mohan S. Diverse applications of artificial intelligence in neuroradiology. Neuroimaging Clin N Am. 2020;30:505–16. https://doi.org/10.1016/j.nic.2020.07.003.
11. Gaidhani BR, Rajamenakshi R, Sonavane S. Brain stroke detection using convolutional neural network and deep learning models. In: 2019 2nd International conference on intelligent communication and computational techniques (ICCT); 2019. p. 242–9.
12. Zaharchuk G, Gong E, Wintermark M, Rubin D, Langlotz CP. Deep learning in neuroradiology. AJNR Am J Neuroradiol. 2018;39:1776–84. https://doi.org/10.3174/ajnr.A5543.
13. Lui YW, Chang PD, Zaharchuk G, Barboriak DP, Flanders AE, Wintermark M, Hess CP, Filippi CG. Artificial intelligence in neuroradiology: current status and future directions. AJNR Am J Neuroradiol. 2020;41:E52–e59. https://doi.org/10.3174/ajnr.A6681.
14. Wichmann JL, Willemink MJ, De Cecco CN. Artificial intelligence and machine learning in radiology: current state and considerations for routine clinical implementation. Investig Radiol. 2020;55:619–27. https://doi.org/10.1097/rli.0000000000000673.
15. Gupta R, Krishnam SP, Schaefer PW, Lev MH, Gilberto Gonzalez R. An East Coast perspective on artificial intelligence and machine learning: part 1: hemorrhagic stroke imaging and triage. Neuroimaging Clin N Am. 2020;30:459–66. https://doi.org/10.1016/j.nic.2020.07.005.
16. Mouridsen K, Thurner P, Zaharchuk G. Artificial intelligence applications in stroke. Stroke. 2020;51:2573–9. https://doi.org/10.1161/strokeaha.119.027479.
17. Fujita H, You J, Li Q, Arimura H, Tanaka R, Sanada S, Niki N, Lee G, Hara T, Fukuoka D, Muramatsu C, Katafuchi T, Iinuma G, Miyake M, Arai Y, Moriyama N. State-of-the-Art of Computer-Aided Detection/Diagnosis (CAD). In: Zhang D, Sonka M, editors. Medical biometrics. Berlin: Springer; 2010. p. 296–305.
18. Sarmento RM, Vasconcelos FFX, Filho PPR, Wu W, de Albuquerque VHC. Automatic neuroimage processing and analysis in stroke-a systematic review. IEEE Rev Biomed Eng. 2020;13:130–55. https://doi.org/10.1109/rbme.2019.2934500.
19. Barber PA, Demchuk AM, Zhang J, Buchan AM. Validity and reliability of a quantitative computed tomography score in predicting outcome of hyperacute stroke before thrombolytic therapy. ASPECTS Study Group. Alberta Stroke Programme Early CT Score. Lancet. 2000;355:1670–4. https://doi.org/10.1016/s0140-6736(00)02237-6.
20. Schröder J, Thomalla G. A critical review of Alberta Stroke Program early CT score for evaluation of acute stroke imaging. Front Neurol. 2016;7:245. https://doi.org/10.3389/fneur.2016.00245.
21. Lee EJ, Kim YH, Kim N, Kang DW. Deep into the brain: artificial intelligence in stroke imaging. J Stroke. 2017;19:277–85. https://doi.org/10.5853/jos.2017.02054.
22. Murray NM, Unberath M, Hager GD, Hui FK. Artificial intelligence to diagnose ischemic stroke and identify large vessel occlusions: a systematic review. J Neurointerv Surg. 2020;12:156–64. https://doi.org/10.1136/neurintsurg-2019-015135.
23. Nagel S, Sinha D, Day D, Reith W, Chapot R, Papanagiotou P, Warburton EA, Guyler P, Tysoe S, Fassbender K, Walter S, Essig M, Heidenrich J, Konstas AA, Harrison M, Papadakis M, Greveson E, Joly O, Gerry S, Maguire H, Roffe C, Hampton-Till J, Buchan AM, Grunwald IQ. e-ASPECTS software is non-inferior to neuroradiologists in applying the ASPECT score to computed tomography scans of acute ischemic stroke patients. Int J Stroke. 2017;12:615–22. https://doi.org/10.1177/1747493016681020.
24. Herweh C, Ringleb PA, Rauch G, Gerry S, Behrens L, Möhlenbruch M, Gottorf R, Richter D, Schieber S, Nagel S. Performance of e-ASPECTS software in comparison to that of stroke physicians on assessing CT scans of acute ischemic stroke patients. Int J Stroke. 2016;11:438–45. https://doi.org/10.1177/1747493016632244.
25. Guberina N, Dietrich U, Radbruch A, Goebel J, Deuschl C, Ringelstein A, Köhrmann M, Kleinschnitz C, Forsting M, Mönninghoff C. Detection of early infarction signs with machine learning-based diagnosis by means of the Alberta Stroke Program Early CT score (ASPECTS) in the clinical routine. Neuroradiology. 2018;60:889–901. https://doi.org/10.1007/s00234-018-2066-5.
26. Do LN, Baek BH, Kim SK, Yang HJ, Park I, Yoon W. Automatic assessment of ASPECTS using diffusion-weighted imaging in acute ischemic stroke using recurrent residual convolutional neural network. Diagnostics (Basel). 2020;10:803. https://doi.org/10.3390/diagnostics10100803.
27. Maegerlein C, Fischer J, Mönch S, Berndt M, Wunderlich S, Seifert CL, Lehm M, Boeckh-Behrens T, Zimmer C, Friedrich B. Automated calculation of the Alberta Stroke Program early CT score: feasibility and reliability. Radiology. 2019;291:141–8. https://doi.org/10.1148/radiol.2019181228.
28. Alom M, Hasan M, Yakopcic, Ch, Tara T, Asari V. Recurrent residual convolutional neural network based on U-Net (R2UNet) for medical image segmentation; 2018. https://arxiv.org//abs/1802.06955.
29. You J, Tsang ACO, Yu PLH, Tsui ELH, Woo PPS, Lui CSM, Leung GKK. Automated hierarchy evaluation system of large vessel occlusion in acute ischemia stroke. Front Neuroinform. 2020;14:13. https://doi.org/10.3389/fninf.2020.00013.
30. Amukotuwa SA, Straka M, Smith H, Chandra RV, Dehkharghani S, Fischbein NJ, Bammer R. Automated detection of intracranial large vessel occlusions on computed tomography angiography: a single center experience. Stroke. 2019;50:2790–8. https://doi.org/10.1161/strokeaha.119.026259.
31. Chatterjee A, Somayaji Nayana R, Kabakis Ismail M. Abstract WMP16: artificial intelligence detection of cerebrovascular large vessel occlusion - nine month, 650 patient evaluation of the diag-

nostic accuracy and performance of the Viz.ai LVO algorithm. Stroke. 2019;50:AWMP16. https://doi.org/10.1161/str.50.suppl_1.WMP16.
32. Olive-Gadea M, Crespo C, Granes C, Hernandez-Perez M, Pérez de la Ossa N, Laredo C, Urra X, Carlos Soler J, Soler A, Puyalto P, Cuadras P, Marti C, Ribo M. Deep learning based software to identify large vessel occlusion on noncontrast computed tomography. Stroke. 2020;51:3133–7. https://doi.org/10.1161/strokeaha.120.030326.
33. Stib MT, Vasquez J, Dong MP, Kim YH, Subzwari SS, Triedman HJ, Wang A, Wang HC, Yao AD, Jayaraman M, Boxerman JL, Eickhoff C, Cetintemel U, Baird GL, McTaggart RA. Detecting large vessel occlusion at multiphase CT angiography by using a deep convolutional neural network. Radiology. 2020;297:640–9. https://doi.org/10.1148/radiol.2020200334.
34. Austein F, Riedel C, Kerby T, Meyne J, Binder A, Lindner T, Huhndorf M, Wodarg F, Jansen O. Comparison of perfusion CT software to predict the final infarct volume after thrombectomy. Stroke. 2016;47:2311–7. https://doi.org/10.1161/strokeaha.116.013147.
35. Huang X, Kalladka D, Cheripelli BK, Moreton FC, Muir KW. The impact of CT perfusion threshold on predicted viable and nonviable tissue volumes in acute ischemic stroke. J Neuroimaging. 2017;27:602–6. https://doi.org/10.1111/jon.12442.
36. Olivot JM, Mlynash M, Thijs VN, Kemp S, Lansberg MG, Wechsler L, Bammer R, Marks MP, Albers GW. Optimal Tmax threshold for predicting penumbral tissue in acute stroke. Stroke. 2009;40:469–75. https://doi.org/10.1161/strokeaha.108.526954.
37. Straka M, Albers GW, Bammer R. Real-time diffusion-perfusion mismatch analysis in acute stroke. J Magn Reson Imaging. 2010;32:1024–37. https://doi.org/10.1002/jmri.22338.
38. Albers GW, Thijs VN, Wechsler L, Kemp S, Schlaug G, Skalabrin E, Bammer R, Kakuda W, Lansberg MG, Shuaib A, Coplin W, Hamilton S, Moseley M, Marks MP. Magnetic resonance imaging profiles predict clinical response to early reperfusion: the diffusion and perfusion imaging evaluation for understanding stroke evolution (DEFUSE) study. Ann Neurol. 2006;60:508–17. https://doi.org/10.1002/ana.20976.
39. Chen L, Bentley P, Rueckert D. Fully automatic acute ischemic lesion segmentation in DWI using convolutional neural networks. Neuroimage Clin. 2017;15:633–43. https://doi.org/10.1016/j.nicl.2017.06.016.
40. Lee H, Lee EJ, Ham S, Lee HB, Lee JS, Kwon SU, Kim JS, Kim N, Kang DW. Machine learning approach to identify stroke within 4.5 hours. Stroke. 2020;51:860–6. https://doi.org/10.1161/strokeaha.119.027611.
41. Yu Y, Guo D, Lou M, Liebeskind D, Scalzo F. The prediction of the hemorrhagic transformation locations after reperfusion therapy in acute stroke patients: a perfusion study using deep learning (P3.212). Neurology. 2018;90:P3.212.
42. Bentley P, Ganesalingam J, Carlton Jones AL, Mahady K, Epton S, Rinne P, Sharma P, Halse O, Mehta A, Rueckert D. Prediction of stroke thrombolysis outcome using CT brain machine learning. Neuroimage Clin. 2014;4:635–40. https://doi.org/10.1016/j.nicl.2014.02.003.
43. Qi D, Hao C, Lequan Y, Lei Z, Jing Q, Defeng W, Mok VC, Lin S, Pheng-Ann H. Automatic detection of cerebral microbleeds from MR images via 3D convolutional neural networks. IEEE Trans Med Imaging. 2016;35:1182–95. https://doi.org/10.1109/tmi.2016.2528129.
44. Flanders AE, Prevedello LM, Shih G, Halabi SS, Kalpathy-Cramer J, Ball R, Mongan JT, Stein A, Kitamura FC, Lungren MP, Choudhary G, Cala L, Coelho L, Mogensen M, Morón F, Miller E, Ikuta I, Zohrabian V, McDonnell O, Lincoln C, Shah L, Joyner D, Agarwal A, Lee RK, Nath J. Construction of a machine learning dataset through collaboration: the RSNA 2019 brain CT hemorrhage challenge. Radiol Artif Intell. 2020;2:e190211. https://doi.org/10.1148/ryai.2020190211.
45. Kaka H, Zhang E, Khan N. Artificial intelligence and deep learning in neuroradiology: exploring the new frontier. Can Assoc Radiol J. 2020;72:35–44. https://doi.org/10.1177/0846537120954293.
46. Wang SH, Tang C, Sun J, Yang J, Huang C, Phillips P, Zhang YD. Multiple sclerosis identification by 14-layer convolutional neural network with batch normalization, dropout, and stochastic pooling. Front Neurosci. 2018;12:818. https://doi.org/10.3389/fnins.2018.00818.
47. Zurita M, Montalba C, Labbé T, Cruz JP, Dalboni da Rocha J, Tejos C, Ciampi E, Cárcamo C, Sitaram R, Uribe S. Characterization of relapsing-remitting multiple sclerosis patients using support vector machine classifications of functional and diffusion MRI data. Neuroimage Clin. 2018;20:724–30. https://doi.org/10.1016/j.nicl.2018.09.002.
48. Ion-Mărgineanu A, Kocevar G, Stamile C, Sima DM, Durand-Dubief F, Van Huffel S, Sappey-Marinier D. Machine learning approach for classifying multiple sclerosis courses by combining clinical data with lesion loads and magnetic resonance metabolic features. Front Neurosci. 2017;11:398. https://doi.org/10.3389/fnins.2017.00398.
49. Yoo Y, Tang LYW, Brosch T, Li DKB, Kolind S, Vavasour I, Rauscher A, MacKay AL, Traboulsee A, Tam RC. Deep learning of joint myelin and T1w MRI features in normal-appearing brain tissue to distinguish between multiple sclerosis patients and healthy controls. Neuroimage Clin. 2018;17:169–78. https://doi.org/10.1016/j.nicl.2017.10.015.
50. Narayana PA, Coronado I, Sujit SJ, Wolinsky JS, Lublin FD, Gabr RE. Deep learning for predicting enhancing lesions in multiple sclerosis from noncontrast MRI. Radiology. 2020;294:398–404. https://doi.org/10.1148/radiol.2019191061.
51. Duong MT, Rudie JD, Wang J, Xie L, Mohan S, Gee JC, Rauschecker AM. Convolutional neural network for automated FLAIR lesion segmentation on clinical brain MR imaging. AJNR Am J Neuroradiol. 2019;40:1282–90. https://doi.org/10.3174/ajnr.A6138.
52. Gessert N, Krüger J, Opfer R, Ostwaldt AC, Manogaran P, Kitzler HH, Schippling S, Schlaefer A. Multiple sclerosis lesion activity segmentation with attention-guided two-path CNNs. Comput Med Imaging Graph. 2020;84:101772. https://doi.org/10.1016/j.compmedimag.2020.101772.
53. Menze BH, Jakab A, Bauer S, Kalpathy-Cramer J, Farahani K, Kirby J, Burren Y, Porz N, Slotboom J, Wiest R, Lanczi L, Gerstner E, Weber MA, Arbel T, Avants BB, Ayache N, Buendia P, Collins DL, Cordier N, Corso JJ, Criminisi A, Das T, Delingette H, Demiralp Ç, Durst CR, Dojat M, Doyle S, Festa J, Forbes F, Geremia E, Glocker B, Golland P, Guo X, Hamamci A, Iftekharuddin KM, Jena R, John NM, Konukoglu E, Lashkari D, Mariz JA, Meier R, Pereira S, Precup D, Price SJ, Raviv TR, Reza SM, Ryan M, Sarikaya D, Schwartz L, Shin HC, Shotton J, Silva CA, Sousa N, Subbanna NK, Szekely G, Taylor TJ, Thomas OM, Tustison NJ, Unal G, Vasseur F, Wintermark M, Ye DH, Zhao L, Zhao B, Zikic D, Prastawa M, Reyes M, Van Leemput K. The multimodal brain tumor image segmentation benchmark (BRATS). IEEE Trans Med Imaging. 2015;34:1993–2024. https://doi.org/10.1109/tmi.2014.2377694.
54. Wu S, Li H, Quang D, Guan Y. Three-plane-assembled deep learning segmentation of gliomas. Radiol Artif Intell. 2020;2:e190011. https://doi.org/10.1148/ryai.2020190011.
55. Tandel GS, Balestrieri A, Jujaray T, Khanna NN, Saba L, Suri JS. Multiclass magnetic resonance imaging brain tumor classification using artificial intelligence paradigm. Comput Biol Med. 2020;122:103804. https://doi.org/10.1016/j.compbiomed.2020.103804.
56. Bangalore Yogananda CG, Shah BR, Vejdani-Jahromi M, Nalawade SS, Murugesan GK, Yu FF, Pinho MC, Wagner BC, Emblem

KE, Bjørnerud A, Fei B, Madhuranthakam AJ, Maldjian JA. A fully automated deep learning network for brain tumor segmentation. Tomography. 2020;6:186–93. https://doi.org/10.18383/j.tom.2019.00026.
57. Lohmann P, Galldiks N, Kocher M, Heinzel A, Filss CP, Stegmayr C, Mottaghy FM, Fink GR, Jon Shah N, Langen KJ. Radiomics in neuro-oncology: basics, workflow, and applications. Methods. 2020;188:112. https://doi.org/10.1016/j.ymeth.2020.06.003.
58. Zeineldin RA, Karar ME, Coburger J, Wirtz CR, Burgert O. DeepSeg: deep neural network framework for automatic brain tumor segmentation using magnetic resonance FLAIR images. Int J Comput Assist Radiol Surg. 2020;15:909–20. https://doi.org/10.1007/s11548-020-02186-z.
59. Chow DS, Khatri D, Chang PD, Zlochower A, Boockvar JA, Filippi CG. Updates on deep learning and glioma: use of convolutional neural networks to image glioma heterogeneity. Neuroimaging Clin N Am. 2020;30:493–503. https://doi.org/10.1016/j.nic.2020.07.002.
60. Jalalifar A, Soliman H, Ruschin M, Sahgal A, Sadeghi-Naini A. A brain tumor segmentation framework based on outlier detection using one-class support vector machine. Annu Int Conf IEEE Eng Med Biol Soc. 2020;2020:1067–70. https://doi.org/10.1109/embc44109.2020.9176263.
61. Nalawade S, Murugesan G, Vejdani-Jahromi M, Fisicaro RA, Bangalore Yogananda CG, Wagner B, Mickey B, Maher E, Pinho MC, Fei B, Madhuranthakam AJ, Maldjian JA. Classification of brain tumor IDH status using MRI and deep learning. bioRxiv. 2019;757344. https://doi.org/10.1101/757344.
62. Nalawade SS, Yu FF, Bangalore Yogananda CG, Murugesan GK, Shah BR, Pinho MC, Wagner BC, Mickey B, Patel TR, Fei B, Madhuranthakam AJ, Maldjian JA. Brain tumor IDH, 1p/19q, and MGMT molecular classification using MRI-based deep learning: effect of motion and motion correction. bioRxiv. 2020;2020.2006.2001.126375. https://doi.org/10.1101/2020.06.01.126375.
63. Charron O, Lallement A, Jarnet D, Noblet V, Clavier JB, Meyer P. Automatic detection and segmentation of brain metastases on multimodal MR images with a deep convolutional neural network. Comput Biol Med. 2018;95:43–54. https://doi.org/10.1016/j.compbiomed.2018.02.004.
64. Grøvik E, Yi D, Iv M, Tong E, Rubin D, Zaharchuk G. Deep learning enables automatic detection and segmentation of brain metastases on multisequence MRI. J Magn Reson Imaging. 2020;51:175–82. https://doi.org/10.1002/jmri.26766.
65. Xue J, Wang B, Ming Y, Liu X, Jiang Z, Wang C, Chen L, Qu J, Xu S, Tang X, Mao Y, Liu Y, Li D. Deep learning-based detection and segmentation-assisted management of brain metastases. Neuro-Oncology. 2020;22:505–14. https://doi.org/10.1093/neuonc/noz234.
66. Kawauchi K, Furuya S, Hirata K, Katoh C, Manabe O, Kobayashi K, Watanabe S, Shiga T. A convolutional neural network-based system to classify patients using FDG PET/CT examinations. BMC Cancer. 2020;20:227. https://doi.org/10.1186/s12885-020-6694-x.
67. Gabelloni M, Faggioni L, Attanasio S, Vani V, Goddi A, Colantonio S, Germanese D, Caudai C, Bruschini L, Scarano M, Seccia V, Neri E. Can magnetic resonance radiomics analysis discriminate parotid gland tumors? A pilot study. Diagnostics (Basel). 2020;10:900. https://doi.org/10.3390/diagnostics10110900.
68. Ma Z, Zhou S, Wu X, Zhang H, Yan W, Sun S, Zhou J. Nasopharyngeal carcinoma segmentation based on enhanced convolutional neural networks using multi-modal metric learning. Phys Med Biol. 2019;64:025005. https://doi.org/10.1088/1361-6560/aaf5da.
69. Inaba A, Hori K, Yoda Y, Ikematsu H, Takano H, Matsuzaki H, Watanabe Y, Takeshita N, Tomioka T, Ishii G, Fujii S, Hayashi R, Yano T. Artificial intelligence system for detecting superficial laryngopharyngeal cancer with high efficiency of deep learning. Head Neck. 2020;42:2581–92. https://doi.org/10.1002/hed.26313.
70. Huang J, Xu J, Kang L, Zhang T. Identifying epilepsy based on deep learning using DKI images. Front Hum Neurosci. 2020;14:590815. https://doi.org/10.3389/fnhum.2020.590815.
71. Hosseini MP, Tran TX, Pompili D, Elisevich K, Soltanian-Zadeh H. Multimodal data analysis of epileptic EEG and rs-fMRI via deep learning and edge computing. Artif Intell Med. 2020;104:101813. https://doi.org/10.1016/j.artmed.2020.101813.
72. Liu Y, Yan Z. A combined deep-learning and Lattice Boltzmann model for segmentation of the hippocampus in MRI. Sensors (Basel). 2020;20:3628. https://doi.org/10.3390/s20133628.
73. Pang S, Lu Z, Jiang J, Zhao L, Lin L, Li X, Lian T, Huang M, Yang W, Feng Q. Hippocampus segmentation based on iterative local linear mapping with representative and local structure-preserved feature embedding. IEEE Trans Med Imaging. 2019;38:2271–80. https://doi.org/10.1109/tmi.2019.2906727.
74. Vlak MH, Algra A, Brandenburg R, Rinkel GJ. Prevalence of unruptured intracranial aneurysms, with emphasis on sex, age, comorbidity, country, and time period: a systematic review and meta-analysis. Lancet Neurol. 2011;10:626–36. https://doi.org/10.1016/s1474-4422(11)70109-0.
75. Kim ST, Brinjikji W, Kallmes DF. Prevalence of intracranial aneurysms in patients with connective tissue diseases: a retrospective study. AJNR Am J Neuroradiol. 2016;37:1422–6. https://doi.org/10.3174/ajnr.A4718.
76. van Gijn J, Kerr RS, Rinkel GJ. Subarachnoid haemorrhage. Lancet. 2007;369:306–18. https://doi.org/10.1016/s0140-6736(07)60153-6.
77. Nakao T, Hanaoka S, Nomura Y, Sato I, Nemoto M, Miki S, Maeda E, Yoshikawa T, Hayashi N, Abe O. Deep neural network-based computer-assisted detection of cerebral aneurysms in MR angiography. J Magn Reson Imaging. 2018;47:948–53. https://doi.org/10.1002/jmri.25842.
78. Sichtermann T, Faron A, Sijben R, Teichert N, Freiherr J, Wiesmann M. Deep learning-based detection of intracranial aneurysms in 3D TOF-MRA. AJNR Am J Neuroradiol. 2019;40:25–32. https://doi.org/10.3174/ajnr.A5911.
79. Stember JN, Chang P, Stember DM, Liu M, Grinband J, Filippi CG, Meyers P, Jambawalikar S. Convolutional neural networks for the detection and measurement of cerebral aneurysms on magnetic resonance angiography. J Digit Imaging. 2019;32:808–15. https://doi.org/10.1007/s10278-018-0162-z.
80. Duan H, Huang Y, Liu L, Dai H, Chen L, Zhou L. Automatic detection on intracranial aneurysm from digital subtraction angiography with cascade convolutional neural networks. Biomed Eng Online. 2019;18:110. https://doi.org/10.1186/s12938-019-0726-2.
81. Hainc N, Mannil M, Anagnostakou V, Alkadhi H, Blüthgen C, Wacht L, Bink A, Husain S, Kulcsár Z, Winklhofer S. Deep learning based detection of intracranial aneurysms on digital subtraction angiography: a feasibility study. Neuroradiol J. 2020;33:311–7. https://doi.org/10.1177/1971400920937647.
82. Park A, Chute C, Rajpurkar P, Lou J, Ball RL, Shpanskaya K, Jabarkheel R, Kim LH, McKenna E, Tseng J, Ni J, Wishah F, Wittber F, Hong DS, Wilson TJ, Halabi S, Basu S, Patel BN, Lungren MP, Ng AY, Yeom KW. Deep learning-assisted diagnosis of cerebral aneurysms using the HeadXNet model. JAMA Netw Open. 2019;2:e195600. https://doi.org/10.1001/jamanetworkopen.2019.5600.
83. Yamanakkanavar N, Choi JY, Lee B. MRI segmentation and classification of human brain using deep learning for diagnosis of Alzheimer's disease: a survey. Sensors (Basel). 2020;20:3243. https://doi.org/10.3390/s20113243.
84. Basaia S, Agosta F, Wagner L, Canu E, Magnani G, Santangelo R, Filippi M. Automated classification of Alzheimer's disease and mild cognitive impairment using a single MRI and deep

neural networks. Neuroimage Clin. 2019;21:101645. https://doi.org/10.1016/j.nicl.2018.101645.
85. Elahifasaee F, Li F, Yang M. A classification algorithm by combination of feature decomposition and kernel discriminant analysis (KDA) for automatic MR brain image classification and AD diagnosis. Comput Math Methods Med. 2019;2019:1437123. https://doi.org/10.1155/2019/1437123.
86. Folego G, Weiler M, Casseb RF, Pires R, Rocha A. Alzheimer's disease detection through whole-brain 3D-CNN MRI. Front Bioeng Biotechnol. 2020;8:534592. https://doi.org/10.3389/fbioe.2020.534592.
87. Li F, Liu M. A hybrid convolutional and recurrent neural network for hippocampus analysis in Alzheimer's disease. J Neurosci Methods. 2019;323:108–18. https://doi.org/10.1016/j.jneumeth.2019.05.006.
88. Liu M, Li F, Yan H, Wang K, Ma Y, Shen L, Xu M. A multi-model deep convolutional neural network for automatic hippocampus segmentation and classification in Alzheimer's disease. NeuroImage. 2020;208:116459. https://doi.org/10.1016/j.neuroimage.2019.116459.
89. Katako A, Shelton P, Goertzen AL, Levin D, Bybel B, Aljuaid M, Yoon HJ, Kang DY, Kim SM, Lee CS, Ko JH. Machine learning identified an Alzheimer's disease-related FDG-PET pattern which is also expressed in Lewy body dementia and Parkinson's disease dementia. Sci Rep. 2018;8:13236. https://doi.org/10.1038/s41598-018-31653-6.
90. Smailagic N, Vacante M, Hyde C, Martin S, Ukoumunne O, Sachpekidis C. ^{18}F-FDG PET for the early diagnosis of Alzheimer's disease dementia and other dementias in people with mild cognitive impairment (MCI). Cochrane Database Syst Rev. 2015;(1):Cd010632. https://doi.org/10.1002/14651858.CD010632.pub2.
91. Klöppel S, Kotschi M, Peter J, Egger K, Hausner L, Frölich L, Förster A, Heimbach B, Normann C, Vach W, Urbach H, Abdulkadir A. Separating symptomatic Alzheimer's disease from depression based on structural MRI. J Alzheimers Dis. 2018;63:353–63. https://doi.org/10.3233/jad-170964.
92. Tong T, Ledig C, Guerrero R, Schuh A, Koikkalainen J, Tolonen A, Rhodius H, Barkhof F, Tijms B, Lemstra AW, Soininen H, Remes AM, Waldemar G, Hasselbalch S, Mecocci P, Baroni M, Lötjönen J, Flier WV, Rueckert D. Five-class differential diagnostics of neurodegenerative diseases using random undersampling boosting. Neuroimage Clin. 2017;15:613–24. https://doi.org/10.1016/j.nicl.2017.06.012.
93. Habes M, Grothe MJ, Tunc B, McMillan C, Wolk DA, Davatzikos C. Disentangling heterogeneity in Alzheimer's disease and related dementias using data-driven methods. Biol Psychiatry. 2020;88:70–82. https://doi.org/10.1016/j.biopsych.2020.01.016.

Foundations of Multiparametric Brain Tumour Imaging Characterisation Using Machine Learning

22

Anne Jian, Kevin Jang, Carlo Russo, Sidong Liu, and Antonio Di Ieva

22.1 Introduction

Advances in neuroradiology have led to improved structural and functional characterisation of brain tumours and their microenvironment. However, accurately characterising subregional changes remains challenging due to temporal variations in tumour dynamics and molecular heterogeneity [1]. Radiomics analysis using high-throughput computational methods increasingly allows extraction of quantitative features from medical images [2]. Combining multiple features from imaging sequences yields superior discriminative power compared to single parameters or visual radiological assessment as it comprehensively captures voxel-based heterogeneity in relation to tumours' anatomical, cellular, metabolic and microvascular patterns. As such, multiparametric analysis may provide a noninvasive means of characterising tumour phenotype to identify diagnostic, prognostic and predictive imaging biomarkers. The high-dimensional data in multiparametric studies, however, poses significant challenges for human interpretation. Machine learning (ML) techniques can be deployed to train computers to recognise patterns and integrate information across thousands of imaging features to make predictions [3]. They can also be trained to improve upon on their performance by selecting the most useful imaging features to build a clinical diagnostic or prognostic model in an automated and efficient manner.

In this paper, we describe the methodological pipeline of developing multiparametric models (Fig. 22.1), focusing on ML- and radiomic-based analysis to characterise brain tumours. We discuss imaging modalities, quantitative parameters and computational tools that have been proposed, with the aim to familiarise clinicians with the pitfalls and opportunities presented by ML-based multiparametric analysis to improve diagnostic and prognostic accuracy in brain tumour patients.

A. Jian
Computational NeuroSurgery (CNS) Lab, Macquarie Medical School, Faculty of Medicine, Health and Human Sciences, Macquarie University, Sydney, NSW, Australia

Royal Melbourne Hospital, Melbourne, VIC, Australia

K. Jang
Computational NeuroSurgery (CNS) Lab, Macquarie Medical School, Faculty of Medicine, Health and Human Sciences, Macquarie University, Sydney, NSW, Australia

Faculty of Medicine and Health, The University of Sydney, Sydney, NSW, Australia

C. Russo · A. Di Ieva (✉)
Computational NeuroSurgery (CNS) Lab, Macquarie Medical School, Faculty of Medicine, Health and Human Sciences, Macquarie University, Sydney, NSW, Australia
e-mail: antonio.diieva@mq.edu.au

S. Liu
Computational NeuroSurgery (CNS) Lab, Macquarie Medical School, Faculty of Medicine, Health and Human Sciences, Macquarie University, Sydney, NSW, Australia

Centre for Health Informatics, Macquarie University, Sydney, NSW, Australia

22.2 Methodological Foundations

Multiparametric Imaging

The selection of imaging sequences for multiparametric assessment of brain tumours should be guided by available facilities, expertise, and the clinical problem at hand. Table 22.1 outlines examples of imaging sequences, features and different computational and ML-based algorithms implemented for different clinical tasks [4–8, 10–21].

Conventional MRI sequences (T1-weighted gradient-echo imaging pre- and post-gadolinium contrast, T2-weighted and T2-weighted fluid-attenuated inversion recovery (FLAIR)) have been most widely investigated in multiparametric studies. They are easily accessible and more robust to different acquisition and analysis methods, however they do not utilise information about tumour tissue fingerprintings

V. E. Staartjes et al. (eds.), *Machine Learning in Clinical Neuroscience*, Acta Neurochirurgica Supplement 134,
https://doi.org/10.1007/978-3-030-85292-4_22

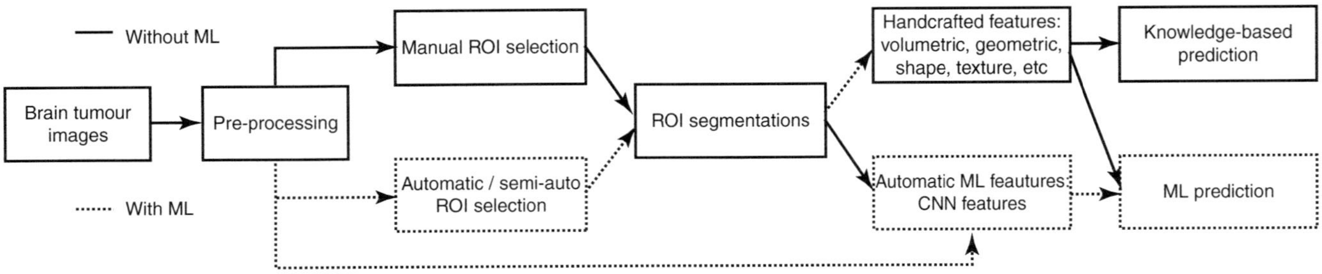

Fig. 22.1 Schematic illustration of brain tumour image characterisation pipeline involving image acquisition, preprocessing, region of interest (ROI) selection and segmentation, feature extraction and prediction

Table 22.1 Examples of multiparametric brain tumour characterisation using computational modelling and machine learning techniques

Application	Imaging sequence and features	Segmentation	Feature selection	Classifier(s)
Diagnosis of brain tumours				
Devos et al. (2005) [4]	Imaging intensities on conventional MRI sequences and metabolic data from MR spectroscopy	Semiautomatic (model-based clustering algorithm)	PCA (prior to LDA only)	LDA, least squares-SVM with linear and radial basis function kernel[a]
Zacharaki et al. (2009) [5]	Shape, statistical, intensity, texture features from T1W, T1C, T2W, FLAIR and relative CBV maps (DSC)	Manual	Ranking-based criterion and recursive feature elimination	LDA, kNN, nonlinear SVM[a]
Di Ieva et al. (2016) [6]	Signal ratio and fractal dimension from SWI-3 Tesla MRI	Manual	–	ROC analysis
Suh et al. (2018) [7]	First-order, shape, texture features from T1C, T2W and FLAIR, tenth percentile ADC value	Semiautomatic (signal intensity threshold, region growing and edge detection)	Univariate filtering using Student's *t*-test and recursive feature elimination	Random forest
Petrujkić et al. (2019) [8]	Euclidean, texture and fractal parameters from T1C, T2, SWI MRI	Manual	Selected combination of parameters that performed best on individual analysis	ROC analysis
Di Ieva et al. (2020) [9]	Fractal parameters from SWI	Manual	PCA	Linear and quadratic discriminant analysis, kNN and SVM[a]
Glioma grading				
Di Ieva et al. (2013) [10]	Fractal dimension from SWI—7 Tesla MRI	Manual	–	Statistical
Zhang et al. (2017) [11]	Histogram and texture features from T1C, FLAIR, and parametric maps from ASL, DWI and DCE	Manual	RFE	25 classifiers incl. SVM[a]
Vamvakas et al. (2019) [12]	Texture and histogram features from conventional, DTI, DSC, mean rCBV and 1H-MRS metabolic ratios	Semiautomatic (clustering method based on DTI parametric maps)	SVM-RFE	SVM
Molecular subtyping				
Alis et al. (2020) [13]	Texture features from FLAIR, T1C and ADC maps	Manual	Wrapper method	Random forest
Bisdas et al. (2018) [14]	Intensity and texture features from FLAIR and DKI	Manual	SVM-RFE	SVM with RBF kernel
Akkus et al. (2017) [15]	Features extracted by deep learning model from T1C and T2W compared with intensity and texture features	Semiautomatic	CNN	CNN compared with SVM
Prognostic biomarkers				

Table 22.1 (continued)

Application	Imaging sequence and features	Segmentation	Feature selection	Classifier(s)
Cui et al. (2016) [16]	Statistical, texture, morphologic, histogram features from T1C and FLAIR	Semiautomatic (hidden Markov random field model, expectation-maximisation algorithm)	Least absolute shrinkage and selection operator (LASSO)	Multivariate regression
Papp et al. (2018) [17]	Tumour-to-background first-order and texture features from ^{11}C-MET PET and clinical information	Semiautomatic	Genetic algorithms	Geometric probability covering algorithm
Zhou et al. (2016) [18]	Texture features from tumour subregions on T1C, FLAIR, T2W	Automatic OTSU thresholding	Supervised forward feature ranking	kNN, Naïve Bayes, SVM with RBF kernel[a]
Distinguishing treatment-induced changes from tumour recurrence				
Nael et al. (2018) [19]	Perfusion parameters from DCE and DSC, ADC	Semiautomatic (voxel-based signal intensity threshold method)	Manual	Logistic regression
Kim et al. (2018) [20]	First-order, volume, shape, texture, wavelet-transformed features from T1C, FLAIR, ADC and CBV data	Semiautomatic (threshold and region-growing algorithm)	LASSO	Generalised linear model
Gao et al. (2020) [21]	Features extracted by DL model from T1W, T1C and T2W	Semiautomatic	DNN (VGG16, VGG19, ResNet50, InceptionV3, InceptionResNetV2)	DNN

ADC apparent diffusion coefficient, *ASL* arterial spin labeling, *CBV* cerebral blood volume, *CNN* convolutional neural network, *DCE* dynamic contrast enhancement, *DKI* diffusion kurtosis imaging, *DNN* deep neural network, *DSC* dynamic susceptibility contrast, *DTI* diffusion tensor imaging, *DWI* diffusion weighted imaging, *FD* fractal dimension, *kNN k*-nearest neighbour, *LASSO* least absolute shrinkage and selection operator, *LDA* linear discriminant analysis, *MET PET* methionine position emission tomography, *mRMR* minimum redundancy maximum relevance, *MRS* magnetic resonance spectroscopy, *PCA* principal component analysis, *RBF* radial basis function, *RFE* recursive feature elimination, *ROC* receiver-operating characteristic, *SWI* susceptibility-weighted imaging, *SVM* support vector machine, *T1C* gadolinium-contrast enhanced T1 sequence
[a]Classifier achieved highest diagnostic performance of all classifiers investigated in the study

such as metabolic, perfusion or diffusion features. Diffusion weighted imaging (DWI) is commonly acquired prior to contrast injection at varying *b*-values from which the apparent diffusion coefficient (ADC) parametric map can be generated to assess tumour cellularity and magnitude of diffusion at a voxel level. However, DWI is sensitive to magnetic field inhomogeneities, and the presence of vasogenic edema and necrosis increases extracellular water diffusivity, possibly falsely elevating ADC even in highly cellular tumours [22]. Diffusion tensor imaging (DTI) further considers the magnitude and direction of water molecules along multiple dimensions, thus disruptions in tissue microstructure can be characterised. There are conflicting results in the literature for diffusion quantification in a number of clinical applications [22].

Both perfusion-weighted imaging (PWI) and magnetic resonance spectroscopy (MRS) have demonstrated superior performance in tasks such as distinguishing treatment-induced changes from tumour progression [23] and determining glioma IDH status [24, 25]. PWI allows characterisation of tumour vascularity and vessel permeability, such as through dynamic susceptibility contrast (DSC)-derived cerebral blood volume (CBV) and K^{trans} from dynamic contrast enhancement (DCE) sequence. Maximal, mean or normalised values of these metrics can be used, with some studies proposing threshold values [19], but these are unlikely to be generalisable across different settings. Radiomic analysis of these parametric maps allows a more comprehensive evaluation of the heterogeneous patterns in microvascular density and permeability [11]. Although not generally used for grading and tumour typing in clinical setting, susceptibility-weighted imaging (SWI) may also be a valuable tool due to its capacity to evaluate intratumoural features such as microvasculature and microbleeds, and thus demonstrating intratumour heterogeneity [10, 26].

MRS is performed using single-voxel and/or multi-voxel point resolved spectroscopy (PRESS) sequences with short and long echo. A number of methodological aspects should be considered, including method of placement of the Region of Interest (e.g. largest area of contrast enhancement? maximal cerebral blood volume (CBV)?), voxel size, spectral fitting and metabolite ratio calculation method, all of which can affect the predictive accuracy of features extracted. The use of hybrid positron emission tomography–magnetic resonance imaging (PET/MRI), particularly with amino acid tracers such as *O*-(2-[18F]fluoroethyl)-L-tyrosine (FET) and 11C-methionine (MET), provides additional valuable metabolic information that enhances the performance of predictive ML models [17, 27], although investigators should be mindful of the distinct challenges presented by PET acquisition and reconstruction variations in radiomics analysis, which are reviewed extensively elsewhere [28].

Advanced MRI exploits a full range of tumour characteristics but presents its own challenges for image preprocessing and analysis. A greater number of sequences incorporated increases the processing time and resources for widespread clinical deployment. Investigators may also select whole tumour volume, single, contiguous or orthogonal slices, and examine peritumoral area and/or tumoral subregions. Thus, considering the benefits and costs, multiparametric assessment requires targeted selection of MRI sequences and data input.

22.3 Image Preprocessing

After image acquisition, preprocessing is usually required to remove bias and artefacts in neuroimaging data generated by inhomogeneous magnetic fields in MRI, and body motions such as head movements and respiratory motions. It follows a number of steps, including resampling image pixel size to reduce resolution variability, skull stripping (i.e. brain segmentation to exclude surrounding structures, such as bone, orbits' contents, etc.), images' co-registration, intensity normalisation and bias field correction. The public software FSL is widely used, integrating components such as the Brain Extraction Tool, a deformable surface modal based algorithm for skull stripping, and FLIRT, an intensity-based image registration tool [29]. However, many artefact removal and image registration algorithms, such as the Brightness Progressive Normalisation algorithm [30, 31], nonparametric nonuniformity normalisation (N3) algorithm [32] and SyN algorithm [33] have been developed. Unlike conventional semiautomated skull stripping algorithms, deep learning (DL)-based methods have also been implemented which are robust to variations in MRI acquisition parameters and applicable to various sequences [34]. A few advanced preprocessing algorithms have been proposed to standardise datasets acquired from multiple sites/ systems using different protocols, such as the spherical coordinates transformation [35] and the multi-atlas region segmentation (MUSE) pipeline [36].

As mentioned above, additional preprocessing is often needed where advanced MRI data are acquired. Raw spectral data from MRS undergo baseline correction, frequency inversion and phase shift before calculation of metabolite signals for *N*-acetyl aspartate, creatine, choline, lipid, glutamine and lipids. Data from DSC, DCE and diffusion imaging are processed on workstations to calculate parametric maps [11, 12, 37].

22.4 Region of Interest (ROI) Selection

Accurate ROI selection of brain tumours is crucial to obtain useful parameters to assist image characterisation. This can be an approximate box surrounding the tumour region, or more precisely, the exact delineation of the tumour contour, namely "tumour segmentation". In some cases, such as CBV maps, investigators may select single or multiple areas of increased perfusion using the "hotspot" method, but this is susceptible to operator-dependent areas. ROI selection on images such as DWI can also be challenging due to poor spatial resolution, thus conventional sequences are required to accurately delineate tumour and exclude areas of necrosis and edema.

Although manual segmentation by experienced clinicians is considered the gold-standard (the "ground truth"), this method is subject to high inter-operator variability, particularly in assessing postoperative tumour volume of glioblastoma, with intraclass correlation coefficient (ICC) reported to be 0.52 [38]. Manual segmentation of non-enhancing part of glioblastoma is also variable, demonstrating an ICC of 0.61 preoperatively, 0.25 postoperatively and 0.53 at progression even among experts [39]. Moreover, it can be time consuming and impractical in providing a large enough dataset for radiomics-based analysis. Thus, automated and semi-automated ML segmentation methods have been explored, such as techniques of contour extraction, grey level threshold [30] and clique propagation [40]. In one study, *k*-medians clustering algorithm based on DTI parametric maps was used to semiautomatically delineate tumour from the surrounding brain tissue [12]. However, surrounding structures could merge with tumour region in the automatic selection process. Automatic grey level-based methods are also prone to errors due to lack of standardisation and different hyperintense-hypointense signal response of tumours in the radiologic images.

Brain tumour segmentation is particularly challenging, above all in diffuse gliomas, due to their infiltrative growth patterns and irregular morphologies which can be visualised as incremental changes in intensity and morphology on MRI. As a result, two distinct lesions may look virtually identical in appearance with similar grey levels, and where the imaging sequence is not specific to the tumour detection, accurate segmentation can be quite difficult. For this reason, a number of automatic DL algorithms [41] have been proposed that overcome the problems associated with manual and conventional automatic methods.

22.5 Feature Extraction and Multiparametric Analysis

Standard radiomic models extract lower- and higher-order features characterising histogram-based properties, intervoxel relationships and grey-scale patterns to evaluate segmented whole tumour or tumour subregions [42], as outlined in Table 22.2. Specifically, first-order features refer to the distribution of individual voxels irrespective of their spatial relationships. Second-order features, known as "textural" features, quantify the spatial relationships between neigh-

Table 22.2 Radiomic parameters used in brain tumour imaging

Parameters and main references	Definition
First-order texture statistics	
Entropy	Measures the inherent randomness in the grey level intensities of an image or ROI
Uniformity	Measures the homogeneity of grey level intensities within an image or ROI
Second- and higher-order texture statistics	
Grey level co-occurrence matrix	Examines the spatial distribution of grey level intensities within an image through a 2D grey tone histogram
Angular second movement	Measures the textural uniformity of an image (also referred to as homogeneity) Captures the two-dimensional complexity of the edge of the tumour abnormalities
Inverse difference moment	Measures local image homogeneity as it assumes larger values for smaller grey tone differences in pair elements
Contrast	Measures spatial tone frequency of an image as the difference between the highest and lowest values of a contiguous set of pixels
Correlation	Measure of grey tone linear dependencies in the image
Bounding ellipsoid volume ratio	Ratio of the tumour volume to the volume of the smallest ellipsoid that entirely encapsulates the tumour. Captures the three-dimensional complexity of tumours
Semi-axis diameter ratios	Ratios of the minor semi-axis length to the longest bounding ellipsoid semi-axis diameter Captures the three-dimensional complexity of tumours
Margin fluctuation	Captures the two-dimensional complexity of the edge of the tumour abnormalities Standard deviation of the difference between the ordered radial distances of the tumour edge from the centroid to all the boundary points, smoothed with an averaging filter of length equal to 10% of tumour boundary
Mean intensity	Average intensity of the pixel values within the ROI
Mean of positive pixel values	Average pixel values of only the positive pixel values within the ROI
Standard deviation (SD)	Quantification of the variance from the mean value (high SD indicating wide variation of pixel values)
Kurtosis	Peakedness (or pointedness) of the histogram of pixel values Positive kurtosis = more peaked distribution Negative kurtosis = flatter distribution
Skewness	Quantifies asymmetry of the histogram Negative skewness = longer tail on left side of histogram Positive skewness = longer tail on right
Grey level run matrix (GLRL)	Number of contiguous voxels that have the same grey level value Characterises the grey level run lengths of different grey level intensities in any direction
Short runs emphasis (SRE)	Measures distributions of short runs. Higher values indicate fine textures
Long runs emphasis (LRE)	Measures distribution of long runs. Higher values indicate course textures
Grey level nonuniformity (GLN)	Measures the distribution of runs over the grey values. Low value when runs are equally distributed along grey levels. Lower value indicates higher similarity in intensity values
Run length nonuniformity (RLN)	Measures distribution of runs over run lengths. Low value when runs are equally distributed over run lengths
Run percentage (RP)	Measures the fraction of the number of realised runs and the maximum number of potential runs Highly uniform ROI volumes produce a low run percentage
Neighbourhood grey tone difference matrix	One dimensional matrix where each grey level entry is the summation of the differences between all the pixels with grey level value and the average grey level value of its neighbourhood
Coarseness	Quantitative measure of local uniformity
Busyness	Rapid intensity changes of neighbourhoods in a given ROI
Complexity	Quantifies the complexity of the spatial information present in an image
Texture strength	Characterising the visual aesthetics of an image
Local binary pattern (LBP)	Quantifies local pixel structures through a binary coding scheme Measures tumour microenvironment
Scale-invariant feature transform (SIFT)	Detects distributed key points with radius on tumour images Measures tumour spatial characteristics
Histogram of oriented gradients (HOG)	Computes block-wise histogram gradients with multiple orientations Measures tumour microenvironment

(continued)

Table 22.2 (continued)

Parameters and main references	Definition
Fractal	
Fractal dimension (box-counting and sand-box algorithms)	A non-integer number between 0 and 2, in a two-dimensional space, or 0 and 3, in a three-dimensional volume, that quantifies the space-filling properties of irregularly shaped objects
Outline box dimension	Evaluates the irregularity in shape of the image. (i.e. how much it deviates from classic geometric figures)
Lacunarity	Pixel distribution of an image at different box sizes and at various grid orientations. Describes the degree of nonhomogeneity within an image
Spatial filtering	
Median filter	Reduces sparse noise. Sets each pixel in ROI equal to the median pixel value of its specified neighbourhood
Entropy filter	Accentuates edges by brightening pixels which have dissimilar neighbours Sets each pixel in the ROI equal to the entropy (measure of disorder) of the pixel values in its specified neighbourhood
Laplacian of Gaussian (LoG) filter	Laplacian filter is a derivative filter used to find areas of rapid change (edges) in an image Images are first smoothed using Gaussian filter before applying the Laplacian

Reprinted with permission [42]

bouring voxels, thus capturing intratumoural heterogeneity [43]. For example, the differential growth patterns of high-grade glioma and other neoplastic lesions result in changes in contrast enhancement patterns and distribution of extracellular fluid that manifest in different spatial distributions of intensities at the voxel level. This can be quantified by texture analysis to differentiate between tumour types [7, 44]. Higher-order features use mathematical filters to identify more abstract patterns including different shades of image texture by suppressing noise or accentuating details.

Apart from texture analysis, the morphological assessment of intracranial neoplasms has been further advanced by the use of fractal analysis, a mathematical tool that quantifies the morphological complexity of objects [45–47]. The fractal dimension (FD), a basic metric in fractal analysis, measures the structural complexity of natural objects. Our previous findings showed that higher FD values of intratumoral SWI patterns (more geometrically complex) were associated with microbleeds and necrosis, and lower values with tumour microvasculature [10]. Applications of fractal-based parameters for differentiation between tumour types [6], tumour segmentation [48], oncological grading [10, 48] and therapeutic monitoring [30, 48] have demonstrated promising results.

A large number of high-dimensional features are generated in multiparametric studies. Thus, feature selection algorithms such as Least absolute shrinkage and selection operator (Lasso) and Elastic Net [49] are commonly used to shrink irrelevant variables and retain the most discriminatory features. Dimension reduction techniques, such as Principal Component Analysis (PCA) [50] which we adopted, reduce feature complexity. Some studies also incorporate feature robustness analysis to select only features that are robust to varying parameters [16, 51]. The feature selection process is important to avoid overfitting, an issue that arises when the number of features exceeds the number of samples, causing model performance to degrade in other patient cohorts not evaluated [2].

Machine Learning Classifiers

Extracted parameters can be input into different ML algorithms to define the scoring automatically for a binary or multiclass classification task, using the "ground truth" or reference standard as class labels for supervised training. Alternatively, parameters can be clustered in an unsupervised fashion, such as using *k*-means clustering of voxels that incorporates multiparametric quantitative measurements to differentiate between radiation necrosis and recurrent glioblastoma [52].

Classic ML methods generally employ handcrafted features and user-defined classification e.g. Support Vector Machine (SVM), Random Forest, and Logistic Regression, and regression algorithms including Linear Regression, Gaussian Process, Tweedie Regressor, etc. The advantages and limitations of several algorithms are summarised in Table 22.3. For any diagnostic or prognostic task, however, the performance of different ML classifiers varies, depending on the combination of imaging sequences and tumour features selected, as well as ML model parameters optimised e.g. kernel types for SVM classifier [11].

22.6 Deep Learning in Brain Tumour Characterisation

Unlike classical ML methods, deep learning is a subset of ML algorithms that uses an end-to-end approach to integrate feature learning and classification. It uses the full amount of information from the original images and features extracted automatically from DL models to directly obtain the final

Table 22.3 Summary of classical machine learning algorithms commonly used for brain tumour classification tasks

	Description	Advantages	Disadvantages
Support Vector Machine (SVM)	Maps feature vectors into a feature space then seeks a hyper-plane that segregates two classes with largest margin	• Less sensitive to amount of data and input dimension • Can generate nonlinear decision boundaries using kernel tricks	• Nonparametric models, support vectors need to be saved as part of the model • Sensitive to imbalanced class distributions
Random forest	Ensemble classifier combining predictions from several decision trees to generate a more stable classifier	• Can integrate large number of input variables • Robust to noise	• A black box, difficult to interpret how the model works
K-nearest neighbour (KNN)	Compares test sample with training samples to find those similar to it then assign it the majority class label	• Simple, no need for train a model • No assumption on data distribution and suitable for nonlinear data	• Nonparametric models, training samples need to be saved and applying the model to new sample is slow • Sensitive to irrelevant /redundant features
Naïve Bayes	Uses prior probabilities of classes and observed feature values of a class to estimate the posterior probability of the test sample belonging to that class	• Computes multiple probability distributions, distinct for each feature of every class • Does not penalise inaccurate probability assignment	• Assumes features are independent
Linear Discriminant Analysis (LDA)	Models each class as a Gaussian distribution and assigns a test sample to the class whose mean is the closest to it	• Closed-form solution, easy to compute decision boundaries • Inherently a multiclass model	• Assumes all the classes have a Gaussian distribution and the Gaussians have the same covariance matrix • Requires significant amount of data for accurate estimation of the Gaussians

result. Therefore, it eliminates dependence on the segmentation step, user-defined feature descriptors and classifiers. DL algorithms have been implemented for glioma genotyping [53] and pseudo-progression detection [21]. We recently developed a Lesion Encoder framework based on the Variational Auto Encoder U-Net [54] to automatically extract features from ROIs using convolutional neural networks (CNN) and then predict overall survival of glioma patients [55]. DL represents the state-of-art ML algorithms and will be increasingly used in multiparametric brain tumour characterisation.

22.7 Performance Evaluation of ML Algorithms

Different metrics are employed to quantitatively evaluate the performance of ML algorithms in different applications. For tumour segmentation, Dice Similarity Coefficient (DSC) and 95% Hausdorff Distance (HD) are commonly used to compare the segmentations of whole tumour or tumour subregions to the ground truth labels. For regression tasks, e.g. determining overall survival, Mean Squared Error (MSE) and Median Standard Deviation can be used to assess the pairwise error between predicted and actual survival; accuracy can also evaluate the number of correctly classified survivors based on their status, e.g. short- (<10 months), mid- (10–15 months) and long-survivors (>15 months). For classification tasks, such as distinction between IDH-wildtype and -mutant glioma, or between tumour recurrence and pseudo-progression, Sensitivity, Specificity, Area Under Curve (AUC) and Accuracy are used as evaluation metrics. While improved accuracy is important, the emphasis is usually given to high sensitivity as clinically, it is more important to be able to reliably predict the genetic profile (e.g. IDH gene status) and true tumour recurrence cases which may have poorer prognosis.

22.8 Clinical Applications

ML models have been investigated for a number of diagnostic and prognostic applications. We recently proposed a radiomics model to merge advanced fractal-based computational modelling with ML methods to objectively discriminate between gliomas and brain metastases [9]. In this study, we acquired preoperative images of 61 patients with grade II–IV gliomas and metastases who underwent conventional MRI protocol and three-dimensional SWI. All sequences were rigidly registered on SWI using the freely available Medical Image Processing, Analysis, and Visualisation (MIPAV) application. This was followed by tumour volume delineation by a neurosurgeon and a neuroradiologist in consensus on each slice of susceptibility-weighted images and

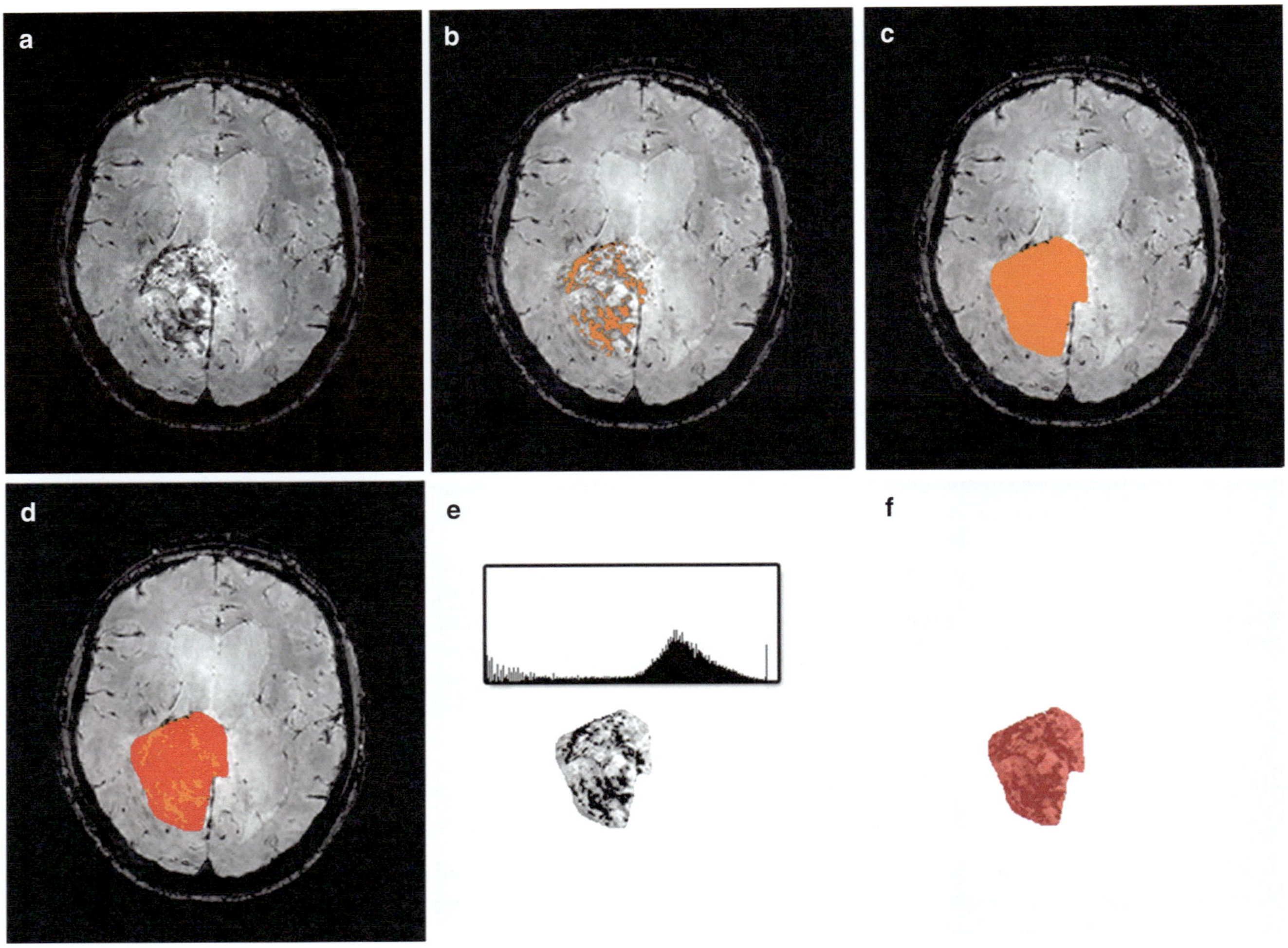

Fig. 22.2 (**a**) SWI of a right-sided glioblastoma. (**b**) Automatic segmentation of the intratumoral SWI pattern for computing of the 3D FD (P2), evaluating the complexity of the heterogeneity of the SWI signal. (**c**) ROI volume (P5) on the entire slices' stack. (**d**) Volume/ROI volume ratio. (**e**) 3D Histogram FD (P1), evaluating the grey levels distribution; (**f**) 3D inner FD (P3), evaluating the grey level and pixels' distribution. (Reprinted with permission [9])

image preprocessing to homogenise the greyscale level of the SWI signals across the dataset using the Brightness Progressive Normalisation algorithm. Several Euclidean parameters and fractal parameters based on the fractal dimension were calculated, as shown in Fig. 22.2. We used the box-counting method implemented in a custom software that we developed in C++ for fractal analysis [56]. Finally, we performed principal component analysis on the transformed variables and selected those components which explained most of the variation for the classification procedure. Linear and quadratic discriminant analysis, *k*-nearest neighbour and support vector machine (SVM) methods were evaluated for the diagnostic task. We found that the SVM classifier achieved the best results, accurately predicting 88% of glioblastomas using quantification of intratumoral SWI features. Differentiation of other glioma grades, particularly grade III gliomas, and metastasis yielded poorer performance.

The distinction of treatment-induced changes from early tumour progression in glioblastoma is also a challenging yet important application. Kim et al. [20] developed a radiomics model using first-order, volume, shape and texture features from contrast-enhanced T1, FLAIR, ADC and CBV data to differentiate pseudo-progression in glioblastoma patients who had newly developed or enlarging contrast-enhancing lesions on MRI within 3 months of completing chemoradiation therapy. They used a segmentation threshold and region-growing algorithm to semiautomatically segment the contrast-enhancing tumour region, and after feature extraction, selected the significant features using the LASSO method, followed by classification using a generalised linear model. Upon both internal and external validation, they found a superior performance by the multiparametric radiomics model (AUC 0.96 and 0.85, respectively) compared to using only conventional MRI, ADC map, CBV map, or any single parameter approaches.

22.9 Conclusions

Multiparametric assessment of brain tumours affords a comprehensive characterisation of the tumour phenotype with the potential to improve diagnostic and prognostic outcomes. Understanding the fundamentals of the methodological workflow, including the applications of various imaging sequences, quantitative parameters and machine learning algorithms will aid clinicians to maximise the performance and utility of a clinical predictive model. Ongoing progress in machine learning such as deep learning algorithms also presents exciting opportunities to improve the accuracy of tumour segmentation and stability of trained models across varying imaging acquisition and preprocessing methods.

Acknowledgements Prof. Antonio Di Ieva acknowledges the Royal Australasian College of Surgeons (RACS) for the 2019 John Mitchell Crouch Fellowship, which allowed the foundation of the Computational NeuroSurgery (CNS) Lab at Macquarie University. Moreover, he is funded by the Australian National Health and Medical Research Council (NHMRC) and by the Australian Research Council (ARC).

Dr. Sidong Liu acknowledges the support of an Australian National Health and Medical Research Council grant (NHMRC Early Career Fellowship).

Conflict of Interest The authors declare that they have no conflict of interest.

References

1. Inda MD-M, Bonavia R, Seoane J. Glioblastoma multiforme:a look inside its heterogeneous nature. Cancers (Basel). 2014;6:226–39. https://doi.org/10.3390/cancers6010226.
2. Lambin P, Leijenaar RTH, Deist TM, Peerlings J, De Jong EEC, Van Timmeren J, Sanduleanu S, Larue RTHM, Even AJG, Jochems A, Van Wijk Y, Woodruff H, Van Soest J, Lustberg T, Roelofs E, Van Elmpt W, Dekker A, Mottaghy FM, Wildberger JE, Walsh S. Radiomics: the bridge between medical imaging and personalized medicine. Nat Rev Clin Oncol. 2017;14:749–62. https://doi.org/10.1038/nrclinonc.2017.141.
3. Senders JT, Arnaout O, Karhade AV, Dasenbrock HH, Gormley WB, Broekman ML, Smith TR. Natural and artificial intelligence in neurosurgery: a systematic review. Neurosurgery. 2018;83:181–92.
4. Devos A, Simonetti AW, Van Der Graaf M, Lukas L, Suykens JAK, Vanhamme L, Buydens LMC, Heerschap A, Van Huffel S. The use of multivariate MR imaging intensities versus metabolic data from MR spectroscopic imaging for brain tumour classification. J Magn Reson. 2005;173:218–28.
5. Zacharaki EI, Wang S, Chawla S, Yoo DS, Wolf R, Melhem ER, Davatzikos C. Classification of brain tumor type and grade using MRI texture and shape in a machine learning scheme. Magn Reson Med. 2009;62:1609–18.
6. Di Ieva A, Le Reste PJ, Carsin-Nicol B, Ferre JC, Cusimano MD. Diagnostic value of fractal analysis for the differentiation of brain tumors using 3-tesla magnetic resonance susceptibility-weighted imaging. Neurosurgery. 2016;79:839–46.
7. Suh HB, Choi YS, Bae S, Ahn SS, Chang JH, Kang SG, Kim EH, Kim SH, Lee SK. Primary central nervous system lymphoma and atypical glioblastoma: differentiation using radiomics approach. Eur Radiol. 2018;28:3832–9. https://doi.org/10.1007/s00330-018-5368-4.
8. Petrujkić K, Milošević N, Rajković N, Stanisavljević D, Gavrilović S, Dželebdžić D, Ilić R, Di Ieva A, Maksimović R. Computational quantitative MR image features - a potential useful tool in differentiating glioblastoma from solitary brain metastasis. Eur J Radiol. 2019;119:108634. https://doi.org/10.1016/j.ejrad.2019.08.003.
9. Di Ieva A, Russo C, Le Reste P-J, Magnussen J, Heller G. Advanced computational and statistical multiparametric analysis of susceptibility-weighted imaging to characterize gliomas and brain metastases. bioRxiv. 2020; https://doi.org/10.1101/2020.04.24.060830.
10. Di Ieva A, Göd S, Grabner G, Grizzi F, Sherif C, Matula C, Tschabitscher M, Trattnig S. Three-dimensional susceptibility-weighted imaging at 7 T using fractal-based quantitative analysis to grade gliomas. Neuroradiology. 2013;55:35–40. https://doi.org/10.1007/s00234-012-1081-1.
11. Zhang X, Yan LF, Hu YC, Li G, Yang Y, Han Y, Sun YZ, Liu ZC, Tian Q, Han ZY, De Liu L, Hu BQ, Qiu ZY, Wang W, Bin CG. Optimizing a machine learning based glioma grading system using multi-parametric MRI histogram and texture features. Oncotarget. 2017;8:47816–30.
12. Vamvakas A, Williams SC, Theodorou K, Kapsalaki E, Fountas K, Kappas C, Vassiou K, Tsougos I. Imaging biomarker analysis of advanced multiparametric MRI for glioma grading. Phys Med. 2019;60:188–98. https://doi.org/10.1016/j.ejmp.2019.03.014.
13. Alis D, Bagcilar O, Senli YD, Yergin M, Isler C, Kocer N, Islak C, Kizilkilic O. Machine learning-based quantitative texture analysis of conventional MRI combined with ADC maps for assessment of IDH1 mutation in high-grade gliomas. Jpn J Radiol. 2020;38:135–43. https://doi.org/10.1007/s11604-019-00902-7.
14. Bisdas S, Shen H, Thust S, Katsaros V, Stranjalis G, Boskos C, Brandner S, Zhang J. Texture analysis-and support vector machine-assisted diffusional kurtosis imaging may allow in vivo gliomas grading and IDH-mutation status prediction: a preliminary study. Sci Rep. 2018;8:1–9.
15. Akkus Z, Ali I, Sedlář J, Agrawal JP, Parney IF, Giannini C, Erickson BJ. Predicting deletion of chromosomal arms 1p/19q in low-grade gliomas from MR images using machine intelligence. J Digit Imaging. 2017;30:469–76.
16. Cui Y, Tha KK, Terasaka S, Yamaguchi S, Wang J, Kudo K, Xing L, Shirato H, Li R. Prognostic imaging biomarkers in glioblastoma: development and independent validation on the basis of multiregion and quantitative analysis of MR images. Radiology. 2016;278:546–53. https://doi.org/10.1148/radiol.2015150358.
17. Papp L, Pötsch N, Grahovac M, Schmidbauer V, Woehrer A, Preusser M, Mitterhauser M, Kiesel B, Wadsak W, Beyer T, Hacker M, Traub-Weidinger T. Glioma survival prediction with combined analysis of in vivo 11 C-MET PET features, ex vivo features, and patient features by supervised machine learning. J Nucl Med. 2018;59:892–9. https://doi.org/10.2967/jnumed.117.202267.
18. Zhou M, Chaudhury B, Hall LO, Goldgof DB, Gillies RJ, Gatenby RA. Identifying spatial imaging biomarkers of glioblastoma multiforme for survival group prediction. J Magn Reson Imaging. 2017;46:115–23. https://doi.org/10.1002/jmri.25497.
19. Nael K, Bauer AH, Hormigo A, Lemole M, Germano IM, Puig J, Stea B. Multiparametric MRI for differentiation of radiation necrosis from recurrent tumor in patients with treated glioblastoma. AJR Am J Roentgenol. 2018;210:18–23. https://doi.org/10.2214/AJR.17.18003.
20. Kim JY, Park JE, Jo Y, Shim WH, Nam SJ, Kim JH, Yoo RE, Choi SH, Kim HS. Incorporating diffusion- and perfusion-weighted MRI into a radiomics model improves diagnostic performance for pseudoprogression in glioblastoma patients. Neuro-Oncology. 2019;21:404–14.

21. Gao Y, Xiao X, Han B, Li G, Ning X, Wang D, Cai W, Kikinis R, Berkovsky S, Di Ieva A, Zhang L, Ji N, Liu S. A deep learning methodology for differentiating glioma recurrence from radiation necrosis using multimodal MRI: algorithm development and validation. JMIR Med Inform. 2020;8(11):e19805. https://doi.org/10.2196/19805.
22. Svolos P, Kousi E, Kapsalaki E, Theodorou K, Fezoulidis I, Kappas C, Tsougos I. The role of diffusion and perfusion weighted imaging in the differential diagnosis of cerebral tumors: a review and future perspectives. Cancer Imaging. 2014;14(1):20.
23. van Dijken BRJ, van Laar PJ, Holtman GA, van der Hoorn A. Diagnostic accuracy of magnetic resonance imaging techniques for treatment response evaluation in patients with high-grade glioma, a systematic review and meta-analysis. Eur Radiol. 2017;27:4129–44. https://doi.org/10.1007/s00330-017-4789-9.
24. Di Ieva A, Choi C, Magnussen JS. Spectrobiopsy in neurodiagnostics: the new era. Neuroradiology. 2018;60:129–31. https://doi.org/10.1007/s00234-017-1957-1.
25. Di Ieva A, Magnussen JS, McIntosh J, Mulcahy MJ, Pardey M, Choi C. Magnetic resonance spectroscopic assessment of Isocitrate dehydrogenase status in gliomas: the new frontiers of spectrobiopsy in neurodiagnostics. World Neurosurg. 2020;133:e421–7. https://doi.org/10.1016/j.wneu.2019.09.040.
26. Di Ieva A, Lam T, Alcaide-Leon P, Bharatha A, Montanera W, Cusimano MD. Magnetic resonance susceptibility weighted imaging in neurosurgery: current applications and future perspectives. J Neurosurg. 2015;123:1463–75. https://doi.org/10.3171/2015.1.JNS142349.
27. Haubold J, Demircioglu A, Gratz M, Glas M, Wrede K, Sure U, Antoch G, Keyvani K, Nittka M, Kannengiesser S, Gulani V, Griswold M, Herrmann K, Forsting M, Nensa F, Umutlu L. Non-invasive tumor decoding and phenotyping of cerebral gliomas utilizing multiparametric 18F-FET PET-MRI and MR fingerprinting. Eur J Nucl Med Mol Imaging. 2019; https://doi.org/10.1007/s00259-019-04602-2.
28. Hatt M, Tixier F, Pierce L, Kinahan PE, Le Rest CC, Visvikis D. Characterization of PET/CT images using texture analysis: the past, the present… any future? Eur J Nucl Med Mol Imaging. 2017;44:151–65. https://doi.org/10.1007/s00259-016-3427-0.
29. Smith SM, Jenkinson M, Woolrich MW, Beckmann CF, Behrens TEJ, Johansen-Berg H, Bannister PR, De Luca M, Drobnjak I, Flitney DE, Niazy RK, Saunders J, Vickers J, Zhang Y, De Stefano N, Brady JM, Matthews PM. Advances in functional and structural MR image analysis and implementation as FSL. NeuroImage. 2004;23(Suppl 1):S208–19.
30. Di Ieva A, Matula C, Grizzi F, Grabner G, Trattnig S, Tschabitscher M. Fractal analysis of the susceptibility weighted imaging patterns in malignant brain tumors during antiangiogenic treatment: technical report on four cases serially imaged by 7 T magnetic resonance during a period of four weeks. World Neurosurg. 2012;77:785.e11–21. https://doi.org/10.1016/j.wneu.2011.09.006.
31. Russo C. Brightness progressive normalization. 2011. http://www.fractal-lab.org/Downloads/bpn_algorithm.html. Accessed 8 Nov 2020.
32. Sled JG, Zijdenbos AP, Evans AC. A nonparametric method for automatic correction of intensity nonuniformity in MRI data. IEEE Trans Med Imaging. 1998;17:87–97.
33. Avants BB, Epstein CL, Grossman M, Gee JC. Symmetric diffeomorphic image registration with cross-correlation: evaluating automated labeling of elderly and neurodegenerative brain. Med Image Anal. 2008;12:26–41. https://doi.org/10.1016/j.media.2007.06.004.
34. Isensee F, Schell M, Pflueger I, Brugnara G, Bonekamp D, Neuberger U, Wick A, Schlemmer HP, Heiland S, Wick W, Bendszus M, Maier-Hein KH, Kickingereder P. Automated brain extraction of multisequence MRI using artificial neural networks. Hum Brain Mapp. 2019;40:4952–64.
35. Russo C, Liu S, Di Ieva A. Spherical coordinates transformation preprocessing in deep convolution neural networks for brain tumor segmentation in MRI. arXiv. 2020. http://arxiv.org/abs/2008.07090.
36. Pomponio R, Erus G, Habes M, Doshi J, Srinivasan D, Mamourian E, Bashyam V, Nasrallah IM, Satterthwaite TD, Fan Y, Launer LJ, Masters CL, Maruff P, Zhuo C, Völzke H, Johnson SC, Fripp J, Koutsouleris N, Wolf DH, Gur R, Gur R, Morris J, Albert MS, Grabe HJ, Resnick SM, Bryan RN, Wolk DA, Shinohara RT, Shou H, Davatzikos C. Harmonization of large MRI datasets for the analysis of brain imaging patterns throughout the lifespan. NeuroImage. 2020;208 https://doi.org/10.1016/j.neuroimage.2019.116450.
37. Sawlani V, Patel MD, Davies N, Flintham R, Wesolowski R, Ughratdar I, Pohl U, Nagaraju S, Petrik V, Kay A, Jacob S, Sanghera P, Wykes V, Watts C, Poptani H. Multiparametric MRI: practical approach and pictorial review of a useful tool in the evaluation of brain tumours and tumour-like lesions. Insights Imaging. 2020;11:84. https://doi.org/10.1186/s13244-020-00888-1.
38. Kubben PL, Postma AA, Kessels AGH, van Overbeeke JJ, van Santbrink H. Intraobserver and interobserver agreement in volumetric assessment of glioblastoma multiforme resection. Neurosurgery. 2010;67:1329–34.
39. Visser M, Müller DMJ, van Duijn RJM, Smits M, Verburg N, Hendriks EJ, Nabuurs RJA, Bot JCJ, Eijgelaar RS, Witte M, van Herk MB, Barkhof F, de Witt Hamer PC, de Munck JC. Inter-rater agreement in glioma segmentations on longitudinal MRI. NeuroImage Clin. 2019;22:101727. https://doi.org/10.1016/j.nicl.2019.101727.
40. Liu S, Song Y, Zhang F, Feng D, Fulham M, Cai W. Clique identification and propagation for multimodal brain Tumor image segmentation. Lect Notes Comput Sci (including Subser Lect Notes Artif Intell Lect Notes Bioinformatics). 2016;9919 LNAI:285–94. https://doi.org/10.1007/978-3-319-47103-7_28.
41. Işin A, Direkoelu C, Şah M. Review of MRI-based brain tumor image segmentation using deep learning methods. Procedia Comput Sci. 2016;102:317–24. https://doi.org/10.1016/j.procs.2016.09.407.
42. Jang K, Russo C, Di Ieva A. Radiomics in gliomas: clinical implications of computational modeling and fractal-based analysis. Neuroradiology. 2020;62:771–90. https://doi.org/10.1007/s00234-020-02403-1.
43. Haralick RM, Dinstein I, Shanmugam K. Textural features for image classification. IEEE Trans Syst Man Cybern. 1973;SMC-3(6):610–21.
44. Artzi M, Bressler I, Ben Bashat D. Differentiation between glioblastoma, brain metastasis and subtypes using radiomics analysis. J Magn Reson Imaging. 2019;50:519–28. https://doi.org/10.1002/jmri.26643.
45. Di Ieva A. The fractal geometry of the brain. New York: Springer; 2016.
46. Di Ieva A, Esteban FJ, Grizzi F, Klonowski W, Martín-Landrove M. Fractals in the neurosciences, part II. Neuroscience. 2015;21:30–43. https://doi.org/10.1177/1073858413513928.
47. Di Ieva A, Grizzi F, Jelinek H, Pellionisz AJ, Losa GA. Fractals in the neurosciences, part I: general principles and basic neurosciences. Neuroscience. 2014;20:403–17. https://doi.org/10.1177/1073858413513927.
48. Iftekharuddin KM, Jia W, Marsh R. Fractal analysis of tumor in brain MR images. Mach Vis Appl. 2003;13:352–62.
49. Li J, Cheng K, Wang S, Morstatter F, Trevino RP, Tang J, Liu H. Feature selection: a data perspective. ACM Comput Surv. 2017;50(6):94.
50. Pearson K. LIII. On lines and planes of closest fit to systems of points in space. Lond Edin Dublin Philos Mag J Sci. 1901;2:559–72. https://doi.org/10.1080/14786440109462720.
51. Cattell R, Chen S, Huang C. Robustness of radiomic features in magnetic resonance imaging: review and a phantom study. Vis Comput Ind Biomed Art. 2019;2(1):19.

52. Yoon RG, Kim HS, Koh MJ, Shim WH, Jung SC, Kim SJ, Kim JH. Differentiation of recurrent glioblastoma from delayed radiation necrosis by using voxel-based multiparametric analysis of MR imaging data. Radiology. 2017;285:206–13. https://doi.org/10.1148/radiol.2017161588.
53. Liu S, Shah Z, Sav A, Russo C, Berkovsky S, Qian Y, Coiera E, Di Ieva A. Isocitrate dehydrogenase (IDH) status prediction in histopathology images of gliomas using deep learning. Sci Rep. 2020;10:7733.
54. Feng Y-Z, Liu S, Cheng Z, Quiroz JC, Rezazadegan D, Chen P, Lin Q, Qian L, Liu X, Berkovsky S, Coiera E, Song L, Qiu X, Cai X. Severity assessment and progression prediction of COVID-19 patients based on the LesionEncoder framework and chest CT. medRxiv. 2020; https://doi.org/10.1101/2020.08.03.20167007.
55. Russo C, Liu S, Di Ieva A. Impact of spherical coordinates transformation pre- processing in deep convolution neural networks for brain tumor segmentation and survival prediction. In: Brain lesion: glioma, multiple sclerosis, stroke and traumatic brain injuries. Berlin: Springer; 2020.
56. Di Ieva A, Russo C. Fractal dimension estimator. 2014. http://www.fractal-lab.org/Downloads/FDEstimator.html. Accessed 18 Nov 2020.

Tackling the Complexity of Lesion-Symptoms Mapping: How to Bridge the Gap Between Data Scientists and Clinicians?

23

Emmanuel Mandonnet and Bertrand Thirion

23.1 Introduction

Large-scale data integration is currently a major trend in neuroscience, where this approach has shown important benefits for standardized measures of the link between brain connectivity and functional scores in the general population [1]. It is yet unclear whether it brings benefit for lesion studies, where the high variability in individual characteristics of both the lesion and its impact potentially overwhelm information gleaned by population-level analysis. More generally, the question arises whether ML algorithms fed by large amounts of data can outperform clinicians acting on a much smaller dataset for predicting unseen cases.

Lesion-symptom mapping addresses the following questions: given a set of behavioural and imaging connectivity measures at the time the lesion occurred in a patient, can we predict what the long-term functional scores will be? For a neurosurgeon, the question becomes: how to predict which cognitive deficits would be induced by a planned extent of resection in a given patient, for whom we have preoperative cognitive scores and functional MRI data? For a neurologist, the most common question is: how to predict the degree of recovery after rehabilitation, given the observed cognitive deficits and functional imaging right after a stroke? While they are related to each other, these two questions are not the same: the timing of patient-data acquisition differs, and different pathophysiological mechanisms underpin the two situations: for example, the well-known phenomenon of prelesional plasticity precedes the surgical resection but not the stroke, explaining the striking difference in outcomes between the two pathologies [2, 3]. Notwithstanding these pathophysiological differences, the overall framework is similar for both situations, and the methods discussed here can, with slight changes, be applied to one or the other. We will refer implicitly to the surgical resection case, but most statements carry over to stroke.

As recently summarized by Price et al. [4] for strokes, outcome prediction is a very hard challenge. This endeavour requires dealing with (1) the complexity of structure-function relationships in the brain, that are only partly common to the population (2) the variability of lesion localization and extent. These two dimensions hamper the accuracy of individual outcome prediction. In this paper, we argue that there is a gap between data scientists and clinicians: while clinicians might have difficulties to leverage the information provided by existing datasets, data scientists might miss the clinical knowledge that would synthesize this information in a unique mechanism that better carries over across individuals than low-level imaging patterns.

In the next sections, we first analyze the problem in greater detail, showing how it relates to other neuroscience questions. Then, following Price et al. [4], we emphasize the distinction between *data-based predictions*—in which ML algorithms learn to make predictions from data only, and *model-based predictions*, in which predictions are derived from a two-step modelling: a first step, inferring how the brain is/was functioning before the lesion, and a second step describing how the lesion will/has impact(ed) brain organization. Finally, we argue that *model-based predictions* can leverage the information provided by extensively explored single cases. We call for a new paradigm to combine insights gained from single-cases analysis with the predictive power of ML algorithms.

E. Mandonnet (✉)
Department of Neurosurgery, Lariboisière Hospital, APHP, Paris, France

Paris University, Paris, France

Paris Brain Institute (ICM), Paris, France

B. Thirion
Inria, CEA, Université Paris-Saclay, Paris, France

V. E. Staartjes et al. (eds.), *Machine Learning in Clinical Neuroscience*, Acta Neurochirurgica Supplement 134,
https://doi.org/10.1007/978-3-030-85292-4_23

23.2 Clarifying the Problem

Several important concepts are implicitly involved in the definition of lesion-symptom mapping proposed above:

- *Predictive personalized* medicine. The main goal is to make predictions at the individual level, i.e. we are not interested in group-level analysis.
- *Multimodal* data-informed approach. The inter-individual variability of brain structural and functional connectivity in relation to anatomical landmarks [5] impedes individual prediction from anatomical MRI alone. Moreover, the weak correlation between structural or functional connectivity and behavioural scores calls for augmenting imaging data. Furthermore, individual outcomes are likely not captured by a single score, but rather by a pattern of deficits, explored through a battery of functional tasks.
- Post-lesional *plasticity*. We are not aiming to predict the behavioural scores right after the lesion, but the functional domains for which plasticity will be overwhelmed, thus limiting patient's recovery.

Lesional Localizationism, Lesional Hodotopism, Functional Localizationism

Despite all the issues related to inter-individual variability in brain organization and lesions characteristics as well, the lesion-symptom mapping problem is well-posed, in the sense that the same pattern of functional deficits should be observed whenever two similarly organized brains undergo the same topographical lesion from the same pathophysiological mechanism—although different plasticity potentials could nonetheless lead to slightly different levels of recovery. In other words, there is a *lesional localizationism*. This grounds the clinicians' knowledge and expertise: in front of a patient with a lesion, the clinician remembers other cases with similar lesion size and location, and infers outcome from those past cases.

This *lesional localizationism* contrasts with the more recent view of *lesional hodotopism* [6], that states that two spatially distant lesions can induce the same dysfunction, because they would impact the same spatially distributed functional network. However, even if a given dysfunction can be caused by two spatially distant lesions, when looking at the whole spectrum of functions, each lesion topography leads to a specific fingerprint. Consequently, *lesional hodotopism* does not help much for clinical practice.

Functional localizationism uses *lesional localizationism* to "assign a functional role to an area" just by taking the "negative" of the deficit [7]. It is inspired from primary (sensory)-motor processing: a lesion to the precentral gyrus leads to a specific motor deficit, hence we assign to the precentral gyrus the functional role of driving voluntary motricity. But this logical shortcut cannot be generalized: the local functional information provided by the consequence of lesions only informs us about the necessary implication of regions into the functional process as a whole. This does not tell us how the entire network would reorganize if the area were damaged, and consequently, one cannot deduce the deficit just by knowing the "functional role of an area".

In summary, there are two separate—albeit closely related—problems [8]:

- Determining, for a given lesion, the set of tasks/scores that will be impacted in the long term.
- Determining the set of areas that are recruited by the performance of a given task, and predicting behavioural scores from network connectivity measures gained from imaging techniques.

From Behavioural Measurements to Cognitive Processes: Leveraging Multidimensional Scores

It is well established that no one-to-one relationship exists between lesion topography and score deficit. In fact, we formulated the questions directly in terms of multiple scores from a set of tasks involving different functions, because these functional scores are not independent from each other. A consequence for lesion-symptom analysis is that behavioural scores should be considered jointly. Specifically, multivariate analytic procedures, such as Principal/Independent Components Analysis PCA/ICA or clustering, attempt to reduce the dimension of the scoring system. The aim of such analysis is twofold: (1) create composite variables that are less noisy than the initial scores; (2) identify elementary cognitive subprocesses that together give rise to behaviour.

An inspiring example is given by language function and its subdivision in (lexico-)semantic, phonological, and motor subsystems. Although this organization has long been recognized (see for example Indefrey & Levelt [9]), it has recently been revisited through a PCA applied to a set of different language testing scores, in order to get a fully data-driven definition of these three components [10, 11]. In these latter studies, the components were reported to be spatially separable (see [7, 12, 13] for definitions of double dissociation and spatial separability). One could thus expect that well-designed compound generally benefit to lesion-symptom mapping.

The Complexity of Lesion-Symptom Mapping

The complexity of lesion mapping is daunting, given the variability of both prelesional brain connectomics and lesional topographies and etiologies: very large multimodal datasets may be necessary to cover all the dimensions of the problem. A possible way forward is to break down the problem, by restricting the analysis to small regions taken e.g. from brain atlases. Yet binding together these unitary pieces of lesion-symptoms mappings for predicting the deficit of a larger lesion remains challenging, given the expected nonlinearity between lesion and deficits. Indeed, whenever two small areas A & B are damaged, the resulting deficit might not be the sum of deficit A + deficit B (neither a linear weighting of the two deficits). Interestingly, some authors have proposed to tackle this nonlinearity by introducing different kinds of interactions between two lesions, and modelling these interactions by a hierarchical tree statistical approach [14].

23.3 Data-Driven vs. Model-Based Approaches

Data-Driven Approaches

The revolution in lesion-symptom mapping came out at the turn of the century, when MRI registration algorithms [15] gave birth to voxel-lesion-symptom mapping (VLSM) techniques [16], that are the lesion-domain counterpart of standard brain mapping techniques. The basic principle is explained in Fig. 23.1. Although perfectly identified from the start, the limitations of this methodology have been overlooked until recently [17, 18]. In VLSM, voxels are treated *independently* from each other, which is problematic in two regards:

- The voxels impacted by a lesion are not randomly distributed within the brain. The laws of the underlying biology of the different pathologies impose strong spatial correlations between voxels. For example, in a stroke, the vascular architecture dictates the probability to find a lesioned voxel in the vicinity of a given voxel. VLSM ignores this important prior information.
- When it comes to functions being supported by spatially distributed networks, the functional consequence of a lesioned voxel is directly related to the extent of the lesion to another part of the network. Here again, voxels cannot be treated independently from each other.

It has been demonstrated in [17] on a sample of stroke lesions with simulated ground-truth lesion-symptoms relationships that VSLM can be heavily biased. The simplest way to circumvent this limitation is to introduce multivariate analysis, through application of ML algorithms (see Fig. 23.2). An important asset of multivariate methods is that they avoid the counterproductive isolation of brain regions, and instead rely on intermediate representations, aka predictive patterns [19, 20]. The statistical maps representing such predictive patterns should not be confused with classical statistical maps based on the univariate approach: the latter test *marginal* associations between voxel-based signal and some information (presence of a lesion), while the former do so, *conditionally* to all other regions considered. This difference has been acknowledged in the field of brain mapping [21, 22], but it turns out to be crucial for lesion mapping: only

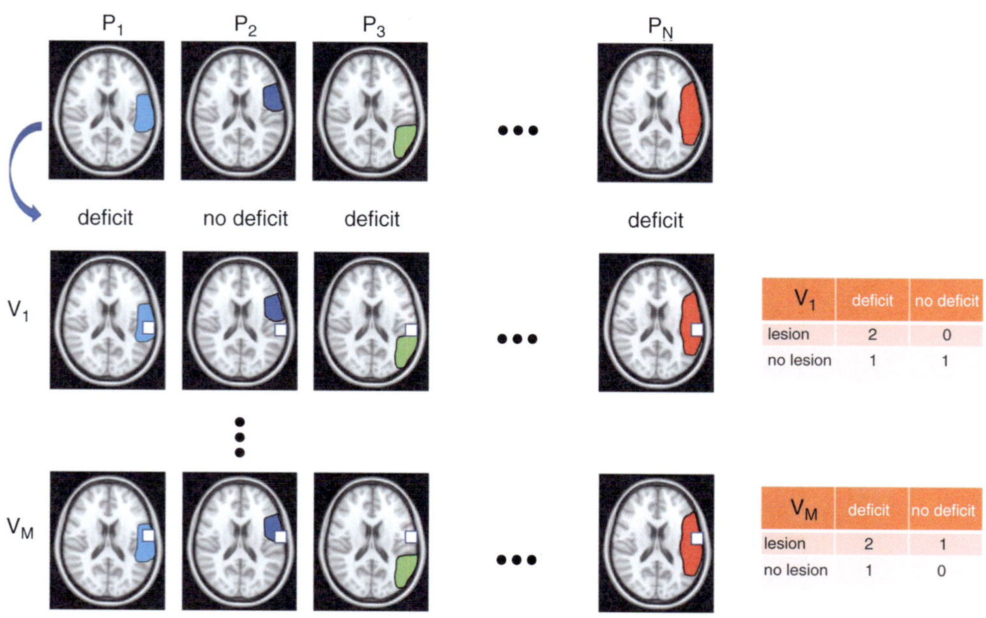

Fig. 23.1 Principle of mass univariate voxel-based lesion-symptoms mapping (VLSM). All patients' images are registered in the same anatomical reference. For each voxel, a contingency table is determined, and a statistical test is applied to decide if the deficit correlates with a higher rate of lesions in this voxel. Classical methods of corrected thresholding for multiple comparison are used, given the high number of voxels (typically between 10^5 and 10^6)

	P_1	P_2	P_3	..	..	P_N	new patient
deficit	no	no	yes	..	..	yes	???
V_1	0	1	0	..	..	0	1
V_2	1	1	0	..	..	1	0
..	..	..	..	..	..	..	..
..	..	..	..	..	..	..	..
V_M	0	1	0	..	..	1	0

Fig. 23.2 Multivariate analysis of lesion-symptoms mapping. Patients are represented in columns and voxels in rows. 0 stands for no lesion in a given voxel for a given patients, and 1 for a lesion. Machine learning algorithms are trained to predict the first row (presence or absence of deficits in each patient), given the following rows. Given the large dimensionality (number of rows), training requires a very large number of patient-cases. Once the algorithm has been trained, it can predict, from the binary values of V_1 to V_M, the presence or absence of deficits in a new patient

multivariate analyses can discount the effect of non-specific associations, such as those induced for example by the vascular tree structure [17, 18].

As these algorithms require training over a large sample of cases, neuropsychological studies should upscale to thousands rather than hundreds of cases [17, 18]. This seems at least challenging, although there exist now some attempts to gather such datasets [23, 24]. The limited datasets available might explain the low predictive accuracy of current ML-based approaches [20, 25, 26]. It is also worth emphasizing that multivariate methods have a hard time dealing with lesion anatomical dependence [27]: if the underlying physiopathological mechanism causes two regions to be either both preserved or damaged, no conclusion can be drawn about the contribution of each area to deficit prediction. The *sample complexity* of ML approaches—i.e. the number of samples that are required to make reliable inference on the behavioural impact of lesions—can be reduced by relying on compressed representations of the data, for instance, using parcellation techniques [28–30]. However, if the true functional unit is a network (distributed over several spatially distant areas) rather than a single area, parcellations might be not the optimal solution for reducing the dimensionality in lesion-symptoms mapping.

Model-Driven (Top-Down) Approaches

Model-driven (top-down) methods constitute a different class of approaches. They leverage prior knowledge about brain functional organization in order to tackle the complexity of lesion-symptom mapping. Even if accurate predictions could be obtained through ML approaches, a certain amount of frustration would remain, as the "black box" nature of some ML algorithms (e.g. deep neural networks) provides only limited evidence about the prediction mechanisms. An alternative approach is to rely on reasoning (including generalizations and analogies) for inferring, even from a few single cases, a phenomenological or, at best, mechanistic model of the lesion-symptom link, that is to *understand* how the lesions changed brain functional organization, and how these changes explain behavioural deficits. In terms of causal reasoning, lesion is an (unwanted) treatment, of which the heterogeneous impacts depend on the prelesional state of the subjects [31]. Such analysis thus requires an in-depth knowledge of the prelesional brain state.

In the first step of the procedure, one should attempt to identify the individual prelesional brain structure and function. The best way is probably to detect deviations to a reference brain. While this is highly challenging in stroke patients (for whom we do not have premorbid data), this is not trivial either in presurgical glioma patients—despite the fact that we can collect in that case both behavioural and imaging data before the surgical lesion: the glioma might have already reshaped the native structural and functional connectivity, rendering the comparison with healthy subjects tricky. In this perspective, current efforts in cognitive neuroscience to build datasets of thousands of people with combined behavioural and imaging data should help to define not only a standard functional brain—by determining group-averaged networks for each cognitive task—but also a population-level distribution of phenotypic variants of structural and functional connectivity for different cognitive task. Such work has already been partly achieved for resting-state functional connectivity [32]. The most well-known example of phenotypic variant to the structuro-functional brain of reference is a left-right flip. Indeed, whereas in most people the left hemisphere is supporting, among other functions, combinatorial phonology for language processing and the right hemisphere is supporting, among other functions, visuospatial and executive processing, about 6% of left-handed and 1% of right-handed people exhibit the reversed pattern of functional organization. Detecting these outliers is of utmost importance, as it has been shown that the reverse pattern of deficits is indeed observed in patients with this left-right flip [33]. However, the importance of phenotypic variants outside of this extreme example remains to be determined.

A second level of modelling aims to describe lesion impact on brain structure and function, that is to determine both how the structural and functional connectivities are modified by the lesion and how these changes reverberate onto behavioural performances. The simplest model that was initially tested by neurosurgeons was the following: if any node of the network evidenced on a task-based functional MRI of a given task is damaged by the lesion, the patient cannot perform the task anymore. It has been clearly demonstrated that this was not valid [34–36]. A refinement consists in computing first how a lesion will impact the connectivity of each cortical area of a brain parcellation, relying on an atlas of tractograms obtained from healthy people. This approach has recently been applied to a large series of stroke patients [37], but the results were rather disappointing, as the prediction did not improve compared to the standard method, in which predictors were defined as lesion-load of each cortical area. A possible reason why this innovative disconnective approach was unsuccessful is the reliance on a brain parcellation that isolates local territories, whereas the relevant functional unit should be a network of spatially distant areas. The importance of a network-level approach in lesion-symptoms mapping has been underlined recently [38], in a work that introduces a method of mapping symptoms to networks, using our current knowledge of resting-state functional connectome. Hence different lesions locations can be bound together, by pointing to a common dedicated network for each functional deficit [39]. For example, tractograms of HCP subjects and a patient's lesion can be registered in the same MNI space, allowing to compute how much a lesion disconnected a functional network (see Fig. 23.3). One would expect these network disconnection indices to provide better predictors than the disconnection indices of each separate area as proposed in [37]. Moreover, selecting a limited number of networks of interest (NOI) can dramatically reduce the number of predictors, thus improving statistical results.

More recently, simulation-based models have been proposed. For example, we can take advantage of the new possibility to compute a patient-specific virtual brain functional connectivity from this patient's structural connectivity [42]. While this approach seems appealing, we note that plasticity is currently not yet included in the model. Moreover, the value of functional connectivity to predict behavioural scores is rather low [43].

In summary, it is anticipated that model-based approaches will inform data-driven predictions, by allowing to reduce the high-dimensional data to a limited number of relevant predictors, that reflect our current knowledge on brain connectivity. By using the right level abstraction to generalize across individuals, the combination of model-based approaches and ML holds the premise of providing efficient prediction of individual outcome [44].

23.4 How to Capitalize on Multimodal Longitudinal Single Cases?

The Value of Multimodal Longitudinal Single Cases

In the big data era, it is tempting to leave apart the knowledge gained from the old-fashioned approach of case reports. In this last part, we would like to demonstrate their value and plead for a renewal of single-cases reports. It should be kept in mind that such single case studies have played an essential role in the past. Most of our current neuropsychological knowledge is deeply rooted in single case studies [45, 46]. It should also be noted that there is a recent trend in neuroscience towards single-case comprehensive approaches. Several studies in healthy individual explored few subjects (typically less than ten), but with extensive measures, ranging from imaging to behavioural scores [47, 48]. Moreover, the degree of universality of a lesion-symptom mechanism from a single case might be higher than expected, especially when considering longitudinal cases, as those offered by surgical glioma patients: the generalizability is not about the correlation between a lesion and a deficit, but rather in the causal impact of a lesion on a pre-resective brain configuration. Indeed *lesional localizationism* states that two similarly organized brains (as established by prelesional non-invasive tools) undergoing the same physiopathological (surgical) lesion will end in the same functional state. Consequently, if the mechanism has been clearly identified, even in a single case, it can help to generate relevant prediction for new cases.

For example, Mandonnet et al. reported a case showing a strong impairment in set-shifting abilities after resection of a glioma in the right temporo-parietal junction [49]. The resection damaged the structural connectivity of the cognitive control network B, resulting in a disrupted functional connectivity of this network. In a second case, the same authors used intraoperative electrical stimulation and axono-cortical evoked potentials to confirm the involvement of the cognitive control network B in set-shifting abilities [50]. The comprehensive analysis of these two single cases led us to infer the general hypothesis that indices of structural disconnection within a given network could provide the most relevant

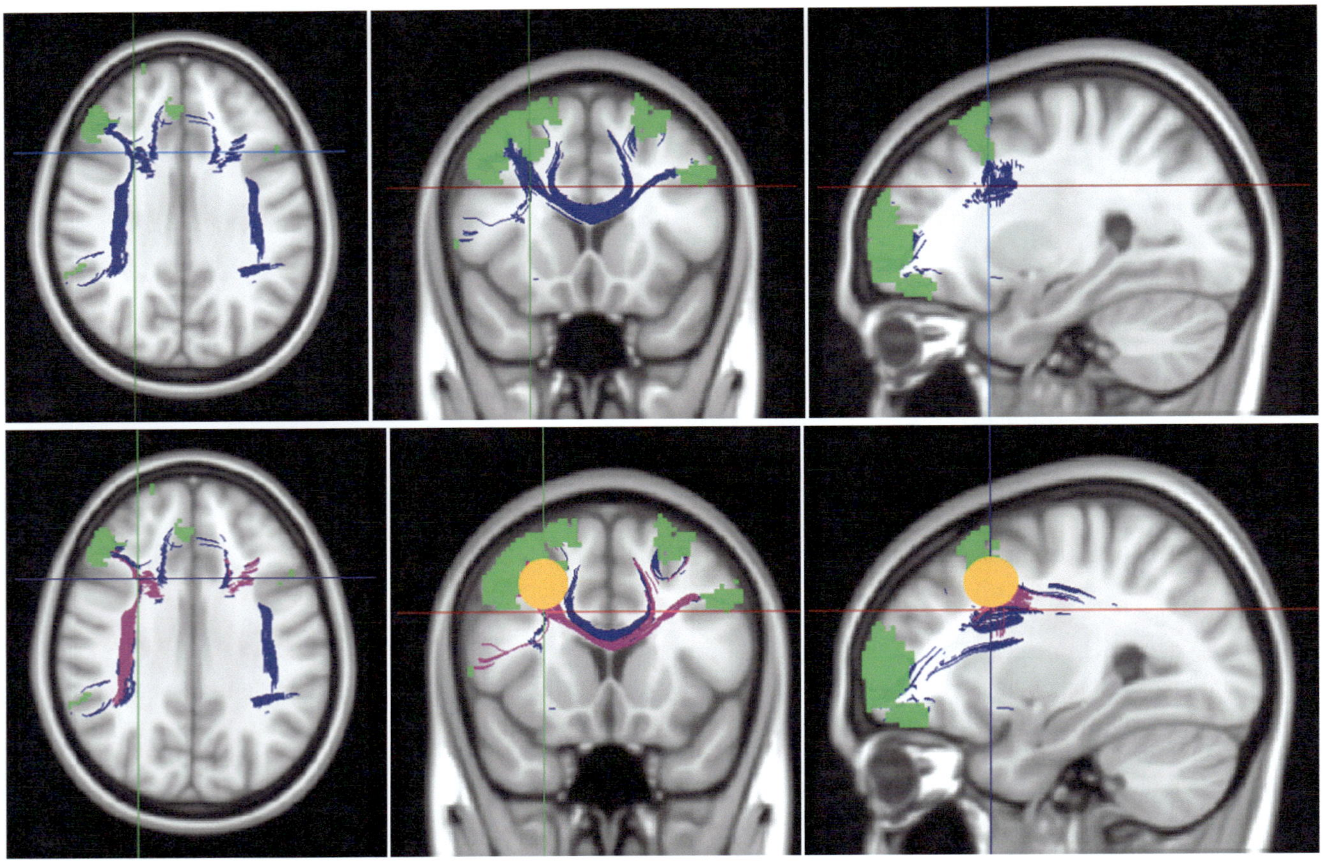

Fig. 23.3 Reducing the dimensionality. Integrity of the "green" network is supposed to be implicated in a given cognitive task. The blue streamlines represent the connectome map of this network, i.e. all the streamlines (either from the patient or from an atlas) linking any of two areas of the network. The magenta streamlines represent the part of the blue streamlines passing through the orange lesion, hence disconnected by the lesion. The ratio between the magenta and blue streamlines provides a predictor reflecting the amount of disconnection induced by the lesion among the green network. Repeating this approach to a restricted set of networks of interest allows to reduce the dimension to the number of selected networks. The method is very generic, in the sense that the networks of cortical areas can be patient-specific (and determined by task-based fMRI or resting-state fMRI) or atlas-based (see for example, the Neurosynth database [40] or the parcellation of Yeo et al. [41])

predictors (see Fig. 23.3 for a detailed explanation). Hence, what was learned from the analysis of these two cases was not some putative area supporting cognitive flexibility, but rather a new way to quantify network-level impact of a lesion for symptom prediction.

A New Paradigm for Combining Single-Case Analysis with the Predictive Power of Machine Learning

Single-case analysis gives the rare opportunity to formulate new hypotheses regarding brain function and the way it is impacted by a lesion. This understanding is naturally integrated in the model-based approach, that can overcome the curse of dimensionality, by downsizing the multidimensional voxels space to a much more restricted set of predictors, on which ML algorithms can be applied efficiently. If the predictive validity is demonstrated, this would constitute a successful generalization from few cases. Nonetheless, it is true that such validation studies still require a relatively large number of cases (typically from 10^2 to 10^3). This highlights the need to find a standardized framework for reporting extensively explored single cases. Building usable databases of image data hinges on the ability to standardize the organization of such data. Fortunately, this bioinformatics endeavour has been taken up by some contributors in the brain imaging community, leading to the BIDS dataset format [51], an extension of which is necessary to handle lesion analysis specifically. This key contribution opens the way towards large data aggregation approaches, probably facilitating in a near future the validation of the paradigm proposed in Fig. 23.4.

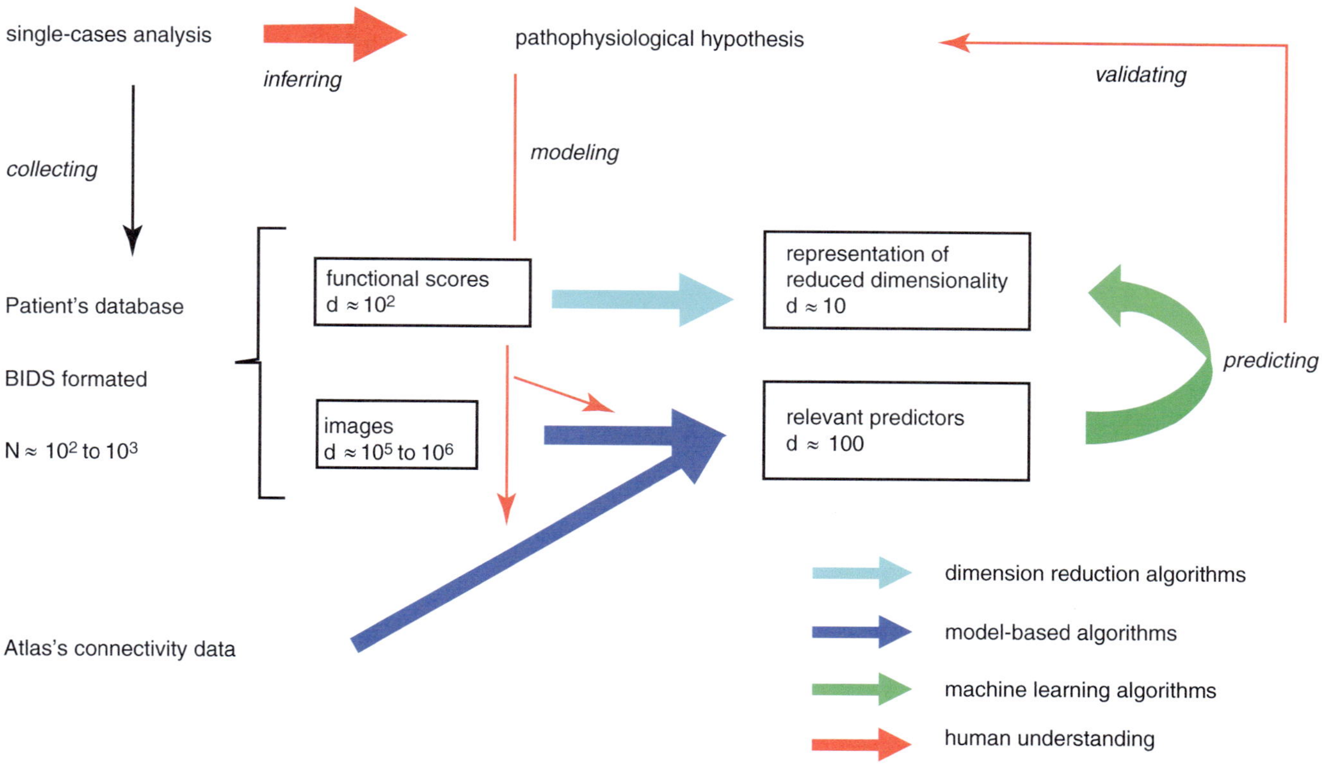

Fig. 23.4 A new paradigm for lesion-symptoms predictions. A new pathophysiological hypothesis about the lesional impact on brain functioning is inferred from a few cases. This hypothesis guides the elaboration of model-based algorithms, allowing to reduce the dimensionality of voxels space to a restricted set of relevant predictors. Functional scores undergo a fully data-based first run of processing, in order to derive a better representation (less noisy, with enhanced separability of cognitive subcomponents). The machine learning algorithms are trained on the patients' database (typical 10^2–10^3 cases). Should the prediction be accurate, this would in turn validate the initial hypothesis

23.5 Conclusion

Data scientists and clinicians need each other: clinicians can be very good at inferring a model allowing data scientists to reduce the high-dimensional anatomical space to a relevant restricted set of predictors, hence providing the adequate level of abstraction for generalization and in turn, data scientists can provide clinicians with optimized predictions powered by ML. We are confident that such collaborative efforts will contribute in a near future to significant advances in symptoms predictions from brain lesion imaging.

Competing Interests The author declares no competing interests.

References

1. Miller KL, Alfaro-Almagro F, Bangerter NK, Thomas DL, Yacoub E, Xu J, Bartsch AJ, Jbabdi S, Sotiropoulos SN, Andersson JLR, Griffanti L, Douaud G, Okell TW, Weale P, Dragonu I, Garratt S, Hudson S, Collins R, Jenkinson M, Matthews PM, Smith SM. Multimodal population brain imaging in the UK Biobank prospective epidemiological study. Nat Neurosci. 2016;19:1523–36. https://doi.org/10.1038/nn.4393.
2. Desmurget M, Bonnetblanc F, Duffau H. Contrasting acute and slow-growing lesions: a new door to brain plasticity. Brain. 2007;130:898–914. https://doi.org/10.1093/brain/awl300.
3. Keidel JL, Welbourne SR, Lambon Ralph MA. Solving the paradox of the equipotential and modular brain: a neurocomputational model of stroke vs slow-growing glioma. Neuropsychologia. 2010;48:1716–24. https://doi.org/10.1016/j.neuropsychologia.2010.02.019.
4. Price CJ, Hope TM, Seghier ML. Ten problems and solutions when predicting individual outcome from lesion site after stroke. NeuroImage. 2017;145:200–8. https://doi.org/10.1016/j.neuroimage.2016.08.006.
5. Duffau H. A two-level model of interindividual anatomo-functional variability of the brain and its implications for neurosurgery. Cortex. 2017;86:303–13. https://doi.org/10.1016/j.cortex.2015.12.009.
6. Catani M, Ffytche DH. The rises and falls of disconnection syndromes. Brain. 2005;128:2224–39. https://doi.org/10.1093/brain/awh622.
7. Shadmehr R, Krakauer JW. A computational neuroanatomy for motor control. Exp Brain Res. 2008;185:359–81. https://doi.org/10.1007/s00221-008-1280-5.
8. Price CJ, Seghier ML, Leff AP. Predicting language outcome and recovery after stroke: the PLORAS system. Nat Rev Neurol. 2010;6:202–10. https://doi.org/10.1038/nrneurol.2010.15.
9. Indefrey P, Levelt WJM. The spatial and temporal signatures of word production components. Cognition. 2004;92:101–44. https://doi.org/10.1016/j.cognition.2002.06.001.
10. Halai AD, Woollams AM, Lambon Ralph MA. Triangulation of language-cognitive impairments, naming errors and their neural

bases post-stroke. Neuroimage Clin. 2018;17:465–73. https://doi.org/10.1016/j.nicl.2017.10.037.

11. Fridriksson J, den Ouden D-B, Hillis AE, Hickok G, Rorden C, Basilakos A, Yourganov G, Bonilha L. Anatomy of aphasia revisited. Brain. 2018;141:848–62. https://doi.org/10.1093/brain/awx363.
12. Henson R. Forward inference using functional neuroimaging: dissociations versus associations. Trends Cogn Sci (Regul Ed). 2006;10:64–9. https://doi.org/10.1016/j.tics.2005.12.005.
13. Rofes A, Mandonnet E, de Aguiar V, Rapp B, Tsapkini K, Miceli G. Language processing from the perspective of electrical stimulation mapping. Cogn Neuropsychol. 2018;36:117–39. https://doi.org/10.1080/02643294.2018.1485636.
14. Godefroy O, Duhamel A, Leclerc X, Saint Michel T, Hénon H, Leys D. Brain-behaviour relationships. Some models and related statistical procedures for the study of brain-damaged patients. Brain. 1998;121(Pt 8):1545–56.
15. Brett M, Leff AP, Rorden C, Ashburner J. Spatial normalization of brain images with focal lesions using cost function masking. NeuroImage. 2001;14:486–500. https://doi.org/10.1006/nimg.2001.0845.
16. Rorden C, Karnath H-O. Using human brain lesions to infer function: a relic from a past era in the fMRI age? Nat Rev Neurosci. 2004;5:813–9. https://doi.org/10.1038/nrn1521.
17. Mah Y-H, Husain M, Rees G, Nachev P. Human brain lesion-deficit inference remapped. Brain. 2014;137:2522–31. https://doi.org/10.1093/brain/awu164.
18. Xu T, Jha A, Nachev P. The dimensionalities of lesion-deficit mapping. Neuropsychologia. 2018;115:134–41. https://doi.org/10.1016/j.neuropsychologia.2017.09.007.
19. Karnath H-O, Sperber C, Rorden C. Mapping human brain lesions and their functional consequences. NeuroImage. 2018;165:180–9. https://doi.org/10.1016/j.neuroimage.2017.10.028.
20. Zhang Y, Kimberg DY, Coslett HB, Schwartz MF, Wang Z. Multivariate lesion-symptom mapping using support vector regression. Hum Brain Mapp. 2014;35:5861–76. https://doi.org/10.1002/hbm.22590.
21. Weichwald S, Meyer T, Özdenizci O, Schölkopf B, Ball T, Grosse-Wentrup M. Causal interpretation rules for encoding and decoding models in neuroimaging. NeuroImage. 2015;110:48–59. https://doi.org/10.1016/j.neuroimage.2015.01.036.
22. Varoquaux G, Schwartz Y, Poldrack RA, Gauthier B, Bzdok D, Poline J-B, Thirion B. Atlases of cognition with large-scale human brain mapping. PLoS Comput Biol. 2018;14:e1006565. https://doi.org/10.1371/journal.pcbi.1006565.
23. Seghier ML, Patel E, Prejawa S, Ramsden S, Selmer A, Lim L, Browne R, Rae J, Haigh Z, Ezekiel D, Hope TMH, Leff AP, Price CJ. The PLORAS database: a data repository for predicting language outcome and recovery after stroke. NeuroImage. 2016;124:1208–12. https://doi.org/10.1016/j.neuroimage.2015.03.083.
24. Weaver NA, Zhao L, Biesbroek JM, Kuijf HJ, Aben HP, Bae H-J, Caballero MÁA, Chappell FM, Chen CPLH, Dichgans M, Duering M, Georgakis MK, van der Giessen RS, Gyanwali B, Hamilton OKL, Hilal S, vom Hofe EM, de Kort PLM, Koudstaal PJ, Lam BYK, Lim J-S, Makin SDJ, Mok VCT, Shi L, Valdés Hernández MC, Venketasubramanian N, Wardlaw JM, Wollenweber FA, Wong A, Xin X, DeCarli C, Fletcher EA, Maillard P, Barnes J, Sudre CH, Schott JM, Ikram MA, Papma JM, Steketee RME, Vernooij MW, Bordet R, Lopes R, Huang C-W, Frayne R, McCreary CR, Smith EE, Backes W, Köhler S, van Oostenbrugge RJ, Staals J, Verhey F, Cheng CY, Kalaria RN, Werring D, Hsu JL, Huang K-L, van der Grond J, Jukema JW, van der Mast RC, Nijboer TCW, Yu K-H, Schmidt R, Pirpamer L, MacIntosh BJ, Robertson AD, de Leeuw F-E, Tuladhar AM, Chaturvedi N, Tillin T, Brodaty H, Sachdev P, Barkhof F, van der Flier WM, Kappelle LJ, Biessels GJ. The Meta VCI Map consortium for meta-analyses on strategic lesion locations for vascular cognitive impairment using lesion-symptom mapping: design and multicenter pilot study. Alzheimers Dement. 2019;11:310–26. https://doi.org/10.1016/j.dadm.2019.02.007.
25. Wiesen D, Sperber C, Yourganov G, Rorden C, Karnath H-O. Using machine learning-based lesion behavior mapping to identify anatomical networks of cognitive dysfunction: spatial neglect and attention. NeuroImage. 2019;201:116000. https://doi.org/10.1016/j.neuroimage.2019.07.013.
26. Thye M, Mirman D. Relative contributions of lesion location and lesion size to predictions of varied language deficits in post-stroke aphasia. Neuroimage Clin. 2018;20:1129–38. https://doi.org/10.1016/j.nicl.2018.10.017.
27. Sperber C. Rethinking causality and data complexity in brain lesion-behaviour inference and its implications for lesion-behaviour modelling. Cortex. 2020;126:49–62. https://doi.org/10.1016/j.cortex.2020.01.004.
28. Thirion B, Varoquaux G, Dohmatob E, Poline J-B. Which fMRI clustering gives good brain parcellations? Front Neurosci. 2014;8:167. https://doi.org/10.3389/fnins.2014.00167.
29. Yourganov G, Fridriksson J, Rorden C, Gleichgerrcht E, Bonilha L. Multivariate connectome-based symptom mapping in post-stroke patients: networks supporting language and speech. J Neurosci. 2016;36:6668–79. https://doi.org/10.1523/JNEUROSCI.4396-15.2016.
30. Pustina D, Avants B, Faseyitan OK, Medaglia JD, Coslett HB. Improved accuracy of lesion to symptom mapping with multivariate sparse canonical correlations. Neuropsychologia. 2018;115:154–66. https://doi.org/10.1016/j.neuropsychologia.2017.08.027.
31. Athey S, Imbens GW. Machine learning for estimating heterogeneous causal effects. Stanford University, Graduate School of Business. 2015. https://econpapers.repec.org/paper/eclstabus/3350.htm. Accessed 4 Sept 2019.
32. Wang D, Buckner RL, Fox MD, Holt DJ, Holmes AJ, Stoecklein S, Langs G, Pan R, Qian T, Li K, Baker JT, Stufflebeam SM, Wang K, Wang X, Hong B, Liu H. Parcellating cortical functional networks in individuals. Nat Neurosci. 2015;18:1853–60. https://doi.org/10.1038/nn.4164.
33. Mandonnet E, Mellerio C, Barberis M, Poisson I, Jansma JM, Rutten G-J. When right is on the left (and vice versa): a case series of glioma patients with reversed lateralization of cognitive functions. J Neurol Surg A Cent Eur Neurosurg. 2020; https://doi.org/10.1055/s-0040-1701625.
34. Giussani C, Roux F-E, Ojemann J, Sganzerla EP, Pirillo D, Papagno C. Is preoperative functional magnetic resonance imaging reliable for language areas mapping in brain tumor surgery? Review of language functional magnetic resonance imaging and direct cortical stimulation correlation studies. Neurosurgery. 2010;66:113–20. https://doi.org/10.1227/01.NEU.0000360392.15450.C9.
35. Kuchcinski G, Mellerio C, Pallud J, Dezamis E, Turc G, Rigaux-Viodé O, Malherbe C, Roca P, Leclerc X, Varlet P, Chrétien F, Devaux B, Meder J-F, Oppenheim C. Three-tesla functional MR language mapping: comparison with direct cortical stimulation in gliomas. Neurology. 2015;84:560–8. https://doi.org/10.1212/WNL.0000000000001226.
36. Mandonnet E, Duffau H. Mapping the brain for primary brain tumor surgery. In: Moliterno Gunel J, Piepmeier JM, Baehring JM, editors. Malignant brain tumors : state-of-the-art treatment. Cham: Springer; 2017. p. 63–79. https://doi.org/10.1007/978-3-319-49864-5_5. Accessed 13 July 2019.
37. Hope TMH, Leff AP, Price CJ. Predicting language outcomes after stroke: is structural disconnection a useful predictor? Neuroimage Clin. 2018;19:22–9. https://doi.org/10.1016/j.nicl.2018.03.037.
38. Fox MD. Mapping symptoms to brain networks with the human connectome. N Engl J Med. 2018;379:2237–45. https://doi.org/10.1056/NEJMra1706158.

39. Boes AD, Prasad S, Liu H, Liu Q, Pascual-Leone A, Caviness VS, Fox MD. Network localization of neurological symptoms from focal brain lesions. Brain. 2015;138:3061–75. https://doi.org/10.1093/brain/awv228.
40. Yarkoni T, Poldrack RA, Nichols TE, Van Essen DC, Wager TD. Large-scale automated synthesis of human functional neuroimaging data. Nat Methods. 2011;8:665–70. https://doi.org/10.1038/nmeth.1635.
41. Yeo BTT, Krienen FM, Sepulcre J, Sabuncu MR, Lashkari D, Hollinshead M, Roffman JL, Smoller JW, Zöllei L, Polimeni JR, Fischl B, Liu H, Buckner RL. The organization of the human cerebral cortex estimated by intrinsic functional connectivity. J Neurophysiol. 2011;106:1125–65. https://doi.org/10.1152/jn.00338.2011.
42. Aerts H, Schirner M, Jeurissen B, Van Roost D, Achten E, Ritter P, Marinazzo D. Modeling brain dynamics in brain tumor patients using the virtual brain. eNeuro. 2018;5:ENEURO.0083-18.2018. https://doi.org/10.1523/ENEURO.0083-18.2018.
43. Vaidya CJ, Gordon EM. Phenotypic variability in resting-state functional connectivity: current status. Brain Connect. 2013;3:99–120. https://doi.org/10.1089/brain.2012.0110.
44. Rahim M, Thirion B, Bzdok D, Buvat I, Varoquaux G. Joint prediction of multiple scores captures better individual traits from brain images. NeuroImage. 2017;158:145–54. https://doi.org/10.1016/j.neuroimage.2017.06.072.
45. When once is enough. Nat Neurosci. 2004;7:93. https://doi.org/10.1038/nn0204-93
46. Rapp B. Case series in cognitive neuropsychology: promise, perils and proper perspective. Cogn Neuropsychol. 2011;28:435–44. https://doi.org/10.1080/02643294.2012.697453.
47. Gordon EM, Laumann TO, Gilmore AW, Newbold DJ, Greene DJ, Berg JJ, Ortega M, Hoyt-Drazen C, Gratton C, Sun H, Hampton JM, Coalson RS, Nguyen AL, McDermott KB, Shimony JS, Snyder AZ, Schlaggar BL, Petersen SE, Nelson SM, Dosenbach NUF. Precision functional mapping of individual human brains. Neuron. 2017;95:791–807.e7. https://doi.org/10.1016/j.neuron.2017.07.011.
48. Pinho AL, Amadon A, Ruest T, Fabre M, Dohmatob E, Denghien I, Ginisty C, Becuwe-Desmidt S, Roger S, Laurier L, Joly-Testault V, Médiouni-Cloarec G, Doublé C, Martins B, Pinel P, Eger E, Varoquaux G, Pallier C, Dehaene S, Hertz-Pannier L, Thirion B. Individual brain charting, a high-resolution fMRI dataset for cognitive mapping. Sci Data. 2018;5:180105. https://doi.org/10.1038/sdata.2018.105.
49. Mandonnet E, Cerliani L, Siuda-Krzywicka K, Poisson I, Zhi N, Volle E, de Schotten MT. A network-level approach of cognitive flexibility impairment after surgery of a right temporo-parietal glioma. Neurochirurgie. 2017;63:308–13. https://doi.org/10.1016/j.neuchi.2017.03.003.
50. Mandonnet E, Vincent M, Valero-Cabré A, Facque V, Dali M, Barberis M, Bonnetblanc F, Rheault F, Volle E, Margulies D. Causal role of the control network B in set-shifting during trail making test part B: a multimodal analysis of a glioma surgery case. Cortex. 2020;132:238–49.
51. Gorgolewski KJ, Auer T, Calhoun VD, Craddock RC, Das S, Duff EP, Flandin G, Ghosh SS, Glatard T, Halchenko YO, Handwerker DA, Hanke M, Keator D, Li X, Michael Z, Maumet C, Nichols BN, Nichols TE, Pellman J, Poline J-B, Rokem A, Schaefer G, Sochat V, Triplett W, Turner JA, Varoquaux G, Poldrack RA. The brain imaging data structure, a format for organizing and describing outputs of neuroimaging experiments. Sci Data. 2016;3:160044. https://doi.org/10.1038/sdata.2016.44.

Part III

Natural Language Processing and Time Series Analysis

24 Natural Language Processing: Practical Applications in Medicine and Investigation of Contextual Autocomplete

Leah Voytovich and Clayton Greenberg

24.1 Introduction

Consider the following thought experiment, known as the Chinese Room Argument [1]: a man who does not speak any Chinese is alone in a room with a book containing questions and their answers written in Chinese characters. A person outside of the room slips the man a note containing a question in Chinese. The man then looks up this question in the book and generates the correct answer, which he then outputs back to the person outside (Fig. 24.1).

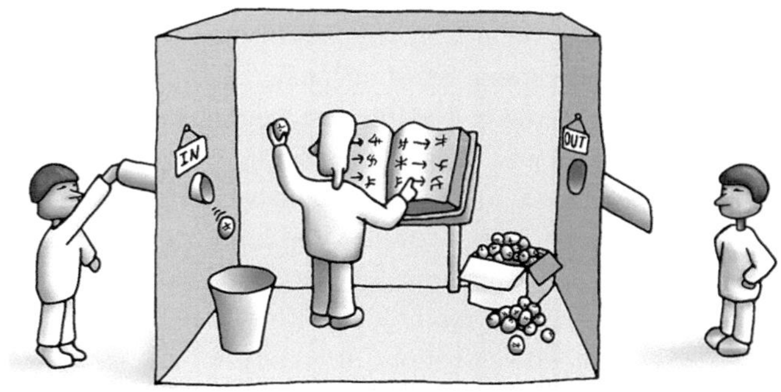

Fig. 24.1 An illustration of the Chinese Room Argument

The question remains, does the man inside the room understand Chinese? To those of us who see the complete picture, we know that the answer is no, but as his output responses make perfect sense to the input questions, he successfully fools those outside the room that he is a fluent Chinese speaker. This example demonstrates the twin goals of natural language processing (NLP) and natural language generation (NLG). An NLP system simulates understanding: natural language in, meaning out. An NLG system moves in the opposite direction: meaning in, natural language out. A sequence-to-sequence framework can be thought of as an NLP and NLG system working together, which gives digital assistants the "ability" to, among other applications, answer spoken questions, retrieve relevant information, and translate novel human utterances.

But just as the man in the room has impoverished knowledge about the questions that he is answering, so too does a computer "fake" understanding. The ideal scenario in applying NLP and NLG is that the system is able to capture the information in the input well enough that the output is correct, relevant, fluent, timely, etc. Since medical professionals are uniquely positioned to evaluate the usefulness and quality of information in medical natural language data, their guidance is essential in developing NLP/NLG tools for medicine.

Autocomplete, in which a small number of suggested completions / corrections for a partially-inputted natural language utterance appear, is now ubiquitous. While the time-saving effect is clear when the suggestions are good, criticism of autocomplete, especially if its suggestions override the user by default, is also ubiquitous. As a running example, let's discuss some basic approaches to autocomplete and their implications for medical applications. The simplest autocomplete system is not much more than a list of words. For some input string, this system would just return all of the words that begin with that string.

Clearly, such a solution is insufficient. An empty input would return the entire list of words. A misspelled input might return no words. Something in between could still return too many suggestions to be useful. So to improve the system, we could reformulate the lookup task into a prediction task. This way, the system not only collects and returns suggestions, but it also computes the probabilities of these suggestions. It should come as little surprise that given perfect data, the most frequently observed suggestion is the most probable suggestion. So, with the recent availability of huge datasets of text and powerful computers to process them, we can make great predictions. In fact, speech recogni-

L. Voytovich (✉) · C. Greenberg
Department of Computer and Information Science, School of Engineering and Applied Science, University of Pennsylvania, Philadelphia, PA, USA
e-mail: leahvoy@seas.upenn.edu

V. E. Staartjes et al. (eds.), *Machine Learning in Clinical Neuroscience*, Acta Neurochirurgica Supplement 134,
https://doi.org/10.1007/978-3-030-85292-4_24

tion has reached its current level of deployment because the predictive models consider increasingly complex contexts: not just the current word but several preceding ones, even high-dimensional representations of the entire document. The cutting edge is now concerned with *which* notion of context provides the most appropriate suggestions. The remainder of this chapter discusses the answer to this question within the particular domain of electronic health records (EHRs).

24.2 Contextual Autocomplete Literature Review

Clinicians spend a significant amount of their time charting information in electronic health records, leading to a notable documentation burden. The taxing process of inefficient EHRs is one of the leading causes of physician stress and burnout [2, 3]. One solution that scientists have begun investigating is contextual autocomplete, which uses natural language processing techniques to provide more efficient charting that will save the clinician substantial time every day [4, 5]. Another motivation for contextual autocomplete in EHRs is the ability to curate prospective clinical data in a manner that does not restrict the clinician to follow a rigid template nor interrupt the clinical workflow [4, 5].

The first study that we will explore is Greenbaum et al. [5], which built an autocomplete model to predict the chief complaint (presenting problem) in the Emergency Department. This model used a multiclass Support Vector Machine (SVM) trained on triage information and represented free text in a Bag-of-Words (BoW) model.[1] The authors motivated their work as a way to reduce documentation burden and streamline data collection, aiding interoperability. The study highlighted the effectiveness of using a contextual autocomplete model over a standard autocomplete model: providing predictive suggestions based on the "context" and a predicted probability rather than simply spelling. They operationalized contextual information as all information gathered when a patient is triaged in the emergency department: initial patient vital signs as well as the triage nurse's description of the patient's state at arrival. In their experiments, "the mean number of keystrokes required to document a presenting problem" was reduced from 11.6 to 0.6, resulting in a 95% improvement. Their system also provided a solution to collecting structured data prospectively, as opposed to using NLP to extract it retrospectively, which they argue is more prone to inaccuracies.

The second study that we will explore is Gopinath et al. [4], which built on the Greenbaum et al. [5] study to provide contextual autocomplete functionality for an entire unstructured clinical note, as opposed to solely the chief complaint. This model extracted clinical concepts from medical notes with the help of named entity recognition (NER). Their application of NER filtered words to only words in the Unified Medical Language System (UMLS), and these filtered words were inserted into a Trie[2] data structure. Then, terms which occurred within a negative context were identified and concepts which appeared fewer than 50 times were pruned out. Concepts were then grouped into two categories: conditions the patient has a history of and symptoms. Finally, they used a TF-IDF[3] encoder to capture a normalized BoW representation of the text.

The main motivations in [4] were to increase documentation efficiency, increase documentation readability by alleviating the need to rely on complicated medical jargon and acronyms for efficiency, and provide some structure to notes that were otherwise free text for use in future applications. The contextual information used in this study included both the patient triage information as well as prior medical notes or history about the patient. Their system grouped clinical terms into "relevancy buckets," which were then used for categorical predictions. They used four concept-specific ranking models: conditions, symptoms, labs, and medications. The machine learning model itself was a shallow, dual-branch neural network architecture that was first trained on the model relevancy buckets and then trained on individual concepts to mention in the note. They combined a context consisting of a TF-IDF representation of triage text and a feature vector indicating the binary presence of each model relevancy bucket in prior EHR notes. The result of this system was a 67% reduction in keystroke burden in a live environment. It is important to note that the 95% improvement in keystroke reduction discussed in [5] is with regards to solely chief complaints, whereas the 67% keystroke reduction in [4] is with respect to the entire free text clinical note.

The studies on contextual autocompletion in EHRs discussed above show promising results with regards to a solution for alleviating documentation burden as well as curating structured data without compromising the clinical workflow. Several technical concepts were mentioned, including inserting and looking up terms in a trie data structure, TF-IDF encodings, BoW models, and multiclass SVMs. The following tutorial will dive deeper into these technical concepts to illustrate how an EHR autocomplete system works and how pieces of this pipeline might be used for related medical applications.

[1] For more information on SVMs and BoW, please refer to the tutorial in the next section.

[2] For more information on Tries, please refer to the tutorial in the next section.

[3] For more information on TF-IDF, please refer to the tutorial in the next section.

24.3 Contextual Autocomplete: Technical Toolkit

In this tutorial, we will review some of the critical NLP techniques mentioned above that are used for contextual autocompletion. Please feel free to follow along and run the code at the following Google Colab link: https://colab.research.google.com/drive/1Fg9CJyoNDb_3yqYBoJhV8TcRomgOW_O2?usp=sharing.

Trie Data Structure

A core data structure used in both studies is the Trie, which is particularly useful in looking up words given a specific prefix. An extremely simple autocomplete model that is solely based on the letters a user types can be implemented using only a Trie data structure. Following is the Python code, heavily inspired by [6], needed to implement a simple Trie-based algorithm that provides predictive suggestions given a prefix (Figs. 24.2 and 24.3):

BoW Model

Text vectorization is the process of converting text into lists (vectors) of numbers. The perhaps simplest, yet still relevant and robust, method for constructing vectors is called the "bag of words." A bag-of-words vector just gives the number of times each unique word occurs. The order of the words in the vector is arbitrary and there are no repeats, so all ordering information from the original text is lost in this model. Therefore, the sole critical implementation choice is which words to include in the vector. Extremely common words

Fig. 24.2 Python implementation of the TrieNode and Trie classes

```
class TrieNode:
 #Constructor
 def __init__(self):
   # Dictionary to contain child nodes
   self.children = {}
   # Boolean indicating whether current node is leaf
   self.isLeaf = False

class Trie():
 #Constructor
 def __init__(self):
   self.root = TrieNode()
   self.word_list = []

 #Form Trie based on list of terms
 def formTrie(self, terms):
   for term in terms:
     self.insert(term)

 # Function to insert word into Trie
 def insert(self, word):

   curr = self.root

   for letter in word:
     # Move to the corresponding child node.
     # If it does not already exist, create it.
     curr = curr.children.setdefault(letter, TrieNode())

   curr.isLeaf = True

 # Search
 def search(self, key):

   root = self.root
   exists = True

   for ltr in key:
     if not (ltr in root.children):
       exists = False
       break
```

Fig. 24.3 Continuation of the Trie class implementation

```
      root = root.children[ltr]

    return (root and root.isLeaf and exists)

  # Get suggestions for given node
  def sugRec(self, node, word):

    if node.isLeaf:
      self.word_list.append(word)

    for (letter, n) in node.children.items():
      self.sugRec(n, word + letter)

    return

  # Print suggestions for given prefix
  def printSug(self, pref):

    self.word_list = []

    n = self.root
    not_exists = False
    temp = ""

    for letter in pref:
      if not letter in n.children:
        not_exists = True
        break

      temp += letter
      n = n.children[letter]

      if not_exists:
        return 0
      elif n.isLeaf and not n.children:
        return -1

      self.sugRec(n, temp)

      for s in self.word_list:
        print(s)

      return 1
```

known as stop words, such as "the," have little discriminative power. They occur everywhere, and more importantly, occurring more or less in some group of interest is quite likely to be an accident rather than a true distinction (Fig. 24.4).

TF-IDF Encoding

While not including stop words in the model's so-called vocabulary (the words that are counted and represented in the BoW vector) is one potential solution, another approach is to scale the numbers in the vector by their predicted usefulness. One way to do that is to use TF-IDF scores rather than simple counts. TF-IDF stands for "Term Frequency" and "Inverse Document Frequency." Term frequency is the number of occurrences of a particular word in a document divided by the total number of words in that document. The equation for term frequency is:

$$\mathrm{TF}_{i,j} = \frac{n_{i,j}}{\sum_k n_{i,j}}$$

Inverse document frequency is the log of the total number of documents divided by the number of documents that contain a particular word. The equation for inverse document frequency is:

$$\text{IDF}(w) = \log\left(\frac{N}{\text{DF}_t}\right)$$

The TF-IDF is simply the product of the term frequency and the inverse document frequency. This process is a useful measure of the relevance of a given word since TF favors words that occur more *frequently* but IDF disfavors words that occur more *widely*. For example, if "the" occurs in every document, then its IDF is zero, which makes its TF-IDF zero as well. The following is a basic TF-IDF implementation that builds on the BoW implementation, above. This code is also heavily inspired by [7] (Figs. 24.5 and 24.6).

Support Vector Machine (SVM)

Support vector machines are a form of supervised machine learning that can be used for both classification and regression tasks. The most simple SVM model is a linear classifier. The following is an implementation of a linear classifier SVM, reproduced from [8] (Fig. 24.7).

Fig. 24.4 Python implementation of the BoW model

```
import pandas as pd

#Create two small documents for demonstration purposes.
documentA = "Pt. complains of traumatic injury on left upper extremity."
documentB = "Pt. complains of nausea but no vomiting."

#Tokenize each word in each document
bagOfWordsA = documentA.split(" ")
bagOfWordsB = documentB.split(" ")

#Create a set of unique words across all documents in the corpus
uniqueWords = set(bagOfWordsA).union(set(bagOfWordsB))

#Create dictionaries that store number of occurrences of each word in each
document
numOfWordsA = dict.fromkeys(uniqueWords, 0)

for word in bagOfWordsA:
 numOfWordsA[word] += 1

numOfWordsB = dict.fromkeys(uniqueWords, 0)

for word in bagOfWordsB:
 numOfWordsB[word] += 1
```

Fig. 24.5 Python implementation of the TF function

```
import math

def computeTF(wordDict, bagOfWords):
   tfDict = {}
   bagOfWordsCount = len(bagOfWords)
   for word, count in wordDict.items():
       tfDict[word] = count / float(bagOfWordsCount)
   return tfDict
```

Fig. 24.6 Python implementation of the IDF and TF-IDF functions

```
tfA = computeTF(numOfWordsA, bagOfWordsA)
tfB = computeTF(numOfWordsB, bagOfWordsB)

def computeIDF(documents):
    N = len(documents)

    idfDict = dict.fromkeys(documents[0].keys(), 0)
    for document in documents:
        for word, val in document.items():
            if val > 0:
                idfDict[word] += 1

    for word, val in idfDict.items():
        idfDict[word] = math.log(N / float(val))
    return idfDict

idfs = computeIDF([numOfWordsA, numOfWordsB])

def computeTFIDF(tfBagOfWords, idfs):
    tfidf = {}
    for word, val in tfBagOfWords.items():
        tfidf[word] = val * idfs[word]
    return tfidf

tfidfA = computeTFIDF(tfA, idfs)
tfidfB = computeTFIDF(tfB, idfs)

df = pd.DataFrame([tfidfA, tfidfB])
```

Confusion Matrix for Visualizing Model Accuracy

Once you have an NLP model built and trained, the next step is to evaluate how well that model is performing. While the range of evaluation methods in NLP is vast and the best method depends on the specific task, a simple yet powerful tool for visualizing model accuracy, particularly for supervised learning classifiers such as the linear SVM above, is called the Confusion Matrix. Each row corresponds to an instance of the predicted class, while each column corresponds to an instance of the actual class. It is easy to visualize the accuracy of the model according to this matrix since all values across the diagonal of the matrix represent correct predictions, while values outside the main diagonal represent prediction errors. This can be implemented directly using the sklearn package as follows (Fig. 24.8).

Fig. 24.7 Python implementation of a linear SVM

```
import matplotlib.pyplot as plt
import numpy as np
from sklearn import svm

# linear data
X = np.array([1, 5, 1.5, 8, 1, 9, 7, 8.7, 2.3, 5.5, 7.7, 6.1])
y = np.array([2, 8, 1.8, 8, 0.6, 11, 10, 9.4, 4, 3, 8.8, 7.5])

# show unclassified data
plt.scatter(X, y)
plt.show()

# shaping data for training the model
training_X = np.vstack((X, y)).T
training_y = [0, 1, 0, 1, 0, 1, 1, 1, 0, 0, 1, 1]

# define the model
clf = svm.SVC(kernel='linear', C=1.0)

# train the model
clf.fit(training_X, training_y)

# get the weight values for the linear equation from the trained SVM model
w = clf.coef_[0]

# get the y-offset for the linear equation
a = -w[0] / w[1]

# make the x-axis space for the data points
XX = np.linspace(0, 13)

# get the y-values to plot the decision boundary
yy = a * XX - clf.intercept_[0] / w[1]

# plot the decision boundary
plt.plot(XX, yy, 'k-')

# show the plot visually
plt.scatter(training_X[:, 0], training_X[:, 1], c=training_y)
plt.legend()
plt.show()
```

Fig. 24.8 Python implementation of a confusion matrix

```
from sklearn.metrics import confusion_matrix

y_true = [0, 1, 0, 1, 0, 1, 1, 1, 0, 0, 1, 1]
y_pred = [0, 1, 0, 1, 0, 1, 1, 1, 0, 0, 1, 1]

confusion_matrix(y_true, y_pred)
```

24.4 Conclusion

NLP is poised to help alleviate clinical documentation burden and the lack of structured EHR data. Contextual autocomplete in electronic medical records shows promising results with respect to improving documentation efficiency and providing a method to curate structured data without interrupting the clinical workflow. This chapter discusses some basic technical methods in NLP that serve as the foundation for building a model for predictive suggestions.

Acknowledgments None.

Disclosures All authors have reviewed and approved this manuscript and have no conflicts of interest in relation to the publication of this study.

References

1. Searle J. Minds, brains, and programs. Behav Brain Sci. 1980;3:417–57. https://doi.org/10.1017/s0140525x00005756.
2. Carayon P, Wetterneck T, Alyousef B, Brown R, Cartmill R, McGuire K, Hoonakker PLT, Slagle J, Roy K, Walker J, Weinger M, Xie A, Wood K. Impact of electronic health record technology on the work and workflow of physicians in the intensive care unit. Int J Med Inform. 2015;84:578–94. https://doi.org/10.1016/j.ijmedinf.2015.04.002.
3. Gardner RL, Cooper E, Haskell J, Harris DA, Poplau S, Kroth PJ, Linzer M. Physician stress and burnout: the impact of health information technology. J Am Med Inform Assoc. 2019;26:106–14.
4. Gopinath D, Agrawal M, Murray L, Horng S, Karger D, Sontag D. Fast, structured clinical documentation via contextual autocomplete. arXiv: 2007.15153; 2020. https://arxiv.org/pdf/2007.15153.pdf.
5. Greenbaum NR, Jernite Y, Halpern Y, Calder S, Nathanson L, Sontag D, Horng S. Contextual autocomplete: a novel user Interface using machine learning to improve ontology usage and structured data capture for presenting problems in the emergency department. 2017. https://www.biorxiv.org/content/biorxiv/early/2017/04/12/127092.full.pdf.
6. Sarkar H. Auto-complete feature using Trie. 2020. https://www.geeksforgeeks.org/auto-complete-feature-using-trie/.
7. Maklin C. TF IDF: TFIDF Python Example. 2019. https://towardsdatascience.com/natural-language-processing-feature-engineering-using-tf-idf-e8b9d00e7e76.
8. McGregor M. SVM machine learning tutorial – what is the support vector machine algorithm, explained with code examples. 2020. https://www.freecodecamp.org/news/svm-machine-learning-tutorial-what-is-the-support-vector-machine-algorithm-explained-with-code-examples/.

Foundations of Time Series Analysis

25

Jonas Ort, Karlijn Hakvoort, Georg Neuloh, Hans Clusmann, Daniel Delev, and Julius M. Kernbach

25.1 Introduction

Data in a temporal resolution consisting of a chronological sequence of observations are referred to as time series (TS). The analysis of temporal data is widespread across scientific disciplines, including finance, marketing, environmental sciences, and medicine. Historically, TS analyses were first applied to physical sciences problems, which account for the strong mathematical and engineering-based flavor permeating the vocabulary and methodological approaches to TS analysis. Based on the data's observed properties, over the last half-century, the primary objective of TS analysis has been the development of a mathematical model capturing these inherent properties to enable forecasting of future events. TS analysis highlighted important mathematical aspects, including trend, seasonality, and residue or noise [1, 2]. *Trend* describes a long-term decrease or increase in the observed data. The mathematical forms these temporal trends can adopt vary, including linear or higher-order patterns. Without an apparent trend, the values' level does not change significantly over time, but the observed data fluctuates around a fixed equilibrium. Thus, a window in the data at timepoint z_t will be on the same level as at timepoint z_{t+k} for any t or k. Temporal data behaving in this static fashion are called *stationary* [1]. A second essential property is *seasonality, which* describes repeating patterns that reoccur in temporal intervals, such as blood pressure (BP) or intracranial pressure (ICP) measurements. Seasonality can encode important morphological features that can be leveraged for forecasting problems. The remaining unsystematic fluctuations in TS are called *residue* or *noise*. Measurement inaccuracies, physiological confounders, or motion artifacts are frequent sources of noise.

Based on the data's assumptions (trends, seasonality, stationarity), a mathematical model can be formulated to capture the existing dynamic relations, understand the data-generating process, and potentially enable forecasting within the limit of the proposed assumptions. Many traditional stochastic methods, including exponential smoothing, moving averages, and autoregressive integrated moving averages (ARIMAS), were successfully applied to forecast future events. More recently, temporal prediction approaches based on machine learning (ML) algorithms gained popularity, due to their potential of leveraging highly nonlinear (complex) patterns and flexible adaption in nonparametric settings [3–6]. Empirically, ML-based methods demonstrated competitive levels of performance and frequently outperformed traditional models [5, 7–9]. In this article, we review classical methods for TS analysis, which, based on historical developments, are rarely considered as typical ML methods, as well as the extension of nonparametric and complex ML methods.

25.2 Foundational Methods

The potential applications of TS analysis are vast but generally adhere to analytical frameworks, with the goals of *forecasting* or *predicting* future events from historical data, recognizing patterns within our data, or sometimes both. However, forecasting—or in ML lingo prediction—and pattern recognition problems should be regarded as rather intertwining than divisional. *Forecasting* evolved in TS analysis long before the recent ML "hype" started [10]. Due to this historically distinct development of TS forecasting and ML prediction approaches, we find a lingual division between classical forecasting methods and ML methods. However,

J. Ort · K. Hakvoort · D. Delev · J. M. Kernbach (✉)
Department of Neurosurgery, Faculty of Medicine, RWTH Aachen University, Aachen, Germany

Neurosurgical Artificial Intelligence Laboratory Aachen (NAILA), RWTH Aachen University Hospital, Aachen, Germany
e-mail: jkernbach@ukaachen.de

G. Neuloh · H. Clusmann
Department of Neurosurgery, Faculty of Medicine, RWTH Aachen University, Aachen, Germany

V. E. Staartjes et al. (eds.), *Machine Learning in Clinical Neuroscience*, Acta Neurochirurgica Supplement 134,
https://doi.org/10.1007/978-3-030-85292-4_25

the classical methods are frequently applied in ML as well. In the following, we review both traditional parametric methods as well as advanced nonparametric approaches.

Parametric Methods

Parametric methods require a priori information about data distribution [3]. Assumptions, including gaussianity or normality, are well recognized in classical statistics. Similar assumptions are pertinent to forecasting methods and include pivotal assumptions about stationarity, trend and seasonality [11]. Additionally, in parametric modeling, we make assumptions regarding the function best describing our data [3].

Autocorrelation is characterized by serial correlation or similarity between two TS with a specified temporal *lag*. Referring to our definition of stationary TS in the introduction, in comparing timepoint z_t and z_{t+k}, the *lag* is expressed by k [1]. Several classical parametric methods thrive on leveraging autocorrelation, highlighting the importance of the prior assumed data distribution [10]. In an ICP TS where the lag equals the time between the ECG's *p*-waves, the linear relationship between two observed parts of the TS will show a strong autocorrelation.

The first set of parametric methods are built on using some form of smoothing. As a popular approach, *moving average* (MA) describes the use of a mean function of past observations to "predict" future values. MA is one of the most simplistic methods and has been applied for almost a century [10, 11]. The traditional MA uses a fixed number of observations to calculate the next value by weighting every observation equally. MA is still frequently used to calculate and visualize trends within the data. However, due to the smoothing effect, that is, averaging over seasonality and other intrinsic patterns of the data, MA performs poorly in predicting actual future values [2, 5, 11]. The extensions of MA include additional weightings to specific features, such as *exponential smoothing* (ES). *Simple exponential smoothing* (SES), also known as first-order exponential smoothing, adds more weight to more recent events [1, 5]. That way, the importance of past observations in predicting the next observation decreases. However, SES demonstrated a limited performance for predicting future observations that inherit trend or seasonality [11]. The limitation in predicting nonstationary data was initially addressed in the 1950s by Charles Holt, introducing a model using three equations and two corresponding smoothing parameters, which better replicated the data's underlying trends [5, 12]. Holt's exponential smoothing method (HESM) was further developed to adjust for seasonality [5, 11, 13] resulting in the Holt-Winter's seasonal exponential smoothing method (HWESM). This parametric approach applies an additional assumption to adjust for seasonality within the smoothing parameters and therefore considers trend, seasonality, and level. The correct selection of smoothing parameters is critical for a well-functioning model and delivering adequate predictions [11].

The second domain of classical forecasting methods are called *ARIMA* methods [11]. As the name suggests, ARIMA models consist of three components: *autoregression (AR)*, *integration (I)*, and *moving average (MA)*. For each component, we need to define the order of the model (p, d, q). The mathematical equations behind the components are well discussed in the literature and can help develop an intuitive understanding of the model order's meaning [11]. *Autoregression* uses autocorrelation (see above, i.e., the similarity between data at different time points) within the data over a chosen number of temporal lags [1, 11]. The order of autocorrelation AR(p) corresponds to the number of chosen lags. In ARIMA, MA can capture the variation based on autocorrelation and uses a regression model on past errors for forecasting. Additionally, we need to specify the order of the applied MA, MA(q). MA(q) can be imagined as the window-length of the MA. Theoretically, AR and MA form an ARMA(p,q) model and can already be used for TS prediction. However, ARMA models assume that the observed TS are stationary [2]. *Integration* (I) is the last component of the ARIMA model and is essential for its applicability to nonstationary TS. This can be achieved by *differencing*, i.e., not calculating the consequential observations of a TS but the differences between them. This procedure is repeated until a stationary dataset is reached. We call this first or second-order differencing, and it enables the application of ARIMA to nonstationary data. It is also possible to extend ARIMA models with seasonality to so-called SARIMA models [5, 11]. Selecting the appropriate model orders and parameters can be challenging in ARIMA-based models. Different approaches have been suggested to optimize the selection process [1, 5, 11, 14]. Thus, ARIMA methods not only resemble ML models in their learning ability but also their general workflow using hyperparameter tuning, training, and testing.

Nonparametric Methods

Nonparametric models do not need a priori information about the data distribution or the function used as a statistical model, respectively [3]. Nonparametric methods scale to complex multidimensional data and nonlinear properties. ML prediction strategies can broadly be categorized as *supervised, unsupervised, or semi-supervised* [3]. When labeled target data are available, supervised models are appropriate. Here, we optimize a model or a function that maps our input features onto the target data (dependent variable). The target's form is important for the model's underlying approach: for *continuous targets, regression models* can be applied (e.g., age, BP, ICP). When the target is *discrete*, the applied models will be based on *classification* (e.g., age-group, outcome-scales, 30-day mortality) [3]. *Unsupervised models* do not require labeled target variables. Applications include cluster analysis by defining groups within the input data that share distinctive properties. Unsupervised models can detect important patterns in the data and help identify relations beyond human comprehension.

Neural Networks (NN) are based on the architecture we attribute to neuronal organization in the brain [11, 15, 16]. For a simple one-directional, so-called *feed-forward* NN, the *input layer* receives the data from the initial features. Following the input layer, an arbitrary number of *hidden layers* follows. Each layer consists of at least one neuron and receives input from neurons of the previous layer. Accordingly, the layers' output is then passed to the next layer. Finally, the *output layer* returns the final output of the function. For the learning process of these constructs, the connections between the layers are essential. Between layers, a *weight* is added to the passed-on output. These weights are modified in the learning process resulting in a model that then maps an output to an input in the testing or validation phase [5, 11, 17]. In brief, every neuron in an artificial neuronal network (ANN) receives inputs and generates outputs. The final result from the output layer is a combination of all weighted inputs from previous layers. ANN can produce models mapping complex input and output relations. The above-described ANN are only moving in one direction, i.e., they are feed-forward. In *recurrent neural networks* (RNN) [18], layers can also feed input into previous layers. These layers are called context layers, and their output is a conditionality depending on prior processed input based on weights *gradients*. In RNNs, a memory effect is created by backpropagation and a so-called vector-state in the hidden layers [18, 19]. Hence, RNNs apply to data with temporal dependencies. However, training RNNs can be computationally intense and be affected by the *gradient problems;* that is, gradients can vanish or explode [5, 20]. A proposed solution for these problems is introducing gate functions as they are implemented in *long short-term memory* networks (LSTM) [21]. In LSTMs, *gates* influence a *cell state,* which resembles a memory function of previously received inputs. This ultimately results in the capability of remembering long-term relationships within the data. LSTM has shown extremely promising results in TS analysis and offer state-of-the-art solutions for distinct problems in deep learning [19, 22–24].

Support vector machines (SVM), albeit not strictly nonparametric, are frequently applied to classification problems. Geometrically, SVM find a plane to separate different classes of data best. In two dimensions, this plane would simply be a line. For the given data, SVM will optimize a separating line that reflects a maximal margin between data observations from different classes [3, 25]. When the dimensions are extended, the line evolves into a hyperplane [3, 25]. SVMs have been among the first ML algorithms applied to TS predictions [6] such as stock markets [26, 27], water-demand in urban distribution centers [28], or meteorological TS [29]. SVMs demonstrated acceptable performance applied to various TS data and frequently outperformed many parametric methods [9, 26].

K nearest neighbor (*k*NN) can be applied in regression and classification. *k*NN is a popular example of instance learning, where the entire dataset is stored, and the distances of new input are compared to already known labeled data points. The new input is then classified toward the k nearest neighbors, that is, the already labeled data points with the smallest distances to the new data point. The *k* determines how many near neighbors are considered in the classification process [3]. The application of *k*NN in TS analysis seems counterintuitive due to the sequential character of TS. However, the recently proposed variant called kNN Time Series Prediction with Invariances (kNN-TSPI) [4] shows promising results in TS forecasting. The kNN-TSPI aims to recognize similarities in TS by utilizing complexity measures, such as permutation entropy, for distance calculation. The applied algorithm performs well compared to established methods and, considering its novelty, remains a promising candidate for future nonparametric TS analytical tools [4, 5].

Clinical Applications

Continuous ICP monitoring plays a pivotal role in the management of neurosurgical ICU patients with traumatic brain injury (TBI) [30, 31], subarachnoid hemorrhage (SAH) [32, 33], and intracranial hemorrhage (ICH) [34, 35]. Early detection of increased ICP is critical to prevent secondary brain injury [36]; thus, predicting ICP events could result in early diagnosis and improved treatment of ICP crisis, thereby preventing secondary brain injury. ML is a suitable choice to predict such harmful events from mined ICP data, as several studies demonstrated the use of ML algorithms for accurate ICP predictions. Using an algorithm called Morphological Clustering and Analysis of Intracranial Pressure (MOCAIP) [37] on ICP waveform morphology, combined with a quadratic classifier, Hamilton and colleagues predicted ICP elevations 5 min before the event, with an accuracy of 0.77, sensitivity of 0.9, and specificity of 0.75 [38]. Modern monitoring systems provide clinicians with constant new information about potential pathophysiological developments and ensure fast notification in critical events. Nevertheless, most monitoring systems operate based on a simple threshold mechanism resulting in high rates of false alarms on ICUs

[39]. Comparing SVM and spectral regression kernel discriminant analysis (SRKDA) in both supervised and semi-supervised models, Scalzo and colleagues used trend and morphological features of 4791 labeled ICP alarms from 108 subjects to reduce the frequency of false alarms. The false alarm rate is reported to be mitigated by 16% using SVMs and 27% using SRKDA respectively, while maintaining a correct alarm recognition rate of 99% [40]. For both models, the semi-supervised version performed better than the supervised version. DL approaches have also been applied to ICP monitoring to detect elevated ICP events: Quachtran et al. used an auto-encoder combined with convolutional neuronal networks (CNN) [41] on ICP data derived from 60 patients. Their model was trained using >70,000 samples and threefold cross-validation, achieving an accuracy of 0.92 in detecting elevated ICP. However, ICP monitoring is rarely used exclusively, but is usually combined with other TS data, such as BP or heart rate (HR), in a multivariate approach to predict ICP. Bonds et al. report successful ICP prediction within a future 5-min timeframe using >5400 h of physiological data from 132 patients (consisting of HR, systolic BP, shock index, mean arterial pressure (MAP), pulse pressure, and ICP) and a model of nearest neighbor regression. Their model showed good consistency with the measured data with a bias of 0.02 (±1.96 SD = 4 mmHg) for the 5-min timeframe and −0.02 (±1.96 SD = 10 mmHg) for 2 h, respectively [42].

Estimating individual prognosis after TBI, ICH, or SAH is difficult, mostly static, and based on initial clinical scores such as Hunt and Hess for SAH [43]. Naturally, outcome prediction is highly complex and entails significant uncertainty for clinical decision making, due to the limited applicability of empirically derived scores for the individual patient. Reliable long-term outcome prediction could benefit the individual patient, clinical caretakers, and the health-care system. Empirically, ML models performed fairly in predicting clinical outcomes in various investigations. Raj and colleagues used two models based on logistic regression predicting 30-day mortality based on multimodal data of 472 patients. The first model used ICP, MAP, and cerebral perfusion pressure (CPP), and the second model added GCS, achieving an AUC of 0.81 and 0.84 respectively [44]. While outcome prediction based on clinical features is usually limited to a snapshot of the observed clinical condition, here, TS is used for the development of dynamic models. Dynamic modeling offers a powerful tool for clinical decision-making and can potentially be adapted for other applications as well.

The acquisition of synchronous extracellular brain potentials by electroencephalography (EEG) is a leading approach for the noninvasive investigation of functional connectivity [45, 46]. The introduction of ML into EEG analysis marked a paradigm shift toward a better diagnosis of epilepsy, localization of epileptic foci, as well as treatment monitoring in epilepsy patients [47–51]. Concurrently, the number of publications using ML in EEG is extensive [52, 53]. Most ML methods enable the user to cluster and automatically detect seizures in EEG data with high accuracy, and generally supervised models perform with higher accuracy than unsupervised models [52]. Zhang and colleagues found an average accuracy of 0.98 or higher using a local mean decomposition algorithm in five different classification models, including a backpropagation neural network, kNN, linear discriminant analysis, SVM, and an SVM with genetic algorithm optimization (GA-SVM). The GA-SVM ultimately outperformed the other models [54]. Feature extraction and dimensionality reduction of highly multidimensional data is a pivotal step for ML modeling. Comparing principal component analysis (PCA) with a modified so-called global modular PCA (GMPCA) for feature extraction and SVM for classification, Jaiswal and Banka report an accuracy of 1.0 (while an accuracy of 1.0 should always warrant careful methodological interpretation) for seizure detection [55]. Besides SVM, ANNs have been frequently used for automated seizure detection [56–58]. Tzallas et al. reported an accuracy ranging from 0.97 to 1.0 using a feed-forward ANN [58] after applying time-frequency processing methods (namely the smoothed pseudo-Wigner-Ville distribution) ahead of classification. Srinivasan et al. use the approximate entropy as input for two ANN (one recurrent and backpropagating, the other feed-forward), achieving an accuracy of up to 1.0 [57]. Both publications, Tzallas 2007 and Srinivasa 2007, demonstrate the use of combined feature extraction and prediction methods. A different approach was applied by Rabbi and Fazel-Rezai using a fuzzy logic method, which is to a certain degree rule-based and can thus mimic "human reasoning" [50]. They obtained a sensitivity of 0.95 for seizure detection, using >112 h of EEG data from 20 patients [50].

25.3 Conclusions

TS data are prevalent in many aspects of clinical medicine and academic neuroscience. Predicting future events from historical data offers us a powerful tool in neurocritical care, and ML has shown highly accurate results in various research objectives ranging from seizure detection in the analysis of electrocorticography data [59–61], massive parallel spike train data (as increasingly recorded with microelectrode arrays) [62], and even in target identification in the surgical treatment of epilepsy [63]. However, flaws in methodology and small sample size can lead to overly optimistic predictive performance [53]. The sheer volume of available methods and existing possibilities can be daunting for clinicians unfamiliar with the methodology. Nevertheless, the adaption of ML for TS analysis can reform old paradigms and can potentially benefit patient care when correctly adopted into the clinical practice. This review introduced the historically used approaches and innovations based on ML methods to ease the implantation into clinical neurosurgery.

Acknowledgments and Disclosure

Funding JMK, and DD are supported by the Bundesministerium für Bildung und Forschung (BMBF COMPLS3-022).

Conflicts of Interest/Competing Interests None of the authors has any conflict of interest to disclose.

References

1. Montgomery DC, Jennings CL, Kulahci M. Introduction to time series analysis and forecasting. 2nd ed (avid J. Balding, N. A. C. Cressie, G. M. Fitzmaurice, G. H. Givens, H. Goldstein, G. Molenberghs, D. W. Scott, A. F. M. Smith, R. S. Tsay, & S. Weisberg, Eds.); 2015. https://doi.org/10.1111/jtsa.12203.
2. Shumway RH, Stoffer DS. Time series analysis and its applications. Springer texts in statistics; 2011. https://doi.org/10.1007/978-1-4419-7865-3.
3. James G, Witten D, Hastie T, Tibshirani R. An introduction to statistical learning, with applications in R. Springer texts in statistics; 2013. https://doi.org/10.1007/978-1-4614-7138-7.
4. Parmezan ARS, Batista GEAPA. A study of the use of complexity measures in the similarity search process adopted by kNN algorithm for time series prediction. In: 2015 IEEE 14th international conference on machine learning and applications (ICMLA); 2015. p. 45–51. https://doi.org/10.1109/icmla.2015.217.
5. Parmezan ARS, Souza VMA, Batista GEAPA. Evaluation of statistical and machine learning models for time series prediction: identifying the state-of-the-art and the best conditions for the use of each model. Inf Sci. 2019;484:302–37. https://doi.org/10.1016/j.ins.2019.01.076.
6. Sapankevych N, Sankar R. Time series prediction using support vector machines: a survey. IEEE Comput Intell Mag. 2009;4(2):24–38. https://doi.org/10.1109/mci.2009.932254.
7. Cortez P. Sensitivity analysis for time lag selection to forecast seasonal time series using neural networks and support vector machines. In: The 2010 international joint conference on neural networks (IJCNN); 2010. p. 1–8. https://doi.org/10.1109/ijcnn.2010.5596890.
8. Grossman RL, Uthurusamy R, Dhillon IS, Koren Y, Ristanoski G, Liu W, Bailey J. Proceedings of the 19th ACM SIGKDD international conference on knowledge discovery and data mining, KDD '13. Undefined. 2013;946–954. https://doi.org/10.1145/2487575.2487655.
9. Kandananond K. A comparison of various forecasting methods for autocorrelated time series. Int J Eng Bus Manage. 2012;4:4. https://doi.org/10.5772/51088.
10. Gooijer JGD, Hyndman RJ. 25 years of time series forecasting. Int J Forecast. 2006;22(3):443–73. https://doi.org/10.1016/j.ijforecast.2006.01.001.
11. Hyndman RJ, Athanasopoulos G. Forecasting: principles and practice. OTEXTS. 2018. https://otexts.com/fpp2/.
12. Holt CC. Forecasting seasonals and trends by exponentially weighted moving averages. Int J Forecast. 2004;20(1):5–10. https://doi.org/10.1016/j.ijforecast.2003.09.015.
13. Winters PR. Forecasting sales by exponentially weighted moving averages. Manag Sci. 1960;6(3):324–42. https://doi.org/10.1287/mnsc.6.3.324.
14. Hyndman RJ, Khandakar Y. Automatic time series forecasting: the forecast package for R. J Stat Softw. 2008;27(3):1–22. https://doi.org/10.18637/jss.v027.i03.
15. Hopfield JJ. Artificial neural networks. IEEE Circuits Dev Mag. 1988;4(5):3–10. https://doi.org/10.1109/101.8118.
16. Jain AK, Mao J, Mohiuddin KM. Artificial neural networks: a tutorial. Computer. 1996;29(3):31–44. https://doi.org/10.1109/2.485891.
17. Bishop CM. Neural networks and their applications. Rev Sci Instrum. 1994;65(6):1803–32. https://doi.org/10.1063/1.1144830.
18. Sherstinsky A. Fundamentals of recurrent neural network (RNN) and long short-term memory (LSTM) network. ArXiv. 2018; https://doi.org/10.1016/j.physd.2019.132306.
19. LeCun Y, Bengio Y, Hinton G. Deep learning. Nature. 2015;521(7553):436–44. https://doi.org/10.1038/nature14539.
20. Bengio Y, Simard P, Frasconi P. Learning long-term dependencies with gradient descent is difficult. IEEE Trans Neural Netw. 1994;5(2):157–66. https://doi.org/10.1109/72.279181.
21. Hochreiter S, Schmidhuber J. Long short-term memory. Neural Comput. 1997;9(8):1735–80. https://doi.org/10.1162/neco.1997.9.8.1735.
22. Choi JY, Lee B. Combining LSTM network ensemble via adaptive weighting for improved time series forecasting. Math Probl Eng. 2018;2018:1–8. https://doi.org/10.1155/2018/2470171.
23. Sagheer A, Kotb M. Time series forecasting of petroleum production using deep LSTM recurrent networks. Neurocomputing. 2019;323:203–13. https://doi.org/10.1016/j.neucom.2018.09.082.
24. Yu Y, Si X, Hu C, Zhang J. A review of recurrent neural networks: LSTM cells and network architectures. Neural Comput. 2019;31(7):1235–70. https://doi.org/10.1162/neco_a_01199.
25. Noble WS. What is a support vector machine? Nat Biotechnol. 2006;24(12):1565–7. https://doi.org/10.1038/nbt1206-1565.
26. Cao LJ, Tay FEH. Support vector machine with adaptive parameters in financial time series forecasting. IEEE Trans Neural Netw. 2003;14(6):1506. https://doi.org/10.1109/tnn.2003.820556.
27. Kim K. Financial time series forecasting using support vector machines. Neurocomputing. 2003;55(1–2):307–19. https://doi.org/10.1016/s0925-2312(03)00372-2.
28. Braun M, Bernard T, Piller O, Sedehizade F. 24-Hours demand forecasting based on SARIMA and support vector machines. Proc Eng. 2014;89:926–33. https://doi.org/10.1016/j.proeng.2014.11.526.
29. Mellit A, Pavan AM, Benghanem M. Least squares support vector machine for short-term prediction of meteorological time series. Theor Appl Climatol. 2013;111(1–2):297–307. https://doi.org/10.1007/s00704-012-0661-7.
30. Abraham P, Rennert RC, Gabel BC, Sack JA, Karanjia N, Warnke P, Chen CC. ICP management in patients suffering from traumatic brain injury: a systematic review of randomized controlled trials. Acta Neurochir. 2017;159(12):2279–87. https://doi.org/10.1007/s00701-017-3363-1.
31. Carney N, Totten AM, O'Reilly C, Ullman JS, Hawryluk GWJ, Bell MJ, Bratton SL, Chesnut R, Harris OA, Kissoon N, Rubiano AM, Shutter L, Tasker RC, Vavilala MS, Wilberger J, Wright DW, Ghajar J. Guidelines for the management of severe traumatic brain injury, fourth edition. Neurosurgery. 2017;80(1):6–15. https://doi.org/10.1227/neu.0000000000001432.
32. Heuer GG, Smith MJ, Elliott JP, Winn HR, Leroux PD. Relationship between intracranial pressure and other clinical variables in patients with aneurysmal subarachnoid hemorrhage. J Neurosurg. 2004;101(3):408–16. https://doi.org/10.3171/jns.2004.101.3.0408.
33. Mack WJ, King RG, Ducruet AF, Kreiter K, Mocco J, Maghoub A, Mayer S, Connolly ES. Intracranial pressure following aneurysmal subarachnoid hemorrhage: monitoring practices and outcome

data. Neurosurg Focus. 2003;14(4):1–5. https://doi.org/10.3171/foc.2003.14.4.3.
34. Elliott J, Smith M. The acute management of intracerebral hemorrhage. Anesth Analg. 2010;110(5):1419–27. https://doi.org/10.1213/ane.0b013e3181d568c8.
35. Rincon F, Mayer SA. Clinical review: critical care management of spontaneous intracerebral hemorrhage. Crit Care. 2008;12(6):237. https://doi.org/10.1186/cc7092.
36. Czosnyka M, Pickard JD. Monitoring and interpretation of intracranial pressure. J Neurol Neurosurg Psychiatry. 2004;75(6):813. https://doi.org/10.1136/jnnp.2003.033126.
37. Hu X, Xu P, Scalzo F, Vespa P, Bergsneider M. Morphological clustering and analysis of continuous intracranial pressure. IEEE Trans Biomed Eng. 2008;56(3):696–705. https://doi.org/10.1109/tbme.2008.2008636.
38. Hamilton R, Xu P, Asgari S, Kasprowicz M, Vespa P, Bergsneider M, Hu X. Forecasting intracranial pressure elevation using pulse waveform morphology. In: 2009 annual international conference of the IEEE engineering in medicine and biology society, 2009; 2009. p. 4331–4. https://doi.org/10.1109/iembs.2009.5332749.
39. Siebig S, Kuhls S, Imhoff M, Gather U, Schölmerich J, Wrede CE. Intensive care unit alarms—how many do we need?*. Crit Care Med. 2010;38(2):451–6. https://doi.org/10.1097/ccm.0b013e3181cb0888.
40. Scalzo F, Hu X. Semi-supervised detection of intracranial pressure alarms using waveform dynamics. Physiol Meas. 2013;34(4):465–78. https://doi.org/10.1088/0967-3334/34/4/465.
41. Quachtran B, Hamilton R, Scalzo F. Detection of intracranial hypertension using deep learning. In: 2016 23rd international conference on pattern recognition (ICPR), 2016; 2016. p. 2491–6. https://doi.org/10.1109/icpr.2016.7900010.
42. Bonds BW, Yang S, Hu PF, Kalpakis K, Stansbury LG, Scalea TM, Stein DM. Predicting secondary insults after severe traumatic brain injury. J Trauma Acute Care Surg. 2015;79(1):85–90. https://doi.org/10.1097/ta.0000000000000698.
43. Rosen DS, MacDonald RL. Subarachnoid hemorrhage grading scales. Neurocrit Care. 2005;2(2):110–8. https://doi.org/10.1385/ncc:2:2:110.
44. Raj R, Luostarinen T, Pursiainen E, Posti JP, Takala RSK, Bendel S, Konttila T, Korja M. Machine learning-based dynamic mortality prediction after traumatic brain injury. Sci Rep. 2019;9(1):17672. https://doi.org/10.1038/s41598-019-53889-6.
45. Essen DCV, Smith SM, Barch DM, Behrens TEJ, Yacoub E, Ugurbil K, WU-Minn HCP Consortium. The WU-Minn Human Connectome project: an overview. NeuroImage. 2013;80:62–79. https://doi.org/10.1016/j.neuroimage.2013.05.041.
46. Michel CM, Koenig T. EEG microstates as a tool for studying the temporal dynamics of whole-brain neuronal networks: a review. NeuroImage. 2017;180(Pt B):577–93. https://doi.org/10.1016/j.neuroimage.2017.11.062.
47. Bagheri E, Jin J, Dauwels J, Cash S, Westover MB. A fast machine learning approach to facilitate the detection of interictal epileptiform discharges in the scalp electroencephalogram. J Neurosci Methods. 2019;326:108362. https://doi.org/10.1016/j.jneumeth.2019.108362.
48. Guo L, Wang Z, Cabrerizo M, Adjouadi M. A cross-correlated delay shift supervised learning method for spiking neurons with application to Interictal spike detection in epilepsy. Int J Neural Syst. 2017;27(03):1750002. https://doi.org/10.1142/s0129065717500022.
49. Montagna F, Buiatti M, Benatti S, Rossi D, Farella E, Benini L. A machine learning approach for automated wide-range frequency tagging analysis in embedded neuromonitoring systems. Methods. 2017;129:96–107. https://doi.org/10.1016/j.ymeth.2017.06.019.
50. Rabbi AF, Fazel-Rezai R. A fuzzy logic system for seizure onset detection in intracranial EEG. Comput Intell Neurosci. 2012;2012:705140. https://doi.org/10.1155/2012/705140.
51. Tsiouris KM, Pezoulas VC, Zervakis M, Konitsiotis S, Koutsouris DD, Fotiadis DI. A long short-term memory deep learning network for the prediction of epileptic seizures using EEG signals. Comput Biol Med. 2018;99:24–37. https://doi.org/10.1016/j.compbiomed.2018.05.019.
52. Hosseini M-P, Hosseini A, Ahi K. A review on machine learning for EEG signal processing in bioengineering. IEEE Rev Biomed Eng. 2021;14:204–18. https://doi.org/10.1109/rbme.2020.2969915.
53. Roy Y, Banville H, Albuquerque I, Gramfort A, Falk TH, Faubert J. Deep learning-based electroencephalography analysis: a systematic review. J Neural Eng. 2019;16(5):051001. https://doi.org/10.1088/1741-2552/ab260c.
54. Zhang T, Chen W. LMD based features for the automatic seizure detection of EEG signals using SVM. IEEE Trans Neural Syst Rehabil Eng. 2016;25(8):1100–8. https://doi.org/10.1109/tnsre.2016.2611601.
55. Jaiswal AK, Banka H. Epileptic seizure detection in EEG signal with GModPCA and support vector machine. Biomed Mater Eng. 2017;28(2):141–57. https://doi.org/10.3233/bme-171663.
56. Sharma A, Rai JK, Tewari RP. Epileptic seizure anticipation and localisation of epileptogenic region using EEG signals. J Med Eng Technol. 2018;42(3):1–14. https://doi.org/10.1080/03091902.2018.1464074.
57. Srinivasan V, Eswaran C, Sriraam N. Approximate entropy-based epileptic EEG detection using artificial neural networks. IEEE Trans Inf Technol Biomed. 2007;11(3):288–95. https://doi.org/10.1109/titb.2006.884369.
58. Tzallas AT, Tsipouras MG, Fotiadis DI. Automatic seizure detection based on time-frequency analysis and artificial neural networks. Comput Intell Neurosci. 2007;2007:80510. https://doi.org/10.1155/2007/80510.
59. Wang X, Gkogkidis CA, Schirrmeister RT, Heilmeyer FA, Gierthmuehlen M, Kohler F, Schuettler M, Stieglitz T, Ball T. Deep learning for micro-Electrocorticographic ({\mu}ECoG) data. ArXiv; 2018.
60. Xie Z, Schwartz O, Prasad A. Decoding of finger trajectory from ECoG using deep learning. J Neural Eng. 2018;15(3):036009. https://doi.org/10.1088/1741-2552/aa9dbe.
61. Zhang X, Xiong Q, Dai Y, Xu X, Song G. An ECoG-based binary classification of BCI using optimized extreme learning machine. Complexity. 2020;2020:1–13. https://doi.org/10.1155/2020/2913019.
62. Leibig C, Wachtler T, Zeck G. Unsupervised neural spike sorting for high-density microelectrode arrays with convolutive independent component analysis. J Neurosci Methods. 2016;271:1–13. https://doi.org/10.1016/j.jneumeth.2016.06.006.
63. Dian JA, Colic S, Chinvarun Y, Carlen PL, Bardakjian BL. Identification of brain regions of interest for epilepsy surgery planning using support vector machines. In: 2015 37th annual international conference of the IEEE engineering in medicine and biology society (EMBC), 2015; 2015. p. 6590–3. https://doi.org/10.1109/embc.2015.7319903.

Overview of Algorithms for Natural Language Processing and Time Series Analyses

26

James Feghali, Adrian E. Jimenez, Andrew T. Schilling, and Tej D. Azad

26.1 Introduction

Natural language processing (NLP) and time series analyses (TSA) have emerged as highly useful computational techniques in modern-day data science and machine learning, with increasingly relevant applications in medicine [1, 2]. NLP is the automatic analysis and representation of human language whereby machines utilize techniques and algorithms to break down text or speech content to extract meaningful and usable information [3]. One immediately recognizable application would be to leverage NLP in order to automate the conversion of free-text patient notes in the electronic medical record into a set of analyzable variables (e.g., tumor size, tumor location, tumor stage), thereby obviating the resource-intensive process of manual chart review [4]. The steps of processing human text rely on a sequence of "low-level tasks," such as assigning parts of speech to words and detection of sentence boundaries, and "high-level tasks" (build on low-level tasks), such as named entity recognition (NER-identifying and categorizing words/phrases into conceptual entities such as "locations" or "diseases") [5].

TSA is used to evaluate repeated measurements for one or more variables taken at uniform time intervals (e.g., hourly, monthly, etc.) and can determine associations with other trends or events as well as forecast the future based on past values in a series (e.g., forecasting the birth rate at all hospitals within a certain city each year or whether an electroencephalogram recording in seconds indicates a patient is experiencing a certain seizure) [1, 6]. Several machine learning algorithms can be used to achieve NLP tasks and perform effective TSA. Herein, we provide a detailed overview of salient deep learning algorithms in the form of a gentle introduction, assuming no prior knowledge in advanced linear algebra or calculus. We also describe relevant techniques in preprocessing data in preparation for modeling. We focus on conceptual underpinnings and basic underlying mathematical operations rather than coding language to ensure accessibility.

J. Feghali · A. E. Jimenez · A. T. Schilling · T. D. Azad (✉)
Department of Neurosurgery, Johns Hopkins University School of Medicine, Baltimore, MD, USA
e-mail: tazad1@jhmi.edu

26.2 Natural Language Processing

Preprocessing

Before applying algorithms on textual data, it must be converted into a mathematical framework that can be modeled. The first step in analyzing a hypothetical website with medical news articles (all the articles as a whole would be denoted as the "corpus" of the project) of different categories for example would be to organize these articles (every individual article would be an "observation") into a dataframe of rows representing individual articles and columns representing various properties of those articles (Table 26.1). This can be achieved by applying specific functions to the HTML content of the website. Then, another series of functions are utilized to standardize variations in the text (Fig. 26.1).

Other preprocessing steps include stemming, lemmatization, and stopword removal. Word stems are essentially the base form of the word with all affixes or inflections removed (Fig. 26.2), and stemming involves truncating a word back into its stem. Stemming is an important normalization step in information retrieval projects but can sometimes produce words that do not exist in the dictionary because it is heuristic or applies a strict set of rules (e.g., convert "his" to "hi" based on the "s" to " " rule or "studies" to "studi" based on the "ies" to "i" rule). Two popular stemming algorithms are the Porter [7] stemmer and the Snowball [8] stemmer. Lemmatization is a more sophisticated process compared to stemming since it resolves words to their basic dictionary form or "lemma" (singular form of nouns, infinitive form of verbs, and positive form of adjective or adverb; e.g., converts "studies" to "study"); however, the part of speech of the

V. E. Staartjes et al. (eds.), *Machine Learning in Clinical Neuroscience*, Acta Neurochirurgica Supplement 134,
https://doi.org/10.1007/978-3-030-85292-4_26

Table 26.1 Basic organization of medical news website articles into a dataframe

Article No.	Title	Content	Category
0	New CT technology…	Researchers have developed a high…	Innovation
1	Novel immunotherapy…	The immunological mechanisms of…	Innovation
2	The first in-utero repair…	Yesterday, surgeons at the hospital…	Innovation
3	Malpractice case in …	Medical malpractice cases have…	Legal

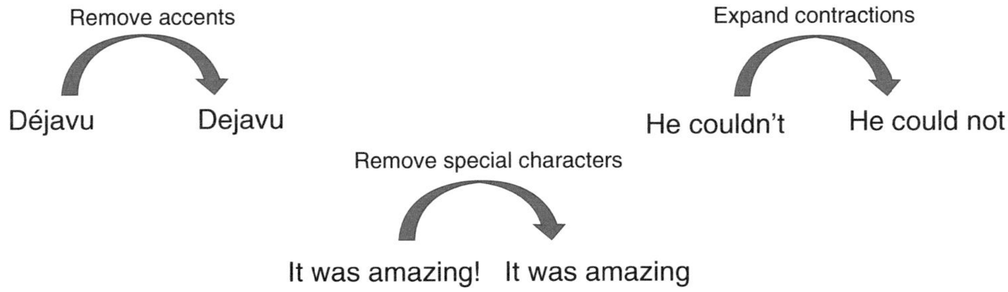

Fig. 26.1 Standardize text

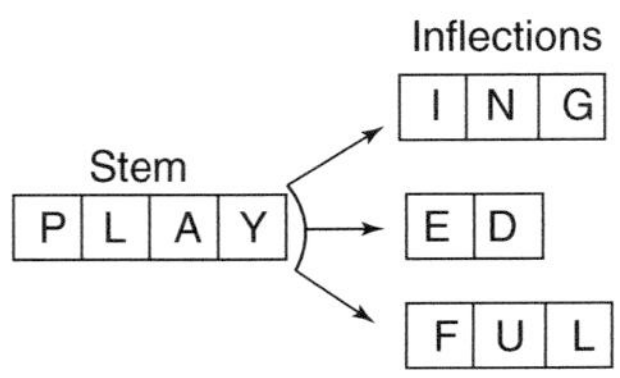

Fig. 26.2 A word stem with examples of inflections

input word would be needed. In that sense, stemming operates independently of context and hence requires less information and runs more rapidly despite the lower accuracy of the output, which may not matter in some applications. The goal of both processes is to normalize different morphological variants into a single item thereby reducing the number of distinct terms or complexity of the text [9]. This makes subsequent tasks run more efficiently. Stopwords are words that do not contribute critical meaning to a sentence such as determiners (e.g., "the", "a", "an" etc.), or prepositions (e.g., "in", "under" etc.), and stopwords happen to be the most commonly encountered words in a textual corpus. Depending on the final objective of an NLP project, these can be removed with little consequence using pre-built lists of stopwords that can be modified by the user.

Tokenization is another fundamental preprocessing step. It involves splitting text into smaller components or "tokens" such as words or characters based on certain delimiters (e.g., spaces). Most often, the tokens are words, and a main goal is to discover the "vocabulary" or set of unique words in a text.

N-grams

N-grams are a series of nearby words represented together, whereby an N-gram is a sequence of N words. For example, "the doctor" is a bigram, and "the doctor administered" is a trigram. Breaking down text into a series of N-grams is a form of tokenization that can be best understood with a sentence example: "The doctor administered the drug". The output of a unigram would be: "The, doctor, administered, the, drug" while the output of a bigram tokenization would be: "The doctor, doctor administered, administered the, the drug". Subsequently, one can calculate the probability of occurrence of each N-gram in the text, which could be useful in certain applications of NLP, including automated sentence completion relying on the most frequent N-gram.

Data Representation

Bag of Words

The bag of words approach is a common way to organize textual data in preparation for analysis. It is a representation of text using a dataframe with columns representing individual words of the complete corpus vocabulary and each row denoting an individual article. The cells would contain the frequency in which the word occurred in each article (Table 26.2). This form of representation has proven to be successful in many NLP pipelines that extract information from radiology reports, including the annotation of head CT reports with important clinical findings (e.g., acute hemorrhage) and the quantification of the number of brain metastases (single vs. 2 or more) in MRI reports [10, 11]. There are two main limitations associated with the bag of words representation. First, it ignores word order and grammar thus completely stripping words of their contextual information. Second, it is biased toward more frequent words which usually contribute less meaning.

One-Hot Encoding

One-hot encodings are an additional way one can convert textual data into numbers amenable for modeling and

Table 26.2 Bag of words representation method

Article No.	Technology	Malpractice	Immunotherapy	Repair	Novel	Category
0	15	0	0	1	5	Innovation
1	0	0	25	0	6	Innovation
2	1	0	0	9	1	Innovation
3	0	10	0	0	0	Legal

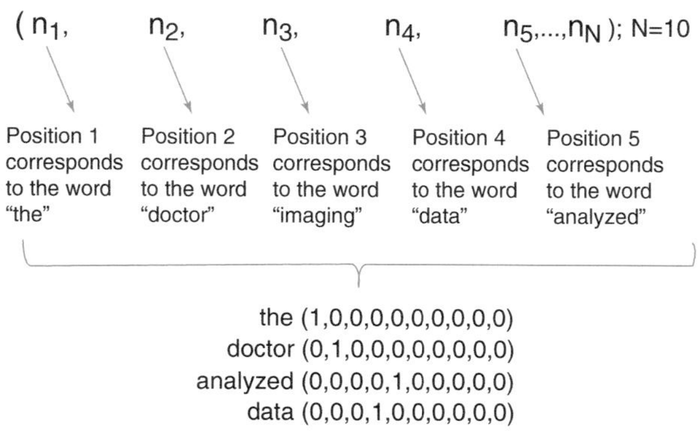

Fig. 26.3 Example of one-hot encoding vectors in a hypothetical project where the total vocabulary is ten words

analysis. A word can be represented by a vector with a length of N = number of words in the complete corpus vocabulary, with a value of zero at all positions except the position corresponding to that word, where a value of 1 is present (Fig. 26.3). A whole observation, or article, can be represented using a one-hot encoding matrix where each row is a unique word in the vocabulary (N number of rows) and the columns are the successive words of the article (Table 26.3). The columns in that matrix would be the one-hot encoding vectors for every word in the article. There are several limitations to one-hot encodings. The contextual or semantic relatedness between words is not communicated by the one-hot vectors. For instance, the vector of the word "cat" would not have more similarity to that of "dog" compared to that of "car" or "restaurant." Similarity between two vectors can be measured with a technique called cosine similarity. Figure 26.4 describes this concept with an example and reviews some algebraic definitions such as vector dot product and magnitude. In one-hot encoded representations, all word vectors are orthogonal to one another, meaning that the dot product of every word pair is zero and similar-meaning words cannot be identified by looking at the vectors. Another limitation of one-hot encoded vectors is the large vector dimensions (as large as the vocabulary) and the large number of zeros in the resultant matrices (such matrices are known as "sparse" matrices).

Word Embeddings: Neural Network Basics

Word embeddings, like one-hot encodings, are vector representations of words. However, they are known as "distributed" representations because the meaning of the word is spread out across all the vector positions rather than having the value "1" only at a single position. Unlike one-hot encoding, the dimension size of the vector is much smaller than the vocabulary size (e.g., can be 300 in a 10,000 word vocabulary). An example of word embeddings is provided in Fig. 26.5. Word analogies can even be represented using arithmetic operations and the embedded word vectors as such: king − man + woman = queen (man is to king as woman is to *queen*) or athens − greece + england = london. The word embeddings are generated based on context, where the meaning of a particular word is derived based on surrounding words. In the two sentences "the *doctor* administered the drug" and "the *nurse* administered the drug," "doctor" and "nurse" could be understood to share certain semantic features just by sharing similar contexts. More specifically, they are more likely to be situated around a similar set of neighboring words. This contextual meaning is what most word embedding algorithms utilize to generate the word vectors.

One widely utilized machine learning neural network algorithm that is used to generate word embeddings is the word2vec algorithm, developed by Tomas Mikolov at Google [12]. To understand how this algorithm works, the basic structure of a neural network should be explained. In the case of supervised learning, where learning occurs on datasets consisting of labeled input-output pairs (e.g., patients with a certain demographic profile [inputs] and whether they actually experienced a complication after surgery [labeled output]), neural networks approximate the function that maps from the inputs to the output by first randomly assigning the function's parameters (or assigning them to zero) and then iteratively adjusting them based on calculated errors between the output predicted by the function and the true output (a process called loss minimization).

We will first explain the terminology and structure of a neural network using the example of a prediction project utilizing a multivariable logistic regression neural network and then extrapolate the concepts to the example of word embeddings. Neural networks are also called "artificial neural networks" or ANNs because they are loosely based on the neuronal structure and connectivity of the brain. The neural network components can be better understood through the logistic regression example in Fig. 26.6, which seeks to predict the probability of a patient experiencing a surgical complication based on some input variables. A neural network is made up of "layers", each consisting of "neurons" or "nodes."

Table 26.3 One-hot encoding representation of an article

	a	surge	of	affected	patients	with	a	…last word in article
a	1	0	0	0	0	0	1	–
Of	0	0	1	0	0	0	0	–
With	0	0	0	0	0	1	0	–
Surge	0	1	0	0	0	0	0	–
Patients	0	0	0	0	1	0	0	–
Affected	0	0	0	1	0	0	0	–
…*N*	–	–	–	–	–	–	–	–

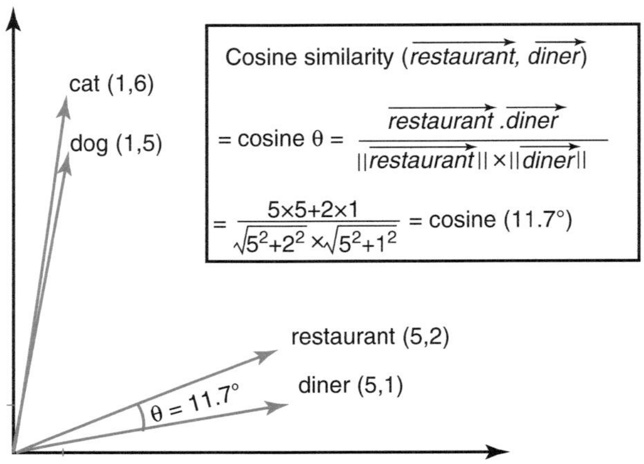

Fig. 26.4 Cosine similarity between vectors. Cosine similarity is used as an index of similarity between two vectors i.e., the higher the cosine similarity, the more similar the two vectors are. Cosine similarity can be calculated geometrically as the cosine of the angle between two vectors or by calculating the dot product ($x_1*x_2 + y_1*y_2 + z_1*z_2$ etc.) and dividing it by the product of the magnitude (square root of the sum of the squared coordinates). Visually, notice how the angle between restaurant and diner is smaller (higher cosine similarity) than the angle between restaurant and dog, or how the dog and cat vectors are more similar to each other compared with those of either restaurant or diner. From this simple example, we can begin to understand the potential of encoding some form of meaning or relatedness in the word vectors. If the same words were encoded with one-hot vectors (e.g., dog (1,0,0,0); diner (0,1,0,0); cat (0,0,1,0); restaurant (0,0,0,1)), the dot product between any two vectors would be 0 and hence no semantic meaning is encoded

The first layer is known as the input layer and the final layer is known as the output layer, and there could be layers in between called hidden layers, where function operations or "transformations" are carried out. The layers are connected to each other by neuron-to-neuron connections known as "arcs", and every arc carries a certain "weight." A "fully connected" neural network is one in which every neuron in a given layer is connected to every neuron in the next layer. Likewise, a "dense" or "fully connected" layer is a type of hidden layer whereby every neuron is connected to every other neuron in the next layer. The goal of an input layer in a logistic regression project is to receive the values of the predictor variables (e.g., age, body mass index, gender) for a certain observation (e.g., neurosurgery patient in the dataset), and the number of neurons composing the input layer would be equal to the number of independent predictor variables (each neuron represents a predictor variable). A neuron in layers other than the input layer computes the weighted sum of the neuron values it is receiving from the previous layer (e.g., age*its weight, body mass index*its weight, gender*its weight, etc.) or in other words, computes a weighted sum of all its inputs, where the weights are those assigned to the connecting arcs. Each neuron also has a "bias" term that it adds to that weighted sum. This bias term can be thought of as a firing threshold for the neuron because it plays a role in determining what output values will be propagated forward; it also functions to add flexibility to the overall model in fitting the given data. Both the weights and the bias terms are what the model is seeking to learn based on the data, as they are the parameters involved in the mapping function. After summing the weighted inputs and the bias term, a neuron feeds the result into an "activation function," which may transform the result into some value between a minimum and a maximum. Two examples of commonly used activation functions are the sigmoid function [$\sigma(x) = \frac{1}{1+e^{-x}}$] and the rectified linear unit function (ReLU) [$f(x) = \max(0, x)$], where x in both cases is the sum of the weighted inputs and the bias term. The sigmoid function converts x into a number between 0 (x values that are relatively large and negative) and 1 (x values that are relatively large and positive). A similar function that converts inputs into a number between −1 and 1 is the tanh function [$\tanh(x) = \frac{2}{1+e^{-2x}} - 1$]. The ReLU function returns zero if x is negative and the actual value of x if it is positive. To further understand the concept of bias and threshold for firing, any negative x is not carried forward by a neuron if it employs the ReLU activation function since 0 signifies a non-firing neuron. For a bias term of +1, the threshold for firing is reduced to −1, because now for example, a weighted sum of −0.99 would result in an x of 0.01 which is positive and hence provides an output to the next layer.

To explain how learning, or the optimization of the function parameters, occurs, some definitions are worth explaining. Unlike epidemiological definitions, the word "sample" in ANNs refers to a single observation or row of data (e.g. one patient) rather than the complete dataset. The word sample is also equivalent to "observation", "input vector", "feature vector" (i.e. a patient is considered a combination of features such as age, BMI, gender, etc.), or an "instance." The algorithm includes "parameters," which are part of the mapping function or final model, and "hyperparameters." Parameters are the weights and the bias term which the model seeks to learn automatically, while hyperparameters are set manually by the user and are external to the model (not dependent on the dataset). They affect the speed and accuracy with which the learning process occurs and are usually fine-tuned by trial and error or by following rules of thumb. After randomly initializing the parameters or setting them to zero, the model subsequently updates those parameters after measuring the loss or error between the predicted output and the true output. One can think of a "loss function" as a function describing the magnitude of the error for an observation. The specific loss function is often chosen by the user based on the predictive model that is being developed (e.g. whether it is predicting a continuous outcome like length of stay or predicting a categorical outcome like complication occurrence). The best loss function for a given model will be one that has a minimum point where specific parameter values minimize the loss and can be approximated (such a function is amenable to being "optimized" or is convex shaped with some "local minima" and a single most minimum point called the "global minimum"). We will take two simple examples to help visualize what the function looks like when plotted. If only one parameter (w) is being optimized, such a loss function plotted as loss on the y-axis versus w on the x-axis would be u-shaped (parabola) for instance. If two parameters, w and b, are being optimized, plotting loss on the z-axis versus w and b on the x- and y-axes respectively would yield a bowl-shaped function in three-dimensional space with a single minimum point. An example of a loss function often used in logistic regression is given in Fig. 26.7. The term "cost function" is often used when evaluating loss with respect to several observations and is the average loss across these observations. The process of learning the correct parameters based on the error between predicted and actual values is known as "gradient descent." A simplified example that can help develop some intuition about the concept as well as general equations involved in the process can be found in Fig. 26.8. Extrapolating these concepts to the case of logistic regression, the derivative

dog (0.90, 0.11, -0.03, 0.20)
cat (0.85, 0.09, -0.02, 0.10)
restaurant (0.22, 0.92, 0.33, -0.50)
diner (0.18, 0.95, 0.28, -0.47)
apple (0.01, 0.52, -0.63, 0.93)

Dot product (dog, cat) = 0.796
Dot product (dog, diner) = 0.164

Fig. 26.5 Example of a word embedding. In this example, five words are encoded using vectors of dimension $d = 4$. Notice how visually, the dog and cat vectors are similar as are the restaurant and diner vectors. Both pairs are very different from the vector of apple. The dot product values (proportional to cosine similarity) confirm the visual comparison

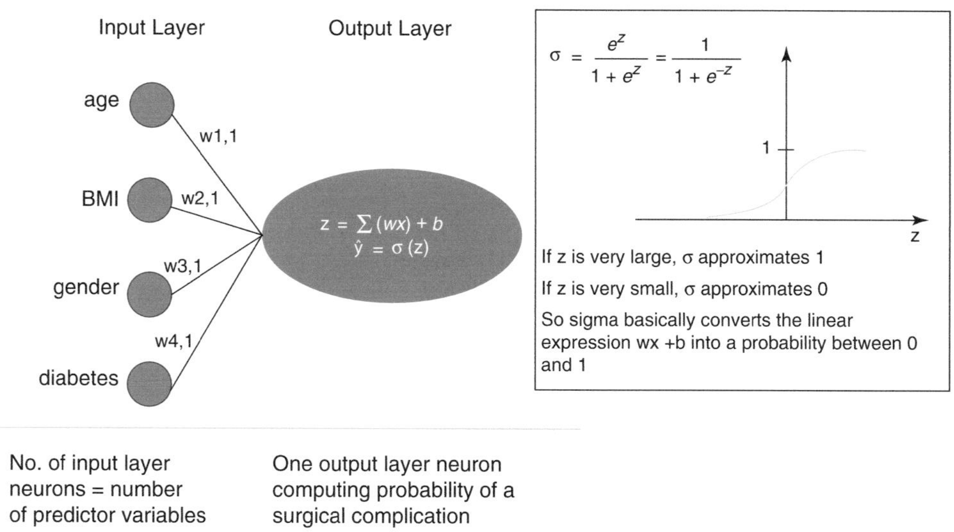

Fig. 26.6 Neural network example for logistic regression. Input layer is made up of four neurons each representing a predictor variable. Initially, before any observations are "seen" by the algorithm, the weights and bias terms are assigned random values or zero values ("initialization"). Output layer neuron computes the weighted sum of its inputs for a patient (e.g. $w_{1,1}$*20 years + $w_{2,1}$*32 kg/m^2 + $w_{3,1}$*1 (1 coded as female and 0 as male) + $w_{4,1}$*1 (patient is diabetic)) and adds a bias term (b) to the result to obtain z for a particular patient. Subsequently, the probability of a complication is computed by the sigmoid activation function (σ). By comparing the error between the predicted probability ($\hat{y}$) and the true output (y), the weights and bias terms are then adjusted, and the process repeats iteratively until the error is minimized. The final optimized weights and bias term will make up the beta values and constant of the predictive model

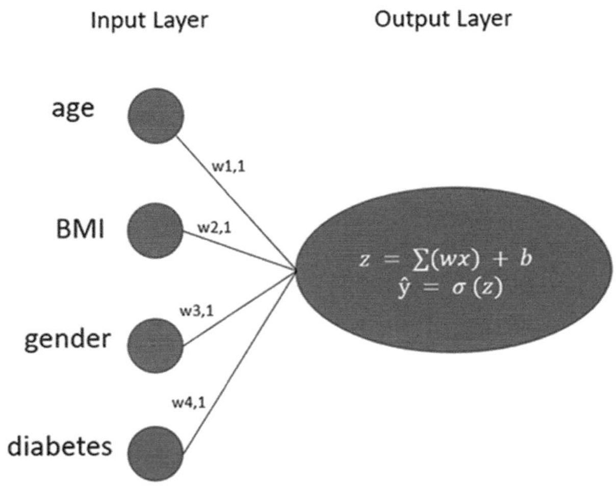

Activation function

$$\sigma = \frac{e^z}{1+e^z} = \frac{1}{1+e^{-z}}$$

Loss function (with respect to an observation)

$L(\hat{y}, y) = -[y \log \hat{y} + (1-y)\log(1-\hat{y})]$; where y is true output value

To make intuitive sense that this is actually measuring loss or discrepancy between predicted and true values, take examples:

1) If y=1, the expression reduces to -logŷ; for this to be minimized, you would want logŷ to be maximized, meaning you want ŷ to be maximized. Since ŷ is a probability value between 0 and 1, the max possible ŷ value is 1, which constitutes a perfect match with y=1
2) If y=0, the expression reduces to -log(1 - ŷ); for this to be minimized, log(1 - ŷ) must be maximized, which means 1 - ŷ must be maximized so ŷ must be zero, which is also a perfect match

Cost function (with respect to all data and the parameters): Average of loss

$$J(w,b) = \frac{1}{N}\sum_{i=1}^{N} L(\hat{y}^{(i)}, y^{(i)})$$

Fig. 26.7 Loss and cost functions for logistic regression

of the loss function with respect to the parameters (weights and bias term) can also be calculated in order to apply gradient descent (Fig. 26.9). Figures 26.8 and 26.9 detail the underlying mathematical operations that characterize learning in any neural network.

The "batch size" is a hyperparameter that determines how many samples should be passed through the algorithm before it updates the parameters (e.g., update parameters after passing five patients through the algorithm). The number of "epochs" is a hyperparameter that determines how many times the algorithm will iterate through the entire dataset. Epoch numbers are relatively large (hundreds or thousands) in order to ensure appropriate error minimization. One can plot the error against the epochs in what is known as a "learning curve" to track learning with progression through the dataset. The term "stochastic gradient descent" denotes a batch size of 1, meaning the parameters update after every observation. "Batch gradient descent" denotes a batch size equal to the size of the training dataset, meaning the parameters update after the algorithm has seen all the data.

At this point, it is useful to mention that a machine learning project with neural networks often utilizes three datasets: the training, validation, and test sets. The training dataset contains the labeled samples that are used to train the model using gradient descent. The validation set is usually a held-out subset of the initial labeled dataset. One can randomly split a large dataset of labeled samples for instance into a training dataset containing 80% of observations and a validation dataset containing the remaining 20%. In practice, as the model is being trained through gradient descent using observations in the training dataset, it is simultaneously being tested for accuracy on observations in the validation dataset. It is important to note that loss in the validation dataset is not used in the training process, and observations in the validation dataset do not contribute to training but are only used to check accuracy as the model is being trained. This process is carried out in order to verify whether there is "overfitting", a situation whereby the accuracy in matching predictions to true values is high in the training dataset but poorer in the validation dataset. This indicates that the model might be overfitted to the training data used to develop the model but might perform poorly on new data. The validation dataset is also used to fine-tune hyperparameters of the model, such as the number of hidden layers in a network. The test set can also be a held-out subset of the initial labeled data and is used to test the predictive accuracy of the final model with its specified hyperparameters.

Word Embeddings: Learning an Embedding Matrix

With an understanding of the structure of a neural network and how it optimizes a set of parameters to minimize loss, the process of word embedding can be discussed in more detail. The task of word embedding can be conceptualized as the process of learning the values of an "embedding matrix" (*E*) of dimensions *d* by *N*, where *d* is the desired size of the

Fig. 26.8 Simplified example of gradient descent when trying to find the intercept (parameter of interest) of the line of best fit for two observed points (assume slope of best fit line is known)

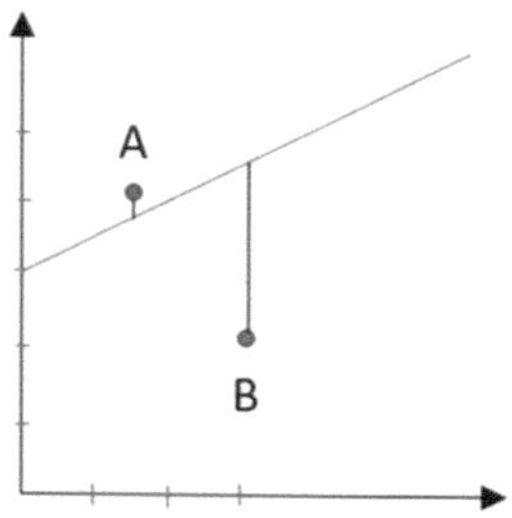

y = ax + b => y = 0.8x + b
initialize b to 3 randomly = > y = 0.8x + 3 (blue line)
degree of fit is judged by the sum of squared residuals, where a residual is the difference between the true y value of a point and the predicted y value by the line. The SSR can be thought of as a loss function. Squaring takes care of negative differences. The lower the SSR, the better the fit.
The squared residual at point A is $[4 - (0.8*1.5 + 3)]^2$
The squared residual at point B is $[2 - (0.8*3 + 3)]^2$
SSR = $[4 - (0.8*1.5 + b)]^2 + [3 - (0.8*3 + b)]^2$ => shape of a parabola

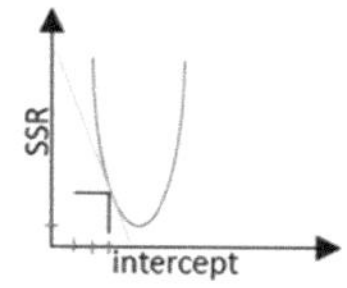

- The goal is to determine which value of the intercept achieves the minimum SSR. Mathematically, that is the point where the slope of the graph (or derivative of SSR with respect to intercept [dL/d(intercept)]) is zero.
- To get closer to this point we must adjust the new intercept into a new value by a certain "step size". That step size should be proportional to our current slope, because we would want to take large steps if we are still far from a slope of zero, but want smaller steps as we get closer to zero.
- Equation for step size = Slope x "learning rate"
  The learning rate is a hyperparameter that we set and is usually between 0.01 and 0.0001 => general equation for step size = dL/d(parameter) x learning rate
  In our example, the parameter is the intercept, and dL/d(intercept) can be derived mathematically (not shown here).
- new parameter = old parameter - step size (move right if slope is negative; move left if slope is positive => both in the direction of the minimum)
- As an example, to move from 3 to the new intercept at a learning rate of 0.01, we first find the step size by plugging in the intercept value of 3 into dL/d(intercept) to get the slope for an intercept = 3 and then multiply by 0.01 => the result will be a negative number since the slope at 3 is negative. From that, we notice that the new parameter becomes 3 - (negative number computed as above) => higher than 3 and closer to the point corresponding to minimum loss. This process repeats iteratively until loss is minimized

embedded word vectors and *N* is the size of the vocabulary. This matrix, when multiplied by the one-hot encoded vector of a word (size *N*), yields the embedded word vector. An example with a cursory review of relevant linear algebra is provided in Fig. 26.10. Learning *E* will consist of randomly initializing its components (the parameters) and then learning them through the process of gradient descent. Word2vec represents a family of algorithms that can set up a supervised prediction task of words in a text, facilitating the learning of *E*. There are two main versions of word2vec that can be used, known as "continuous bag of words" (CBOW), where we try to predict a target word given its surrounding context, and "skip-gram", where we try to predict the surrounding context given a target or focus word (Fig. 26.11). In general, CBOW is more suitable for generating word embeddings from a small corpus while skip-gram works better in a large corpus. To understand some of the algorithms involved in word2vec, we will take a simplified setup of skip-gram where word embeddings are generated by predicting a single context word from a given focus word in a hypothetical small vocabulary of 5 words. Moving from the input layer to the hidden layer is described in Fig. 26.12, and moving from the hidden layer to the output layer is described in Fig. 26.13. These are meant to provide a general intuition on how word embeddings are generated by setting up a supervised learning task of prediction. Note that the goal is really not to predict nearby words if given a specific word, but this setup appears to be a very effective way to generate word embeddings with contextual meaning. From Fig. 26.13, we notice that the softmax function will require summing up dot products across the vocabulary in the denominator, and in practice, this operation is inefficient or computationally expensive. Word2vec utilizes "hierarchical softmax" or "negative sampling" to render the algorithm more efficient, but these processes are beyond the scope of this chapter [12]. Aside from word2vec, GloVe (global vectors for word representations) represents an even simpler algorithm for generating word embeddings that is also commonly used [13].

Word Embeddings: Implementation

In practice, a user does not have to generate word embeddings for every NLP project. There are several pre-trained word embeddings that were generated from very large vocabularies and text corpora, some of which are clinic notes [14]. Such word embeddings are expected to generalize and work well in NLP projects utilizing the same type of input text (e.g., clinic notes).

Recurrent Neural Networks

Recurrent neural networks (RNNs) are neural networks that are suited for tasks dealing with sequential data. In NLP, that would mean a task where the sequence of the words is a fundamental piece of information for completing the task (e.g., information about previous words feeding in as input to

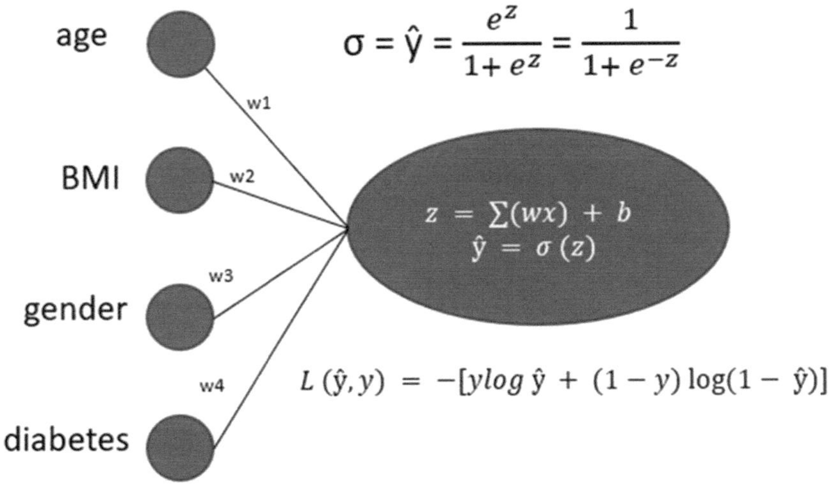

To apply gradient descent, the derivative of the loss function should be calculated with respect to every parameter. That way, the step size can be determined in order to move from the old parameters to the new parameters.

Some mathematical rules must be known:

1) chain rule: $\frac{dy}{dx} = \frac{dy}{du} * \frac{du}{dx}$

e.g. $y = \frac{1}{1+e^x}$; $\frac{dy}{dx} = \frac{dy}{d(1+ex)} * \frac{d(1+ex)}{dx} = -\frac{1}{(1+e^x)^2} * e^x$; In this example: $u = 1 + e^x$

2) derivative of log ŷ is 1/ŷ

3) derivative of 1/x = $-1/x^2$

Take w1 as an example:

$\frac{dL}{dw1} = \frac{dL}{d\hat{y}} * \frac{d\hat{y}}{dz} * \frac{dz}{dw1}$ (chain rule) => process of derivative traveling backwards through the algorithm is known as "backpropagation"

a) $\frac{dL}{d\hat{y}}$ (use chain rule) = $\frac{-y}{\hat{y}} + \frac{1-y}{1-\hat{y}}$

b) $\frac{d\hat{y}}{dz}$ (use chain rule) = $-\frac{1}{(1+e^{-z})^2} * -e^{-z}$ => add 1 and subtract 1 in the numerator:

$$-\frac{-e^{-z}+1-1}{(1+e^{-z})^2} = \frac{e^{-z}+1-1}{(1+e^{-z})^2} = \frac{1+e^{-z}}{(1+e^{-z})^2} - \frac{1}{(1+e^{-z})^2} = \frac{1}{1+e^{-z}} - \frac{1}{(1+e^{-z})^2} = \hat{y} - \hat{y}^2 = \hat{y}\,(1-\hat{y})$$

c) $\frac{dz}{dw1} = x1$

$\Rightarrow \frac{dL}{dw1} = (\hat{y} - y) * x1$

$\Rightarrow$ extrapolate to w2: $\frac{dL}{dw2} = (\hat{y} - y) * x2$

$\Rightarrow$ extrapolate to w3: $\frac{dL}{dw3} = (\hat{y} - y) * x3$

$\Rightarrow$ extrapolate to w4: $\frac{dL}{dw4} = (\hat{y} - y) * x4$

$\Rightarrow \frac{dL}{db} = (\hat{y} - y)$ [since $\frac{dz}{db}$ =1]

recall: step size = slope * learning rate
new parameter = old parameter - step size
e.g. to apply gradient descent on w1 after seeing one observation, compute dL/dw1 based on formula, then multiply it by learning rate and subtract result from old w1 to obtain new w1

Fig. 26.9 Gradient descent applied to the loss function of logistic regression

functions working on downstream words). One such task can be word prediction, where an algorithm can predict the next most likely word given a sequence of words. Another application is machine translation from one language into another. NER, predicting whether a word falls under a certain category (e.g., a person's name), represents another task that can leverage RNNs. An example that demonstrates how sequences can help with entity recognition is the following sentence: "The surgeon who previously took care of the patient Mr. Keys was Dr. Rivers." The words "surgeon" and "Dr." help identify "Rivers" as a person's name, and "patient" as well as "Mr." help identify "Keys" as a person. The structure of a basic RNN is represented in Fig. 26.14. If the same task was modeled with a standard feed-forward neural network (multilayer perceptron) where the input word vectors are stacked on top of each other in an input layer followed by a dense hidden layer then an output layer, one can imagine how difficult it would be to go through different samples. That is because each sample has a different number of inputs and hence the input layer cannot have a fixed number of neurons (unless the input layer is "padded" with zero-value neurons as large as the largest sample—not feasible). In addition, if an RNN learns that "Harry" is a person's name in position 1 of a sequence, it can easily identify "Harry" as a name in any position (learned features generalize across different positions of text). That is not possible in a standard feed-forward network because of the difference in architecture. If words are used as inputs, these can be one-hot vectors or word embeddings. The potential advantage of using word embeddings becomes clear if you take the sentences: "The surgeon on the case was John Fisher" and "The doctor on the case was William Madison." If an RNN uses word embeddings to learn that John Fisher is the name of a person, the similarity between the embedded vectors of "surgeon" and "doctor" will make it easier for the network to recognize that William Madison is also a name. The type of RNN used in NER has a many-to-many (inputs-to-outputs) structure with equal numbers of inputs and outputs (each input word has a predicted probability as an output). Other structures can be used for different tasks. For sentiment classification (e.g., determining whether a patient's free-text review of a doctor is positive or negative), a many-to-one RNN with only a single "$\hat{y}$" coming after the last input word in a sequence can be used.

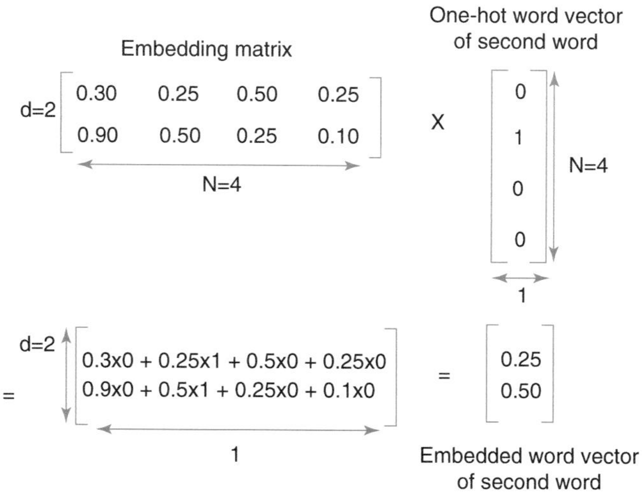

Fig. 26.10 Word embedding matrix example. A vector can be thought of as a matrix of dimensions: vector size by 1. Matrices can be multiplied together when the number of columns in the first matrix equal the number of rows in the second matrix. The number of rows (*d*) of an embedding matrix "*E*" is set to the desired size of the final embedded word vector. The number of columns is equal to the size of the vocabulary (*N*). To get the embedded word vector, the embedding matrix is multiplied by the one-hot vector of the word (in this case, the second word in a hypothetical vocabulary of four words). The resulting matrix from a matrix multiplication has dimensions: no. of rows = no. of rows of first matrix (e.g., 2); no. of columns = no. of columns of second matrix (e.g., 1). The 1 by 1 value of the resultant matrix is obtained by the dot product of the first row in matrix *E* with the first and only column in the one-hot matrix. The 2 by 1 value is the dot product of second row in *E* with the column in the one-hot matrix. Notice how multiplying by the embedding matrix simply picks out the values of a certain column: here for example, the second word in the vocabulary picks out the second column of *E*. Every column in *E* represents the corresponding embedded word vector. Word embedding consists of learning the values inside that embedding matrix, which are the parameters of the learning task

Before moving on to more sophisticated RNNs, it is worthwhile discussing the limitations of the simplest RNN architectures. One limitation is unidirectionality, which becomes clear in the example "Keys was the surgeon on the case." In a unidirectional RNN, the algorithm cannot use

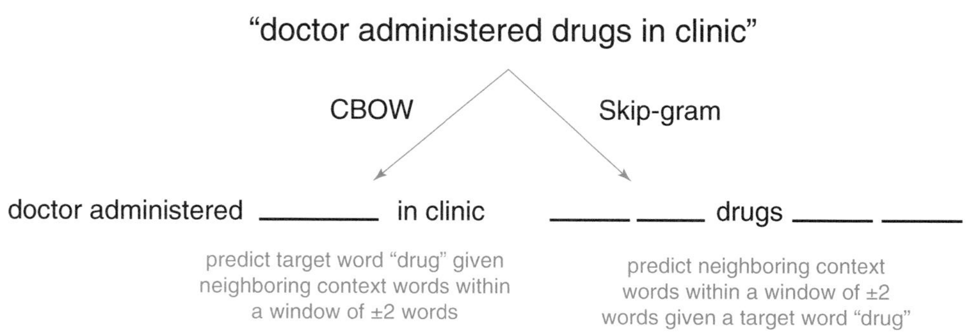

Fig. 26.11 CBOW and skip-gram approaches of setting up a prediction task. The window of words constitutes a hyperparameter that can be set to a desired number

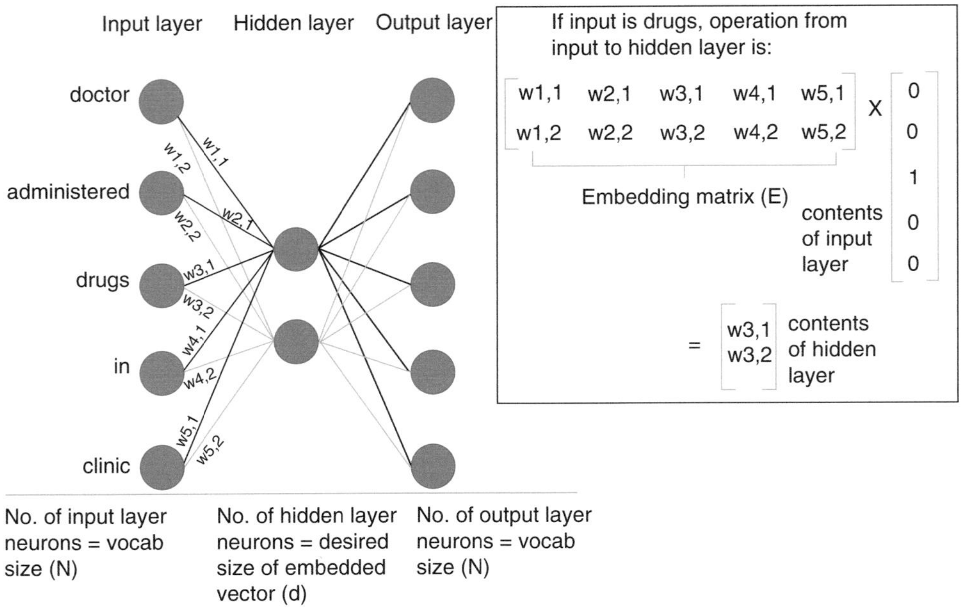

Fig. 26.12 Skip-gram predicting one context word "clinic" given the word "drugs" in a vocabulary of five words: from input to hidden layer. The input layer has no. of neurons equal to the corpus vocabulary (*N*) where each neuron represents a word. The input to that layer is a one-hot encoded vector representing the focus word (drugs in this one-sample example). The hidden layer has a size equal to the desired dimension of the embedded word vectors (in this case: 2). The neurons compute the weighted sum of their inputs. This can be represented by a matrix-vector multiplication where the embedding matrix contains the weights that the algorithm is seeking to optimize. *E* has dimensions *d* by *N*, and every column is the embedded vector of a word. The multiplication picks out the embedded vector of the corresponding input word

information from "surgeon" to figure out that "Keys" is a name. Hence, bidirectional RNNs are better suited for NER tasks [15]. Another major limitation of simpler RNNs is the vanishing gradient problem which limits the ability of RNNs to process long-term dependencies (e.g., how a word very early on in a sentence affects a word located very far downstream). The vanishing gradient problem can be understood by looking at how backpropagation works to modify early parameters. By closely looking at the chain rule, the gradient of the loss with respect to the parameters in the early layers (e.g., first time-step) is a product of derivatives that depend on components situated at later layers. If some of the terms in this product are small (less than 1), then the resulting gradient of the early parameters will be even smaller. In some instances, it is too small to cause a meaningful update in the weights after a certain batch, especially after being multiplied by a learning rate. The weight is hence "stuck" and cannot be optimized due to this vanishingly small gradient. A similar problem that occurs less often in RNNs is the exploding gradient problem, whereby many of the terms are large (>1), and the resulting gradient is exponentially large, complicating the optimization process. RNNs processing data over thousands of time-steps and feed-forward ANNs that are very deep (several hidden layers) can suffer from these unstable gradients.

Gated Recurrent Units

Gated recurrent units (GRUs) are a modification of the standard RNNs that mitigates the vanishing gradient problem by employing gate mechanisms that determine which word elements are worth retaining from time-step to time-step [16, 17]. That way, they are able to learn long-term dependencies between words. They can be thought of as an RNN framework that prioritizes the memory of certain words and word elements over others (e.g., the words "doctor" and "drug" are more important than articles and prepositions; retaining whether a subject is singular or plural helps in predicting whether the verb downstream is singular or plural). The structure of a simplified GRU and the underlying mathematical operations are summarized in Fig. 26.15.

Long Short-Term Memory (LSTM) Network

Another neural network structure capable of mitigating the vanishing gradient problem and of learning long-term dependencies is the LSTM, which came before GRUs and is more flexible but more computationally expensive [18]. The repeating unit of an LSTM has a cell state (*c*) that flows through the unit and that can be modified with only some minor linear (i.e., can be modeled with a straight line) interactions according to the values of different gates. The structure of a basic LSTM is represented in detail in Fig. 26.16. Certain variants of that structure can be used, including the

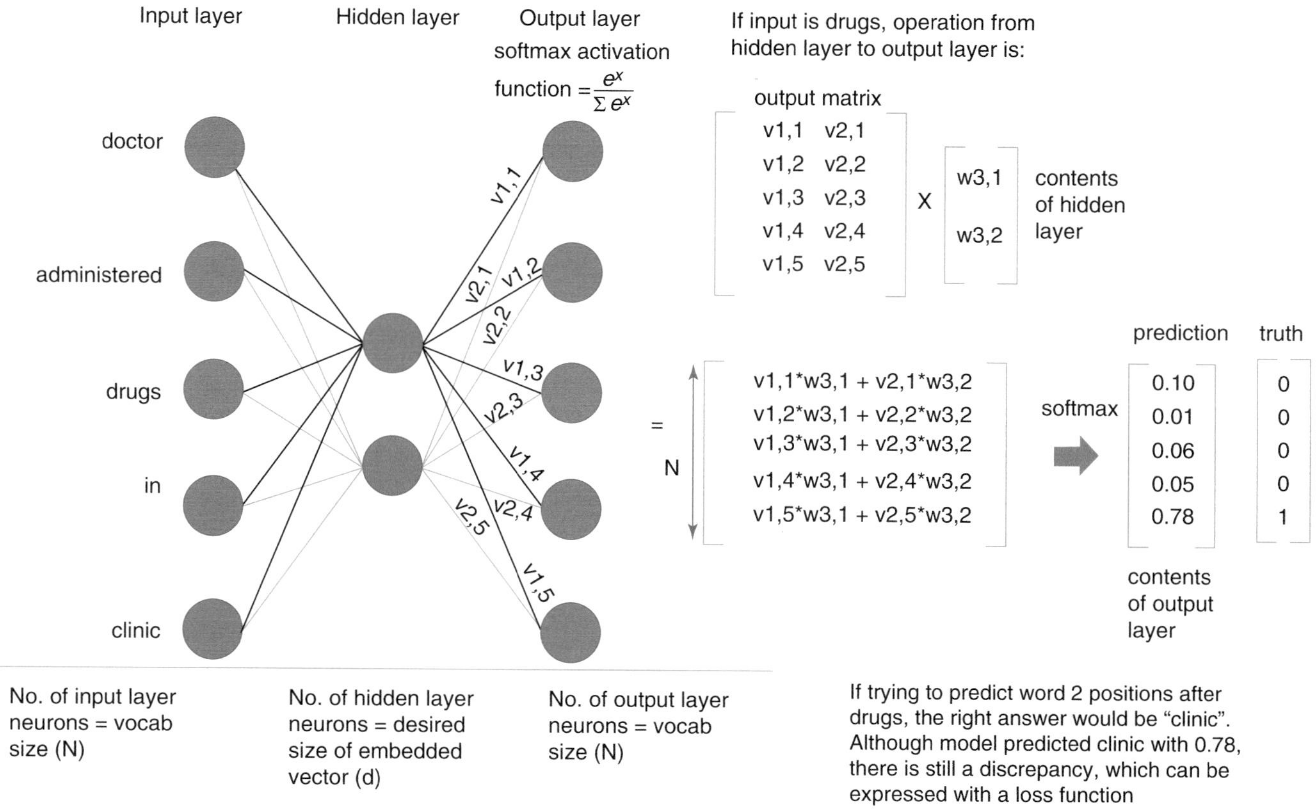

Fig. 26.13 Skip-gram predicting one context word "clinic" given the word "drugs" in a vocabulary of five words: from hidden to output layer. An output matrix, of dimensions *N* by *d*, is multiplied by the embedded vector to produce an output vector of dimension *N*. The rows of the output matrix can be thought of as containing embedded vectors for context words. To convert the contents of the output layer into a probability distribution, a softmax activation function, which resembles the sigmoid function, is assigned to the output neurons, converting the output contents into a probability of occurrence for different words in the vocabulary as a context word two positions down from "drugs". Note that sigmoid activation functions are typically used in binary classification problems (two possible outcomes) while the softmax is used in *k*-possible classifications (*k*-possible outcomes). Discrepancy between the probability assigned to "clinics" (the right word at that position) and "1" can be represented by a loss function. The process of stochastic gradient descent can optimize the embedding matrix to minimize that loss and hence provide word embeddings of size "*d*" for words in the vocabulary

addition of a "peephole" element, which is basically allowing the gates to take a peek at the cell state of the previous cell to compute their values [19]. There is no universally better algorithm when comparing GRUs and LSTM variants, and both have achieved favorable results in a variety of tasks.

Convolutional Neural Networks

Convolutional neural networks (CNNs) are models that utilize filters (also known as kernels) to extract features from the input by an operation known as convolution. CNNs were first developed to solve tasks that relied on processing visual input (e.g., classify picture of an animal as a cat vs. a dog or a handwritten number as the correct intended number by determining shared features between different pictures of the class "cat" or the number "9" for instance) or what is known as "computer vision" [20]. Hence, we will explain the basic concepts of a CNN using examples from computer vision and then generalize to NLP. First, the building blocks of a CNN will be discussed individually followed by a description of the complete CNN architecture.

In visual input processing, a grayscale image can be thought of as a 2-dimensional (2D) matrix of pixel values that represent brightness (higher values = brighter or more white pixels). One possibility to process such an image would be to convert it into a flattened vector of pixel values and feed it to a standard feed-forward ANN (Fig. 26.17). Several limitations become apparent with this approach. First, if one is starting with an 800 by 680 pixel image for example, the flattened input vector size and hence input layer neurons would be 544,000. With a subsequent dense hidden layer of 1000 neurons for example, the weight matrix operating on the inputs would be of size 1000 by 544,000 (544 million parameters). With such a large number of parameters to learn, the computational process would be impractical, and an immense amount of data would be required to build a model that does not suffer from overfitting. Moreover, col-

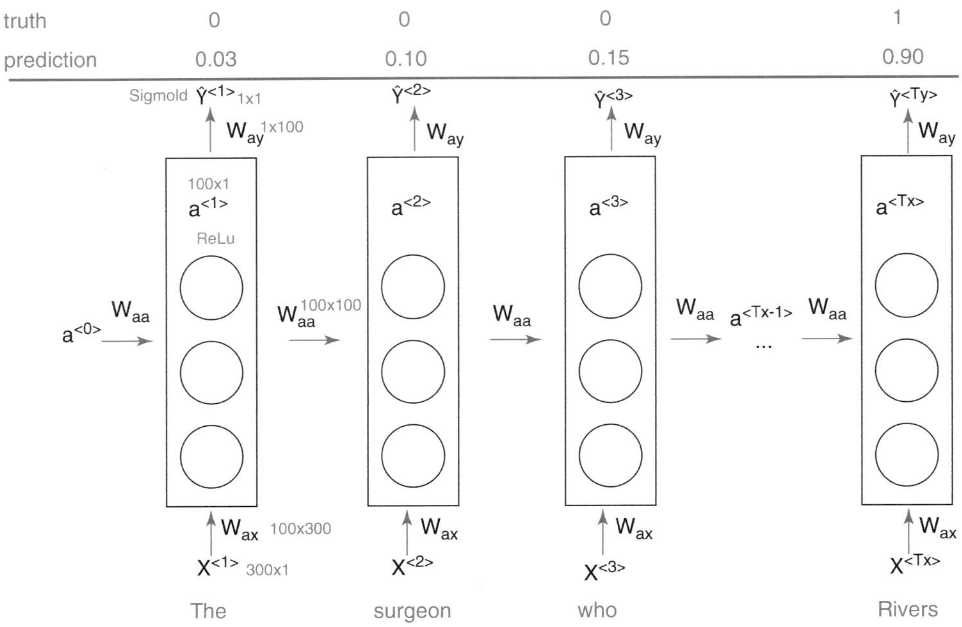

Fig. 26.14 Recurrent neural network structure with NER example. A sentence is being fed into the network to predict how likely each word represents a person's name. This is an example of a many-to-many RNN structure where the number of outputs $\hat{y}^{\langle i \rangle}$ equals the number of inputs $x^{\langle i \rangle}$. The letter "*a*" represents hidden layers and every $x^{\langle i \rangle}$ is a word fed sequentially into an input layer, whereby every $x^{\langle i \rangle}$ in the sequence is referred to as the "*ith time-step*". $a^{\langle 0 \rangle}$ is a starting point and is just an all-zero vector. An example of possible dimensions of every layer and weight matrix are provided in the figure and can be set by the user. Here for instance, pre-trained 300-dimension word embeddings are used as inputs, and hidden layers of 100 neurons and a ReLU activation function (tanh is another function that is commonly used) are used. The hidden layer also adds a bias term (b_a). The output layer in this case is a single neuron with a sigmoid function and a bias term (b_y). Notice how information from the hidden layer of a word is fed to a downstream hidden layer with a W_{aa} matrix transformation. This represents a form of "memory" for the network. The words can be one-hot vectors or word embeddings for example, and W_{ax} is the weight matrix that is multiplied by the input word vector. Putting this all together, the operations in the hidden and output layers can be summarized by: $a^{\langle 1 \rangle} = \mathrm{ReLU}\,(W_{aa}\, a^{\langle 0 \rangle} + W_{ax}\, x^{\langle 1 \rangle} + b_a)$ & $\hat{y}^{\langle 1 \rangle} = \sigma(W_{ay}\, a^{\langle 1 \rangle} + b_y)$. The discrepancy between the predicted probabilities ($\hat{y}$) and the labeled truth (y) can be modeled with a loss function typically used for sigmoid functions: $L(\hat{y},y) = -[y\log \hat{y} + (1 - y) \log (1 - \hat{y})]$. Backward propagation "through time" (since passes through different time-steps) subsequently optimizes the weights and bias terms as sentences are fed into the network

lapsing the 2D pixel matrix into a single vector eliminates valuable spatial information from the image. In CNN, the input can take on more than one dimension, such as the example of a 2D, N by N matrix representation of pixel values of a grayscale image. The filter or kernel is a 2D, n by n matrix of a smaller size that can "convolve" over the image pixels or overlap them sequentially to extract certain features that are registered in a resultant matrix called a feature map. This process of convolution is described in Fig. 26.18. If the filter contains some specific values, it can systematically extract a certain feature from the image, such as vertical edges (Fig. 26.19). There are different filters for different features, including horizontal edges and diagonal edges. While one can design the filter to extract a specific feature, the values of a filter are actually weights that are learnable in the context of a visual processing task (e.g., determining the value of a handwritten number). When CNNs are set up with randomly initialized filters, the network can learn specific weights that end up extracting important features, such as vertical or horizontal edges, that are relevant to the task at hand. A potential issue to think about is that the corner and edge pixels in the input image are included in much less convolution steps than central pixels, so they contribute less information. One way to address this would be to "pad" the input image with zero-value pixels (Fig. 26.20). The padding can also be used to take care of stride values that may cause the filter to "fall off" the input image while convolving. "Same padding" is when padding is applied to yield a feature map with the same size as the unpadded image, such as in Fig. 26.20, where a pad of size 1 applied to a 4 × 4 image yields a 4 × 4 feature map. In addition to convolving over a 2D input, it is also possible for CNNs to receive 3D input volumes, such as an RGB image with three stacked pixel matrices for every channel (red-green-blue). The convolution process in this case is described in Fig. 26.21.

With this knowledge, a convolution layer of a CNN can now be described (Fig. 26.22). Each filter essentially yields a feature map that gets summed with a bias term, and the result is fed through an activation function such as ReLU. One can rely on certain notations to describe any convolution layer

$$\tilde{h}^{<t>} = tanh(W_{hh}(r^{<t>} \odot h^{<t-1>}) + W_{hx}x^{<t>} + b_h)$$ practically a gate with the value 0 or 1 due to the sigmoid output

$$u^{<t>} = \sigma(W_{uh}h^{<t-1>} + W_{ux}x^{<t>} + b_u)$$

$$r^{<t>} = \sigma(W_{rh}h^{<t-1>} + W_{rx}x^{<t>} + br)$$ a measure of the relevance of $h^{<t-1>}$ in computing $\tilde{h}^{<t>}$

$$h^{<t>} = u^{<t>} \odot \tilde{h}^{t} + (1 - u^{<t>}) \odot h^{<t-1>}$$ If gate value u is 0, then keep h like previous time-step. If gate value u is 1, then update h to $\tilde{h}$

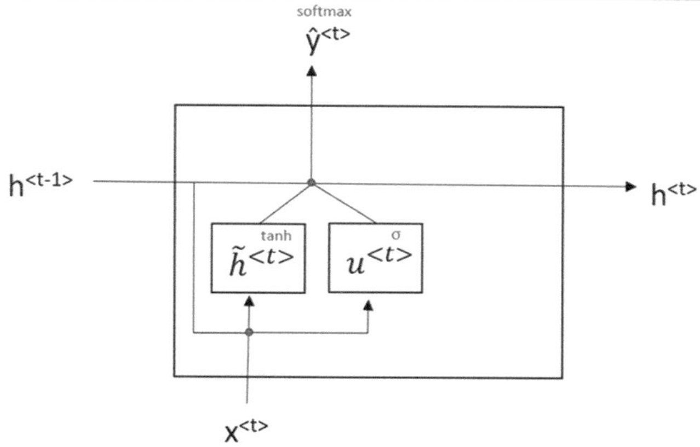

Fig. 26.15 Gated recurrent unit cell structure. In essence, one can think of a GRU as an RNN framework containing a hidden state ($h^{(t)}$) that could either stay the same as that of the previous time-step ($h^{(t-1)}$) or update into a new one if the model learns that important information worth "memorizing" is encoded in the particular input word. The candidate hidden state that can replace the previous one is denoted by $\tilde{h}^{(t)}$. The update gate ($u^{(t)}$)is a sigmoid function that can be conceptualized as yielding 0 or 1 depending on the importance or relevance of the input. The hidden state of the current memory cell ($h^{(t)}$) consequently keeps the same value from the previous time-step if $u^{(t)} = 0$ (check equation of $h^{(t)}$) or takes on the value of the candidate hidden state if $u^{(t)} = 1$. When the gate value is 1 (i.e., cell will replace the previous hidden state with a candidate hidden state), we pay attention to a reset gate or relevance term ($r^{(t)}$) which reflects how relevant the previous hidden state is to computing the candidate hidden state (if it is zero, the candidate hidden state is reset to a value completely independent from the previous time-step). The resultant $h^{(t)}$ is fed forward to the next cell and possibly to an output layer, as in standard RNNs. Note that $\tilde{h}^{(t)}$, $h^{(t-1)}$, $u^{(t)}$, and $r^{(t)}$ are vectors of the same size, so the "⊙" symbol denotes element-wise rather than matrix multiplication. So in effect, there is gating for retention of individual features or elements of the input

(l). The input to that layer can be denoted by: $N_H^{[l-1]} \times N_W^{[l-1]} \times d^{[l-1]}$, which are the height, width, and depth dimensions. The generated output can be similarly denoted by: $N_H^{[l]} \times N_W^{[l]} \times d^{[l]}$, where $d^{[l]}$ is the number of filters. Each filter is denoted by: $n^{[l]} \times n^{[l]} \times d^{[l-1]}$, where the filter depth is equivalent to the input depth. The size of the output can be calculated with the following formula: $N_H^{[l]} = \frac{N_H^{[l-1]} - n^{[l]} + 2p^{[l]}}{s^{[l]}} + 1$, where "$p$" and "$s$" are the padding size and stride size, respectively. The width can also be calculated with the same formula. The number of filters, stride, and padding size at each layer are all hyperparameters of the CNN.

In addition to convolution layers, CNNs contain pooling layers, which reduce the spatial size of the representation, thereby decreasing the number of parameters and increasing the computational speed. One type of pooling is referred to as "max pooling," and this process is described in Fig. 26.23. Pooling layers only have hyperparameters, such as dimension size and stride. Padding is rarely employed, except in some specific circumstances. Commonly used hyperparameters include 2 × 2 max pooling with a stride of 2, which halves the height and width in the absence of padding. In pooling, there are no parameters to be learned by backpropagation. Pooling works by capturing local regions of high activation from the input and preserving them which shrinks the representation while maintaining valuable information. Another type of pooling is known as "average pooling," where the average of values in a certain window of cells, rather than the maximum value, is calculated. Pooling also works on volume inputs, whereby the pooling process is applied separately to every channel of the input. The output would hence have the same depth as the input.

Toward the end of the network, the third type of layer that is encountered is the fully connected layer. The volume produced by a series of convolution and pooling operations is typically flattened into a vector (a column of neurons) that is subsequently fed into fully connected layers (dense connections) prior to reaching the output layer. Putting all this information together, the complete architecture of a CNN can be visualized (Fig. 26.24). With progression through the layers, the height and width dimensions typically decrease while the depth increases. The selection of the hyperparameters is often guided by previously published literature.

CNNs Applied to NLP

Having discussed the structure of a CNN as it relates to visual input processing, the information can be readily

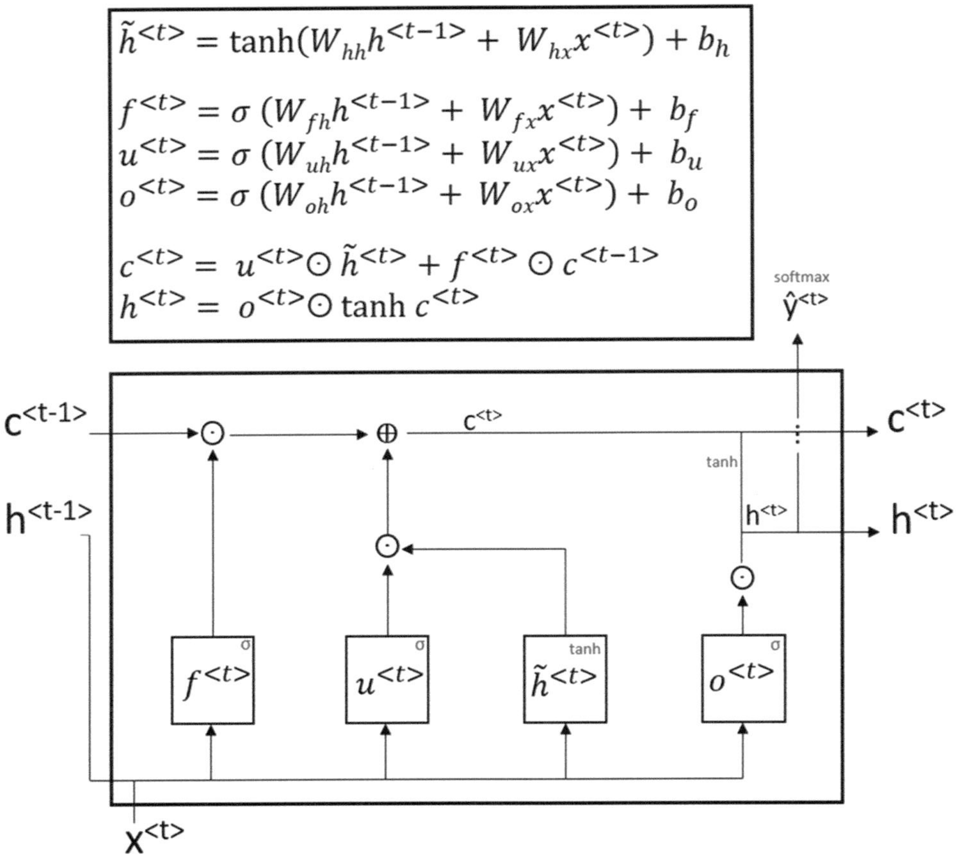

Fig. 26.16 Long short-term memory (LSTM) cell structure. As the cell state flows through the unit ($c^{\langle t-1\rangle}$ to $c^{\langle t\rangle}$), it can be modified with linear interactions according to the contents of different gates, which are all sigmoid functions operating on the input of the current unit $x^{\langle t\rangle}$ and the hidden state from the previous time-step $h^{\langle t-1\rangle}$ to determine how best to modify the cell state. The first gate is the forget gate $f^{\langle t\rangle}$ which determines what information from the previous cell state will be dumped or forgotten (0 = discard; 1 = retain). For example, when encountering a new subject, the network might need to forget the properties (gender; singular vs. plural) of the past subject. In the subsequent steps, the network determines what new information is going to be stored in the cell state. A vector of candidate values $\tilde{c}^{\langle t\rangle}$ is generated from a tanh operation on $x^{\langle t\rangle}$ and $h^{\langle t-1\rangle}$, and it is then multiplied element-wise with an update gate that determines what portion of each candidate element will be added to the cell state. The resultant state is passed on to the next cell. A filtered version of this cell state, created by a tanh activation function and multiplication by an output gate (decides which elements to output), is also fed into an output layer and the next cell

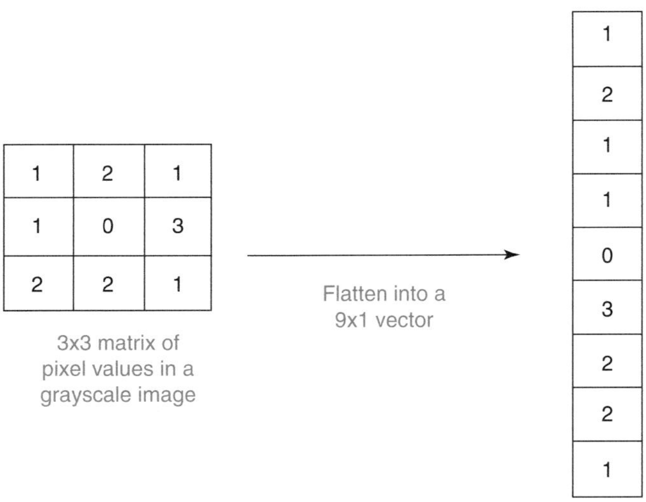

Fig. 26.17 Processing visual input by flattening the image matrix into a vector

extrapolated to NLP. The same basic principles apply except for some considerations regarding input structure and filter dimensions. CNNs can achieve good results in several NLP tasks, especially those that involve classification, including sentiment analysis (e.g., is an online review of a doctor positive or negative) and topic categorization [21]. The input can be in the form of embedded word vectors such as those generated by word2vec or GloVe. An example of a CNN applied in the context of NLP is provided in Fig. 26.25.

26.3 Time Series Analysis

With a general understanding of how a variety of neural networks process data in order to optimize model parameters in the context of NLP, the application of these same algorithms in TSA can be readily appreciated. Neural networks have

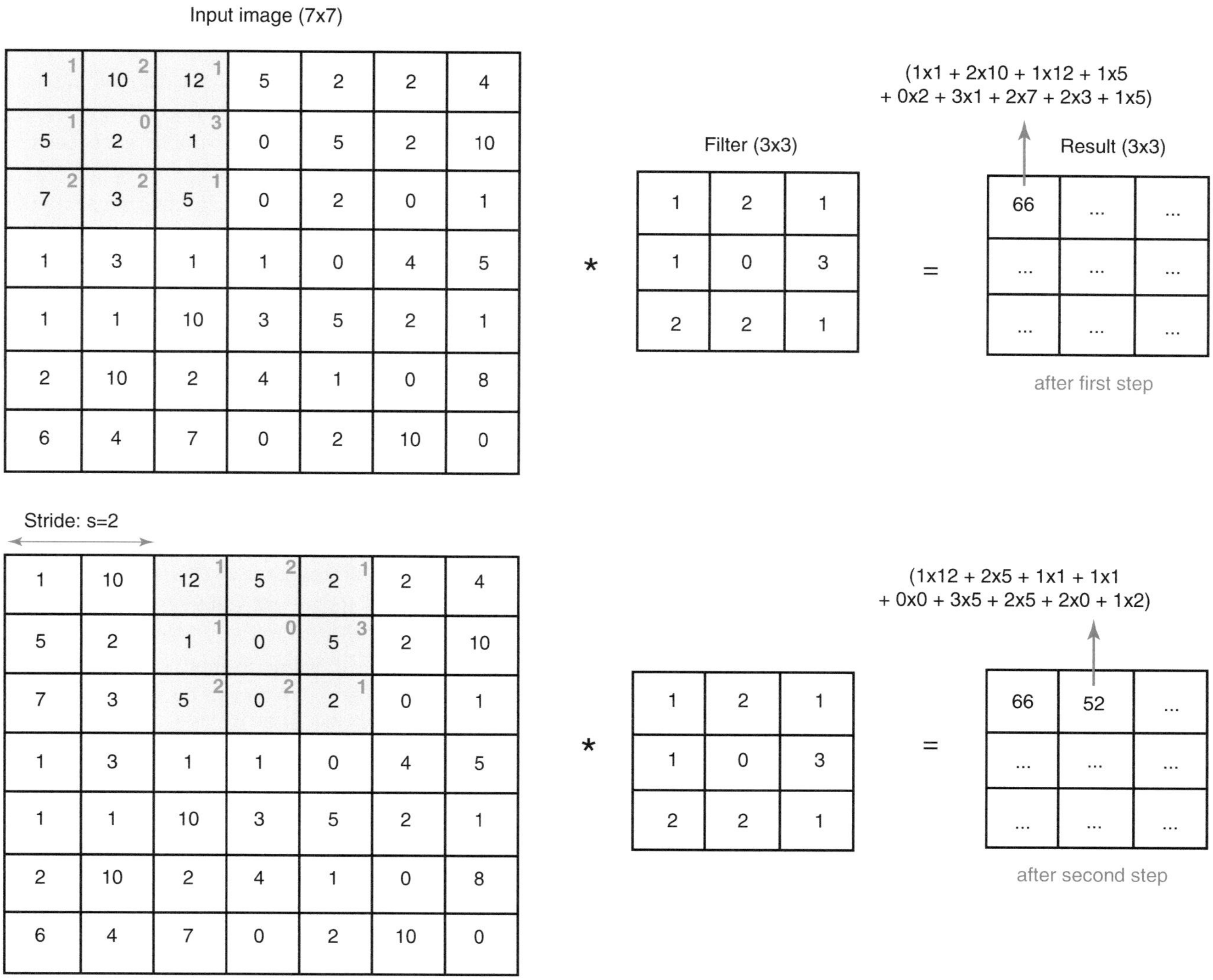

Fig. 26.18 Convolution process. The n by n filter is overlapped with an N by N input image matrix, and the element-wise products are summed together to compute the corresponding value in the resultant matrix, called a feature map, at the first position (66). The filter then "convolves" to the next position by moving to the right by a "stride" of squares set by the user (here $s = 2$) and computes the sum of element-wise products to yield the next value of the feature map (52). A similar process occurs for the third step. At the fourth step, the filter moves back to the left-most edge of the input image and displaces downwards by the stride value (top left corner of filter would overlap with "7" from the input image) and the process continues until all the feature map is filled. The formula used to compute the size of the feature map is: $\frac{N-n}{s}+1$. If the result is a decimal, then it is rounded down. The asterisk in this figure denotes the convolution operation

achieved favorable results in many TSA tasks, especially forecasting [22]. In the remaining part of this chapter, we present some neural network architectures used in forecasting.

Preprocessing

Prior to implementing algorithms, the time series data is often explored to identify general trends, which are a long-term increase or decrease of values in a series (e.g., decrease in cigarette sales over time), and seasonality, which is a fixed repeating short-term cycle in the series (e.g., fixed increase in alcohol sales every weekend). Seasonality can be additive (fixed magnitude of variation) or multiplicative (fixed percentage of variation) as demonstrated in Fig. 26.26. Moreover, the series can be analyzed for the presence of autocorrelation, which is the significant correlation between values at a time (t) and preceding values with a certain lag (t − 1, t − 2, t − 3, etc.). To measure autocorrelation, lag variables of the measurement of interest can be created (Table 26.4), and the association between the original variable and the lag variable can be evaluated with a Pearson correlation test for example. One can also produce an autocorrelation plot (correlation coefficient vs. lag value), also known as an autocorrelation function, which can also help

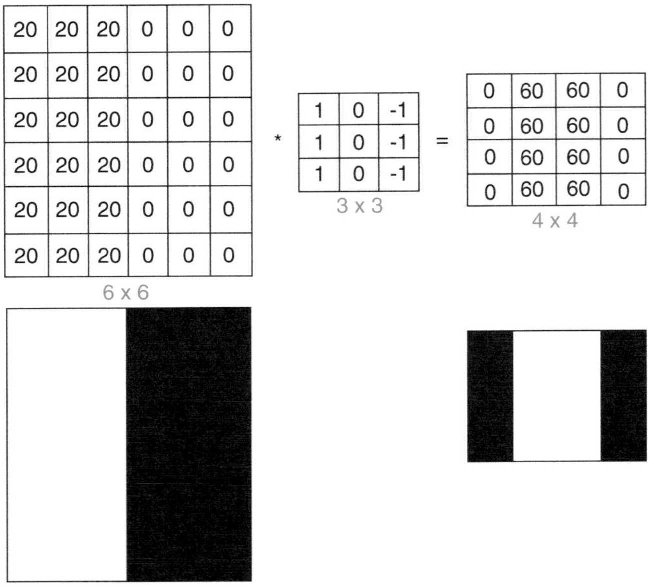

Fig. 26.19 Vertical edge detection filter. This filter is designed to capture vertical edges in an image. Notice how the resultant 4 × 4 matrix is maximally activated at its center, indicating that the input image had a vertical edge in its center. This is only a simplified example. With a larger and more complex input image, the feature map would also be an image containing white vertical edges at the same places where the initial image had vertical edges

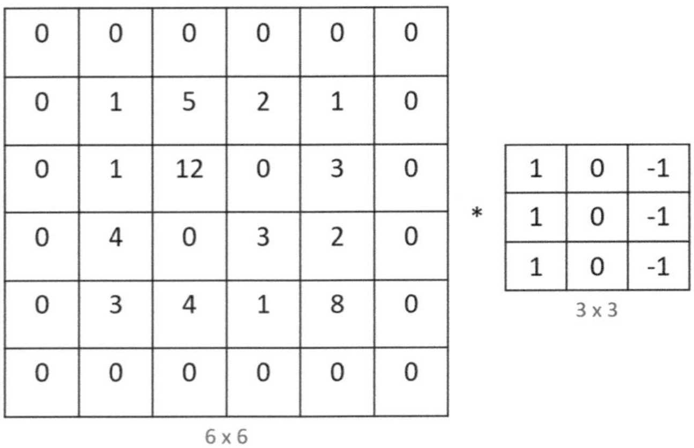

Fig. 26.20 Padding example of a 4 × 4 input image with a pad size = 1. Even for a stride value of 2, the filter matrix can now convolve over the input without falling off on the right edge. Note that if the input image was not padded, no computations would have been performed for filter positions that do not completely overlap the input. To compute the size of the resultant feature map with padding involved, the following equation can be used: $\frac{N-n+2p}{s}+1$, where p is the padding size (here $p = 1$)

identify seasonality (Fig. 26.27). Commonly encountered autocorrelations are a positive correlation and a negative correlation between values at time (t) and values from the previous time-step ($t - 1$), known as "stickiness" and "swings," respectively. All these data exploration steps and others are often guided by some domain knowledge or expertise in the specific topic. In this phase, it is also necessary to identify unusual periods or outliers to avoid training the network on these nonsystematic components of the time series. In TSA, it is imperative to note that splitting up the data into training and validation cannot be done randomly because the values are not independent. Successive observations are needed to train and test a model, so typically, the first $n\%$ of successive observations are selected for training, leaving the next 100-$n\%$ for validation.

Neural Networks: Multilayer Perceptron

A standard feed-forward ANN with an input layer, hidden layers, and an output layer is also referred to as a multilayer perceptron. This neural network can be used to forecast the next value in a time series (y_{t+1}) using current (y_t) and previous ($y_{t-1}, y_{t-2}, \ldots, y_{t-n}$) values. Every prediction will be made according to a window or sequence size of previous time-steps (e.g. in a training dataset of 100 values and a window of 4, use first 4 successive values as input ($y_{t-3}, y_{t-2}, y_{t-1}, y_t$) to predict the fifth value (y_{t+1}); then in the second sample, use second to fifth values as input ($y_{t-3}, y_{t-2}, y_{t-1}, y_t$) to predict the sixth value (y_{t+1}), and so on iteratively). The architecture of such a network in TSA is provided in Fig. 26.28. One preprocessing step that might help the activation functions work better is to convert the numerical input data into proportional values between 0 and 1 (maximum value becomes 1, minimum value becomes zero, and all values in between become proportional decimals between 0 and 1), a process known as normalization, since activation functions are sensitive to the magnitude of continuous variables (e.g., can work poorly with very large numbers). This transformation can be achieved with different functions in various softwares (e.g., "MiniMaxScaler" in Python). After the model is trained/validated and predictions are made, these predictions can be "inverse-transformed" into the original input scale (e.g., from 0–1 to \$0–\$950) to evaluate predictive accuracy. In time series forecasting applications, the multilayer perceptron models commonly include a single hidden layer. With an increase in the number of hidden layers and their neurons, the risk of overfitting and the computational time increase. To capture seasonality in the model, an additional input (y_{t-k}; k = seasonality; e.g., 12 in a monthly time series with a seasonal cycle every year) can be provided.

Neural Networks: LSTM

Given their suitability for sequence type data, RRNs in general and LSTMs in particular represent other commonly used algorithms in time series forecasting. Similarly to the multilayer perceptron, the time series

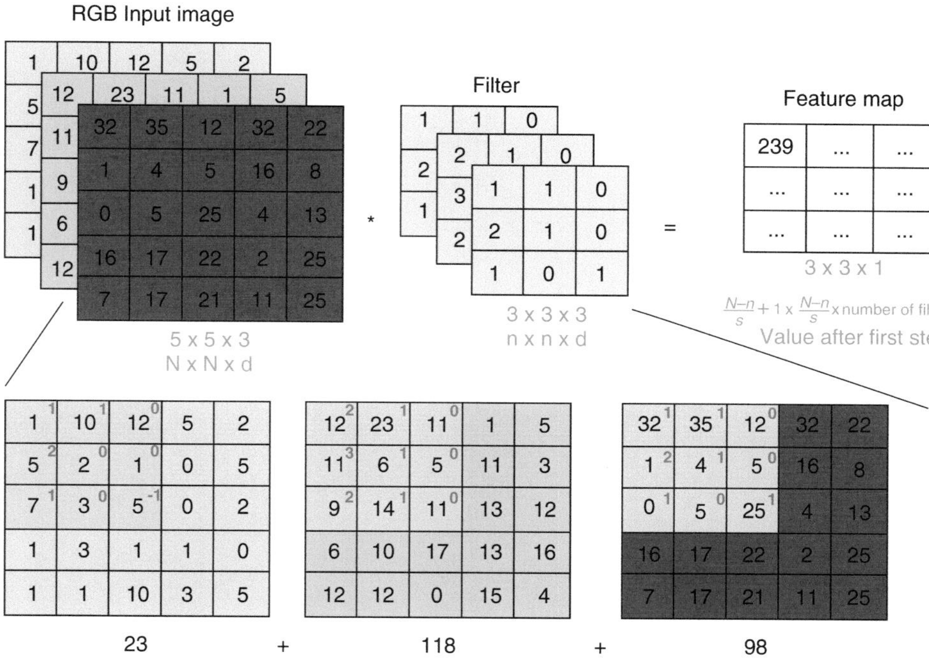

Fig. 26.21 Convolving over a volume (e.g., RGB image with three channels). This is a convolution operation over a volume, in this case stacked matrices of pixels in an RGB (red-green-blue) image. Shown here is the example of one filter, which should also be a volume with the same "depth" (d) as the input. The depth is also known as the "number of channels." Notice that the filter channels need not have the same values, but the overall filter can be thought of as extracting a certain feature from corresponding channels in the input. The filter channels are simultaneously overlapped over their corresponding input channels. As a result, a sum of element-wise products is produced in every channel, and the summed total would be the first value in the feature map. The remaining values are calculated by the same convolutional process described in the 2D input example, with the filters moving together simultaneously. Notice that the feature map has a size calculated by the same formula: $\frac{N-n}{s}+1$, but now the depth would equate to the number of filters. Here, only one filter of three dimensions was used, so the depth of the feature map is one. If an x number of three-dimensional filters were used to extract several features, then the feature map would have a depth of x

data can be preprocessed according to a certain window or sequence size to create input-output pairs (e.g., four successive values in the time series predicting the fifth value). The successive values can be fed to LSTM cells, and the output can be a single predicted value which is compared to the true value. Mean squared error can also be used as a loss function. Several LSTM layers can be stacked on top of each other in addition to using subsequent dense layers before the single predicted output. As with other neural networks, risk of overfitting increases as the network increases in depth. The initial time series does not require preprocessing in terms of seasonality since the LSTM is designed to capture that component during the modeling process.

Neural Networks: CNNs

CNNs can also be used in time series forecasting and are employed in similar fashion to NLP applications, whereby a one-dimensional sequence of values (in univariable cases) is taken as input to predict the next output. Like all algorithms used for forecasting, the data must be preprocessed into input-output pairs (e.g., using six successive values to predict the seventh value). As in NLP, the filters must have the same width as the input (width = 1 in a univariable time series). The filters convolve vertically over the time series input according to a stride value and feed the data forward into the network (Fig. 26.29). In time series forecasting, the output usually contains a linear activation function.

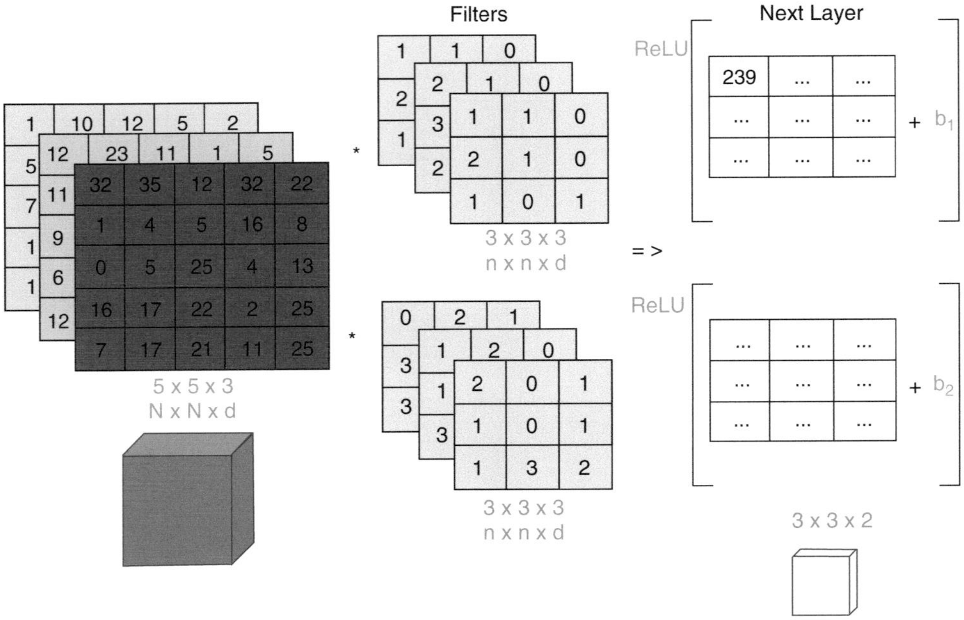

Fig. 26.22 CNN convolutional layer. First, a bias term (b_1) is added to all the values of the output from the first filter and then the resultant values are passed through a ReLU activation function for example. Another bias term (b_2) is added to the output values of the second filter followed by a ReLU activation. The resultant 3 × 3 × 2 volume represents the activation in the next layer. The values in the filters can be thought of as weights that are to be learned. The bias terms are the other parameters that need to be learned. In a hypothetical example involving 50 3 × 3 × 3 filters (for 50 features), the number of parameters to be learned would be: 3 × 3 × 3 × 50 + 50 = 1400. Notice that no matter how large the input image is, the number of parameters would remain the same (dependent on the number and size of filters), which is a favorable property of CNNs

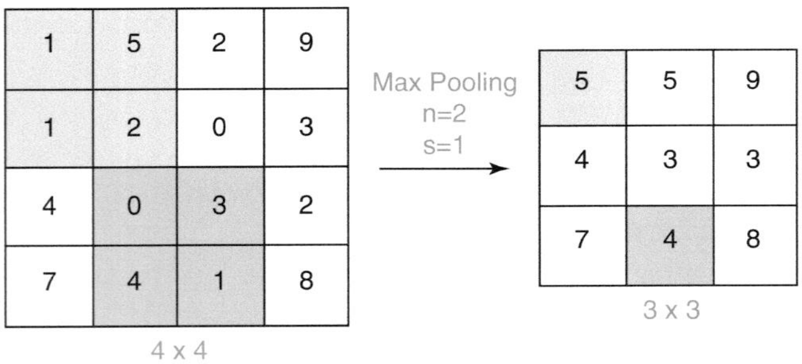

Fig. 26.23 Max pooling. Max pooling sequentially goes through a window of cells and selects out the maximum value. In this example, the hyperparameters are set to 2 × 2, 1-stride max pooling, so a 2 × 2 window overlaps sequentially over the input matrix and chooses the maximum value at every step. The first and eighth steps are colored in this example. The output dimensions are calculated using the same formula of convolution layers: $\frac{N-n+2p}{s}+1$

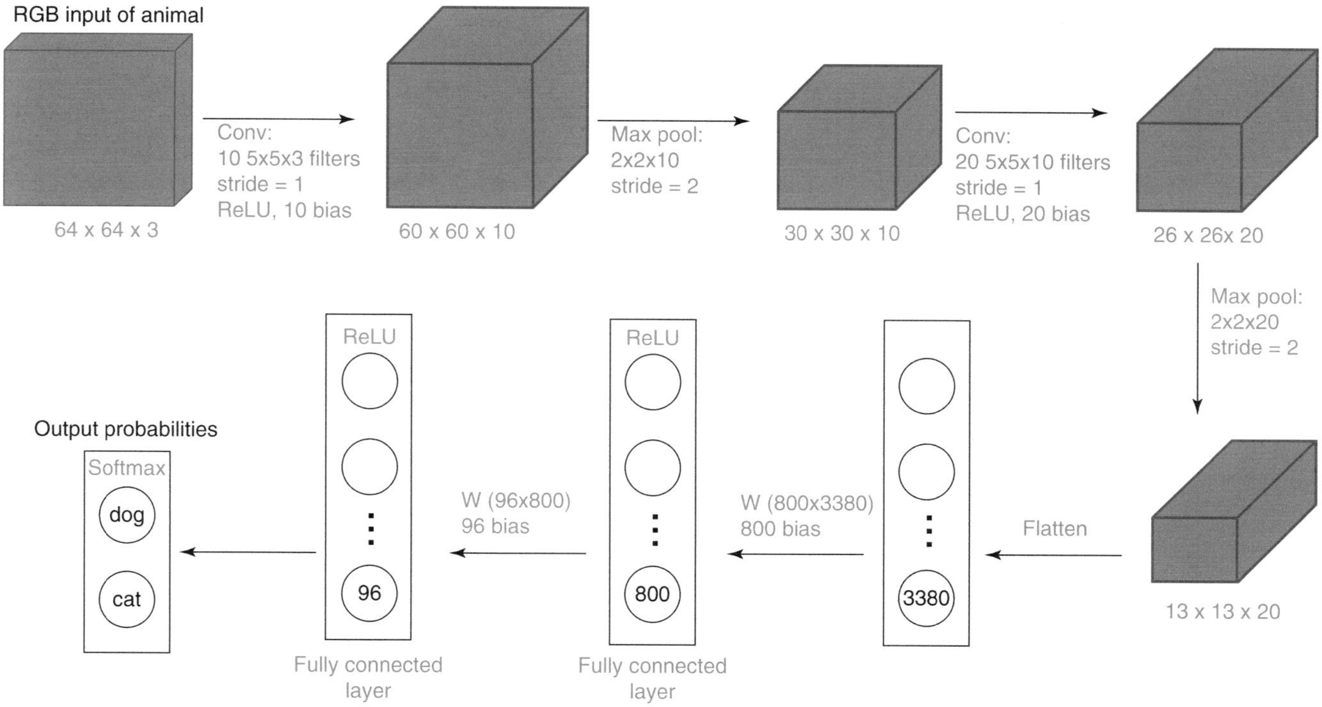

Fig. 26.24 Complete CNN architecture: example of predicting the class of an input image. Architecture usually consists of alternating convolution and pooling layers, after which the volume of features is flattened and fed through a series of fully connected layers

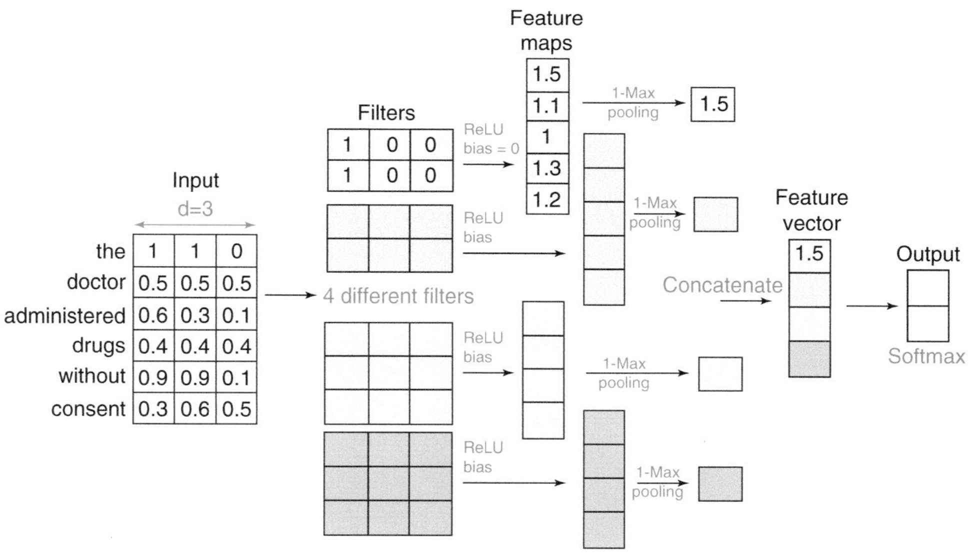

Fig. 26.25 Example of CNN as applied to NLP. In NLP, the input can be successive words encoded as word embedding vectors of size $d = 3$ for instance. The width of the filters should equate to the size of the word embedding because the embeddings constitute discrete symbols (i.e., words). Encoding information from partial embeddings across many words (e.g., 2 by 2 filter with stride 1 moving across the example input) would not work well. The filters hence start at the top of the input and compute the resultant sum of element-wise products; they then move downward by a stride value which is often set to 1. Example values are provided for the first filter to facilitate visualization. Activation functions, such as ReLU, and a bias are also added to the computation. Here, four different filters are used, some with a different length, to capture a variety of word relations (between nearby words for length = 2 and far away words for length = 3). Pooling provides the single highest value for every feature map, and the resultant values are concatenated into a feature vector. This is subsequently fed into an output layer through a matrix transformation

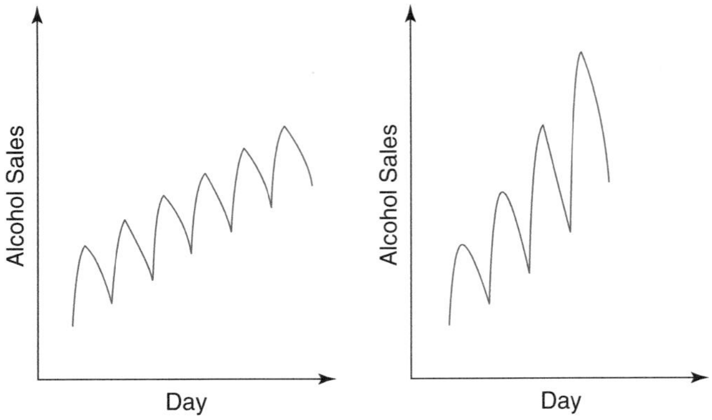

Fig. 26.26 Time series with an increasing trend and seasonal variation. Additive seasonality (left) versus multiplicative seasonality (right)

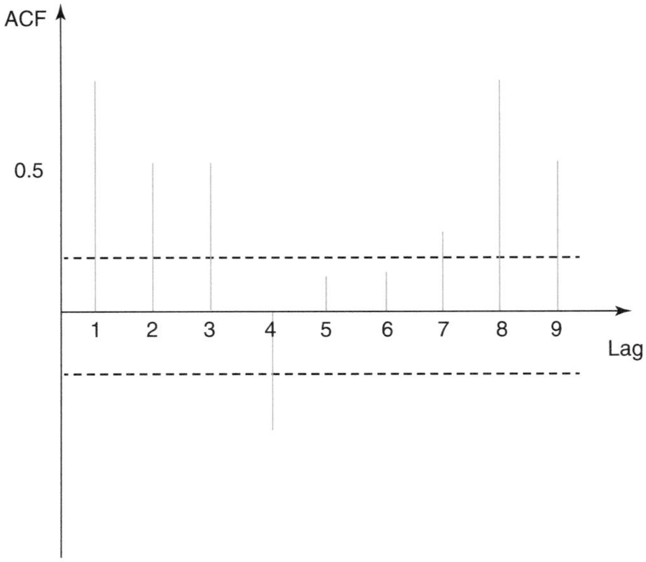

Fig. 26.27 Autocorrelation plot. Bars surpassing the threshold represent statistically significant autocorrelations. A negative autocorrelation is observed for lag value 4 (t vs. $t - 4$), and seasonality is evident every seven time-steps (e.g., 1 week if measurements are daily)

Table 26.4 Daily alcohol sales with lag variables

Day	Sales ($)	Lag-1 sales ($)	Lag-2 sales ($)	Lag-1 sales ($)
1	423.2	–	–	–
2	445.1	423.2	–	–
3	456.3	445.1	423.2	–
4	461.4	456.3	445.1	423.2
5	652.2	461.4	456.3	445.1
6	821.4	652.2	461.4	456.3
7	450.4	821.4	652.2	461.4
8	432.7	450.4	821.4	652.2

If the series has N periods, N lag variables can be created, but they will become successively shorter

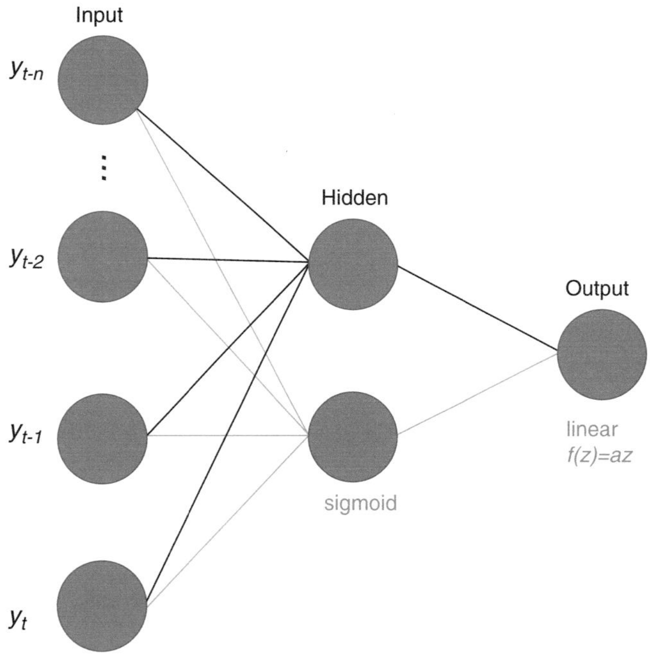

Fig. 26.28 Simplified multilayer perceptron with one hidden layer of two neurons applied to time series forecasting. The input consists of a series of consecutive values, and the hidden layer consists of an activation function such as sigmoid or ReLU. The output layer is a single neuron with a linear activation function that outputs the next predicted value (e.g., $452.1 predicted alcohol sales on the next day). The discrepancy between predicted values and the actual values is modeled with a loss function, suitable for the prediction of continuous variables (e.g., mean squared error), which is minimized by learning the parameters (weights and bias terms) of the model

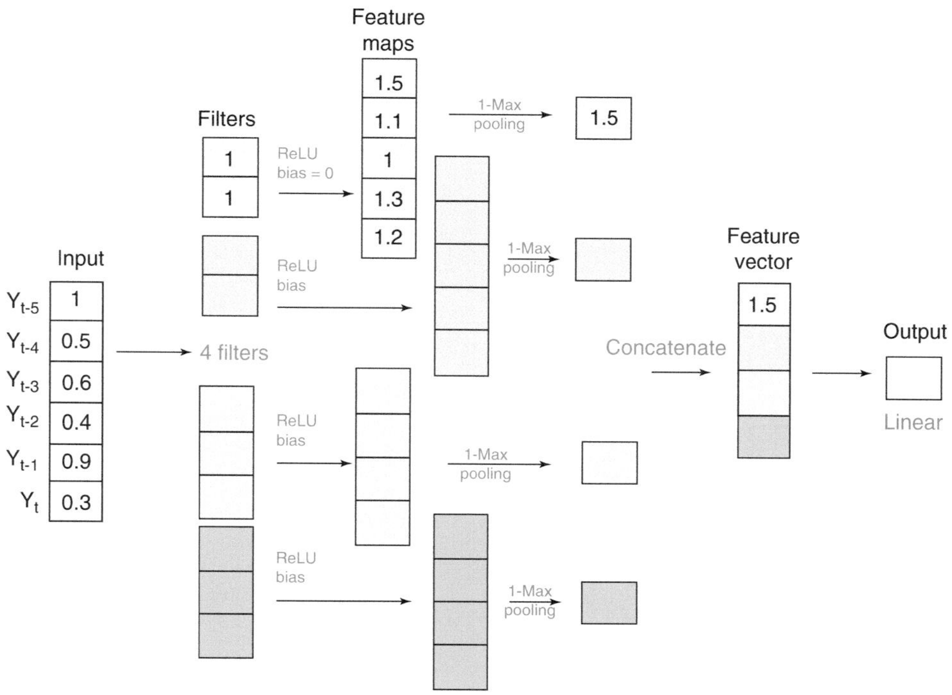

Fig. 26.29 Example of CNN as applied to time series forecasting. As in NLP, the width of the filters should equate to the size of the input (e.g., width = 1 in a univariable time series). The filters hence start at the top of the input and compute the resultant sum of element-wise products; they then move downward by a stride value which is often set to 1. Example values are provided for the first filter to facilitate visualization. In this example, six successive values in the sequence are used to predict the seventh value. Activation functions, such as ReLU, and a bias are also added to the computation. Here, four different filters are used, some with a different length. Pooling provides the single highest value for every feature map, and the resultant values are concatenated into a feature vector. This is subsequently fed into an output layer through a matrix transformation

26.4 Conclusion

A host of machine learning algorithms have been used to perform several different tasks in NLP and TSA. Prior to implementing these algorithms, some degree of data preprocessing is required. Deep learning approaches utilizing multilayer perceptrons, RNNs, and CNNs represent commonly used techniques. In supervised learning applications, all these models map inputs into a predicted output and then model the discrepancy between predicted values and the real output according to a loss function. The parameters of the mapping function are then optimized through the process of gradient descent and backward propagation in order to minimize this loss. This is the main premise behind many supervised learning algorithms. As experience with these algorithms grows, increased applications in the fields of medicine and neuroscience are anticipated.

Acknowledgments None.

Funding None.

Disclosure of Funding None.

Financial Disclosure The authors received no financial support for the research, authorship, and/or publication of this chapter.

Conflict of Interest The authors have no conflicts of interest to disclose.

References

1. Beard E, Marsden J, Brown J, Tombor I, Stapleton J, Michie S, West R. Understanding and using time series analyses in addiction research. Addiction. 2019;114(10):1866–84.
2. Chen X, Xie H, Wang FL, Liu Z, Xu J, Hao T. A bibliometric analysis of natural language processing in medical research. BMC Med Inform Decis Mak. 2018;18(1):14.
3. Cambria E, White B. Jumping NLP curves: a review of natural language processing research. IEEE Comput Intell Mag. 2014;9(2):48–57.
4. Yim W-W, Yetisgen M, Harris WP, Kwan SW. Natural language processing in oncology: a review. JAMA Oncol. 2016;2(6):797–804.
5. Nadkarni PM, Ohno-Machado L, Chapman WW. Natural language processing: an introduction. J Am Med Inform Assoc. 2011;18(5):544–51.

6. Wang H, Preston SH. Forecasting United States mortality using cohort smoking histories. Proc Natl Acad Sci U S A. 2009;106(2):393–8.
7. Porter MF. An algorithm for suffix stripping. Program. 1980;14(3):130–7.
8. Bird S. NLTK: the natural language toolkit. In: Proceedings of the COLING/ACL 2006 Interactive Presentation Sessions. Sydney: Associaton for Computational Linguistics; 2006. p. 69–72.
9. Liu H, Christiansen T, Baumgartner WA Jr, Verspoor K. BioLemmatizer: a lemmatization tool for morphological processing of biomedical text. J Biomed Semantics. 2012;3:3.
10. Senders JT, Karhade AV, Cote DJ, et al. Natural language processing for automated quantification of brain metastases reported in free-text radiology reports. JCO Clin Cancer Informatics. 2019;3:1–9.
11. Zech J, Pain M, Titano J, Badgeley M, Schefflein J, Su A, Costa A, Bederson J, Lehar J, Oermann EK. Natural language-based machine learning models for the annotation of clinical radiology reports. Radiology. 2018;287(2):570–80.
12. Mikolov T, Chen K, Corrado G, Dean J. Efficient estimation of word representations in vector space. arXiv Prepr. arXiv1301.3781; 2013.
13. Pennington J, Socher R, Manning CD. Glove: global vectors for word representation. In: Proceedings of 2014 conferences on empirical methods in natural language processing; 2014. p. 1532–43.
14. Khattak FK, Jeblee S, Pou-Prom C, Abdalla M, Meaney C, Rudzicz F. A survey of word embeddings for clinical text. J Biomed Informatics X. 2019;4:100057.
15. Chowdhury S, Dong X, Qian L, Li X, Guan Y, Yang J, Yu Q. A multitask bi-directional RNN model for named entity recognition on Chinese electronic medical records. BMC Bioinformatics. 2018;19(17):499.
16. Cho K, Van Merriënboer B, Bahdanau D, Bengio Y. On the properties of neural machine translation: encoder-decoder approaches. arXiv Prepr. arXiv1409.1259; 2014.
17. Chung J, Gulcehre C, Cho K, Bengio Y. Empirical evaluation of gated recurrent neural networks on sequence modeling. arXiv Prepr. arXiv1412.3555; 2014.
18. Hochreiter S, Schmidhuber J. Long short-term memory. Neural Comput. 1997;9(8):1735–80.
19. Gers FA, Schmidhuber J. Recurrent nets that time and count. In: Proceedings of IEEE-INNS-ENNS international joint conference on neural networks. IJCNN 2000. Neural computing. New challenges and perspectives new millennium, vol. 3; 2000. p. 189–94.
20. LeCun Y, Bottou L, Bengio Y, Haffner P. Gradient-based learning applied to document recognition. Proc IEEE. 1998;86(11):2278–324.
21. Kim Y. Convolutional neural networks for sentence classification. arXiv Prepr. arXiv1408.5882; 2014.
22. Zhang GP. Neural networks in business forecasting. Hershey: IGI Global; 2004.

Part IV

Ethical and Historical Aspects of Machine Learning in Medicine

A Brief History of Machine Learning in Neurosurgery

27

Andrew T. Schilling, Pavan P. Shah, James Feghali, Adrian E. Jimenez, and Tej D. Azad

Abbreviations

ANN	Artificial neural network
CNN	Convolutional neural network
CT	Computed tomography
FCM	Fuzzy c-means
ML	Machine learning
MRI	Magnetic resonance imaging
N^2QOD	National Neurosurgery Quality and Outcome Database
NIS	National Inpatient Sample
NLP	Natural language processing

27.1 Introduction

Machine learning (ML) is a subfield of artificial intelligence that involves algorithms which can dynamically learn from data to make predictions or decisions. The promise of ML is algorithms capable of automated self-improvement without the need for iterative programming [1]. Ideally, this enables the algorithms to accommodate for complexity in data or prediction beyond human comprehension [2]. These algorithms are typically trained on sample data before deployment. Broadly, ML can be categorized as supervised learning, unsupervised learning, or reinforcement learning according to the feedback provided throughout training. The data analyzed can be structured, like a tabular database, or unstructured, such as clinical imaging or an electronic health record. ML algorithms typically perform as a function of the scale of their training dataset; large and rich training data is likely to yield a more robust algorithm [3]. While ML is increasingly part of modern applications, its role within medicine and neurosurgery continues to evolve [4]. Clinical neurosurgery encompasses a highly diverse set of disease processes, inspiring the development of a variety of unique ML applications for clinical prediction, diagnosis, and prognosis. Here, we present a brief history of the use of machine learning in neurosurgery over the past three decades, highlighting contemporary applications and the near future.

27.2 The Evolution of Machine Learning in Neurosurgery

1990s: Early Applications in Neurosurgery

It is well-appreciated that the principles underlying machine learning emerged from early attempts by physiologists and mathematicians to model the brain [5]. Donald O. Hebb's discoveries in the field of neural plasticity were soon implemented in silico [6, 7]. The origins of neural networks date back to foundational efforts by Frank Rosenblatt in the 1950s to create the perceptron, an algorithm designed for image recognition inspired by the natural organization of neurons [8, 9]. While many fields benefited from these neurologically-informed advancements in computing over the subsequent decades, the initial application of machine learning in neurosurgery began in the 1990s. Throughout this decade, clinical prediction and preoperative planning were the predominant applications of machine learning [10]. Commonly, these tasks were examples of supervised learning as researchers began pitting computers against radiologists and neurosurgeons in mock battles of clinical decision-making [1].

Early endeavors to apply ML to unstructured data in neurosurgery were met with modest success. Researchers commonly compared artificial neural networks (ANN) to the performance of clinicians on a variety of image identification tasks. An early proof-of-concept emerged in 1992 when

Andrew T. Schilling and Pavan P. Shah contributed equally with all other contributors.

A. T. Schilling · P. P. Shah · J. Feghali · A. E. Jimenez
T. D. Azad (✉)
Department of Neurosurgery, Johns Hopkins University School of Medicine, Baltimore, MD, USA
e-mail: tazad1@jhmi.edu

V. E. Staartjes et al. (eds.), *Machine Learning in Clinical Neuroscience*, Acta Neurochirurgica Supplement 134,
https://doi.org/10.1007/978-3-030-85292-4_27

Floyd et al. demonstrated that an ANN could outperform human observers at detecting circular lesions in simulated single-photon emission computed tomography images [11]. However, this signal detection task was conducted using computer-generated images with significant noise, meant to resemble a brain or liver lesion. A few years later, machine learning was explored more broadly on neurosurgical clinical imaging. In 1995, Christy et al. developed a neural network developed for grading supratentorial astrocytomas [12]. The study compared feature detection in magnetic resonance imaging (MRI). The neural network correctly distinguished between high- and low-grade tumors with an accuracy of 61% relative to a 57% for a neuroradiologist, though this modest improvement did not reach statistical significance. By the end of the decade, researchers developed ANNs that could outperform clinical experts at glioma grading from MRIs [13]. Forays into unsupervised machine learning methods such as fuzzy c-means (FCM) clustering for tumor volume estimation on MRI similarly yielded similarly promising results [14].

2000s: Refinement and Expansion

After the potential for machine learning in neurosurgery was first widely demonstrated in the 1990s, incremental advancements were steadily made in the 2000s. Neurosurgical publications featuring machine learning rose from 3–4 per year in 2000–2001 to 12–13 per year by the end of the decade [10]. The role of unsupervised learning in brain tumor detection and segmentation was further developed. FCM algorithms continued to outperform clinical experts at glioma segmentation [15]. With the success of tumor detection and segmentation using MRI, machine learning was subsequently applied to the radiologic diagnosis of brain tumors. Several ANNs outperformed radiologists at distinguishing between the imaging characteristics of various intra-axial cerebral tumors, pediatric posterior fossa tumors, and suprasellar masses on MRI [16–18]. Additional machine learning algorithms were also introduced in the neurosurgical literature throughout this time including support vector machines and naïve Bayes classifiers [19]. Notably, the use of ML for outcome prediction in neurosurgery was largely neglected in this decade [10].

Furthermore, the stage was set in the 2000s for the advent of "big data." With the passage of legislation such as Health Information Technology for Economic and Clinical Health Act in 2009, the American medical industry saw a paradigm shift from paper records to electronic health records [20]. Interest in "big data" rapidly grew, as these electronic health records enabled clinicians to search and process clinical data at a larger scale than before. This trend, along with a growing awareness and interest in machine learning among medical researchers, led to a marked increase in the application of ML within neurosurgery that defined the subsequent decade [1].

2010s: Exponential Growth and Adoption of Machine Learning

Around the start of the 2010s, ML began to see explosive growth within the neurosurgical community. This coincided with the rapid expansion of both structured and unstructured data throughout medicine secondary to the widespread adoption of electronic health records [21]. Databases, such as the National Inpatient Sample (NIS) and the National Neurosurgery Quality and Outcome Database (N^2QOD), increased access to large-scale neurosurgical datasets [22]. The number of neurosurgery ML publications rose from less than 15 per year in 2010–2011 to greater than 40 per year in 2015–2016, and by the end of this period ML was being applied to all stages of neurosurgical care: preoperative planning, intraoperative guidance, postoperative outcome prediction, and neurophysiological monitoring [10]. By the end of the decade, one survey study of neurosurgeons demonstrated that 28.5% of respondents were utilizing ML in their clinical practice, and 31.1% in their research [23].

As the initial excitement surrounding ML led to widespread utilization, it became evident that certain applications of ML algorithms would be more successful than others. For example, ML proved to be particularly effective at analyzing unstructured data, as these data sources often contain valuable information that is difficult to characterize using traditional statistical methods. A majority of these efforts were directed toward clinical imaging, but other applications included interpretation of electroencephalography and free-text clinical notes [10]. ML studies demonstrated promising results for a variety of clinical tasks, including preoperative characterization of lesions on imaging [24, 25]. intraoperative classification of tumors [26], and advanced prediction of epileptic seizures based on EEG signals [27]. The development of deep learning algorithms led to unprecedented breakthroughs in machine vision when provided with large training datasets [28]. On the other hand, the application of ML to structured data forms, such as tabular data regarding clinical features and patient outcomes, generated mixed results. Although some studies demonstrated that ML outperformed traditional statistical modeling for clinical outcome prediction [29–31], a multitude of other neurosurgical publications found no difference between ML and regression modeling [32–34]. Toward the end of the decade, critical analysis of ML performance was also garnering attention in the greater medical literature. One systematic review across multiple specialties even demonstrated that there was no overall difference between ML and logistic regression model performance for binary outcomes [35].

Overall, this decade saw a great increase in the awareness and utilization of ML in neurosurgical research and clinical practice. As seen with many new technologies, the use of ML within neurosurgery followed a trajectory well-characterized by the Gartner Hype Cycle; initial excitement resulted in extensive utilization, which was followed by a critical analysis of the capabilities of the technology and its appropriate use [36]. While ML can offer powerful advantages over traditional statistics in certain scenarios, care must be taken in selecting the appropriate applications for ML.

27.3 Contemporary and Novel Applications

In recent years, there has been a surge of new machine learning implementations seeking to address challenging questions within neurosurgery. In this section, we highlight a group of studies that appropriately apply ML to derive clinically meaningful data from generally imperceptible patterns and features.

ML has demonstrated promise in brain tumor management through a wide variety of applications. Current clinical workflows for neurosurgical tumor care require multiple imaging studies for surgical planning and follow-up. These studies provide a rich source of data to which ML can readily be applied to gain clinically valuable information. For instance, several studies have applied ML to cranial imaging for tumor diagnosis and characterization as well as glioma grading [15, 17, 18, 37, 38], and some have demonstrated similar or better diagnostic performance when directly compared to radiologists [37, 38]. Notably, two of the studies that evaluated radiologists assisted by ML versus radiologists alone both demonstrated a significant improvement in classification of intracranial tumors when aided by ML [17, 18]. This shift from ML-versus-clinician to ML-plus-clinician will be crucial in future research, as initial clinical implementation is more likely to follow the latter framework [39].

Additional applications of ML to brain tumor imaging highlight its ability to derive clinically meaningful data from features that are not easily discernible by visual inspection. One common phenomenon that often complicates neurosurgical tumor care is pseudoprogression of brain tumors after treatment with stereotactic radiosurgery. Pseudoprogression is simply a sequela of radiosurgical treatment involving tumor necrosis, inflammation, and vascular injury, but it is often visually indistinguishable from true tumor progression on follow-up magnetic resonance imaging. Thus, the current gold standard for differentiating pseudoprogression from true progression is pathologic examination. However, researchers have demonstrated that ML models hold promise for differentiating pseudoprogression from true tumor progression for both brain metastases and glioblastoma [40, 41].

Another neurosurgical question that has been difficult to resolve with conventional imaging interpretation is peritumoral glioblastoma invasion. It is well known that glioblastoma extends beyond visible enhancing tumor on MRI, but it has been extremely difficult to differentiate infiltrating tumor from vasogenic edema in the peritumoral region on imaging. One study by Akbari et al. demonstrated that ML algorithms applied to multiparametric MRI images were able to estimate the extent of tumor infiltration and even predict locations of future tumor recurrence [42]. This novel application of ML demonstrates how future integration into clinical workflows may improve preoperative tumor targeting by informing boundaries for supratotal tumor resection.

Intraoperatively, ML promises to dramatically alter surgical workflow through the real-time diagnosis of brain tumors. When compared to pathologist-confirmed histology, deep convolutional neural networks (CNNs) predicted brain tumor diagnosis using stimulated Raman histology with commensurate accuracy in under 150 s [43]. Finally, ML algorithms have also demonstrated promise in predicting molecular subtype and even survival for glioblastoma patients based on complex radiographic patterns [44]. Overall, novel applications of ML modeling to neurosurgical tumor management have shown how the technology has the potential to advance each stage of care, from initial diagnosis to long-term outcomes.

While the above examples illustrate the utility of ML in brain tumor management, ML has also been applied within a variety of other neurosurgical domains. For neurosurgical emergencies such as stroke, hemorrhage, and hydrocephalus, time to diagnosis and treatment has a drastic impact on treatment success and patient outcomes. One study demonstrated that a three-dimensional convolutional neural network was able to accurately screen computed tomography (CT) head imaging for acute neurological illnesses and reduce time to diagnosis from minutes to seconds in a randomized, double-blinded, prospective trial [45]. Within the field of spine surgery, ML models have been developed for automated spine segmentation for computer-assisted surgery and automated detection of vertebral body compression fractures on CT imaging [46, 47]. Functional neurosurgeons have utilized ML to predict treatment outcomes for patients undergoing surgical treatment for epilepsy based on perioperative brain imaging, demonstrating how ML can aid clinical decision-making by identifying which patients are most likely to benefit from surgical intervention [48–50].

Although the majority of ML research thus far within neurosurgery has been related to image analysis, additional studies have also demonstrated its effectiveness with other unstructured data sources. ML has also demonstrated promise in rudimentary EEG analysis, such as differentiating normal from abnormal signals and detecting epileptic seizures [51–54]. Natural language processing (NLP) has been applied to clinical notes to extract key information from unstructured text, such as identifying incidental durotomies in spine surgery and extracting key radiographic variables from radiology reports [55–57]. These initial applications demonstrate how NLP is a powerful way for clinicians to quickly and accurately extract data from notes, and its promise as a potential tool for retrospective analysis of key clinical outcomes.

Despite the success of novel ML applications within neurosurgical research, significant barriers remain to its widespread clinical implementation. Many ML models are mechanistically impossible to interpret, and thus referred to as "black box" models. While they can still be assessed based on their output, the lack of comprehensible information regarding how the model derived that output may cause reluctance in implementation [58, 59]. Furthermore, ML models are highly dependent on the quantity and quality of data they are trained on and applied to, which can further limit generalizability and reproducibility [60]. This means that (1) ML models may underperform in real world applications, as research data may be of higher quality and (2) large training data sets will be essential to advanced ML modeling. Current access to patient data across institutions and regions remains quite limited. While considerable challenges still impede the widespread clinical adoption of ML, recent studies detailing novel applications of ML within neurosurgery demonstrate how proper development and deployment has the potential to shift the paradigm of both clinical research and patient care.

27.4 Conclusion

The rapid growth of machine learning in neurosurgery over the past three decades has been catalyzed by the digitization of medicine and the democratization of data science tools. While the benefit of machine learning may be comparable to conventional regression techniques when analyzing structured data, it offers an unprecedented potential to revolutionize the analysis of unstructured data. Amidst the quantitative expansion of machine learning in neurosurgery, there is an increased need for qualitative improvement and judicious deployment thereof.

Financial Disclosure The authors received no financial support for the research, authorship, and/or publication of this article.

References

1. Jordan MI, Mitchell TM. Machine learning: trends, perspectives, and prospects. Science. 2015;349(6245):255–60.
2. Obermeyer Z, Emanuel EJ. Predicting the future—big data, machine learning, and clinical medicine. N Engl J Med. 2016;375(13):1216.
3. Yu K-H, Beam AL, Kohane IS. Artificial intelligence in healthcare. Nat Biomed Eng. 2018;2(10):719–31.
4. Beam AL, Kohane IS. Big data and machine learning in health care. JAMA. 2018;319(13):1317–8.
5. McCulloch WS, Pitts W. A logical calculus of the ideas immanent in nervous activity. Bull Math Biophys. 1943;5(4):115–33.
6. Farley B, Clark W. Simulation of self-organizing systems by digital computer. Trans IRE Prof Group Inf Theory. 1954;4(4):76–84.
7. Hebb DO. The organization of behavior: a neuropsychological theory. London: Wiley; Chapman & Hall; 1949.
8. Kononenko I. Machine learning for medical diagnosis: history, state of the art and perspective. Artif Intell Med. 2001;23(1):89–109.
9. Rosenblatt F. The perceptron: a probabilistic model for information storage and organization in the brain. Psychol Rev. 1958;65(6):386.
10. Senders JT, Zaki MM, Karhade AV, Chang B, Gormley WB, Broekman ML, Smith TR, Arnaout O. An introduction and overview of machine learning in neurosurgical care. Acta Neurochir. 2018;160(1):29–38.
11. Floyd CE Jr, Tourassi GD. An artificial neural network for lesion detection on single-photon emission computed tomographic images. Investig Radiol. 1992;27(9):667–72.
12. Christy PS, Tervonen O, Scheithauer BW, Forbes GS. Use of a neural network and a multiple regression model to predict histologic grade of astrocytoma from MRI appearances. Neuroradiology. 1995;37(2):89–93.
13. Abdolmaleki P, Mihara F, Masuda K, Buadu LD. Neural networks analysis of astrocytic gliomas from MRI appearances. Cancer Lett. 1997;118(1):69–78.
14. Clarke LP, Velthuizen RP, Clark M, Gaviria J, Hall L, Goldgof D, Murtagh R, Phuphanich S, Brem S. MRI measurement of brain tumor response: comparison of visual metric and automatic segmentation. Magn Reson Imaging. 1998;16(3):271–9.
15. Emblem KE, Nedregaard B, Hald JK, Nome T, Due-Tonnessen P, Bjornerud A. Automatic glioma characterization from dynamic susceptibility contrast imaging: brain tumor segmentation using knowledge-based fuzzy clustering. J Magn Reson Imaging. 2009;30(1):1–10.
16. Bidiwala S, Pittman T. Neural network classification of pediatric posterior fossa tumors using clinical and imaging data. Pediatr Neurosurg. 2004;40(1):8–15.
17. Kitajima M, Hirai T, Katsuragawa S, Okuda T, Fukuoka H, Sasao A, Akter M, Awai K, Nakayama Y, Ikeda R. Differentiation of common large Sellar-Suprasellar masses: effect of artificial neural network on radiologists' diagnosis performance. Acad Radiol. 2009;16(3):313–20.
18. Yamashita K, Yoshiura T, Arimura H, Mihara F, Noguchi T, Hiwatashi A, Togao O, Yamashita Y, Shono T, Kumazawa S. Performance evaluation of radiologists with artificial neural network for differential diagnosis of intra-axial cerebral tumors on MR images. Am J Neuroradiol. 2008;29(6):1153–8.
19. Buchlak QD, Esmaili N, Leveque J-C, Farrokhi F, Bennett C, Piccardi M, Sethi RK. Machine learning applications to clinical decision support in neurosurgery: an artificial intelligence augmented systematic review. Neurosurg Rev. 2020;43:1235–53.
20. Adler-Milstein J, Jha AK. HITECH Act drove large gains in hospital electronic health record adoption. Health Aff. 2017;36(8):1416–22.
21. Raju B, Jumah F, Ashraf O, Narayan V, Gupta G, Sun H, Hilden P, Nanda A. Big data, machine learning, and artificial intelligence: a field guide for neurosurgeons. J Neurosurg. 2020;1(aop):1–11.
22. McGirt MJ, Speroff T, Dittus RS, Harrell FE, Asher AL. The National Neurosurgery Quality and Outcomes Database (N2QOD): general overview and pilot-year project description. Neurosurg Focus. 2013;34(1):E6.
23. Staartjes VE, Stumpo V, Kernbach JM, Klukowska AM, Gadjradj PS, Schröder ML, Veeravagu A, Stienen MN, van Niftrik CHB,

Serra C, Regli L. Machine learning in neurosurgery: a global survey. Acta Neurochir. 2020;162:3081–91.
24. Akbari H, Macyszyn L, Da X, Wolf RL, Bilello M, Verma R, O'Rourke DM, Davatzikos C. Pattern analysis of dynamic susceptibility contrast-enhanced MR imaging demonstrates Peritumoral tissue heterogeneity. Radiology. 2014;273(2):502–10.
25. Juan-Albarracín J, Fuster-Garcia E, Manjon JV, Robles M, Aparici F, Martí-Bonmatí L, Garcia-Gomez JM. Automated glioblastoma segmentation based on a multiparametric structured unsupervised classification. PLoS One. 2015;10(5):e0125143.
26. Eberlin LS, Norton I, Dill AL, Golby AJ, Ligon KL, Santagata S, Cooks RG, Agar NYR. Classifying human brain tumors by lipid imaging with mass spectrometry. Cancer Res. 2012;72(3):645–54.
27. Moghim N, Corne DW. Predicting epileptic seizures in advance. PLoS One. 2014;9(6):e99334.
28. Zhou M, Scott J, Chaudhury B, Hall L, Goldgof D, Yeom KW, Iv M, Ou Y, Kalpathy-Cramer J, Napel S. Radiomics in brain tumor: image assessment, quantitative feature descriptors, and machine-learning approaches. Am J Neuroradiol. 2018;39(2):208–16.
29. Karhade AV, Ahmed AK, Pennington Z, Chara A, Schilling A, Thio QCBS, Ogink PT, Sciubba DM, Schwab JH. External validation of the SORG 90-day and 1-year machine learning algorithms for survival in spinal metastatic disease. Spine J. 2020;20:14–21. https://doi.org/10.1016/j.spinee.2019.09.003.
30. Oermann EK, Kress M-AS, Collins BT, Collins SP, Morris D, Ahalt SC, Ewend MG. Predicting survival in patients with brain metastases treated with radiosurgery using artificial neural networks. Neurosurgery. 2013;72(6):944–52.
31. Rughani AI, Dumont TM, Lu Z, Bongard J, Horgan MA, Penar PL, Tranmer BI. Use of an artificial neural network to predict head injury outcome. J Neurosurg. 2010;113(3):585–90.
32. Gravesteijn BY, Nieboer D, Ercole A, Lingsma HF, Nelson D, Van Calster B, Steyerberg EW, Åkerlund C, Amrein K, Andelic N. Machine learning algorithms performed no better than regression models for prognostication in traumatic brain injury. J Clin Epidemiol. 2020;122:95.
33. Van Os HJA, Ramos LA, Hilbert A, Van Leeuwen M, van Walderveen MAA, Kruyt ND, Dippel DWJ, Steyerberg EW, van der Schaaf IC, Lingsma HF. Predicting outcome of endovascular treatment for acute ischemic stroke: potential value of machine learning algorithms. Front Neurol. 2018;9:784.
34. Panesar SS, D'Souza RN, Yeh F-C, Fernandez-Miranda JC. Machine learning versus logistic regression methods for 2-year mortality prognostication in a small, heterogeneous glioma database. World Neurosurg X. 2019;2:100012.
35. Christodoulou E, Ma J, Collins GS, Steyerberg EW, Verbakel JY, Van Calster B. A systematic review shows no performance benefit of machine learning over logistic regression for clinical prediction models. J Clin Epidemiol. 2019;110:12–22.
36. Chen JH, Asch SM. Machine learning and prediction in medicine—beyond the peak of inflated expectations. N Engl J Med. 2017;376(26):2507.
37. Juntu J, Sijbers J, De Backer S, Rajan J, Van Dyck D. Machine learning study of several classifiers trained with texture analysis features to differentiate benign from malignant soft-tissue tumors in T1-MRI images. J Magn Reson Imaging. 2010;31(3):680–9.
38. Rauschecker AM, Rudie JD, Xie L, et al. Artificial intelligence system approaching neuroradiologist-level differential diagnosis accuracy at brain MRI. Radiology. 2020;295(3):626–37.
39. Senders JT, Arnaout O, Karhade AV, Dasenbrock HH, Gormley WB, Broekman ML, Smith TR. Natural and artificial intelligence in neurosurgery: a systematic review. Neurosurgery. 2018;83(2):181–92.
40. Akbari H, Rathore S, Bakas S, et al. Histopathology-validated machine learning radiographic biomarker for noninvasive discrimination between true progression and pseudo-progression in glioblastoma. Cancer. 2020;126(11):2625–36.
41. Peng L, Parekh V, Huang P, et al. Distinguishing true progression from radionecrosis after stereotactic radiation therapy for brain metastases with machine learning and Radiomics. Int J Radiat Oncol. 2018;102(4):1236–43.
42. Akbari H, Macyszyn L, Da X, Bilello M, Wolf RL, Martinez-Lage M, Biros G, Alonso-Basanta M, O'Rourke DM, Davatzikos C. Imaging surrogates of infiltration obtained via multiparametric imaging pattern analysis predict subsequent location of recurrence of glioblastoma. Neurosurgery. 2016;78(4):572–80.
43. Hollon TC, Pandian B, Adapa AR, Urias E, Save AV, Khalsa SSS, Eichberg DG, D'Amico RS, Farooq ZU, Lewis S. Near real-time intraoperative brain tumor diagnosis using stimulated Raman histology and deep neural networks. Nat Med. 2020;26(1):52–8.
44. Macyszyn L, Akbari H, Pisapia JM, Da X, Attiah M, Pigrish V, Bi Y, Pal S, Davuluri RV, Roccograndi L. Imaging patterns predict patient survival and molecular subtype in glioblastoma via machine learning techniques. Neuro-Oncology. 2015;18(3):417–25.
45. Titano JJ, Badgeley M, Schefflein J, Pain M, Su A, Cai M, Swinburne N, Zech J, Kim J, Bederson J. Automated deep-neural-network surveillance of cranial images for acute neurologic events. Nat Med. 2018;24(9):1337–41.
46. Burns JE, Yao J, Summers RM. Vertebral body compression fractures and bone density: automated detection and classification on CT images. Radiology. 2017;284(3):788–97.
47. Vania M, Mureja D, Lee D. Automatic spine segmentation from CT images using convolutional neural network via redundant generation of class labels. J Comput Des Eng. 2019;6(2):224–32.
48. Gleichgerrcht E, Munsell B, Bhatia S, Vandergrift WA III, Rorden C, McDonald C, Edwards J, Kuzniecky R, Bonilha L. Deep learning applied to whole-brain connectome to determine seizure control after epilepsy surgery. Epilepsia. 2018;59(9):1643–54.
49. Munsell BC, Wee C-Y, Keller SS, Weber B, Elger C, da Silva LAT, Nesland T, Styner M, Shen D, Bonilha L. Evaluation of machine learning algorithms for treatment outcome prediction in patients with epilepsy based on structural connectome data. NeuroImage. 2015;118:219–30.
50. Taylor PN, Sinha N, Wang Y, Vos SB, de Tisi J, Miserocchi A, McEvoy AW, Winston GP, Duncan JS. The impact of epilepsy surgery on the structural connectome and its relation to outcome. NeuroImage Clin. 2018;18:202–14.
51. Gemein LAW, Schirrmeister RT, Chrabąszcz P, Wilson D, Boedecker J, Schulze-Bonhage A, Hutter F, Ball T. Machine-learning-based diagnostics of EEG pathology. NeuroImage. 2020;220:117021.
52. van Leeuwen KG, Sun H, Tabaeizadeh M, Struck AF, van Putten MJA, Westover MB. Detecting abnormal electroencephalograms using deep convolutional networks. Clin Neurophysiol. 2019;130(1):77–84.
53. Roy S, Kiral-Kornek I, Harrer S. ChronoNet: a deep recurrent neural network for abnormal EEG identification. In: Conference on artificial intelligence in medicine, Europe. Cham: Springer; 2019. p. 47–56.
54. Siddiqui MK, Morales-Menendez R, Huang X, Hussain N. A review of epileptic seizure detection using machine learning classifiers. Brain Informatics. 2020;7(1):1–18.
55. Ehresman J, Pennington Z, Karhade AV, et al. Incidental durotomy: predictive risk model and external validation of natural language process identification algorithm. J Neurosurg Spine. 2020;33(3):342–8.
56. Karhade AV, Bongers MER, Groot OQ, Kazarian ER, Cha TD, Fogel HA, Hershman SH, Tobert DG, Schoenfeld AJ, Bono CM. Natural language processing for automated detection of incidental durotomy. Spine J. 2020;20(5):695–700.

57. Senders JT, Cho LD, Calvachi P, McNulty JJ, Ashby JL, Schulte IS, Almekkawi AK, Mehrtash A, Gormley WB, Smith TR. Automating clinical chart review: an open-source natural language processing pipeline developed on free-text radiology reports from patients with glioblastoma. JCO Clin Cancer Informatics. 2020;4:25–34.
58. Shortliffe EH, Sepúlveda MJ. Clinical decision support in the era of artificial intelligence. JAMA. 2018;320(21):2199–200.
59. Vayena E, Blasimme A, Cohen IG. Machine learning in medicine: addressing ethical challenges. PLoS Med. 2018;15(11):e1002689.
60. Azad TD, Ehresman J, Ahmed AK, Staartjes VE, Lubelski D, Stienen MN, Veeravagu A, Ratliff JK. Fostering reproducibility and generalizability in machine learning for clinical prediction modeling in spine surgery. The Spine Journal. 2020 (In press). https://doi.org/10.1016/j.spinee.2020.10.006.

Machine Learning and Ethics

28

Tiit Mathiesen and Marike Broekman

28.1 Introduction

Machine learning (ML) has a unique capacity to structure and analyze data in amounts beyond a human scale. The complexity and size of data surpasses detailed oversight and accountability by humans. Human ethical duties and responsibilities may become occluded or altered when ML is used. Subsequently, novel ethical dilemmas arise when ML handles very large data sets or calculates statistical correlations and covariation in such sets for medical decision-making. Three ethically sensitive areas include (1) personal integrity in cases of data leakage in a wide sense, (2) justice in resource reallocation from care-cost to cost for information technology (it), and (3) ethical accountability in ML-assisted medical decision-making. In this essay, we will discuss these areas and attempts to ameliorate the ethical risk. This essay is intended to introduce these themes of ethical challenges in medical applications of AI.

28.2 Personal Integrity

A prerequisite for and hallmark of ML is an ability to rapidly systematize or analyze large data sets. Such sets contain enormous amounts of personal information, both sensitive and insensitive. This creates a potential source for leakage, as these data sets can never be completely anonymous or inaccessible to misuse [1–3].

Indeed, each individual dataset may become large enough to be unique and over-determined: it will be possible to remove information such as names and personal identification-numbers without compromising uniqueness of the set. Thus, everyone is theoretically identifiable even if overt personal identification is removed in a process of "anonymization." In principle, everybody in the database can be identified and thus personal information is accessible with enough efforts. The same argument goes with data protection in general. Security analysts equal data protection with making access to stored data too complex to be cost-effective while data is never completely protected [4]. In reality, data security breaches are common large-scale events [5, 6]. Democratically elected political leaders advocate it should be commercialized and made available to external partners to improve care but also to generate revenue [7]. Commercialization is only possible if legal protection is attenuated: new legislation needs to change protection of personal integrity. Data security breaches can have serious consequences.

In addition to the inherent risks related to the collection and storage of data, there will be weaknesses related to the use and ownership of data [8]. For example, personal data has become a business asset [9]. Private companies sell data for identification and targeting of customers or, even worse, to manipulate populations [10]. Although tech companies sell data with users' explicit consent, but a different trend has emerged during the last years. Apparently, a market for population biological- and health data has arisen. The prime example is Iceland, where a private company owns data on genetic codes and health on two-third of the population [2]. Policy makers have come to think of individual, population data as an asset. Political leaders in Sweden advocate for changes in legislation to allow large-scale export of population health data with a double aim. The major argument is disruptive, beneficial knowledge of health to "revolutionize

T. Mathiesen (✉)
Department of Neurosurgery, Copenhagen University Hospital, University of Copenhagen, Copenhagen, Denmark

Department of Clinical Medicine, Copenhagen University Hospital, University of Copenhagen, Copenhagen, Denmark

Department of Clinical Neuroscience, Karolinska Institutet, Stockholm, Stockholm, Sweden
e-mail: tiit.illimar.mathiesen@regionh.dk

M. Broekman
Department of Neurosurgery, Leiden University Medical Center, Leiden, Zuid-Holland, The Netherlands

V. E. Staartjes et al. (eds.), *Machine Learning in Clinical Neuroscience*, Acta Neurochirurgica Supplement 134,
https://doi.org/10.1007/978-3-030-85292-4_28

healthcare." The second aim is commercialization to finance hospitals, support novel technology and generate revenue [7, 11]. There is an obvious disagreement between the values that lead to our prevailing legal protection of personal data, including some degree of individual ownership, and the politics behind realization of commercial values. Apart from the conflict of values, large-scale data-mining projects for health-care solutions have a history of failure to deliver expected results.

Given the above, it is not realistic to believe that sensitive personal information will always be stored and used in a safe way and they will probably always be accessible for an attacker with sufficient zeal and resources.

28.3 Justice and Investments in Information Technology

Justice is one of the four biomedical principles suggested by Childress and Beauchamp [12] to facilitate ethical decision-making in medicine. Justice addresses resource allocation and comprises an imperative to design distributions that maximize equality in care and health. Health care spending has increased constantly, and measures to limit spending and cut down health-care budgets appear to become increasingly important for political management of society. Political resource allocation and choice between different budget areas such as healthcare, education, police and infrastructure comprise horizontal prioritization of resources, while prioritization within a field is "vertical"; e.g., the choice between allocating more resources for pediatric oncology or ventilators for Covid-19 patients. Horizontal prioritization of novel information technology for healthcare will leave less money available for biomedical research, staff, buildings, instruments, and material for care. Investments to improve productivity become attractive when healthcare budgets are strained, and prioritization of information technology is typically promulgated as a means to increase productivity. Marketing of new technology is strong. Technological inventions are part of a thriving entrepreneurial industry of skilled engineers and salesmen. However, we will see below that large tenders have led to enormous public investments in untested technological solutions.

Information technology has been successful in pattern recognition in large data sets such as radiological images and biological molecular files. We have also seen spectacular examples that AI can overpower humans in strategic games like Go, Chess and Jeopardy. Enthusiasm from such applications has fostered hopes of comprehensive it-solutions of "the future healthcare challenge." The IBM Watson employed spectacular advanced natural- language processing in playing Jeopardy. The system was tested in a laboratory setting and produced show case examples demonstrated how IBM Watson outperformed clinicians in diagnoses of rare diseases. Given such promising IT achievements, business models for AI-assisted healthcare and management of huge datasets developed rapidly and attracted investments. For example, the IBM Watson programs were expected to improve complex medical decisions in real life or even replace human medical experts for diagnostics and therapy. Systematic tracking of healthcare procedures, including strategies, indications and results would improve therapies and research. Investments were made by large tech companies, start-up companies and public partners. Money that would have been available to deliver care or investments in already validated technologies was redistributed to tech companies and entrepreneurs. Today, AI has unfortunately not lived up to its promise.

Indeed, many spectacular and widely published projects have turned into scandals, especially when public actors such as governmental regions and hospitals have made large investments in unproven technology. One can even argue that money moved from healthcare to industry in a "reverse Robin Hood"-like process. Health care expenditure has increased massively in the last decades, and lead to a reactive call for rationing and prioritization to curb costs. Hence, health care is increasingly under-financed in relation to population expectations and demands; rich countries such as Sweden even reported that they were not able to meet legitimate healthcare needs under normal conditions [13]. In contrast, tech industry is already fed with huge investments in the hope of financial return.

One example is implementation of the comprehensive health records, that do not involve AI per se, but have been bought as potential platforms for future ML applications. The capital region in Denmark invested in a system from Epic. "Sundhetsportalen" (SP) was bought by elected politicians as a comprehensive platform for communication, research, analysis and documentation, although health-care personnel criticized its lack of intuitive support of daily work. It soon became evident that expected functionalities had not been developed and could thus not be delivered. The program worked well for tracking cost and accounting of patients, but workflows and communication met obstacles as the system was primarily designed for accounting and created obstacles when used by nursing staff and physicians for daily delivery of healthcare; hopes for research support and data analyses were never met. The Danish national auditors concluded that money intended for healthcare had been badly invested for untested technology, which decreased productivity by 30% and created new costs to maintain safety and research [14, 15]. Interestingly, this negative information has not been disclosed as the system is sold on in the US, Holland, Sweden and Finland as a fully successful solution to future health-care management.

Another scandal is related to the IBM Watson. IBM Watson had been described to "almost understand the meaning of language, rather than just recognizing patterns of words" [16]. It was aggressively marketed "is real, it's mainstream, it's here, and it can change almost everything about health care" [17]. One application was developed as a comprehensive oncology tool: "*Watson for Oncology was supposed to learn by ingesting the vast medical literature on cancer and the health records of real cancer patients. The hope was that Watson, with its mighty computing power, would examine hundreds of variables in these records—including demographics, tumor characteristics, treatments, and outcomes—and discover patterns invisible to humans. It would also keep up to date with the bevy of journal articles about cancer treatments being published every day*" [16]. Large institutions like Cleveland Clinic, MD Andersson and Memorial Sloan Kettering Cancer Center entered into largely published partnerships with large investments [16]. It soon became clear that Watson was unable to independently mine and process medical news or published knowledge, retrieve relevant patient info from charts, compare individual patients to the "big data" of previous patients, or even suggest therapies beyond simple guidelines. The flagship collaborations were discontinued within a few years after large spending. The MD Anderson cancer center spent $62 million on the project before canceling it 2016 according to the University audit [16].

A third example was the locally largely published GVD-project in Stockholm City council [18, 19]. This was also an IT-system for unified documentation of all care related-data and single portal access with extensive hopes for data analyses. The project was expended to be running in 2004. Responsible personnel left or were fired, and the project was finally discontinued in 2007 after having exceeded the budget of 200 million SEK with 1.4 billion SEK "of taxpayers money." It was very delayed and delivered nothing that was clinically useful or applicable [19]. The auditors had then since 2003 criticized poor anchoring in actual care-processes, lack of cost control and nebulous chains of command. The analytic capacity of AI is indispensable for metabolomics and analyses of gene- or epigenetic panels, but such successes cannot be freely extrapolated to analyses of complex, ambiguous or vague data and outcomes.

The investment decisions appear to have been fueled by spectacular examples of pattern recognition and performance in games with fixed rules where analogy with "other complex tasks" has been taken to guarantee similar abilities in categorically different challenges, such as health care delivery. It appears that the public investors, typically third-party payers, confidently made strategic decisions while lacking sufficient knowledge of healthcare and AI to analyze necessary performance of products. Confidence without correlation to competence was described by Kruger and Dunning [20]. The decision-makers were probably particularly vulnerable when attracted by bandwagon-style marketing of "future technology" and "disruptive novelty." This moderately informed desire to join cutting-edge development paired with a need to decrease direct health-care cost has been toxic to health care performance and budgets. The good intentions paired with limited economic accountability and the Dunning–Kruger effect lead to redistribution of money from healthcare to an already thriving entrepreneurial IT industry. This reversed Robin Hood effect creates injustice in vertical prioritization of societal and health-care resources.

28.4 Accountability: Who Decides and What Is the Decision Based On?

Health care delivery entails a social contract between expert caregivers and society. Essential elements include expert skills, professional ethics and accountability among care givers, which are the only guarantees that professional experts fulfil their contract obligations. Expertise has elements that can only be understood by experts, which is why external regulation cannot fully grasp or regulate professional activity [21]. Moreover, every medical decision combines medical facts and values. Medical facts require medical knowledge and must be differentiated from values. Values belong to the realm of ethics. For accountability, value judgments and medical facts must be transparent and the process from values and facts to a decision must be traceable [22]. This is challenged by the introduction of AI into healthcare.

Values and AI

The classic example of values and artificial intelligence is the hypothetical case of an automatically driving car that faces collision when a child suddenly steps into the road: to we want the car to guarantee driver safety and run over the child, or do we prefer a drastic maneuver that saves the child but may hurt the driver. The dilemma must either be solved with programing measures or one must consider that machine learning will allow the program to make an autonomous choice independent of human deliberation? For this kind of problem, Goodall [23] concluded: "*The study reported here investigated automated vehicle crashing and concluded the following: (a) automated vehicles would almost certainly crash, (b) an automated vehicle's decisions that preceded certain crashes had a moral component, and (c) there was no obvious way to encode complex human morals effectively in software.*"

With todays' AI, deliberate programming of ethical parameters is still necessary for machine learning of this kind of dilemma. The explicit definition of values is a prerequisite. In analogy, games where AI excel like chess, go or Jeopardy comprise explicit definitions of success. In contrast to moral decisions, the concept of winning a game is free of any ambiguity and does not include involvement of meta-level judgment. An algorithm for machine learning from a training cohort of past instances is probably too complex for success. Even a hypothetical case of successful ML is, however, problematic, regardless of whether supervised or unsupervised learning is employed. With a supervised strategy, ML is instructed by the programmer of what is right and wrong. In contrast, an unsupervised strategy would discern patterns of deliberate human action and thereby perpetuate bias of human performance without any meta-level ethical evaluations or critical analyses.

Another narrative involves the concept of independent artificial intelligence. Moore's law expresses that processors increase processing capacity exponentially. Moore's law and the postulate that consciousness will arise as a necessary result of sufficient complexity foster a belief that any sufficiently complex computer can achieve independent cognition and moral agency like a human individual—but with a superior capacity. The theme of "AI taking over" is frequently evoked in popular culture, not least "a Space Odyssey 2001" by Arthur C Clarke and the subsequent film by Stanley Kubrick. The dystopic suggestion is that AI, if "conscious," will protect itself and the hardware while allowing children and passengers or even all of mankind to succumb. Nick Bostrom has developed philosophical analyses and warned for independent and unaccountable AI [24]. Philosophy of consciousness holds the postulate above as a simplification with limited support, but it still does not appear that we can expect ML or AI to provide accountable human moral deliberation.

Traceability of Decisions and Recommendations

A main feature of ML is its capacity to learn from data without explicit programming [25]. In other words, data is handled without an explicit instruction of how data is to be evaluated and grouped. Even the programmer of ML or neuronal networks is ignorant of the exact steps that lead to a result. Results of a calculation are thus displayed without any explanation of which calculation, evaluation, comparison or strategy led to the specific result. In reality, input is transformed in a "black box" to generate an answer to the programmed task. For example, in neural networks a middle layer is inserted between input and output. The weights connecting input variables to the middle variables and those connecting the middle variables to the output variable are being adjusted in several iterations. The end model is a result of these iterations, but cannot be interpreted as to how much the various input variables contribute to the outcome [26].

Under this condition, accountable ethical decision-making can be a problematic. One can argue that at least one person must be the responsible moral agent, i.e., the person that makes an ethical decision [27, 28]. One could speculate that the real moral agent is the manufacturer of the device, the owner of the system or a responsible professional. The traditional framework of healthcare identifies a responsible physician as the ultimate moral agent; the physician will be asked to make a decision based on a recommendation from a machine learning process that he cannot oversee or fully interpret [29]. The difficulty to interpret ML data is illustrated by abundant examples of bias or misleading decision-making. It is important to realize that one or several correct result from an ML program can never guarantee the next question will be correctly answered. Machine learning can, as it works today, not outstep boundaries of its training cohort and the basis or its judgment are not explicit when a response is delivered. The training cohort may be biased, comprise an irrelevant population, fail to differentiate objective and man-made qualities that can be influenced by the results of ML or make decisions based on covariates that in reality represent epiphenomena.

Ribeiro et al. [30] made the" Wolf vs. husky" study, which illustrates the importance of a classifier in ML. In this study, they used a training set with images of wolves and huskies for supervised learning and soon came up with an algorithm that made a number of consecutive classifications of images not used for training correctly before classifying some very clear images wrongly. The researchers suspected a bug but found out that the model learned to classify an image based on whether there was snow in it. All images of wolves used for training had snow in the background, while the ones of huskies did not. Subsequently, wolves without snow in the background were classified as huskies and vice versa.

Moreover, in real life other animals than those in the training set can be encountered. Ribeiro et al. continue: "*We know our wolf vs. husky model doesn't know a bear when it sees one. It will try to classify it as either a wolf or a husky.*" The neural model assigns a probability to a given output, but the probability does not reflect the confidence in the output. Predictions are confident even if they make no sense at all: "*When the model encounters the image of a bear, the output can be anything from 100% wolf to 100% husky.*" Sending a pet-dog to play with a "husky" may kill the dog if the creature is a mis-classified wolf or a bear.

In analogy, moral medical and ethical decisions based on ML or AI can have catastrophic results if the algorithm has made mistakes of a kind a human cannot vision or understand.

28.5 Discussion

We have described several of the ethical dilemmas inherent in big data and Machine learning: lack of guaranteed privacy, risk of unjust horizontal resource allocations and a fundamental lack of ethical accountability. These must be acknowledged and addressed when implementing support and benefits of ML and AI.

Protection of privacy is dependent on regulation and prevention. Privacy and implementations of data are already legally governed. In Europe, the data protection law (GDPR) limits storage and use of individual data and EU-guidelines require use of data to be lawful, ethical and robust [31]. Still, whenever AI. ML or Big Data are employed for future benefits past proven or even necessary utility, massive amounts of personal information are potentially available for "predators" and may be utilized providing cost is lower than benefit. For this reason, active prevention of very large sets of individual data is fundamental. The need to prevent access and formation of very large sets is unfortunately seen by some policymakers and entrepreneurs as an unnecessary obstacle of necessary progress and neglected for the enthusiastic promises of benefit and revenue from large-scale "future comprehensive access," such that were exemplified as misuse of public money in the "justice" section. Regardless, a major factor for reasonable vertical prioritization is awareness of the Kruger–Dunning effect and delegation of decisions that involve professionals and requires professional knowledge to those with bona fide competence of the area affected. Probably, stricter legal requirements for accountability and personal responsibility of public spending can limit ignorance-fed well intended projects that turned into financial scandals.

Human judgment is necessary even if artificial intelligence may develop autonomous ethical judgment, much like alpha-zero learned to play chess by playing games against itself. Such judgments must be evaluated, and Alan Winfield suggested an "Ethical Turing Test." This test would have multiple judges to decide if the AI's decision is ethical or unethical [32]. Another, but ethically unacceptable, solution for the ethical governance of computational systems is to bypass human ethics and imagine "the construction of ethics, as an outcome of machine learning rather than a framework of values" [33]. An unethical robot is just as likely as an ethical robot [34].

We conclude that the ability to make an accountable ethical decision depends on how AI results can be interpreted. We must modulate our expectations of which kind of ML results are traceable enough to be interpreted and that can support human ethical deliberation [35]. The need for a moral agent to be informed is, however, not unique for AI and ML related decisions, this is a prerequisite for all ethical decisions. Still, we can never be informed of all facts nor independently analyze all underlying information for any decision in ethics and healthcare. The lack of complete traceability is thus not unique to AI it is a difference of degree and magnitude. The novel and unique situation arises when potential computing possibilities and size of data create a situation where inherent or unique AI-related bias leads to recommendations and support that is profoundly perverted and misleading, while appreciated by the human decision-maker as a high-quality result of objective, advanced technology. The moral agent needs to retain moral integrity. In addition to moral competence, knowledge of how AI and ML work to produce output is crucial. Critical analyses must always be exercised. Precaution is necessary to rely only on AI output that has resulted from an explicit interpretable analytic task in a relevant population.

Acknowledgments This study was supported by a grant from The Swedish Medical Association (Sveriges Läkarförbund).

Conflict of Interest The authors declare that they have no conflict of interest.

References

1. Floridi L, Taddeo M. What is data ethics? Philos Trans A Math Phys Eng Sci. 2016;374(2083):20160360. https://doi.org/10.1098/rsta.2016.0360.
2. Merz JF, McGee GE, Sankar P. 'Iceland Inc.'?: On the ethics of commercial population genomics. Soc Sci Med. 2004;58:1201–9.
3. Mittelstadt BD, Floridi L. The ethics of big data: current and foreseeable issues in biomedical contexts. Sci Eng Ethics. 2016;22(2):303–41. https://doi.org/10.1007/s11948-015-9652-2.
4. Adams RL. Identity theft protection: 10 ways to secure your personal data. Forbes website. 2017. https://www.forbes.com/sites/robertadams/2017/05/05/identity-theft-protection-10-ways-to-secure-your-personal-data/#55cc87f62fde. Accessed 19 Apr 2018.
5. https://en.wikipedia.org/wiki/List_of_data_breaches. Accessed 19 Jan 2021.
6. Paul K. Even the CEO of Equifax has had his identity stolen—3 times. 2019. https://www.marketwatch.com/story/even-the-ceo-of-equifax-has-had-his-identity-stolen-3-times-2019-02-27
7. Mathiesen T, Sandlund M. Chapter 30. Etik och ehälsa 419-428. In: Petersson G, Rydmark M, Thurin A, editors. Medicinsk informatik. Stockholm: Liber; 2021.
8. Smolan S. The human face of Big Data. PBS Documentary. 2016. Accessed 24 Feb 2016.
9. Morris J, Lavendera E. Why big companies buy, sell your data. CNN website. 2012. https://www.cnn.com/2012/08/23/tech/web/big-data-acxiom/index.html. Accessed 19 Apr 2018.
10. Cadwalladr C. Fresh Cambridge Analytica leak 'shows global manipulation is out of control'. The Observer. The Guardian; 2020. Accessed 13 Jan 2020.
11. Röstlund L, Gustavsson A. Konsulterna. Stockholm: Mondial; 2019.
12. Beauchamp TL, Childress JF. Principles of biomedical ethics. 6th ed. Oxford: Oxford University Press; 2009.
13. Mathiesen T, Arraez M, Asser T, Balak N, Barazi S, Bernucci C, Bolger C, Broekman MLD, Demetriades AK, Feldman Z, Fontanella MM, Foroglou N, Lafuente J, Maier AD, Meyer B, Niemelä M, Roche PH, Sala F, Samprón N, Sandvik U, Schaller

K, Thome C, Thys M, Tisell M, Vajkoczy P, Visocchi M, EANS Ethico-Legal Committee. A snapshot of European neurosurgery December 2019 vs. March 2020: just before and during the Covid-19 pandemic. Acta Neurochir. 2020;162(9):2221–33. Epub 2020 Jul 8. PMID: 32642834; PMCID: PMC7343382. https://doi.org/10.1007/s00701-020-04482-8.
14. http://www.rigsrevisionen.dk/media/2104845/sr1717.pdf. Accessed 19 Jan 2021.
15. Larsen B. Sundhetsplatfoemn er den storste skandale. POV. International. 2017. https://pov.international/sundhedsplatformen-er-den-storste-skandale/. Accessed 20 Jan 2021.
16. Strickland E. How IBM Watson overpromised and underdelivered on AI health care. In: IEEE Spectrum: Technology, Engineering, and Science News; 2019. Accessed 4 Apr 2019.
17. Saxena M. IBM Watson Progress and 2013 roadmap (slide 7). Armonk, NY: IBM; 2013. Accessed 12 Nov 2013.
18. https://itivarden.idg.se/2.2898/1.130869/missarna-som-knackte-gvd. Accessed 25 Jan 2021.
19. Öberg F. IT-projekt i vården har blivit miljardcirkus. Svenska Dagbladet. 2019. https://www.svd.se/it-projekt-i-varden-har-blivit-miljardcirkus. Accessed 20 Jan 2021.
20. Kruger J, Dunning D. Unskilled and unaware of it: how difficulties in recognizing one's own incompetence lead to inflated self-assessments. J Pers Soc Psychol. 1999;77(6):1121–34.
21. Cruess SR. Professionalism and medicine's social contract with society. Clin Orthop Relat Res. 2006;449:170–6.
22. Eijkholt M, Broekman M, Balak N, Mathiesen T, EANS Ethico-Legal Committee. Three pitfalls of accountable healthcare rationing. J Med Ethics. 2021:medethics-2020-106943. Epub ahead of print. https://doi.org/10.1136/medethics-2020-106943.
23. Goodall NJ. Ethical decision making during automated vehicle crashes. Transp Res Rec. 2014;2424(1):58–65. https://doi.org/10.3141/2424-07.
24. Bostrom N. Superintelligence. Oxford: Oxford University Press; 2016. p. 126–30. ISBN 978-0-19-873983-8. OCLC 943145542.
25. Samuel AL. Some studies in machine learning using the game of checkers. IBM J Res Dev. 1959;3:210–29.
26. Kianpour M, Wen S-F. Timing attacks on machine learning: state of the art. In: Intelligent systems and applications. Advances in intelligent systems and computing, vol. 1037; 2020. p. 111–25. ISBN 978-3-030-29515-8. https://doi.org/10.1007/978-3-030-29516-5_10.
27. Adams JR, Drake RE. Shared decision-making and evidence-based practice. Community Ment Health J. 2006;42(1):87–105.
28. Christman J. Autonomy in moral and political philosophy. Stanford Encyclopedia of Philosophy. 2003 [2018]. https://plato.stanford.edu/archives/spr2018/entries/autonomy-moral/
29. Nissenbaum H. Accountability in a computerized society. Sci Eng Ethics. 1996;2:25–42.
30. Ribeiro MT, Singh S, Guestrin C. "Why should I trust you?": explaining the predictions of any classifier. In: Proceedings of the 22nd ACM SIGKDD international conference on knowledge discovery and data mining (KDD '16). Association for Computing Machinery, New York, NY, USA; 2016. p. 1135–44. https://doi.org/10.1145/2939672.2939778.
31. https://ec.europa.eu/digital-single-market/en/news/ethics-guidelines-trustworthy-ai. Accessed 10 Jan 2021.
32. Winfield AF, Michael K, Pitt J, Evers V. Machine ethics: the design and governance of ethical AI and autonomous systems [scanning the issue]. Proc IEEE. 2019;107(3):509–17.
33. Ganesh MI. Entanglement: machine learning and human ethics in driver-less car crashes. APRJA; 2017. http://www.aprja.net/entanglement-machine-learning-and-human-ethics-in-driver-less-car-crashes/.
34. Vanderelst D, Winfield A. The dark side of ethical robots. In: Proceedings of the 2018 AAAI/ACM conference on AI, ethics, and society. New Orleans, LA: ACM; 2018. p. 317–22. https://doi.org/10.1145/3278721.3278726.
35. De Laat PB. Algorithmic decision-making based on machine learning from big data: can transparency restore accountability? Philos Technol. 2018;31:525–41. https://doi.org/10.1007/s13347-017-0293-z.

The Artificial Intelligence Doctor: Considerations for the Clinical Implementation of Ethical AI

29

Julius M. Kernbach, Karlijn Hakvoort, Jonas Ort, Hans Clusmann, Georg Neuloh, and Daniel Delev

29.1 Introduction

The field of medicine has become increasingly data-driven, with artificial intelligence (AI) and machine learning (ML) attracting much interest across disciplines [1–4]. While the implementation in patient care still lags behind, almost every type of clinician is predicted to use some form of AI technology in the foreseeable future [3]. Evolving with the industrialization of AI, where the academic and industrial boundaries of AI-associated research are increasingly blurred, the number of ML-based algorithms developed for clinical and commercial application within health care is continuously increasing. Realizing the accompanying rising ethical concerns, many institutions, governments, and companies alike have since formulated sets of rules and principles to inform research and guide the implementation into clinical care [5]. More than 80 policies on "Ethical AI" have since been proposed [6], including popular examples such as the European Commission's AI strategy [7], the UK's Royal College of Physicians' Task Force Report [8], the AI Now Institute's Report [9], as well as statements from major influences form the industry (e.g., Google, Amazon, IBM) [10]. Collectively, there appears to be a widespread agreement between the distinct proposals regarding meta-level aims, including the use of AI for the common good, preventing harm while upholding people's rights, and following widely-respected values of privacy, fairness, and autonomy. Demonstrating considerable overlap, the suggested pillars building Ethical AI converge to the principles of autonomy, beneficence, non-maleficence, justice and fairness, privacy, responsibility, and transparency [6]. While certain principles, generally describing the four bioethical principles of autonomy, beneficence, non-maleficence, and justice, are well-known in healthcare, AI-specific concerns arise regarding the autonomy, accountability, and need of explicability of AI-based systems.

Until now, there are relatively few neurosurgical papers implementing AI. However, the recent trend demonstrates the growing interest in ML and AI in neurosurgery [11, 12]. From a clinician's point of view, AI can be untransparent, and without methodological foundations, pose a severe risk to patients' care. How can we make AI transparent for clinicians and patients? How do we choose which clinical decisions are going to be delegated to AI? How do we prevent adverse events caused by AI algorithms? When the AI agent makes wrong decisions—who can be held responsible? There is a clear increase of directives and papers on AI ethics [6, 10] offering guidelines to these critical questions. This article non-exhaustively covers basic practical guidelines regarding AI-specific ethical aspects that will be useful for every ML or AI researcher, author, and reviewer aiming to ensure ethical innovation in AI-based medical research.

29.2 Transparency and Explicability

Research in AI systems rapidly advances across medical disciplines; however, the trust placed in developed applications lags behind [13]. Many proposals on ethical AI guidelines acknowledge the lack of algorithmic transparency and accountability as the most prevalent problems to address [6]. As humans and responsible clinicians, we must understand and interpret the outcome of an AI or ML model. With the European Union being at the forefront of shaping the

Julius M. Kernbach and Karlijn Hakvoort have contributed equally to this work.

J. M. Kernbach (✉) · K. Hakvoort · J. Ort · D. Delev
Neurosurgical Artificial Intelligence Laboratory Aachen (NAILA), RWTH Aachen University Hospital, Aachen, Germany

Department of Neurosurgery, Faculty of Medicine, RWTH Aachen University, Aachen, Germany
e-mail: jkernbach@ukaachen.de

H. Clusmann · G. Neuloh
Department of Neurosurgery, Faculty of Medicine, RWTH Aachen University, Aachen, Germany

V. E. Staartjes et al. (eds.), *Machine Learning in Clinical Neuroscience*, Acta Neurochirurgica Supplement 134,
https://doi.org/10.1007/978-3-030-85292-4_29

international debate on Ethical AI, the General Data Protection Regulation (GDPR) was introduced in 2018. Herein, articles 13–14 mandates "meaningful information about the logic involved" for all decisions made by artificially intelligent systems [14]. This *right to an explanation* of the directive implies that any clinician using AI-based decision-making is legally bound to convey patients with explanations to the applied ML and AI models' inner workings. Suppose the AI-based decision cannot be explained. In that case, the clinician ends up in the uncomfortable position of vouching for the application's trustworthiness without being able to interpret its methodology and outcome. Unfortunately, many ML and AI models are considered "black boxes" that do not explain their predictions in a comprehensible way. The consequent lack of transparency and explicability of predictive models in medicine can have severe consequences [15, 16].

The precise lack of interpretability has been exacerbated with the rise and popularity of deep learning (DL) models. As a form of representation learning with multiple layers of abstraction, DL methods are extremely good at discovering intricate patterns in high-dimensional data [17, 18] that are beyond the human scope of perception. DL methods have produced promising results in speech recognition, visual object recognition, object detection, and many other domains such as drug discovery and genomics. They frequently outperformed different ML algorithms in image recognition and computer vision [19–21], speech recognition [22, 23] and more. DL methods, including deep neural networks, are increasingly complex and challenging—if not impossible—to interpret because the function relating the input data through multiple complex layers of neurons to the final outcome vector is far too complex to comprehend. Fortunately, in the spirit of "Explainable AI" [24–26], approaches have been developed to address the black box problem. Broadly, Explainable AI involves creating a second (post hoc) model to explain the first black box model [26]. Successful analytical approaches to "open the black box" have since been proposed. One example are local interpretable model-agnostic explanations (LIME), which can explain the predictions of a classifier in a comprehensible manner by learning an interpretable model locally around the prediction [27]. Other implementations primarily rely on assessing variable importance, such as RISE (Randomized Input Sampling for Explanation), which probes deep image classification modes with a randomly masked version of the input image [28]. However, particularly in the clinical context, evidence to whether post hoc approximations can adequately explain deep models remains very limited [27, 29, 30].

With the increasing success of AI and, in particular, DL, a "myth of accuracy-interpretability trade-off" arise, meaning that complicated deep models are necessary for excellent predictive performance [26]. However, more complex models are often not more accurate, particularly when the data are structured with a good representation in terms of naturally meaningful features. In DL, the inherent complexity scales to large datasets [17, 31]. Particularly successful examples of employed DL include studies on electronic health records, as demonstrated by Rajkomar and colleagues in >200,000 adult patients cumulating a total of >46.8 billion data points [32], and large prospective population cohort studies of >500,000 participants from the UK Biobank [33]. But even in the big-data omics fields, such as imaging or genomics, investigations in part question the superiority of DL compared to simple models based on available data. Schulz and colleagues showed that the increase in performance of linear models in brain imaging does not saturate at the limit of current data availability, and DL is not beneficial at the currently exploitable sample sizes such as those based on the UK Biobank (>10,000 3D multimodal brain images [34]. In the prediction of genomic phenotypes, DL performance was competitive to linear models but did not outperform linear models by a sizable margin (>100,000 participants with >500,000 features) [35]. Historically, linear models have long dominated data analysis, as complex transformations into rich high-dimensional spaces were computationally infeasible. In small sample sizes particularly, complex methods with high variance such as many DL methods tend to overfit: the algorithm performs "too well" on training data to the extent that it negatively impacts the interpretation of new data. Less complex models such as general linear models are generally less prone to overfitting—especially with regularization strategies applied [36, 37].

The best practice recommendations on predictive modeling hence include considerations of the given structure on the input data, the choice of feature engineering, sample size and model complexity, and more [38–40] and should always be considered when selecting the appropriate models for a given predictive modeling task.

29.3 Fairness and Bias

There is global agreement that AI should be fair and just [6]. Herein, unfairness relates explicitly to the effect of unwanted *bias* and *discrimination*. While biased decision-making is hardly unique to AI and ML, research demonstrated that ML models tend to amplify societal bias in the available training data [41, 42]. Skewed training data is a major influence on bias amplification and can lead to severe adverse events arising from the lack of inclusion of ethical minorities. Esteva and colleagues used DL to identify skin cancer from photographs using 129,450 images (with only 5% of dark-skinned participants). While the classification works en par with expert knowledge on light skin, it fails to diagnose melanoma in people with dark skin colors [3, 43]. This highlights the importance of deliberate data acquisition that is representable and diverse (e.g., regarding race, gender), focusing on including minorities. Many of the ML applications available today can be considered "narrow AI," that is, they help with specific tasks on specific types of data. An AI system trained on a certain patient cohort cannot unconsciously be used on an entirely different population. Therefore, the limits of generalizability should always be kept in mind. However, even in balanced data sets, bias may be amplified due to spurious (mostly unlabeled) correlations. For example, in a balanced picture data set of 50% men cooking and 50% women cooking, unlabeled influences, e.g., children, which co-occur more often with women, can be labeled cooking as well. Hence, more women will be associated with cooking [30]. To counteract unwanted bias in balanced data sets, adversarial debiasing was proposed [30, 44, 45]. Models are trained adversarially to preserve task-specific information while eliminating, e.g., gender-specific cues in images. The removal of features associated with the protected variable (gender, ethnicity, age, or others) within the intermediate representation leads to less biased predictions in balanced data sets. Protected variables include gender, race, and socioeconomic status. Failure to address the societal bias could ultimately widen the present gap in health outcome [3, 46].

We welcome increasing diversity within a research group itself, which increases detection of possible (unconsciousness) biases. Nowadays, diversity is an important factor in obtaining European and national research funding [47]. For every AI application, it should clearly be outlined which patient characteristics within training were available. An extensive table with patient characteristics, including sex, age, ethical background, length, weight, and BMI, as well as detailed disease information should be included. Major sources of bias should be described within the limitation section as well. It is important to realize that most biases are unintended and do not arise deliberately. Despite attempts to reduce biases, these can occur when not expected at all.

29.4 Liability and Legal Implications

While the important ethical issues mentioned above are still a matter of intensive and critical debate, the first steps toward structured and transparent software legalization using ML have been successfully made. The Medical Device Regulation (MDR, EU Regulation 2017/745) is an essential step toward better software use regulation, aiming at improved safety and transparency. MDR and the Guidance on Qualification and Classification of Software in Regulation (EU) 2017/745, which was endorsed by the Medical Device Coordination Group (MDCG), accurately address the definition of software. Herein, software is regarded as a medical device, meaning that medical device software (MDSW) is any software that is intended to be used alone or in combination for any purpose mentioned by the definition of medical device, i.e., used for diagnostic, prevention, prediction, prognosis or treatment of a disease (for a full report, c.f. to the EU 2017/745). MDSW can be independent and still qualifies as such regardless of its physical localization (i.e., cloud).

Furthermore, the MDR defines software as a set of instructions that processes input data and creates output data. Thus, MDR encompasses to a full extend any use of AI technology. One needs to look more precisely at the decision steps assisting the qualification as MDSW. Here, one will unmistakably find that if the software is not acting for the individual patient's benefit, it is not covered by the MDR. A more critical interpretation of this part could suggest that software or AI technology, which is not used in a clinical setup, is not considered by the MDR. This is indeed the usual case when AI technology is used in an experimental and scientific setting. However, in this setting, any discoveries or assistance by the AI technology should not be directly used to influence patients' diagnostics or treatment. In the case of IBM Watson's AI for Oncology program [15], the developed algorithm for the recommendation of treatment choices for patients with cancer frequently suggested harmful and erroneous treatment regimes. If the harmful algorithm were to be integrated into the actual clinical routine, many patients would have suffered preventable harm. Compared to errors on the single doctor-patient level, the faulty AI recommender would have inflicted harm on an exponentially higher level. Following this line of thought and embracing the ethical axiom of "primam non nocere," one can argue that any software, AI technology, or ML algorithm, which is intended to be used for clinical decision-making of any kind, needs to be CE or FDA approved. Although this is inevitably associated with considerable effort, it will guarantee that every software life cycle will include all the steps of paramount importance, such as hazard management and quality management. Although the software does not directly harm a patient, it still can create harmful situations by providing incorrect information. This gap has been successfully addressed by the Rule 11 of the MDR. Consequently, many software applications (including AI, ML, and statistical tools like risk calculators) will fall into Class IIa or Class IIb. Indeed, all these regulating measures may seem less progressive. Still, they try to solve the legal question of liability by introducing terms as the *intended purpose* and the use outside of it.

One further problem in AI liability is that the law, including tort law, "is built on legal doctrines that are focused on human conduct, which when applied to AI, may not function" [48]. Moreover, until now, there is no clear legal definition of AI that can be used as a foundation for new laws regarding its use since existing definitions were created to understand AI instead of regulating it. The legal definitions are, therefore, often circular and/or subjective [49].

Additionally, *adopting* AI applications that might influence clinical decision-making may "evolve dynamically in ways that are at times unforeseen by system designers" [50]. With adaptation, the AI system gains *autonomy*. But our definition of what is considered autonomous or intelligent is still ill-defined and will likely change over time due to rapid developments within the field of AI [49].

Until AI definitions and regulations are clearly defined, care should be warranted to use AI-assisted tools. Clinical decision-making algorithms could be allocated to research purposes only, which demands the approval of an ethical commission, patient insurance, and patients' consent before its use. AI has already been proven very helpful—especially in making diagnoses and predicting prognosis and outcome—also within the field of neurosurgery [11]. In the end, every outcome from an AI algorithm should be checked against the current medical gold-standard and clinical guidelines. For future considerations, the development of concise AI definitions and regulations is relevant to deflect potential harm.

29.5 Conclusion

With the continuously advancing field of AI, fostering trust in the clinical implementation of AI applications becomes imperative. Almost every type of clinician is predicted to use some form of AI technology in the foreseeable future, hence, shaping the ethical and regulatory use of AI becomes increasingly important. In the article, we reviewed *transparency and algorithmic explicability* as the trade-off between complexity and available data, the *mitigation of unwanted biases* that even affect balanced data sets, and the *legal considerations* when advancing AI in health care. We introduce approaches, including post hoc models and adversarial attacks, to combat the above problems and foster Ethical AI.

Acknowledgments and Disclosure *Funding:* J. M. K. and D. D. are supported by the Bundesministerium für Bildung und Forschung (BMBF COMPLS3–022).

Conflicts of Interest/Competing Interests None of the authors has any conflict of interest to disclose.

References

1. Deo RC. Machine learning in medicine. Circulation. 2015;132(20):1920–30. https://doi.org/10.1161/CIRCULATIONAHA.115.001593.
2. Jordan MI, Mitchell TM. Machine learning: trends, perspectives, and prospects. Science. 2015;349:255–60. https://doi.org/10.1126/science.aaa8415.
3. Topol EJ. High-performance medicine: the convergence of human and artificial intelligence. Nat Med. 2019;25(1):44–56.
4. Vellido A. Societal issues concerning the application of artificial intelligence in medicine. Kidney Dis. 2019;5(1):11–7.
5. Whittlestone J, Alexandrova A, Nyrup R, Cave S. The role and limits of principles in AI ethics: towards a focus on tensions. In: AIES 2019—Proceedings of the 2019 AAAI/ACM conference on AI, ethics, and society; 2019. p. 195–200.
6. Jobin A, Ienca M, Vayena E. Artificial intelligence: the global landscape of ethics guidelines. arXiv; 2019.
7. European Commision. Artificial intelligence: commission takes forward its work on ethics guidelines; 2019.
8. Reznick RK, Harris K, Horsley T. Artificial intelligence (AI) and emerging digital technologies; 2020.
9. Crawford K, Dobbe R, Dryer T, et al. AI now 2019 report. New York: AI Now Institute; 2019.
10. Floridi L. Establishing the rules for building trustworthy AI. Nat Mach Intell. 2019;1(6):261–2.
11. Bonsanto MM, Tronnier VM. Artificial intelligence in neurosurgery. Chirurg. 2020;91(3):229–34.
12. Senders JT, Arnaout O, Karhade AV, Dasenbrock HH, Gormley WB, Broekman ML, Smith TR. Natural and artificial intelligence in neurosurgery: a systematic review. Clin Neurosurg. 2018;83(2):181–92.
13. Dreiseitl S, Binder M. Do physicians value decision support? A look at the effect of decision support systems on physician opinion. Artif Intell Med. 2005;33(1):25–30. https://doi.org/10.1016/j.artmed.2004.07.007.
14. Goodman B, Flaxman S. European Union regulations on algorithmic decision making and a "right to explanation". AI Mag. 2017;38(3):50–7. https://doi.org/10.1609/aimag.v38i3.2741.
15. Ross C, Swetlitz I. IBM's Watson supercomputer recommended 'unsafe and incorrect' cancer treatments, internal documents show. Stat+; 2018.
16. Varshney KR, Alemzadeh H. On the safety of machine learning: cyber-physical systems, decision sciences, and data products. Big Data. 2016;5:246–55.
17. Goodfellow I, Bengio Y, Courville A, Bengio Y. Deep learning. Cambridge, MA: The MIT Press; 2016.
18. LeCun Y, Bengio Y, Hinton G. Deep learning. Nature. 2015;521(7553):436.
19. Djuric U, Zadeh G, Aldape K, Diamandis P. Precision histology: how deep learning is poised to revitalize histomorphology for personalized cancer care. NPJ Precis Oncol. 2017;1:22. https://doi.org/10.1038/s41698-017-0022-1.
20. Farabet C, Couprie C, Najman L, Lecun Y. Learning hierarchical features for scene labeling. IEEE Trans Pattern Anal Mach Intell. 2013;35(8):1915–29. https://doi.org/10.1109/TPAMI.2012.231.
21. Krizhevsky A, Sutskever I, Hinton GE. ImageNet classification with deep convolutional neural networks. Adv Neural Inf Proces Syst. 2012. https://doi.org/10.1061/(ASCE)GT.1943-5606.0001284.
22. Hinton G, Deng L, Yu D, et al. Deep neural networks for acoustic modeling in speech recognition. IEEE Signal Process Mag. 2012;29(6):82–97. https://doi.org/10.1109/MSP.2012.2205597.
23. Mikolov T, Deoras A, Povey D, Burget L, Černocký J. Strategies for training large scale neural network language models. In: 2011 IEEE workshop on automatic speech recognition and understanding, ASRU 2011, PRO; 2011. https://doi.org/10.1109/ASRU.2011.6163930.
24. Albers DJ, Levine ME, Stuart A, Mamykina L, Gluckman B, Hripcsak G. Mechanistic machine learning: how data assimilation leverages physiologic knowledge using Bayesian inference to forecast the future, infer the present, and phenotype. J Am Med Inform Assoc. 2018;25(10):1392–401. https://doi.org/10.1093/jamia/ocy106.

25. Lundberg SM, Nair B, Vavilala MS, et al. Explainable machine-learning predictions for the prevention of hypoxaemia during surgery. Nat Biomed Eng. 2018;2(10):749–60. https://doi.org/10.1038/s41551-018-0304-0.
26. Rudin C. Stop explaining black box machine learning models for high stakes decisions and use interpretable models instead. Nat Mach Intell. 2019;1:206–15. https://doi.org/10.1038/s42256-019-0048-x.
27. Ribeiro MT, Singh S, Guestrin C. "Why should i trust you?" Explaining the predictions of any classifier. In: Proceedings of the ACM SIGKDD International Conference on Knowledge Discovery and Data Mining; 2016. https://doi.org/10.1145/2939672.2939778.
28. Petsiuk V, Das A, Saenko K. RISE: randomized input sampling for explanation of black-box models. arXiv; 2018.
29. Mittelstadt B. Principles alone cannot guarantee ethical AI. Nat Mach Intell. 2019;1(11):501–7.
30. Wang T, Zhao J, Yatskar M, Chang KW, Ordonez V. Balanced datasets are not enough: Estimating and mitigating gender bias in deep image representations. In: Proceedings of the IEEE International Conference on Computer Vision 2019-October; 2019. p. 5309–18.
31. Esteva A, Robicquet A, Ramsundar B, Kuleshov V, DePristo M, Chou K, Cui C, Corrado G, Thrun S, Dean J. A guide to deep learning in healthcare. Nat Med. 2019;25(1):24–9. https://doi.org/10.1038/s41591-018-0316-z.
32. Rajkomar A, Oren E, Chen K, et al. Scalable and accurate deep learning for EHR—supplement. NPJ Digit Med. 2018;1:18.
33. Weng SF, Vaz L, Qureshi N, Kai J. Prediction of premature all-cause mortality: a prospective general population cohort study comparing machine-learning and standard epidemiological approaches. PLoS One. 2019;14:e0214365. https://doi.org/10.1371/journal.pone.0214365.
34. Schulz MA, Thomas Yeo BT, Vogelstein JT, Mourao-Miranada J, Kather JN, Kording K, Richards B, Bzdok D. Deep learning for brains?: different linear and nonlinear scaling in UK biobank brain images vs. machine-learning datasets. In: bioRxiv; 2019. https://doi.org/10.1101/757054.
35. Bellot P, de los Campos G, Pérez-Enciso M. Can deep learning improve genomic prediction of complex human traits? Genetics. 2018;210(3):809–19. https://doi.org/10.1534/genetics.118.301298.
36. Hastie T, Tibshirani R, Friedman J. Springer series in statistics the elements of statistical learning—data mining, inference, and prediction. Berlin: Springer; 2009.
37. James G, Witten D, Hastie T, Tibshirani R. An introduction to statistical learning. Curr Med Chem. 2000. https://doi.org/10.1007/978-1-4614-7138-7.
38. Kuhn M, Johnson K. Applied predictive modeling. New York: Springer; 2013. https://doi.org/10.1007/978-1-4614-6849-3.
39. Neeman T. Clinical prediction models: a practical approach to development, validation, and updating by Ewout W. Steyerberg. Int Stat Rev. 2009;77(2):320–1. https://doi.org/10.1111/j.1751-5823.2009.00085_22.x.
40. Poldrack RA, Huckins G, Varoquaux G. Establishment of best practices for evidence for prediction: a review. JAMA Psychiat. 2020;77(5):534–40. https://doi.org/10.1001/jamapsychiatry.2019.3671.
41. Hardt M, Price E, Srebro N. Equality of opportunity in supervised learning. In: Advances in neural information processing systems; 2016.
42. Yao S, Huang B. Beyond parity: fairness objectives for collaborative filtering. In: Advances in neural information processing systems; 2017.
43. Esteva A, Kuprel B, Novoa RA, Ko J, Swetter SM, Blau HM, Thrun S. Dermatologist-level classification of skin cancer with deep neural networks. Nature. 2017;542(7639):115–8.
44. Xie Q, Dai Z, Du Y, Hovy E, Neubig G. Controllable invariance through adversarial feature learning. In: Advances in neural information processing systems; 2017.
45. Zhang BH, Lemoine B, Mitchell M. Mitigating unwanted biases with adversarial learning. In: AIES 2018—Proceedings of the 2018 AAAI/ACM conference on AI, ethics, and society; 2018. https://doi.org/10.1145/3278721.3278779.
46. Stringhini S, Carmeli C, Jokela M, et al. Socioeconomic status and the 25 × 25 risk factors as determinants of premature mortality: a multicohort study and meta-analysis of 1.7 million men and women. Lancet. 2017;389(10075):1229–37.
47. European Commission E. Work Programme 2018–2020: Science with and for society; 2018.
48. Bathaee Y. The artificial intelligence black box and the failure of intent and causation. Harv J Law Technol. 2018;31(2):889–936.
49. Buiten MC. Towards intelligent regulation of artificial intelligence. Eur J Risk Regul. 2019;10(1):41–59.
50. Gasser U, Almeida VAF. A layered model for AI governance. IEEE Internet Comput. 2017;21(6):58–62.

30 Predictive Analytics in Clinical Practice: Advantages and Disadvantages

Hendrik-Jan Mijderwijk and Hans-Jakob Steiger

30.1 Introduction

Predictive analytics are daily used by clinical neuroscientists, mainly for nonclinical purposes. Google algorithms for example pave the way for rapid access to our personal interests and needs. Predictive analytics applied to daily clinical patient care are however less used. Ironically, clinical neuroscientists increasingly report on predictive algorithms specifically developed to support daily clinical care [1, 2]. The availability of electronic health record (EHR) systems and user-friendly statistical packages has fueled model development approaches by many clinical neuroscientists.

The overarching aim of predictive analytics in clinical practice is to improve patient outcomes in terms of quality, safety, and efficiency [3]. Nowadays, predictive analytics have become inevitable because stakeholders (policy makers, funders, and patients themselves) want to participate in decision making on which treatment to choose that provides maximal benefit together with minimal costs and patient burden.

Although it is known that predictive analytics can outperform the predictions made by clinical neuroscientists themselves [4], it has been hard to include predictive analytics in current clinical workflows. The increasing amount of available predictive algorithms induces uncertainty by potential end-users (e.g., clinical neuroscientists) which model to use, if any. Their potentiality is often not recognized by end-users.

Herein, we describe and tabulate advantages and disadvantages of predictive analytics in clinical practice (Table 30.1). We highlight the application of predictive analytics and address potential endeavors that might foster the inclusion of these tools into clinical workflows.

Table 30.1 Several advantages and disadvantages of predictive analytics in clinical practice

Advantages	Disadvantages	Potential remedy
The toolbox of predictive analytics is expanding	Predictive analytics can become more "engineering" than science resulting in research waste	We should not go for analyzing available data, but for analyzing clinical conditions in equipoise regarding the optimal management
Advanced predictive analytic techniques are able to model complex predictor-outcome associations	Models may become opaque for end-users resulting in a decline in user trust and usage	Developers should be transparent in model reporting and give sufficient detailed background information
Sophisticated analyses can be executed easily	Interpretability and generalizability can be jeopardized	Keep analysis simple, but not simplistic
Risk estimations are increasingly based on large patient cohorts	Individual patients and confounding may still not be captured by the model	Clinical neuroscientists should have basic scientific knowledge on how to interpret a model and should understand that risks provided by a model are still conditional
Predictive analytics may aid decision making and clinical workflow	Overreliance on predictive analytics may induce de-skilling of (clinical) competencies	Regular reflection by end-users
The rise of EHRs and other data sources have made predictive analytics available to clinical neuroscientists and modeling commonplace	Using immature tools may harm many patients	Regulatory approval including certification labels

H.-J. Mijderwijk (✉)
Department of Neurosurgery, Heinrich Heine University, Medical Faculty, Düsseldorf, Germany
e-mail: Hendrik-Jan.Mijderwijk@med.uni-duesseldorf.de

H.-J. Steiger
Department of Neurosurgery, Kantonsspital Aarau, Aarau, Switzerland
e-mail: hsteiger@uni-duesseldorf.de

V. E. Staartjes et al. (eds.), *Machine Learning in Clinical Neuroscience*, Acta Neurochirurgica Supplement 134,
https://doi.org/10.1007/978-3-030-85292-4_30

30.2 Data Considerations: What to Put into a Predictive Tool?

Quantity Versus Quality

Large sample sizes are highly desirable when prediction models are generated, especially when highly flexible methods are used [5, 6]. However, the quantity of the available data does not guarantee high quality of the data. This is nicely demonstrated in the Google Flu Trends (GFT) analysis in 2013. Google search-term data were used to predict the seasonal flu. Some predictors identified by the Google algorithm had no (biological) relation with the flu. The GFT prediction was unreliable and a simple model from the *Centers for Disease Control and Prevention* outperformed the GFT model [7]. Theory-free studies and theory-free driven algorithms are prone to provide biased results since they rely too much on the data.

Hypothesis based studies use subject matter knowledge to mitigate bias, resulting in more quality and structured data sets. These data sets are therefore more tailored to the studied clinical condition. However, such data collection is often manually executed and therefore time consuming, which may result in lower sample sizes.

In 2020, Google published a predictive analytic tool that was trained on a big data set that was of high clinical quality [8]. The predictive analytic tool outperformed clinicians in diagnosing malignancies on radiological studies. Thus, to flourish and reach its potential, predictive analytics need a combination of data quantity and data quality—that may come from different data sources—to aid clinical neuroscientists in understanding and controlling complex conditions in neuroscience such as subarachnoid hemorrhage (SAH) [9].

Theoretical Construct and Empirical Construct

Predictive analytics in clinical practice are normally based on the results of empirical data. Clinical neuroscientists try to better understand theoretical constructs through empirical data. However, do the study variables (predictors and outcomes) adequately represent the condition that is aimed to be unraveled? For example, do empirical surrogate markers such as health insurance status adequately represent a tested theoretical construct such as social economic status? [10]. Other observational data from a national registry have shown that functional outcome (empirical construct) may not be a valid indicator for quality of care (theoretical construct) when comparing stroke centers [11]. Thus, measurement instruments may not fully capture the theoretical construct and may not be comparable across cases and centra.

The array of data resources that are being used for predictive analytics is increasing. Next to (national) registry data, other data sources like EHRs, open sources (such as meteorological data), and claim data have been used for analyses. Nowadays, neurosurgical procedures and diagnoses are coded in EHRs for billing purposes. These codes can be easily used for predictive analytics. For example, ICD codes have been used to predict spontaneous subarachnoid hemorrhage admissions to evaluate the gut feeling of clinical neuroscientists that SAH admissions appear in clusters [9]. Such data collection (covering a long time period, i.e., data from a decade) would not have been possible so easily with traditional manual data collection by researchers. The rationale for documentation of this kind of data is not for scientific purposes but rather for administrative purposes which may result in several data anomalies and incomplete patient information. First, confounding variables are normally not documented, and clinical outcomes are omitted. Patient frailty, for example, is not routinely assessed and documented, but is a robust predictor of poor surgical outcomes [12, 13]. Second, miscoding of variables may emerge. It has been shown that postoperative complications have been miscoded as comorbidities [14]. Using such data may create bias in effect estimation of predictor-outcome associations and ultimately in prediction. Third, coding behavior varies between hospitals and among health care professionals. If no one codes a SAH, the patient does not have a SAH and will be wrongly excluded from analysis. Fourth, different EHR software is currently being used between hospitals, such as HiX and Epic. Thus, currently, patient data is spread across multiple inter-institutional and intra-institutional data sources. The lack of an integral EHR system makes it hard to include all the relevant data from a patient into a predictive analytic tool.

Clinical empirical data can also be noisy and threaten the theoretical construct studied. For example, cardiopulmonary variables such as pulse oximetry, capnography, and heart rate are prone for artifacts. Blood samples taken from a patient may be hemolytic and hence subjected to artifacts such as falsely elevated potassium levels. A predictive tool is only able to provide sensible predictions if the input is adequate. In general: *garbage in, garbage out.*

Analyzing Available Data or Analyzing Clinical Equipoise

Intraarterial nimodipine therapy and norepinephrine infusions for symptomatic vasospasm in patients suffering from aneurysmal subarachnoid hemorrhage are highly predictive for poor functional outcome and patient mortality. Although such a predictive model may be highly accurate, it does not provide an option to reduce the risk for the patient. Such predictive models do not influence clinical decision making by clinical neuroscientists and will not improve clinical outcomes. The model is not able to provide interventions to prevent patients from becoming poor grade patients. In other words, the actionability of such models is low. A much more interesting question is to predict rebleeding prior to cerebral aneurysm treatment (microsurgical clipping or neuroendovascular treatment) when an aneurysmal SAH patient arrives at the hospital at 22:00 hours, because there is equipoise regarding the optimal management. Can we wait for another 12 h to treat the aneurysm at daytime leaving the patient at risk for a rebleeding? Or should we intervene immediately and expose the patient to a probably fatigued and less experienced team? A predictive tool that accurately classifies those patients into high and low rebleeding risks will help the clinical neuroscientist to make informed decisions and will influence patient outcomes accordingly.

Another example: predicting readmissions after brain surgery with data automatically drawn from EHR has become of increasing interest [15]. These noble predictive analyses often overfit the small number of patients however. Furthermore, the local EHR will not notice a readmission in another hospital. The actionability is again supposed to be low, because providing the risk of a readmission in 30 days is unlikely to change the behavior of the clinical neuroscientist. The model might be useful for just informing patients, however. The performance measures of such models is generally low, likely due to the fact that clinical data alone is insufficient and other factors such as social determinants of health are not considered, yet more appropriate for predicting hospital readmission [16].

30.3 Interpreting the Model's Output: An Essential Role for the Clinical Neuroscientist

Clinical and Scientific Competencies

Clinical decision making on new patients currently still involves clinical judgment and personal preferences extrapolated from our previous experiences. In contrast to the number of patients predictive models are exposed to (models are commonly trained on hundreds, thousands or even bigger numbers of patients), the number of patients a clinical neuroscientist is exposed to is relatively small. Therefore, clinical decision making based on our own clinical experience can be moot.

To interpret a model adequately, basic knowledge on quantitative predictive analysis is needed for clinical neuroscientists to understand and integrate probabilistic data in their patient work-up. Predictive analytics using logistic regression for example, will provide a probability of an event to occur. The probability provided will likely be incorrect, because either the patient will undergo the event or not. In clinical practice, a patient cannot be 75% shunt-dependent after aneurysmal SAH after 30 days. The patient will be judged as shunt-dependent and will have a permanent shunt inserted or will be judged as not shunt-dependent. Another important aspect to be aware of is statistical overfitting. Overfitting is a common problem due to complex modeling relative to the effective sample size. Using an overfitted model on new patients may be harmful. Overfitted models likely provide overestimated risks for high-risk patients and underestimated risks for a low-risk patient, which can be observed in a calibration plot. Therefore, clinical neuroscientist should be aware of the model's performance. Discrimination and calibration are well-known model performance measures. Discrimination refers to the ability of a prediction model to discriminate between patients with and without the event of interest and is quantified using the *c*-statistic. The *c*-statistic ranges from 0.5 to 1, where 0.5 means that the prediction model is equivalent to a coin toss and 1 refers to perfect discrimination. Calibration refers to the agreement between predicted and observed outcome and is highly consequential to medical decision making—it has been labeled as the Achilles heel of predictive analytics [17].

Methodological aspects such as study bias should be considered as well. Confounding is a critical aspect in translating results from predictive analytics into clinical decision making. Predictive analytics are often hampered by confounding by indication. Causal inferences can therefore not be drawn. An example in which confounding by indication matters is the use of predictive analytics based on retrospective glioblastoma patient data. Predictive analytics for patient survival often include treatment effects such as extent of surgical resection and type of post-surgical therapy. Drawing conclusions on the effectiveness of therapies should be done cautiously. Exemplifying this, it is likely that glioblastoma patients with a good general condition as reflected in the Karnofsky performance score (KPS) with a relatively good prognosis for survival will get standard post-surgical therapy (radiotherapy plus concomitant and maintenance temozolomide) and that glioblastoma patients with a poor general condition with a worse survival prognosis have a greater probability to receive subparts of standard therapy and/or experimental designs. However, if bias is adequately taken into account, such models can be well used for shared decision making with relatives or patients themselves.

Thus, interpreting results from predictive analytics urge for an adequate risk communication to patients and their relatives across all educational levels, especially in shared decision making situations. This will be a vital new skill that clinical neuroscientists should master in the future, because—at least for now—a computer cannot take over this skill.

Clinical neuroscientists are also at risk of de-skilling of their clinical competencies. Overreliance on predictive analytics may negatively affect the ability of making firm interpretations of signs and symptoms [18]. In addition, it may induce stereotyping of patients and decrease clinical knowledge and self-confidence [18–20]. In unforeseen situations, such as the local shutdown of the academic hospital in Düsseldorf in 2020, neurosurgeons and other clinical neuroscientists should be able to provide adequate patient care without the use of modern predictive analytics, which may be difficult for younger professionals as a result of de-skilling [21]. We should be aware of de-skilling due to overreliance which can be controlled by regular reflections of end-users.

Clinical Neuroscientist's Vigilance

The imperfect nature from predictive analytics should be considered and is highly consequential. Predictive analytics are dynamic processes. The lifetime of a prediction tool may be limited. It is known that the performance of predictive tools wane over time if the tool is exposed to more data or to new promising prognostic variables.

Another vital aspect to consider is the condition of the investigated patients. For example, the course of the aneurysmal SAH disease may be complicated by meningitis which in a worst-case scenario progresses into a meningitis-sepsis. Clinical neuroscientists may consult predictive analytic tools that are trained to identify (meningitis)-sepsis. Likely, those tools have learned from patients diagnosed with a sepsis [22]. Utilizing such a tool for clinical decision making should be done cautiously in patients without a diagnosed sepsis, since those tools are commonly not trained on patients that are—although they were at risk for a sepsis—prevented from a sepsis due to adequate medical care at the neurointensive care unit.

Sometimes the inclusion or exclusion of interesting variables into a predictive tool can make the model impractical. Recently, a predictive analytic approach for predicting shunt-dependency after aneurysmal SAH showed an impressive performance [23]. The use of prognostic variables that may emerge in the course of the disease, such as delayed cerebral ischemia, make application of the tool by clinical neuroscientists, however, complex. Another example: surgical resection of a recurrent glioblastoma during the course of the disease in glioblastoma patients is difficult to include in a predictive analytic tool because this data is not available at baseline or at the moment the model is intended to be used. However, this may alter survival time. Thus, if a predictive tool is used for prognostication, the clinical neuroscientist should critically evaluate if his/her patient resembles the patients used for model generation.

30.4 Integrating the Model into the Clinical Workflow: Reporting Is Imperative

User Trust

Why do we trust our patient interview? Why do we trust our clinical patient examination? Why do we trust the additional investigations—such as laboratory results from our lumbar puncture and radiological results of the MRI scan—of our patient? One of the reasons is that we know they are reliable at most of the time. We trust them, because we observe the glioblastoma in the left temporal lobe as we perform the surgical procedure. We see that our liquor tap is purulent, and that it becomes clearer during therapy with antibiotics. Furthermore, we are able to (re)weight the strength of our observations in the light of the clinical course of the patient. Although the literature provides many reports of predictive analytics that should have promising effects for our daily clinical routine, why don't we use them regularly in our daily clinical practice? Do we not trust these tools? One of the reasons might be that we are not familiar we these techniques, and probably the lack of technical know-how. Clinicians are commonly not trained in statistics and scientific methodology like epidemiologists and statisticians—understanding the structure of algorithms from machine learning methods can be challenging even for experts, however. End-users remain wary, especially when machine learning algorithms are used, as they cannot directly and exactly see, control, and understand how the patient data is weighted and modeled by the developers in opaque predictive analytic tools. End-users want to know how a predictive tool got the results provided [3].

Transparency

To make predictive analytics convincing for the clinical neuroscientist, model transparency is imperative. Transparency is key to trust and application of the predictive tool. Transparent reporting according to the Transparent Reporting of a multivariable prediction model for Individual Prognosis or Diagnosis (TRIPOD) guidelines is needed for transparency in model development and for external validation and impact study attempts [24]. Caveats for clinical use of the model should be clearly explained and readily available. For example, is the model for shared decision making and confounding by indication should be taken into account, then the clinical neuroscientist should be aware of that. Trust in predictive analytics by clinical neuroscientists will further enhance if models are regularly updated as more data becomes available, since patient populations may evolve over time and the half-life of clinical data can be short [25]. Recently, an innovative calibration drift detection system identifying the need for model updating has been proposed [26]. Such reporting systems are important because miscalibration may lead to severely flawed predictions. For example, patients identified by a miscalibrated model as having low risk of postoperative complication may be falsely withdrawn from preventive treatment.

Safe Use and Regulatory Approval

It is known that clinicians may incorrectly interpret the results of predictive analytics, and many biases may have to be taken into account [6, 27]. Applying a predictive tool to patients not taking into account methodological shortcomings can harm many patients and is unethical. Developers should ideally provide online calculators, apps or desktop applications that possibly can be embedded within EHRs to aid uptake in the clinical workflow together with sufficient detailed background information of the model development including its caveats.

Merely presenting a clinical predictive tool without a clear recommended action will likely not survive in clinical practice. However, a clinical predictive tool with a clear recommendation that disrupts the workflow of a clinical neuroscientist will also not survive. The variables needed for the predictive tool should be easily accessible and being measurable without minimal measurement error [1]. The predictive tools provided should offload the clinical neuroscientists and not load them with additional work. Ideally, clinical neuroscientists should not have to open additional packages next to their EHR to use a predictive tool. Re-entering patient data into a model to obtain individual prognosis estimates should be avoided if these data can be derived directly from the EHR, such as age, patient gender, and KPS.

Clinical neuroscientists need impact studies that show the benefits, harms, and sustainability of the clinical prediction models used. Unfortunately, these studies are clearly underrepresented in the literature. There is an over-emphasis on model development studies and a focus on increasing model performances measures. Model performance measures are likely not convincing enough for end-users; yet the impact of predictive tools on the outcomes—i.e., effectiveness of the model—tracked over time will increase model trust and usability [3]. In addition, a label that certifies a prediction model to be deployed in clinical practice might be a next step to enhance clinical uptake. Attempts to estimate the value of predictive analytics in clinical practice, such as the "number needed to benefit" have been suggested [28]. Regulatory approval endeavors have been underway [22]. Food and Drug Administration (FDA) approval or Conformité Européenne (CE) approval may ultimately help to convince clinical neuroscientists that a particular predictive tool meets clinical quality standards and can be applied safely.

30.5 Concluding Remarks

In this relatively new era of predictive analytics, clinical neuroscientists play a critical role in outlining the clinical problems the predictive analytics have to solve. In addition, clinical neuroscientists play a critical role in interpreting the output of predictive analytics in light of the clinical scenario of the individual patient. Only clinicians can discuss the results with the patients and activate treatment regimes. Clinical neuroscientists should be therefore ideally trained and skilled on how to integrate a model in their patient work-up. To fully use the potential of predictive analytics, clinical neuroscientists need to understand at the one hand the difference between his/her patient and the ones included in the predictive algorithm, and the available resources that might be considered to intervene in the course of the patients' disease.

Combining predictive analytics with the knowledge clinical neuroscientists have of the pathophysiology and patient's preferences will have a positive synergistic effect on individual patient care what neither can do alone. Ultimately, if used sensibly, predictive analytics have the potential to be an additional component in the *history taking—clinical examination—additional investigations—(predictive analytics)—diagnosis/treatment plan* patient work-up of clinical neuroscientists. It can enhance this clinical process by making better informed decision together with their patients.

To foster the progress of predictive analytics into the clinical workflow of the clinical neuroscientist, (1) the used data sets should be more refined to the clinical scenario studied, (2) predictive analytics should ideally be used to study patients in equipoise regarding optimal management, not to study the available data, and (3) clinical neuroscientists should have knowledge on effective implementation of the designed predictive tools for the right patients.

Conflict of Interest On behalf of all authors, the corresponding author states that there is no conflict of interest.

References

1. Mijderwijk H-J, Steyerberg EW, Steiger H-J, Fischer I, Kamp MA. Fundamentals of clinical prediction modeling for the neurosurgeon. Neurosurgery. 2019;85:302–11.
2. Senders JT, Staples PC, Karhade AV, Zaki MM, Gormley WB, Broekman MLD, Smith TR, Arnaout O. Machine learning and neurosurgical outcome prediction: a systematic review. World Neurosurg. 2018;109:476–86.
3. Benda NC, Das LT, Abramson EL, Blackburn K, Thoman A, Kaushal R, Zhang Y, Ancker JS. "How did you get to this num-

ber?" stakeholder needs for implementing predictive analytics: a pre-implementation qualitative study. J Am Med Inform Assoc. 2020;27:709–16.
4. Saposnik G, Cote R, Mamdani M, Raptis S, Thorpe KE, Fang J, Redelmeier DA, Goldstein LB. JURaSSiC: accuracy of clinician vs risk score prediction of ischemic stroke outcomes. Neurology. 2013;81:448–55.
5. Obermeyer Z, Emanuel EJ. Predicting the future—big data, machine learning, and clinical medicine. N Engl J Med. 2016;375:1216–9.
6. Rajkomar A, Dean J, Kohane I. Machine learning in medicine. N Engl J Med. 2019;380:1347–58.
7. Lazer D, Kennedy R, King G, Vespignani A. Big data. The parable of Google Flu: traps in big data analysis. Science. 2014;343:1203–5.
8. McKinney SM, Sieniek M, Godbole V, Godwin J, Antropova N, Ashrafian H, Back T, Chesus M, Corrado GS, Darzi A, Etemadi M, Garcia-Vicente F, Gilbert FJ, Halling-Brown M, Hassabis D, Jansen S, Karthikesalingam A, Kelly CJ, King D, Ledsam JR, Melnick D, Mostofi H, Peng L, Reicher JJ, Romera-Paredes B, Sidebottem R, Suleyman M, Tse D, Young K, de Fauw J, Shetty S. International evaluation of an AI system for breast cancer screening. Nature. 2020;577:89–94.
9. Steiger H-J, Petridis AK, Tortora A, Mijderwijk H-J, Beseoglu K, van Lieshout JH, Kamp MA, Fischer I. Meteorological factors for subarachnoid hemorrhage in the greater Düsseldorf area revisited: a machine learning approach to predict the probability of admission of patients with subarachnoid hemorrhage. Acta Neurochir. 2019;162:187–95.
10. Fischer I, Mijderwijk HJ, Kahlert UD, Rapp M, Sabel M, Hänggi D, Steiger HJ, Forster MT, Kamp MA. Association between health insurance status and malignant glioma. NeuroOncol Pract. 2020;7:531–40.
11. Amini M, van Leeuwen N, Eijkenaar F, Mulder MJHL, Schonewille W, Lycklama A, Nijeholt GL, Hinsenveld WH, Goldhoorn RJ, van PJ D, Jenniskens S, Hazelzet J, DWJ D, Roozenbeek B, Lingsma HF, and on behalf of the MR Clean Registry Investigators. Improving quality of stroke care through benchmarking center performance: why focusing on outcomes is not enough. BMC Health Serv Res. 2020;20:1723–10.
12. Huq S, Khalafallah AM, Patel P, Sharma P, Dux H, White T, Jimenez AE, Mukherjee D. Predictive model and online calculator for discharge disposition in brain tumor patients. World Neurosurg. 2020:1–24.
13. Robinson TN, Wu DS, Pointer L, Dunn CL, Cleveland JC Jr, Moss M. Simple frailty score predicts postoperative complications across surgical specialties. Am J Surg. 2013;206:544–50.
14. Hannan EL, Racz MJ, Jollis JG, Peterson ED. Using Medicare claims data to assess provider quality for CABG surgery: does it work well enough? Health Serv Res. 1997;31:659–78.
15. Lohmann S, Brix T, Varghese J, Warneke N, Schwake M, Suero Molina E, Holling M, Stummer W, Schipmann S. Development and validation of prediction scores for nosocomial infections, reoperations, and adverse events in the daily clinical setting of neurosurgical patients with cerebral and spinal tumors. J Neurosurg. 2020;1:1–11.
16. Chen JH, Asch SM. Machine learning and prediction in medicine—beyond the peak of inflated expectations. N Engl J Med. 2017;376:2507–9.
17. Van Calster B, McLernon DJ, van Smeden M, Wynants L, Steyerber EW, On behalf of Topic Group 'Evaluating Diagnostic Tests and Prediction Models' of the STRATOS Initiative. Calibration: the Achilles heel of predictive analytics. BMC Med. 2019;17:230.
18. Cabitza F, Rasoini R, Gensini GF. Unintended consequences of machine learning in medicine. JAMA. 2017;318:517–2.
19. Hoff T. Deskilling and adaptation among primary care physicians using two work innovations. Health Care Manage Rev. 2011;36:338–48.
20. Panesar SS, Kliot M, Parrish R, Fernandez-Miranda J, Cagle Y, Britz GW. Promises and perils of artificial intelligence in neurosurgery. Neurosurgery. 2019;87:33–44.
21. Ausman J. The transition of neurosurgeons through the technology and information age. Surg Neurol Int. 2012;3:45–3.
22. Parikh RB, Obermeyer Z, Navathe AS. Regulation of predictive analytics in medicine. Science. 2019;363:810–2.
23. Muscas G, Matteuzzi T, Becattini E, Orlandini S, Battista F, Laiso A, Nappini S, Limbucci N, Renieri L, Carangelo BR, Mangiafico S, Della Puppa A. Development of machine learning models to prognosticate chronic shunt-dependent hydrocephalus after aneurysmal subarachnoid hemorrhage. Acta Neurochir. 2020;162:3093–105.
24. Collins GS, Reitsma JB, Altman DG, Moons K. Transparent reporting of a multivariable prediction model for individual prognosis or diagnosis (TRIPOD): the TRIPOD statement. BMC Med. 2015;13:1–10.
25. Chen JH, Alagappan M, Goldstein MK, Asch SM, Altman RB. Decaying relevance of clinical data towards future decisions in data-driven inpatient clinical order sets. Int J Med Inform. 2017;102:71–9.
26. Davis SE, Greevy RA Jr, Lasko TA, Walsh CG, Matheny ME. Detection of calibration drift in clinical prediction models to inform model updating. J Biomed Inform. 2020;112:103611–0.
27. Rajkomar A, Hardt M, Howell MD, Corrado G, Chin MH. Ensuring fairness in machine learning to advance health equity. Ann Intern Med. 2018;169:866–8.
28. Liu VX, Bates DW, Wiens J, Shah NH. The number needed to benefit: estimating the value of predictive analytics in healthcare. J Am Med Inform Assoc. 2019;26:1655–9.

Part V

Clinical Applications of Machine Learning in Clinical Neuroscience

31 Big Data in the Clinical Neurosciences

G. Damian Brusko, Gregory Basil, and Michael Y. Wang

31.1 Introduction

The clinical neurosciences have always been at the forefront of research innovation, adopting the most innovative and novel technologies to enhance understanding of the neural axis. Two important and increasingly utilized concepts that evolved together over time are big data and machine learning.

Machine learning models have been applied in a growing number of areas and across scientific disciplines, especially within neuroscience. One of the first studies to mention "machine learning" as a predictive modeling tool was a 1967 article fittingly published in the *Journal of Theoretical Biology*. Reed et al. described a series of experiments carried out by "high speed computers" that successfully predicted evolutionary patterns based on hereditary changes and the natural selection process outlined by Darwin [1]. Interestingly, the study conclusions were the result of computer simulations of a poker game, equating game strategy to evolutionary survival strategy. Driven by advances in computing software, machine learning and the coevolution of big data collection methods transitioned from theory into practice.

Defining big data is more challenging. Commonly, big data is described as a large, complex set of data requiring advanced computational analysis to identify trends or associations. Machine learning models often augment these analyses, which can be too complex and time consuming for human processing power alone. Therefore, machines are needed to find patterns hidden within big data, but clinicians or researchers must still determine which associations are most clinically relevant. Examining relationships identified from big datasets and machine learning is one of the current frontiers in clinical neuroscience.

This chapter will discuss the initial development of big data within neurosurgery and how early adopters set the standards for accurate data collection and reporting. Additional focus will be placed on the more recently developed national databases and registries which aim to elicit real world quality improvements in neurosurgical practice. Finally, machine learning's influence on the current and future states of clinical research across subspecialties will also be discussed.

31.2 Historical Context Within Neurosurgery

One of the earliest studies in the neurosurgical literature to specifically mention machine learning as a predictive tool was for traumatic brain injury (TBI). Beginning in the 1970s, several studies describe various prediction algorithms for TBI outcomes. The rationale for using these innovative machine learning models was the need to more accurately guide management plans while also balancing difficult family discussions for patients with severe TBI. Numerous clinical factors such as Glasgow Coma Scale (GCS) and pupillary response were known to be important clinical prognostic factors, but accuracy of long-term clinical outcome predictions were enhanced when predictive modeling was applied. Choi et al. described decision-tree models in which patients are split into smaller and smaller subsets based on clinical characteristics [2] and logistic regression modeling where the study sample is split into test and validation groups [3]. The authors concluded that the decision-tree and logistic regression models provided the most accurate predictions for patients with severe TBI and that decision-trees in particular enhanced bedside decision-making owing to the simple visual representation.

As the statistical methodologies for predicting clinical outcomes began to evolve, so too did the way in which data was managed. Improvements in computing technology enabled collection of larger amounts of data and the ability to

G. D. Brusko (✉) · G. Basil · M. Y. Wang
Department of Neurological Surgery, University of Miami Miller School of Medicine, Lois Pope Life Center, Miami, FL, USA
e-mail: g.brusko@med.miami.edu

V. E. Staartjes et al. (eds.), *Machine Learning in Clinical Neuroscience*, Acta Neurochirurgica Supplement 134,
https://doi.org/10.1007/978-3-030-85292-4_31

aggregate similar data from other institutions. Thus, the concept of a clinical database was formed. Again, the earliest neurosurgical implementation of large databases began in neurotrauma. Jennett et al. first reported on the creation of a database in 1968 for severe TBI patients in Scotland that was eventually expanded to also include a total of 700 patients from the Netherlands and the United States (US) [4]. Like many of the national registries today which will be discussed, the Jennett data bank required trained persons to enter the clinical data, ensuring consistency across sites.

Citing Jennett's trauma database as the origin, in 1979 the National Traumatic Coma Data Bank (TCDB) pilot phase began, which collected a more comprehensive set of variables that included pre-hospital data such as injury mechanism, alcohol or drug use at time of injury, and whether the patient had been wearing a helmet or seatbelt [5]. In addition to addressing predictive factors for clinical outcomes, the study discussed the importance of the TCDB as a tool for multicenter and interdisciplinary collaboration, which would provide the foundations for continued research. The TCDB proved to be successful in contributing significantly to the neurosurgical literature. Perhaps, the most enduring aspect of the TCDB though was the methodology devised to ensure accuracy. Intensive care unit data was prospectively collected via standardized forms at least every 8 h. Data was then entered into a "microcomputer" within each hospital that transmitted all data to the central repository at one center and was programmed to prevent erroneous entry of values. Furthermore, staged data audits occurred at individual sites and training sessions for those responsible for data collection, entry, and monitoring were frequently held. The use of standardized data collection forms, microcomputers and computer-based editing, all innovative at the time, have become the basic procedural standards that are familiar to researchers today.

One additional concept that has become increasingly important today in discussing clinical studies is the common data element (CDE). These standardized terms and validated collection tools create a core framework around which investigators can develop a study. Importantly, use of CDEs allows for more reliable comparisons between studies on the same topic and thus can help facilitate meta-analyses. CDEs are often consensus-driven and provide a quick and cost-effective way to identify which variables and data instruments should be included for a specific research topic [6]. For example, the National Institute of Neurological Disorders and Stroke (NINDS) defined 980 data elements across nine content areas to serve as a guideline for variables to be included in stroke studies [7]. Another example is the Patient-Reported Outcomes Measurement Information System (PROMIS), which provides a validated set of tools often utilized in spine studies to assess quality of life metrics. Use of CDEs becomes especially important when developing a clinical database and helps to guide decisions regarding which variables are most important to collect.

31.3 Evolution of Clinical Neurosurgical Databases

During the past decade, numerous national databases, registries, and international collaborations have facilitated trends in literature primarily toward an outcome-based analysis of current neurosurgical practice. This is in part a direct result of the analytic opportunities big data affords, particularly when combined with machine learning. As multicenter participation grows over time, the sample size and follow-up periods increase, enabling stronger and more accurate predictions of how specific treatments affect patient outcomes. More importantly, the relevant data becomes actionable and often elicits a change in practice leading to quality improvement (QI).

One of the most notable QI efforts is the National Surgical Quality Improvement Program (NSQIP) which was developed within the Veteran's Administration in the US during the 1990s. Its aim was to stratify morbidity and mortality risks of numerous surgical procedures and subsequently improve care for veterans undergoing surgery [8]. With data from over 400,000 cases, the program defined a median benchmark for acceptable risks and identified outlier hospitals performing both better and worse than the average. Some argued that these distinctions would harbor punitive actions against the low-performing institutions, or even the surgeons themselves. Conversely, lessons learned from institutions who consistently demonstrate a lower rate of adverse events could be applied broadly, and thus lead to national quality improvements.

The most successful of the national surgical databases, however, is the Society of Thoracic Surgeons (STS) National Database, first established in the late 1980s and now with over 90% participation of US thoracic surgeons [9, 10]. Results from the database enabled the STS to set their own national benchmarks for performance and allowed surgeons to compare their individual outcomes and foster quality improvement. In addition, utilization of big data provided robust support for the true value of thoracic procedures with respect to reimbursements.

Citing the success of the STS database in achieving wide-reaching quality improvements and policy reforms, the National Neurosurgery Quality Outcomes Database (N^2QOD), presently QOD, sought to build a similar model for neurosurgical outcomes. Additionally, the Affordable Care Act led to Centers for Medicare and Medicaid Services (CMS) reforms that allowed specialty groups such as neurosurgery to create Qualified Clinical Data Registries (QCDRs). Partnering with national leaders in national quality improvement and computer software designed with a focus on collection of clinical data, QOD developed predictive models for quality of life (QOL) outcomes in patients undergoing spine surgery. The models aimed to enhance shared decision-making with patients through expectation setting and modifiable risk factor adjustments [11, 12]. A significant number of high impact studies have been published as a direct result of QOD analyses. However, the greater success of QOD has been confirmation that the undertaking is feasible and worthwhile across all clinical settings from academic to community-based and lends supports for its continued expansion [13].

Since its inception, the QOD spine module has expanded to include registries for lumbar, cervical and spinal deformity surgeries. Most recently, QOD and the American Academy of Orthopaedic Surgeons (AAOS) Registry Program announced a collaboration with the goal of creating a more encompassing and impactful database called the American Spine Registry (ASR). While the results of this partnership are yet to be elucidated, the ASR will likely enhance spine surgeons' efforts to offer highly competitive value-based healthcare in today's evolving market. Although the ASR will become the largest spine registry, there are other highly productive databases that further highlight the importance of this growing area of data science. For example, the International Spine Study Group (ISSG) has published primarily on treatment of adult spinal deformity (ASD) over the past decade and have recently begun to examine long-term outcomes in minimally invasive ASD surgery [14]. Surgical innovation and new technology may drive these evolutions in practice initially, but ultimately favorable long-term outcomes lead to broad acceptance within the field, which now is often augmented by analysis of large surgical databases.

Other neurosurgical subspecialties have developed national databases as well. Similar to the ASR model, in 2019 the NeuroVascular Quality Initiative (NVQI) merged with the QOD vascular module to form the NVQI-QOD registry for stroke, aneurysm, and arteriovenous malformations. The Neuropoint Alliance, which oversees QOD, also manages the Stereotactic Radiosurgery Registry and the Registry for the Advancement of Deep Brain Stimulation in Parkinson's Disease (RAD-PD), both of which aim to improve quality within functional neurosurgery. A timeline highlighting the foundation of each of the national neurosurgical databases discussed in this chapter is shown in Fig. 31.1.

However, limitations exist for large multicenter databases and machine learning models used to analyze them. The accuracy of predicted outcomes and impact on clinical practice is directly related to the quality and accuracy of the granular data inputted. Presently, the electronic health record is designed to allow easier charting of clinical data and extrapolation for coding and billing purposes, often making data extraction difficult when conducting research. Thus, it is critical that efficient data collection methods such as natural language processing (NLP) are established [15]. Loss to follow-up during multi-year study periods, particularly in select spine cohorts, also presents a common problem and affects prediction accuracy of long-term outcomes [16]. To mitigate these challenges, the resources needed to ensure extensive data collection can be costly and may limit the scalability of databases to the larger centers with enough human and economic capital. Furthermore, the rapid increase in machine learning modeling to explore large datasets created a lack of reporting standardization, making results less reproducible and limiting validity [17]. The Transparent Reporting of a multivariate prediction model for Individual Prognosis Or Diagnosis (TRIPOD) Statement attempts to improve reporting and offers a 22-item checklist for reference [18]. Finally, the questions posited and answered with data from these registries should be actionable in clinical practice, driving the quality improvement process forward.

Additional efforts are now being directed at collecting patient outcome data in a real-time manner. The potential exists for patient function to be tracked algorithmically. This would allow for data collection to be performed without such

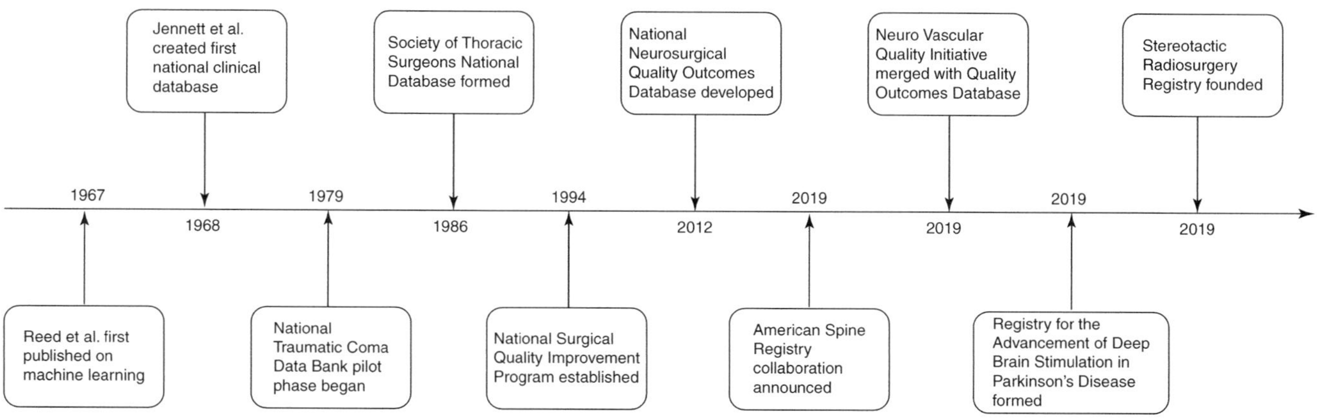

Fig. 31.1 Timeline highlighting the development of the national surgical databases and registries

discrete time points (e.g.,: preoperatively and postoperatively at 3, 6, 12, and 24 months). Rather, the patient could be assessed on any given day or week, minimizing sampling bias. This would also allow for the detection of declining function, to allow for continuous prospective patient monitoring as shown in Fig. 31.2.

31.4 Future Directions

Despite some limitations, big data will continue to play an important role in clinical research. Today's world is data-driven in nearly every facet, and new computing technology will undoubtedly improve the ability to collect data, analyze

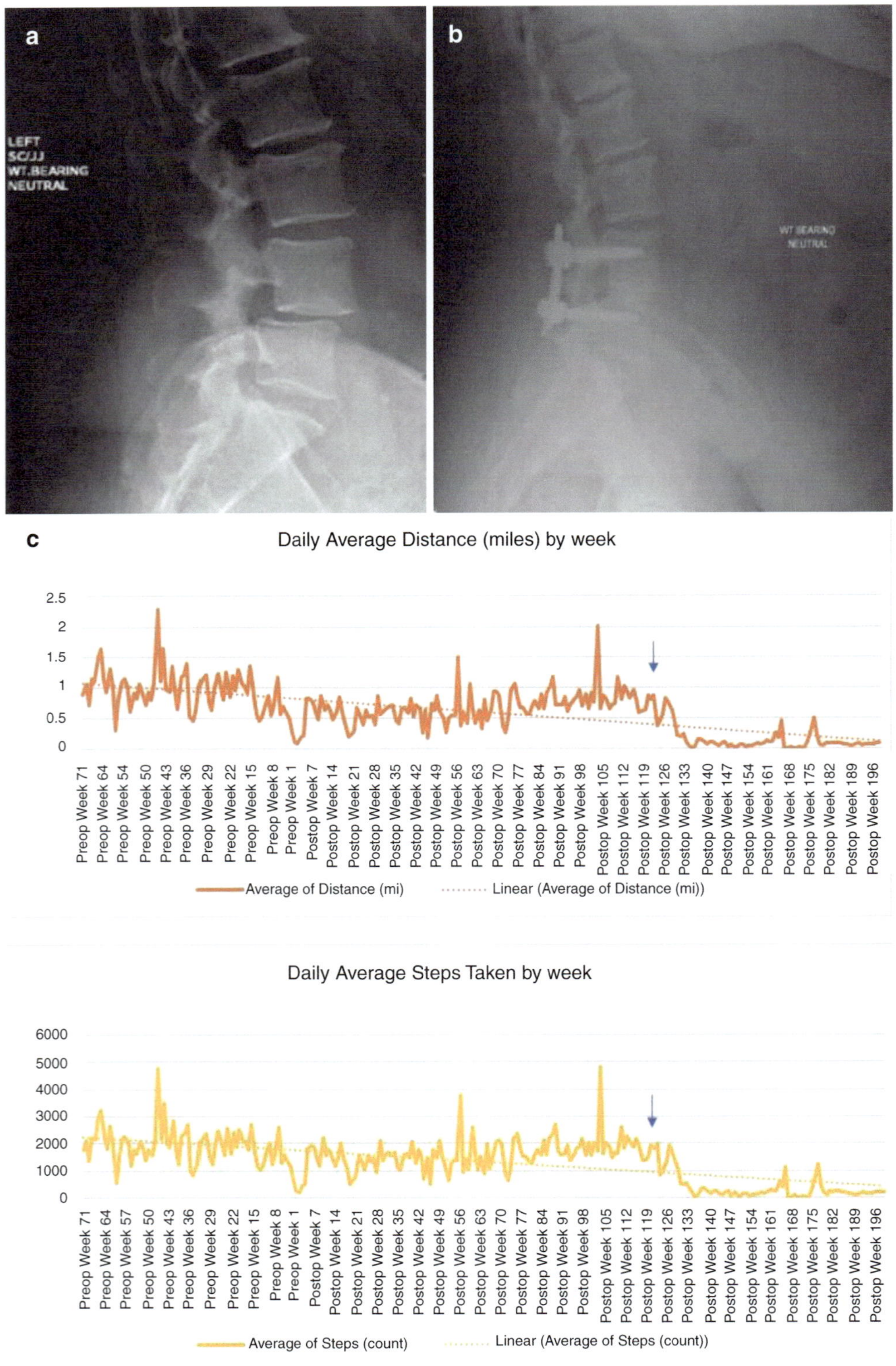

Fig. 31.2 A 61-year-old female with leg and back pain diagnosed with a degenerative anterolisthesis of L4 on L5 (Panel **a**) who underwent an L4–5 minimally invasive, endoscopic transforaminal lumbar interbody fusion (TLIF) (Panel **b**). At her 3-month postoperative visit, the patient reported complete resolution of her preoperative symptoms. The patient's activity data collected from her iPhone demonstrated a progressive decline in activity level leading up to surgery (Panel **c**). Her 1-year preoperative average daily physical activity was 1905 ± 1474 steps taken. Two months prior to surgery her average daily steps taken had fallen to 1450 ± 1243 steps ($p < 0.001$). Her average weekly steps taken exceeded her 1-year preoperative baseline at 6 weeks (1911 ± 1320 steps), demonstrating rapid improvement. Her activity remained relatively stable until about 130 weeks postoperatively (as indicated by the blue arrow), which coincided with a new diagnosis of pancreatic cancer

results, and evolve clinical practice as first occurred decades ago. The foundations within neurosurgery for national databases and predictive analytics already exist so the question remains—where will the field go from here?

Within spine surgery, one possible application is international collaboration and merging of quality improvement concepts to foster real-time changes in healthcare standards. Enhanced Recovery After Surgery (ERAS) programs have become an international QI project over the past two decades, through which iterative improvements in standardized perioperative protocols aim to fully optimize outcomes [19]. Neurosurgery has become a recent implementer of ERAS programs and has a history of developing successful national data banks as previously discussed. Therefore, creation of an international ERAS outcomes database that prospectively tracks all patients enrolled in pathways may provide a revolutionary way in patient care is developed and implemented worldwide.

Other subspecialties have adapted machine learning tools to not only predict various outcome measures but enhance preoperative surgical planning. For example, the role of connectomics in cranial neurosurgery has become increasingly popular. While concepts like the Human Connectome Project have many decades, if not generations, until complete, other more readily available applications have been examined [20, 21]. Recent studies have demonstrated promising results that connectome analysis with machine learning tools can be used to predict clinical outcomes after temporal lobe epilepsy and deep brain stimulation surgeries [22, 23]. For neuro-oncologists, predicting particular genotype mutations like IDH in gliomas based on MRI and connectome sequences may prove useful for adjuvant treatment planning [24]. Algorithms that analyze diffusion tensor imaging sequences have been recently developed to augment preoperative surgical planning for intracranial lesions as well [25]. Machine learning models have also been shown to predict the development of delayed cerebral ischemia in subarachnoid hemorrhage patients more accurately than standard models or clinicians [26]. As the national registries in each of the subspecialties develop over time, machine learning applications will continue to identify solutions for improving neurosurgical care.

31.5 Conclusion

In summary, big data and the machine learning tools used for analyses clearly have an important role in the development of neurosurgical care. The origins of big data in neurosurgery trace back to the TBI databases developed in the 1960s and 1970s and set standards for the ways in which data should be collected and managed. The continued development of robust clinical databases used today can enhance the shared decision-making process between patient and surgeon and set expectations for outcomes. Furthermore, the databases aim to set national benchmarks within neurosurgery that provide leverage as the US transitions to a value-based care model. The QOD spine modules have been the most successful to date, but newer collaborations such as the ASR and NVQI-QOD will likely become the new standards for which neurosurgical care is compared. Lastly, machine learning models will further support the utility of big data within the clinical neurosciences as advances in theory and technology simultaneously evolve.

Conflict of Interest Statement The authors declare the following conflicts of interest:

G. Damian Brusko: None.

Gregory Basil: Stockholder (Kinesiometrics).

Michael Wang: Consultant (Depuy-Synthes Spine, Spineology, Stryker); Royalties (Children's Hospital of Los Angeles, Depuy-Synthes Spine, Springer Publishing, Quality Medical Publishing); Speaker's Bureau (Medtronic, Globus); Stock (Innovative Surgical Devices, Kinesiometrics, Medical Device Partners).

References

1. Reed J, Toombs R, Barricelli NA. Simulation of biological evolution and machine learning. I. Selection of self-reproducing numeric patterns by data processing machines, effects of hereditary control, mutation type and crossing. J Theor Biol. 1967;17:319–42. https://doi.org/10.1016/0022-5193(67)90097-5.
2. Choi SC, Muizelaar JP, Barnes TY, Marmarou A, Brooks DM, Young HF. Prediction tree for severely head-injured patients. J Neurosurg. 1991;75:251–5. https://doi.org/10.3171/jns.1991.75.2.0251.
3. Choi SC, Barnes TY, Bullock R, Germanson TA, Marmarou A, Young HF. Temporal profile of outcomes in severe head injury. J Neurosurg. 1994;81:169–73. https://doi.org/10.3171/jns.1994.81.2.0169.
4. Jennett B, Teasdale G, Galbraith S, Pickard J, Grant H, Braakman R, Avezaat C, Maas A, Minderhoud J, Vecht CJ, Heiden J, Small R, Caton W, Kurze T. Severe head injuries in three countries. J Neurol Neurosurg Psychiatry. 1977;40:291–8. https://doi.org/10.1136/jnnp.40.3.291.
5. Marshall LF, Becker DP, Bowers SA, Cayard C, Eisenberg H, Gross CR, Grossman RG, Jane JA, Kunitz SC, Rimel R, Tabaddor K, Warren J. The National Traumatic Coma Data Bank. Part 1: design, purpose, goals, and results. J Neurosurg. 1983;59:276–84. https://doi.org/10.3171/jns.1983.59.2.0276.
6. Whyte J, Vasterling J, Manley GT. Common data elements for research on traumatic brain injury and psychological health: current status and future development. Arch Phys Med Rehabil. 2010;91:1692–6. https://doi.org/10.1016/j.apmr.2010.06.031.
7. Saver JL, Warach S, Janis S, Odenkirchen J, Becker K, Benavente O, Broderick J, Dromerick AW, Duncan P, Elkind MS, Johnston K, Kidwell CS, Meschia JF, Schwamm L. Standardizing the structure of stroke clinical and epidemiologic research data: the National Institute of Neurological Disorders and Stroke (NINDS) stroke common data element (CDE) project. Stroke. 2012;43:967–73. https://doi.org/10.1161/strokeaha.111.634352.
8. Khuri SF, Daley J, Henderson W, Hur K, Demakis J, Aust JB, Chong V, Fabri PJ, Gibbs JO, Grover F, Hammermeister K, Irvin G III, McDonald G, Passaro E Jr, Phillips L, Scamman F, Spencer J, Stremple JF. The Department of Veterans Affairs' NSQIP:

the first national, validated, outcome-based, risk-adjusted, and peer-controlled program for the measurement and enhancement of the quality of surgical care. National VA Surgical Quality Improvement Program. Ann Surg. 1998;228:491–507. https://doi.org/10.1097/00000658-199810000-00006.
9. Clark RE. The development of the Society of Thoracic Surgeons voluntary national database system: genesis, issues, growth, and status. Best Pract Benchmarking Healthc. 1996;1:62–9.
10. Thourani VH, Badhwar V, Shahian DM, O'Brien S, Kitahara H, Vemulapalli S, Brennan JM, Habib RH, Fernandez F, D'Agostino RS, Lobdell K, Rankin JS, Gammie JS, Higgins R, Sabik J, Schwann TA, Jacobs JP. The Society of Thoracic Surgeons adult cardiac surgery database: 2019 update on research. Ann Thorac Surg. 2019;108:334–42. https://doi.org/10.1016/j.athoracsur.2019.05.001.
11. Asher AL, McCormick PC, Selden NR, Ghogawala Z, McGirt MJ. The National Neurosurgery Quality and outcomes database and NeuroPoint Alliance: rationale, development, and implementation. Neurosurg Focus. 2013;34:E2. https://doi.org/10.3171/2012.10.Focus12311.
12. McGirt MJ, Bydon M, Archer KR, Devin CJ, Chotai S, Parker SL, Nian H, Harrell FE Jr, Speroff T, Dittus RS, Philips SE, Shaffrey CI, Foley KT, Asher AL. An analysis from the quality outcomes database, part 1. Disability, quality of life, and pain outcomes following lumbar spine surgery: predicting likely individual patient outcomes for shared decision-making. J Neurosurg Spine. 2017;27:357–69. https://doi.org/10.3171/2016.11.Spine16526.
13. Asher AL, Knightly J, Mummaneni PV, Alvi MA, McGirt MJ, Yolcu YU, Chan AK, Glassman SD, Foley KT, Slotkin JR, Potts EA, Shaffrey ME, Shaffrey CI, Haid RW, Fu KM, Wang MY, Park P, Bisson EF, Harbaugh RE, Bydon M. Quality outcomes database spine care project 2012–2020: milestones achieved in a collaborative north American outcomes registry to advance value-based spine care and evolution to the American spine registry. Neurosurg Focus. 2020;48:E2. https://doi.org/10.3171/2020.2.Focus207.
14. Wang MY, Tran S, Brusko GD, Eastlack R, Park P, Nunley PD, Kanter AS, Uribe JS, Anand N, Okonkwo DO, Than KD, Shaffrey CI, Lafage V, Mundis GM, Mummaneni PV. Less invasive spinal deformity surgery: the impact of the learning curve at tertiary spine care centers. J Neurosurg Spine. 2019:1–8. https://doi.org/10.3171/2019.6.Spine19531.
15. Staartjes VE, Stienen MN. Data mining in spine surgery: leveraging electronic health records for machine learning and clinical research. Neurospine. 2019;16:654–6. https://doi.org/10.14245/ns.1938434.217.
16. Schröder ML, de Wispelaere MP, Staartjes VE. Predictors of loss of follow-up in a prospective registry: which patients drop out 12 months after lumbar spine surgery? Spine J. 2019;19:1672–9. https://doi.org/10.1016/j.spinee.2019.05.007.
17. Azad TD, Ehresman J, Ahmed AK, Staartjes VE, Lubelski D, Stienen MN, Veeravagu A, Ratliff JK. Fostering reproducibility and generalizability in machine learning for clinical prediction modeling in spine surgery. Spine J. 2020. https://doi.org/10.1016/j.spinee.2020.10.006.
18. Moons KG, Altman DG, Reitsma JB, Ioannidis JP, Macaskill P, Steyerberg EW, Vickers AJ, Ransohoff DF, Collins GS. Transparent reporting of a multivariable prediction model for individual prognosis or diagnosis (TRIPOD): explanation and elaboration. Ann Intern Med. 2015;162:W1–73. https://doi.org/10.7326/m14-0698.
19. Ljungqvist O, Scott M, Fearon KC. Enhanced recovery after surgery: a review. JAMA Surg. 2017;152:292–8. https://doi.org/10.1001/jamasurg.2016.4952.
20. Markram H. The blue brain project. Nat Rev Neurosci. 2006;7:153–60. https://doi.org/10.1038/nrn1848.
21. Toga AW, Clark KA, Thompson PM, Shattuck DW, Van Horn JD. Mapping the human connectome. Neurosurgery. 2012;71:1–5. https://doi.org/10.1227/NEU.0b013e318258e9ff.
22. Gleichgerrcht E, Keller SS, Drane DL, Munsell BC, Davis KA, Kaestner E, Weber B, Krantz S, Vandergrift WA, Edwards JC, McDonald CR, Kuzniecky R, Bonilha L. Temporal lobe epilepsy surgical outcomes can be inferred based on structural connectome hubs: a machine learning study. Ann Neurol. 2020;88:970–83. https://doi.org/10.1002/ana.25888.
23. Shang R, He L, Ma X, Ma Y, Li X. Connectome-based model predicts deep brain stimulation outcome in Parkinson's disease. Front Comput Neurosci. 2020;14:571527. https://doi.org/10.3389/fncom.2020.571527.
24. Kesler SR, Harrison RA, Petersen ML, Rao V, Dyson H, Alfaro-Munoz K, Weathers SP, de Groot J. Pre-surgical connectome features predict IDH status in diffuse gliomas. Oncotarget. 2019;10:6484–93. https://doi.org/10.18632/oncotarget.27301.
25. Yeung JT, Taylor HM, Young IM, Nicholas PJ, Doyen S, Sughrue ME. Unexpected hubness: a proof-of-concept study of the human connectome using pagerank centrality and implications for intracerebral neurosurgery. J Neurooncol. 2021;151(2):249–56. https://doi.org/10.1007/s11060-020-03659-6.
26. Savarraj JP, Hergenroeder GW, Zhu L, Chang T, Park S, Megjhani M, Vahidy FS, Zhao Z, Kitagawa RS, Choi HA. Machine learning to predict delayed cerebral ischemia and outcomes in subarachnoid hemorrhage. Neurology. 2021;96(4):e553–62. https://doi.org/10.1212/wnl.0000000000011211.

32 Natural Language Processing Applications in the Clinical Neurosciences: A Machine Learning Augmented Systematic Review

Quinlan D. Buchlak, Nazanin Esmaili, Christine Bennett, and Farrokh Farrokhi

32.1 Introduction

Natural language processing (NLP) is a subfield of computer science, artificial intelligence (AI) and linguistics. It encompasses a set of computational techniques underpinned by machine learning that have been designed to represent, model and analyze human language [1–3]. NLP involves converting unstructured text data into structured datasets that can be readily analyzed by computers and used to predict and classify [4]. NLP application in medicine may be rule-based or statistical [5, 6] and can be used to process high-volume text datasets for information extraction, dimensionality reduction, pattern analysis, keyword identification, anonymization, topic modeling, document classification, sentiment analysis, translation, text generation and question answering [7–9].

The number of studies applying NLP in medicine has been growing steadily [8]. NLP has been used to classify health records [10], detect adverse drug reactions [11–13], facilitate medication reconciliation [14], develop and annotate radiology reports [15], automate the diagnostic process [16–21], develop clinical decision support tools [22], enable risk stratification [23, 24], identify cohorts of patients [25–27], facilitate immunohistochemical analysis [28], guide the administration of intravenous contrast [29] and monitor for infection [30–33] and infection risks [34]. Buchlak et al. applied NLP to facilitate the systematic review process [35]. Electronic medical records (EMR) have been widely implemented and the volume of text data captured in the course of routine clinical practice is immense and growing. Text-based clinical notes provide rich and detailed clinical data that may not be gleaned from other parts of the EMR [36]. These factors have spurred research into more advanced and capable NLP methods [37] to facilitate clinical research.

NLP is increasingly being used to predict clinical outcomes. It has been applied to the automated detection of postoperative complications [38] and to predict patient length of stay and discharge disposition [39]. Murff et al. applied NLP to automate the identification of 30-day postoperative complications in patients undergoing major surgery [40]. Karhade et al. applied NLP to automate the detection of postoperative infections after lumbar discectomy surgery [41]. Rajkomar et al. used NLP to develop a system to automatically chart patient symptoms using transcribed medical history conversations [42]. Liang et al. applied NLP to automate the diagnosis of childhood diseases, analyzing EMR text data from more than 1.3 million pediatric patient visits [43]. Galetta et al. used NLP to analyze clinical trial documentation and predict the likelihood of study termination [44].

NLP research has benefited from the development and release of deep transformer [45] models and transfer learning. Transfer learning involves pretraining a model on a data-rich problem, allowing it to develop relevant associations that can then be transferred to generate appropriate solutions to subsequent tasks [46]. The Text-to-Text Transfer Transformer (T5) [46], Generative Pre-trained Transformer 3 (GPT-3) [47], Bidirectional Encoder Representations from Transformers (BERT) [48], XLNet [49] and RoBERTa [50] models are deep transformer language models, each incorporating many millions of parameters, which have been pretrained on vast text datasets. The Collossal Clean Crawl Corpus (C4) dataset used to train the T5 model stands at 750 gigabytes of text data. These models can be used to effec-

Q. D. Buchlak (✉) · C. Bennett
School of Medicine, The University of Notre Dame Australia, Sydney, NSW, Australia
e-mail: quinlan.buchlak1@my.nd.edu.au

N. Esmaili
School of Medicine, The University of Notre Dame Australia, Sydney, NSW, Australia

Faculty of Engineering and Information Technology, University of Technology Sydney, Ultimo, NSW, Australia

F. Farrokhi
Neuroscience Institute, Virginia Mason Medical Center, Seattle, WA, USA

V. E. Staartjes et al. (eds.), *Machine Learning in Clinical Neuroscience*, Acta Neurochirurgica Supplement 134,
https://doi.org/10.1007/978-3-030-85292-4_32

tively perform a wide array of NLP functions including the generation of news articles [47] and text summaries [51, 52] that are indistinguishable from those written by humans. Pretrained deep language models can be used for high performance document classification without necessitating text preprocessing or feature engineering [48]. The exploration and application of pretrained language models may be beneficial to research and practice in the clinical neurosciences.

The primary objective of this study was to provide a systematic, up-to-date review of NLP applications in the clinical neurosciences. Its secondary objective was to explore some basic NLP use cases to facilitate literature synthesis and provide a sample of clear examples for a clinical audience. This study was guided by two research questions: (1) How has NLP been applied in the clinical neurosciences? (2) Can NLP be applied to facilitate the systematic review process?

32.2 Method

Our method was informed by the Preferred Reporting Items for Systematic Reviews and Meta-Analyses (PRISMA) guidelines [53]. A comprehensive search strategy was developed [54] and applied to the following databases in accordance with recommended practice [55]: PubMed, ScienceDirect, Embase, Ovid, Ebsco, Google Scholar and Scopus. The PROBAST (prediction model risk of bias assessment tool) was used to assess risk of bias [56, 57].

Study Identification

The literature search was conducted between September and October, 2020. The search strategy employed comprehensive combinations of search terms, including methodological and clinical domain keywords and MeSH terms (Table 32.1). The following search query used as an input to PubMed and generated 213 results: [(nlp OR "natural language processing" OR "text classification" OR "topic modeling" OR "topic modelling") AND (neurosurgery OR "spine surgery" OR neuroscience)]. All clinical neuroscience journals indexed by Scimago were individually searched for articles that had applied NLP. The reference lists of each included study were searched to identify additional relevant papers [58]. Reference lists of relevant review articles were also mined.

Table 32.1 MeSH terms and keywords used in the search strategy

	Methods	Clinical neurosciences
Keywords and MeSH terms	• Natural language processing • Gensim • Latent Dirichlet allocation • NLTK • SpaCy • Topic modeling • Text/document classification • Transformer model • Language model	• Brain • Neurology • Neurosciences • Neurosurgery • Spine • Spine surgery • Brain surgery

Inclusion and Exclusion Criteria

Inclusion criteria were: original research published in a peer-reviewed journal; applied NLP methods; research question was relevant to clinical neuroscience (e.g., neurosurgery, spine surgery, or neurology); and published in English. Reviews that applied NLP were included. Exclusion criteria were: described NLP but did not apply it; research protocol; published abstract only; and research that focused on psychiatric disorders, cognitive neuroscience or neurophysiology. Articles were selected for inclusion by QDB and selections were verified by NE. Articles classified as meeting inclusion and exclusion criteria independently by both researchers were included in the analysis, with disagreements resolved by discussion.

Data Collection and Extraction

Numerous datapoints from each included study were collected and coded. Data included: abstract, reference, purpose, study design, NLP input, NLP output, software and data resources used and performance metrics. Authors of each included paper were recorded, along with the lead author's institution and country.

Analysis

Quantitative and qualitative analyses were conducted. Data extracted from each article was used to calculate descriptive statistics. Abstracts were used to feed an NLP analysis that consisted of three phases: (1) keyword identification, (2) text summarization, and (3) training and testing document classifiers. The text was tokenized and converted to lower case, numeric characters and English stop words were removed and remaining tokens were lemmatized [35]. Text summarization was achieved by using the large (770 million parameters) and small (60 million parameters) forms of the T5 transformer model [46]. Multiple document classifiers were trained to explore the development of a system to facilitate automated article screening and selection. The classification outcome was article inclusion in this systematic review, after completion of manual selection and coding. A transfer learning approach for text classification was applied using the BERT [48], RoBERTa [50], and XLNet [49] pretrained deep language models. These models enabled the use of raw, unprocessed text as input. Model classification performance was assessed using threefold cross-validation, with the accuracy, area under the receiver operating characteristic curve (AUC), precision, recall, F1 and Matthew's correlation coefficient (MCC) metrics. The MCC ranges from negative-one to one, while other metrics range between zero and one, with higher numbers indicating better performance. Analyses were conducted using custom Python scripts and the SciPy [59], Scikit-learn [60], NLTK [61], gensim [62, 63], Keras [64], transformers [65], and simpletransformers [66] packages.

32.3 Results

The search resulted in the retrieval of 1131 records. We assessed 142 full-text articles; 94 were excluded, which left 48 for analysis (Fig. 32.1). Study characteristics are displayed in Table 32.2. The most prevalent institutions (affiliated with the first author) were Harvard Medical School ($n = 5$) and Cincinnati Children's Hospital ($n = 3$). The number of publications applying NLP to the clinical neurosciences has increased substantially over the past 5 years (Fig. 32.2).

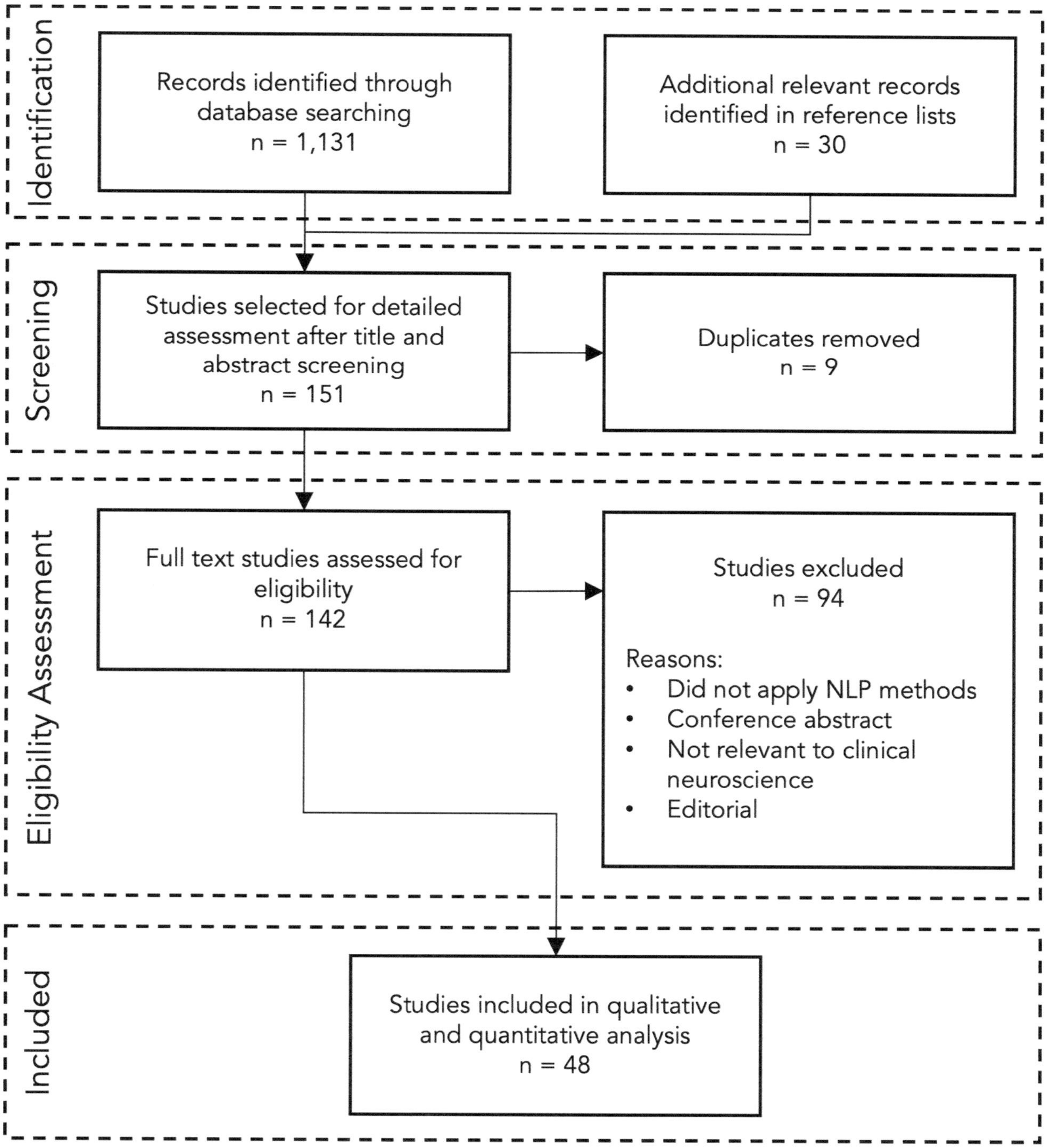

Fig. 32.1 Overview of study screening and selection

Table 32.2 A summary of included study characteristics

Study characteristic	Descriptive statistics
Design	45 (94%) retrospective 3 (6%) prospective
Article type	45 (92%) original research 3 (8%) review
Clinical domain	21 (45%) neurology 16 (33%) neurosurgery 8 (16%) spine surgery 3 (6%) clinical neuroscience
Country	32 (65%) USA 4 (8%) France 2 (4%) UK 2 (4%) Canada 2 (4%) China 2 (4%) Russia 1 (2%) Australia 1 (2%) Japan 1 (2%) Germany 1 (2%) Netherlands

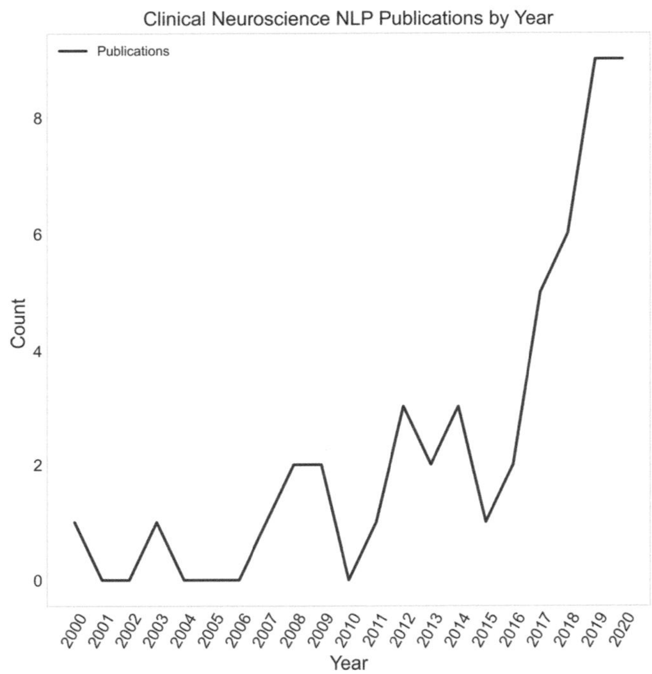

Fig. 32.2 The number of included publications that have applied NLP within the clinical neurosciences by year

NLP Application Domains

NLP has been applied in the clinical neurosciences to facilitate literature synthesis, data extraction, patient identification, automated clinical reporting, and outcome prediction (Table 32.3).

NLP for Patient Cohort Identification

NLP enabled the identification of groups of patients at scale. Zhang et al. processed 4.2 million patient records, identifying 5589 patients with potential cerebral artery aneurysms for inclusion in their study [67]. Zanaty et al. used NLP to retrospectively analyze health records and identify patients for inclusion in their study on decreasing the rate of intracranial aneurysm growth by administering aspirin [27].

NLP for Automated Reporting

NLP was applied to facilitate automated reporting. Karhade et al. [41] developed a system that processed clinical notes of patients who underwent spine surgery to identify those who required reoperation for wound infection within 90 days. Karhade et al. also developed NLP-based systems that processed clinical notes to automatically identify intraoperative vascular injuries [68] and incidental durotomies [69] associated with spine surgery. Wissel et al. incorporated their NLP-based system into a hospital EMR. It analyzed clinical notes and sent alerts to neurologists when epilepsy patients who could potentially benefit from surgery had an upcoming visit. To maximize performance and safety, the algorithm was retrained weekly [70].

NLP for Data and Information Extraction

NLP was used to extract structured data from text. Senders et al. developed an open-source NLP pipeline for variable extraction from clinical text and used it to extract salient features associated with glioblastoma from MRI reports [71]. Knapp et al. [72] used NLP to extract clinical data from the medical records of 3075 Alzheimer's patients. Palacios et al. [73] extracted topics from the text and metadata of a patient support community website.

NLP for Literature Synthesis

NLP was deployed to analyze and synthesize academic literature. Sing et al. [74] derived 100 topics from over 25,000 spine surgery abstracts. Buchlak et al. [35] used NLP to facilitate the systematic review process by modeling topics.

NLP for Outcome Prediction

Only a few studies used NLP to predict clinical outcomes. Danilov et al. [75] used NLP to process 101,654 operative reports and predict the duration of a patient's postoperative hospital stay. Monsour et al. developed an NLP-based tool to predict non-home discharge subsequent to craniotomy for meningioma resection using preoperative clinical notes and radiology reports. This tool appears to be the first publicly available NLP-driven clinical decision support tool implemented in the clinical neurosciences [76].

NLP Analysis

Keywords extracted using NLP techniques highlighted primary clinical practice domains (epilepsy and surgery), data sources and analysis methods used across the corpus

Table 32.3 Summaries of included studies

Reference	Clinical neuroscience subdomain	NLP algorithm inputs	NLP algorithm outputs	NLP purpose/ application type	Risk of bias
Barbour et al. (2019) [82]	Neurology	Electronic medical records	Risk factors for sudden unexpected death in epilepsy	Patient/cohort identification, risk stratification	+
Buchlak et al. (2019) [35]	Neurosurgery	Research abstracts	Topics	Topic modeling	+
Campillo-Gimenez et al. (2012) [77]	Neurosurgery	Clinical notes from 5010 patients (radiology and pathology reports, discharge summaries, consultation notes)	Surgical site infections after neurosurgery within 30 days (no implant) or within 1 year (implant)	Outcome prediction	+
Castro et al. (2017) [94]	Neurology	Electronic medical records	Identification of patients with cerebral aneurysms and controls	Patient/cohort identification	+
Chase et al. (2017) [95]	Neurology	Enriched set of clinical notes from patients with well-established MS ($n = 165$) and controls ($n = 545$)	MS diagnosis	Patient/cohort identification	+
Cohen et al. (2016) [96]	Neurosurgery	Clinical notes	Identification of potential surgical candidates	Patient/cohort identification	+
Connolly et al. (2014) [97]	Neurology	Epilepsy progress notes	Epilepsy type and treating hospital	Patient/cohort identification, data/information extraction	+
Crasto and Shepherd (2007) [98]	Clinical neuroscience	177 Journal of Neuroscience abstracts	Identification of an article as citable or not	Document classification	+
Crasto et al. (2003) [99]	Clinical neuroscience	177 Journal of Neuroscience abstracts	Identification of an article as citable or not	Document classification	+
Cui et al. (2014) [100]	Neurology	Discharge summaries	Extracting epilepsy phenotypes and correlated anatomical locations	Data/information extraction, document classification	+
Dang et al. (2009) [101]	Spine surgery	Radiology reports	Descriptive statistics and trends	Data/information extraction	?
Danilov et al. (2020) [75]	Neurosurgery	101,654 operative reports	Duration of postoperative hospital stay	Outcome prediction	+
Danilov et al. (2020) [102]	Neurosurgery	Preoperative clinical text for 1167 glial tumor resection patients	Muscle weakness (paresis)	Outcome prediction, data/ information extraction	+
Dergachyova et al. (2018) [103]	Neurosurgery	103 postoperative reports (anterior cervical discectomy and fusion, lumbar disc herniation, and pituitary adenoma). 62,489 PubMed abstracts. 32,271 full-text articles	The next activity in a surgical process—a verb describing the movement performed by the surgeon, an instrument used, and an operated anatomical structure	Outcome prediction	+
Elkins et al. [104]	Neurology	471 neuroradiology reports	Coding report for stroke	Document classification	+
Fonferko-Shadrach et al. (2019) [105]	Neurology	Epilepsy clinic letters	Extract clinical information from clinic letters to enrich routinely collected data	Data/information extraction	+
Fraser et al. (2014) [106]	Neurology	Transcriptions of speech for patients with semantic dementia and progressive nonfluent aphasia, and healthy controls	Syntactic and semantic features	Patient/cohort identification, document classification	+
Gaebel et al. (2015) [107]	Neurosurgery	Clinical documentation (in German) in electronic health records	Identification of adverse events documented in the EMR that occurred during treatment	Data/information extraction, document classification	–
Hamid et al. (2013) [18]	Neurology	Clinical notes of 742 Iraq and Afghanistan veterans	Psychogenic nonepileptic seizure diagnosis	Document classification	+

(continued)

Table 32.3 (continued)

Reference	Clinical neuroscience subdomain	NLP algorithm inputs	NLP algorithm outputs	NLP purpose/ application type	Risk of bias
Hoogenboom et al. (2014) [108]	Neurology	EMR notes	Identification of patients with MDD for inclusion in the study	Patient/cohort identification	+
Huhdanpaa et al. (2018) [5]	Spine surgery	Lumbar spine MRI radiology reports	Extracted reported presence of type 1 Modic endplate changes	Document classification	?
Karhade et al. (2019) [69]	Spine surgery	Operative notes	Detection of incidental durotomies	Document classification	+
Karhade et al. (2020) [41]	Spine surgery	Free-text notes of patients who underwent surgery	Reoperation for wound infection within 90 days	Automated reporting/ document classification	+
Karhade et al. (2020) [68]	Spine surgery	Operative notes	Automated identification of intraoperative vascular injury	Automated reporting/ document classification	+
Knapp et al. (2016) [72]	Neurology	3075 Alzheimer's patient clinical records	Observational data	Data/information extraction	+
Lin et al. (2008) [109]	Neurology	Abstracts from the Society for Neuroscience annual meeting 2001–2006	Topics	Topic modeling	+
Marcotte et al. (2017) [76]	Neurology	Clinical notes (25 patients)	Extraction of linguistic features (fluency, lexical, syntactic complexity and semantic)	Data extraction	–
Monsour et al. (2020) [76]	Neurosurgery	Preoperative clinical notes and radiology reports	Discharge disposition	Outcome prediction	+
Naud and Usui (2008) [110]	Clinical neuroscience	Research posters presented at the Society for Neuroscience annual meeting	Topics	Topic modeling	+
Noorbakhsh-Sabet et al. (2018) [111]	Neurology	Brain MRI reports	Patients with cerebral microbleeds	Document classification, patient/cohort identification	+
Palacios et al. (2020) [73]	Neurology	Text and metadata from a patient community website	Topics	Topic modeling	+
Pantazatos et al. (2009) [112]	Neurology	Neuroimaging and microarray datasets	Coding of phenotypes	Data/information extraction	+
Pons et al. (2019) [113]	Neurology	CT reports and clinical notes	Extraction of indication, Glasgow Coma Scale score, and CT outcome	Data/information extraction	+
Senders et al. (2020) [71]	Neurosurgery	MRI reports for 562 patients with glioblastoma	Extraction of 15 radiologic characteristics	Data/information extraction	+
Sing et al. (2017) [74]	Spine surgery	25,805 spine research abstracts	Derived 100 topics	Topic modeling	+
Speier et al. (2013) [114]	Neurology	Electrocorticography signals	Improved spelling performance	Data processing	+
Tan et al. (2018) [115]	Spine surgery	413 X-ray reports and 458 MRI reports	Clinical findings associated with back pain	Information/data extraction	+
Thirukumaran et al. (2019) [116]	Spine surgery	Clinical notes from 172 patients with SSI and 1407 controls	Identification of surgical site infections	Reporting, patient/ cohort identification	+
Titano et al. (2018) [20]	Neurology	Cranial imaging reports	Acute neurologic events	Reporting, patient/ cohort identification	+
Tvardik et al. (2018) [33]	Neurosurgery	Clinical records	Hospital acquired infections	Reporting, patient/ cohort identification	+

Table 32.3 (continued)

Reference	Clinical neuroscience subdomain	NLP algorithm inputs	NLP algorithm outputs	NLP purpose/ application type	Risk of bias
Weng et al. (2017) [36]	Neurology	Clinical notes	Medical specialty classification (e.g., cardiology, neurology, etc.)	Document classification	+
Wissel et al. (2020) [117]	Neurosurgery	Clinical notes from patients with epilepsy and a history of surgery and patients who were seizure-free without surgery	Identification of candidates for epilepsy surgery	Risk stratification, patient/cohort identification	+
Wissel et al. (2019) [70]	Neurosurgery	Clinical notes	Assign surgical candidacy scores to patients	Patient/cohort identification	+
Xu et al. (2020) [118]	Neurology	Diagnostic text or codes	Patients with neurological disorders	Patient/cohort identification	+
Yang et al. (2012) [119]	Neurosurgery	PubMed abstracts	Identification of 1168 glioma-related molecules	Data/information extraction	+
Yarkoni et al. (2011) [120]	Neurology	Research articles	Functional mapping	Data/information extraction	+
Zanaty et al. (2019) [27]	Neurosurgery	Clinical notes	Identification of patients with intracanial aneurysms	Patient/cohort identification	+
Zhang et al. (2019) [67]	Neurosurgery	4.2 million patient records	5589 patients with potential cerebral aneurysms	Patient/cohort identification	+

EMR electronic medical record, *CT* computed tomography, *MDD* major depressive disorder, *MRI* magnetic resonance imaging, *MS* multiple sclerosis, *SSI* surgical site infection

Table 32.4 Keywords identified across the abstracts of all included articles using NLP

Keyword	Frequency
Patient	126
Data	76
NLP	67
Algorithm	62
Clinical	61
Study	56
Note	46
Epilepsy	45
Language	43
Model	43
Processing	39
Analysis	39
Report	37
Natural	36
Medical	35
Learning	35
Surgical	35

(Table 32.4). Document classifiers demonstrated moderate performance, with XLNet slightly outperforming BERT and RoBERTa (Figure 32.3). The T5 transformer model yielded credible abstract summaries with only a few errors. The larger 770 million parameter T5 model appeared to yield better summaries than the smaller 60 million parameter model (Table 32.5)

NLP Resources

Various tools and resources have been developed and used to facilitate NLP research. Those applied in the identified clinical neuroscience corpus included guidelines, software packages and datasets (Table 32.6).

32.4 Discussion

This study provided a systematic overview and synthesis of NLP applications within the clinical neurosciences. To this point, these applications have been diverse but limited. It was evident that NLP use cases coalesced primarily into five main themes: automated reporting, patient cohort identification, clinical data and information extraction, research literature synthesis and clinical outcome prediction. NLP has demonstrated the potential to facilitate quality and safety improvement, clinical coding and automated prospective monitoring and reporting for adverse events and clinical outcomes at the organizational and health system levels [77, 78]. NLP designed to predict outcomes has the potential to improve clinical decision making and facilitate the development of personalized medicine [79]. Analysis of included articles suggested that the number of published studies applying NLP to the clinical neurosciences is increasing rap-

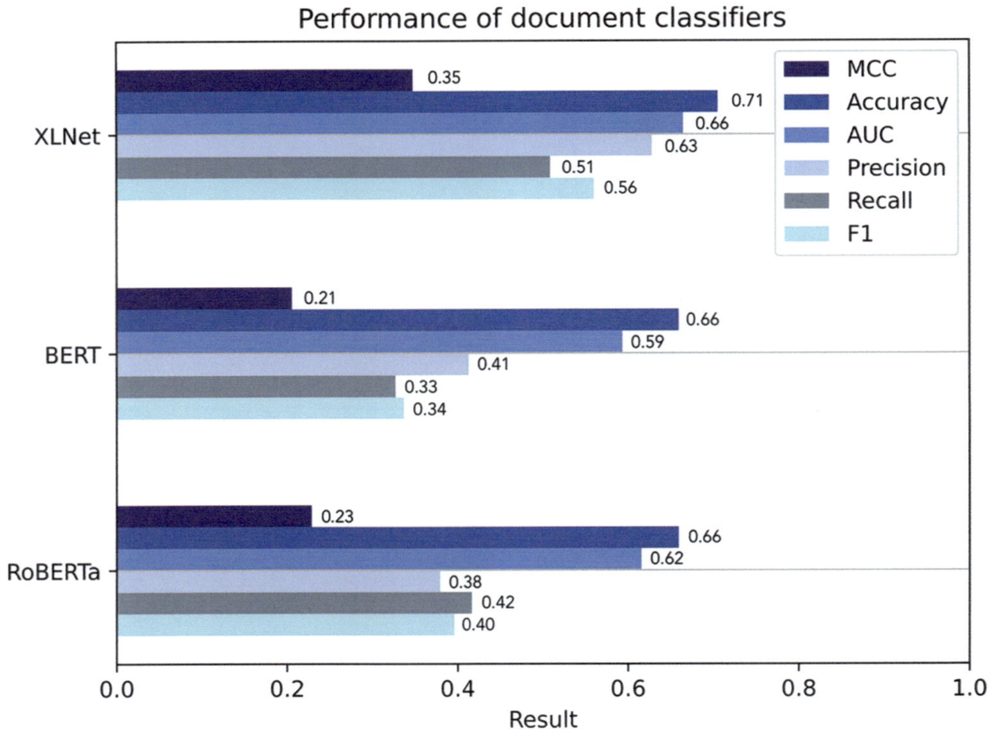

Fig. 32.3 Performance of document classifiers trained to differentiate articles included in this review from those that were excluded. Article abstracts were used as input

Table 32.5 Text summarization results for selected abstracts

Abstract used as NLP input	NLP-generated summary using the small 60 million parameter T5 model	NLP-generated summary using the large 770 million parameter T5 model
Karhade et al. (2020)	Background: Surgical site infections are a major driver of morbidity, study says. The aim of this study was to develop natural language processing (NLP) algorithms for automated reporting of postoperative wound infection requiring reoperation after lumbar discectomy	Surgical site infections are a major driver of morbidity and increased costs in the postoperative period after spine surgery. This study developed natural language processing (NLP) algorithms for automated reporting of wound infection requiring reoperation after lumbar discectomy
Senders et al. (2020)	The aim of this study was to develop an open-source natural language processing pipeline. The pipeline allows for text mining of narratively written clinical reports. Small sample sizes and class imbalance should not be considered as absolute contraindications	Study developed an open-source natural language processing (NLP) pipeline for text mining. Model extracted radiologic characteristics from free-text radiology reports for patients with glioblastoma. Report-level classification accuracy was not associated with the number of words in the distinct text documents
Wissel et al. (2020)	A natural language processing application was trained on notes from patients with epilepsy and history of resective surgery. The testing set included all patients who were seizure-free without surgery and an upcoming neurology visit. Training and testing sets were updated weekly for 1 year. One- to three-word phrases contained in patients' notes were used as features	Natural language processing (NLP) application uses provider notes to assign epilepsy surgery candidacy scores. Training set [sic] was updated weekly and included notes from a mean of 519 67 [sic] patients. Of the 6395 patients who visited the neurology clinic, 4211 (67%) were evaluated by the model
Zhang et al. (2019)	Intracranial aneurysms and surrounding vasculature could affect risk of rupture. Morphological parameters correlated with ruptured middle cerebral artery (MCA)	Five hundred sixty-one patients with 638 MCA aneurysms diagnosed between 1990 and 2016 were included in this study. Greater bottleneck and size ratio, and irregular, multilobed, temporally projecting, are [sic] associated with higher rupture risk, according to a statistical analysis
The present study	Natural language processing (NLP) is a domain of artificial intelligence that models human language. It has been used to automate the diagnostic process, detect adverse events, develop decision support tools and predict clinical outcomes. However, applications to the clinical neurosciences appear to be limited. NLP has recently matured with the implementation of deep transformer models and transfer learning	Natural language processing (NLP) has been used to automate the diagnostic process, detect adverse events and predict clinical outcomes. Applications to the clinical neurosciences have so far been limited, but research is underway to enhance research and practice in the neurosciences

Sentences output by the models were capitalized
Errors in model-generated text have been marked

Table 32.6 NLP resources used by clinical neuroscience researchers

Domain	Tools
Guidelines and standards	• Velupillai et al. (2018) [37]
Software	• BERT [48] • Cancer Text Information Extraction System (caTIES) [121] • General architecture for text engineering (GATE) framework [88] • GloVe [122] • Health Information Text Extraction (HITEx) [123] • Medical Knowledge Analysis Tool (MedTAS/P) [124] • NeuroText • NOMINDEX [125, 126] • pyLDAvis • quanteda (R) • RoBERTa [50] • tidytext (R) • tidyverse (R) • word2vec [127] • Yale cTAKES Extension (YTEX) [128]
Datasets	• CLEF eHealth datasets [129] • Columbia Open Health Data (COHD) [130] • iDASH repository [131] • Japanese clinical documents [132] • National Surgical Quality Improvement Program (NSQIP) registry • Spoken clinical handover transcriptions [133] • Transcribed medical reports (www.mtsamples.com)

idly. This trend is likely driven by the recent development and open release of mature NLP technologies, along with the accumulation of rich text datasets within health system EMRs. EMR systems and the corresponding accumulation of large text-based datasets in the course of routine clinical practice have set the scene for the effective application of NLP technologies. NLP enables further beneficial use of clinical notes, beyond the immediate patient care lifecycle. It can be used to rapidly acquire additional data from large clinical text corpora, facilitating research and the development of clinical interventions.

Few studies deployed pretrained deep language models (e.g., XLNet, BERT, RoBERTa, T5, etc.). These models can be used for successful document classification and summarization. A salient benefit of these models is that they remove the need for feature engineering, resulting in a more efficient and replicable classifier training and validation process. The automated generation of NLP features is more scalable and efficient and less labor intensive [41]. These deep learning models, however, require much more training data than shallower machine learning models that necessitate feature engineering. Limited datasets, like the one used to train the classifiers in this study to differentiate between included and excluded articles, appear to be associated with only moderate performance when using pretrained deep learning models. Future research may investigate the deployment of other machine learning models to facilitate systematic review article screening. Improved deep learning model performance may be achieved by exploring text dataset augmentation techniques. There is substantial potential to further explore the application of deep language models to classify and summarize documents in the clinical neurosciences.

As clinical NLP matures, multiple issues require close consideration by researchers including model interpretability, research replicability, the development of personalized models, the delivery of time sensitive predictions [37], and ethical system implementation to facilitate clinical practice [80]. The potential for bias should be considered and mitigated [81]. Challenges facing the implementation of NLP include variations in EMR systems, clinical practice and clinical language and access to sufficiently sized clinical datasets [82]. Integrating NLP-based decision support systems into comprehensive perioperative care processes may serve to improve patient safety [83]. The continued development of guidelines [37] and principles [80] will facilitate the efficacious development and implementation of beneficial and safe machine learning driven clinical tools.

NLP research is often underpinned by powerful open-source software. NLP resources are continually developing and becoming more usable for clinicians. Resources applied in the body of literature reviewed here were summarized to facilitate future research. Because NLP research in the neurosciences appears to be in the early stages of development, this list is incomplete. NLP software packages include gensim [62, 63], SpaCy [84], the Natural Language Toolkit (NLTK) [61], pyLDAvis [85], Simple Transformers [66], Stanza (formerly known as StanfordNLP) [86, 87] and the General Architecture for Text Engineering (GATE) [88]. We focus primarily on packages that can be used with Python because our team has specialized in this language. Gensim is a fast and widely used library that facilitates unsupervised topic modeling and other NLP functions for large volumes of text [63]. SpaCy is a library designed for production use and has a reputation for rapid parsing [89]. It enables natural language understanding, information extraction and preprocessing to facilitate deep learning [84]. NLTK is a platform that facilitates both symbolic and statistical NLP. It interfaces with annotated corpora and offers access to text processing libraries for tokenization, stemming, tagging, parsing, semantic reasoning and classification [90]. pyLDAvis enables topic visualization and interpretation [85]. Simple Transformers facilitates access to, and the implementation of, deep transformer models [66]. It does not yet, however, support some custom weighted models like ClinicalBERT [91]. Stanza interfaces with CoreNLP and offers a broad range of tools for various NLP functions (e.g., linguistic annotation), supporting more than 60 languages [86, 87]. It now incorporates clinical and biomedical models to enable named entity recognition and syntactic analysis in specialist literature [92]. GATE, developed over a 20-year period, provides a collection of text analysis tools and processes for various aspects of language engineering [88]. While some of these packages are designed to perform specific and distinct functions, there is substantial overlap between many of them and many cater for numerous languages. Comparisons of NLP software packages, reviewing performance and documentation quality, are rare. StanfordNLP (Stanza) appears to demonstrate strong named entity recognition performance when compared with other packages [93]. Further development of open-source software systems by engineers that make the application of mature NLP technologies easier for clinicians will facilitate translational research and clinical innovation. Further adoption of these kinds of tools by clinical neuroscience practitioners is likely to result in additional useful research outputs and clinical decision support tools that may deliver benefits to patients. Future research evaluating and quantifying the impact of NLP systems on the overall time it takes to complete systematic reviews would be informative.

The majority of included studies came from the United States. While a small number of studies were identified from non-English speaking countries, NLP is inherently tied to language and some articles applying NLP to the neurosciences published in languages other than English may not have been captured by this review.

32.5 Conclusion

The application of NLP in the clinical neurosciences has so far been limited, but this field of research appears to be snowballing. As NLP technologies mature, the potential for them to generate clinical benefits for patients and providers grows. NLP and machine learning appear to be enhancing research and practice in the clinical neurosciences.

Disclosures All authors have reviewed and approved this manuscript and have no conflicts of interest in relation to the publication of this study.

References

1. Cambria E, White B. Jumping NLP curves: a review of natural language processing research. IEEE Comput Intell Mag. 2014;9:48–57.
2. Pons E, Braun LMM, Hunink MGM, Kors JA. Natural language processing in radiology: a systematic review. Radiology. 2016;279:329–43.
3. Young T, Hazarika D, Poria S, Cambria E. Recent trends in deep learning based natural language processing. IEEE Comput Intell Mag. 2018;13:55–75.
4. Friedman C, Elhadad N. Natural language processing in health care and biomedicine. In: Biomedical informatics. Berlin: Springer; 2014. p. 255–84.
5. Huhdanpaa HT, Tan WK, Rundell SD, Suri P, Chokshi FH, Comstock BA, et al. Using natural language processing of free-text radiology reports to identify type 1 modic endplate changes. J Digit Imaging. 2018;31:84–90.
6. Taggart M, Chapman WW, Steinberg BA, Ruckel S, Pregenzer-Wenzler A, Du Y, et al. Comparison of 2 natural language processing methods for identification of bleeding among critically ill patients. JAMA Netw Open. 2018;1:e183451.
7. Cardinal RN. Clinical records anonymisation and text extraction (CRATE): an open-source software system. BMC Med Inform Decis Mak. 2017;17:50.
8. Chen X, Xie H, Wang FL, Liu Z, Xu J, Hao T. A bibliometric analysis of natural language processing in medical research. BMC Med Inform Decis Mak. 2018;18:14.
9. Panesar SS, Kliot M, Parrish R, Fernandez-Miranda J, Cagle Y, Britz GW. Promises and perils of artificial intelligence in neurosurgery. Neurosurgery. 2020;87:33–44.
10. Zheng L, Wang Y, Hao S, Shin AY, Jin B, Ngo AD, et al. Web-based real-time case finding for the population health Management of Patients with diabetes mellitus: a prospective validation of the natural language processing–based algorithm with statewide electronic medical records. JMIR Med Inform. 2016;4:e37.
11. Li F, Yu H. An investigation of single-domain and multidomain medication and adverse drug event relation extraction from electronic health record notes using advanced deep learning models. J Am Med Inform Assoc. 2019;26:646–54.
12. Sarker A, Gonzalez G. Portable automatic text classification for adverse drug reaction detection via multi-corpus training. J Biomed Inform. 2015;53:196–207.
13. Wei Q, Ji Z, Li Z, Du J, Wang J, Xu J, et al. A study of deep learning approaches for medication and adverse drug event extraction from clinical text. J Am Med Inform Assoc. 2020;27:13–21.
14. Li Q, Spooner SA, Kaiser M, Lingren N, Robbins J, Lingren T, et al. An end-to-end hybrid algorithm for automated medication discrepancy detection. BMC Med Inform Decis Mak. 2015;15:37.
15. Zech J, Pain M, Titano J, Badgeley M, Schefflein J, Su A, et al. Natural language–based machine learning models for the annotation of clinical radiology reports. Radiology. 2018;287:570–80.
16. Fiszman M, Chapman WW, Aronsky D, Evans RS, Haug PJ. Automatic detection of acute bacterial pneumonia from chest X-ray reports. J Am Med Inform Assoc. 2000;7:593–604.
17. Goff DJ, Loehfelm TW. Automated radiology report summarization using an open-source natural language processing pipeline. J Digit Imaging. 2018;31:185–92.
18. Hamid H, Fodeh SJ, Lizama AG, Czlapinski R, Pugh MJ, LaFrance WC Jr, et al. Validating a natural language processing tool to exclude psychogenic nonepileptic seizures in electronic medical record-based epilepsy research. Epilepsy Behav. 2013;29:578–80.
19. Jain NL, Knirsch CA, Friedman C, Hripcsak G. Identification of suspected tuberculosis patients based on natural language processing of chest radiograph reports. In: Proceedings of the AMIA Annual Fall Symposium. American Medical Informatics Association; 1996. p. 542.
20. Titano JJ, Badgeley M, Schefflein J, Pain M, Su A, Cai M, et al. Automated deep-neural-network surveillance of cranial images for acute neurologic events. Nat Med. 2018;24:1337–41.
21. Yadav K, Sarioglu E, Smith M, Choi H. Automated outcome classification of emergency department computed tomography imaging reports. Acad Emerg Med. 2013;20:848–54.
22. Wagholikar KB, MacLaughlin KL, Henry MR, Greenes RA, Hankey RA, Liu H, et al. Clinical decision support with automated text processing for cervical cancer screening. J Am Med Inform Assoc. 2012;19:833–9.

23. Liao KP, Ananthakrishnan AN, Kumar V, Xia Z, Cagan A, Gainer VS, et al. Methods to develop an electronic medical record phenotype algorithm to compare the risk of coronary artery disease across 3 chronic disease cohorts. PLoS One. 2015;10:e0136651.
24. McCoy TH, Castro VM, Cagan A, Roberson AM, Kohane IS, Perlis RH. Sentiment measured in hospital discharge notes is associated with readmission and mortality risk: an electronic health record study. PLoS One. 2015;10:e0136341.
25. Cui L, Bozorgi A, Lhatoo SD, Zhang G-Q, Sahoo SS. EpiDEA: extracting structured epilepsy and seizure information from patient discharge summaries for cohort identification. In: AMIA Annual Symposium Proceedings, vol. 2012. Washington, DC: American Medical Informatics Association; 2012. p. 1191.
26. Shivade C, Raghavan P, Fosler-Lussier E, Embi PJ, Elhadad N, Johnson SB, et al. A review of approaches to identifying patient phenotype cohorts using electronic health records. J Am Med Inform Assoc. 2014;21:221–30.
27. Zanaty M, Roa JA, Nakagawa D, Chalouhi N, Allan L, Al Kasab S, et al. Aspirin associated with decreased rate of intracranial aneurysm growth. J Neurosurg. 2019;1:1–8.
28. Chang J-F, Popescu M, Arthur GL. Automated extraction of precise protein expression patterns in lymphoma by text mining abstracts of immunohistochemical studies. J Pathol Inform. 2013;4:20.
29. Trivedi H, Mesterhazy J, Laguna B, Vu T, Sohn JH. Automatic determination of the need for intravenous contrast in musculo-skeletal MRI examinations using IBM Watson's natural language processing algorithm. J Digit Imaging. 2018;31:245–51.
30. Branch-Elliman W, Strymish J, Kudesia V, Rosen AK, Gupta K. Natural language processing for real-time catheter-associated urinary tract infection surveillance: results of a pilot implementation trial. Infect Control Hosp Epidemiol. 2015;36:1004–10.
31. Gundlapalli AV, Divita G, Redd A, Carter ME, Ko D, Rubin M, et al. Detecting the presence of an indwelling urinary catheter and urinary symptoms in hospitalized patients using natural language processing. J Biomed Inform. 2017;71:S39–45.
32. Hu Z, Simon GJ, Arsoniadis EG, Wang Y, Kwaan MR, Melton GB. Automated detection of postoperative surgical site infections using supervised methods with electronic health record data. Stud Health Technol Inform. 2015;216:706.
33. Tvardik N, Kergourlay I, Bittar A, Segond F, Darmoni S, Metzger M-H. Accuracy of using natural language processing methods for identifying healthcare-associated infections. Int J Med Inform. 2018;117:96–102.
34. Jones M, DuVall SL, Spuhl J, Samore MH, Nielson C, Rubin M. Identification of methicillin-resistant Staphylococcus aureus within the nation's veterans affairs medical centers using natural language processing. BMC Med Inform Decis Mak. 2012;12:1–8.
35. Buchlak QD, Esmaili N, Leveque J-C, Farrokhi F, Bennett C, Piccardi M, et al. Machine learning applications to clinical decision support in neurosurgery: an artificial intelligence augmented systematic review. Neurosurg Rev. 2020;43:1235–53. https://doi.org/10.1007/s10143-019-01163-8.
36. Weng W-H, Wagholikar KB, McCray AT, Szolovits P, Chueh HC. Medical subdomain classification of clinical notes using a machine learning-based natural language processing approach. BMC Med Inform Decis Mak. 2017;17:1–13.
37. Velupillai S, Suominen H, Liakata M, Roberts A, Shah AD, Morley K, et al. Using clinical natural language processing for health outcomes research: overview and actionable suggestions for future advances. J Biomed Inform. 2018;88:11–9.
38. D'Avolio LW, Nguyen TM, Goryachev S, Fiore LD. Automated concept-level information extraction to reduce the need for custom software and rules development. J Am Med Inform Assoc. 2011;18:607–13.
39. Bacchi S, Gluck S, Tan Y, Chim I, Cheng J, Gilbert T, et al. Prediction of general medical admission length of stay with natural language processing and deep learning: a pilot study. Intern Emerg Med. 2020;15:989–95.
40. Murff HJ, FitzHenry F, Matheny ME, Gentry N, Kotter KL, Crimin K, et al. Automated identification of postoperative complications within an electronic medical record using natural language processing. JAMA. 2011;306:848–55.
41. Karhade AV, Bongers MER, Groot OQ, Cha TD, Doorly TP, Fogel HA, et al. Can natural language processing provide accurate, automated reporting of wound infection requiring reoperation after lumbar discectomy? Spine J. 2020;20(10):1602–9.
42. Rajkomar A, Kannan A, Chen K, Vardoulakis L, Chou K, Cui C, et al. Automatically charting symptoms from patient-physician conversations using machine learning. JAMA Intern Med. 2019;179:836–8.
43. Liang H, Tsui BY, Ni H, Valentim CCS, Baxter SL, Liu G, et al. Evaluation and accurate diagnoses of pediatric diseases using artificial intelligence. Nat Med. 2019;25:433–8.
44. Geletta S, Follett L, Laugerman M. Latent Dirichlet allocation in predicting clinical trial terminations. BMC Med Inform Decis Mak. 2019;19:242.
45. Vaswani A, Shazeer N, Parmar N, Uszkoreit J, Jones L, Gomez AN, et al. Attention is all you need. In: Advances in neural information processing systems; 2017. p. 5998–6008.
46. Raffel C, Shazeer N, Roberts A, Lee K, Narang S, Matena M, et al. Exploring the limits of transfer learning with a unified text-to-text transformer. In: ArXiv Prepr ArXiv191010683; 2019.
47. Brown TB, Mann B, Ryder N, Subbiah M, Kaplan J, Dhariwal P, et al. Language models are few-shot learners. In: ArXiv Prepr ArXiv200514165; 2020.
48. Devlin J, Chang M-W, Lee K, Toutanova K. Bert: pre-training of deep bidirectional transformers for language understanding. In: ArXiv Prepr ArXiv181004805; 2018.
49. Yang Z, Dai Z, Yang Y, Carbonell J, Salakhutdinov RR, Le QV. XLNet: Generalized autoregressive pretraining for language understanding. In: Advances in neural information processing systems; 2019. p. 5753–63.
50. Liu Y, Ott M, Goyal N, Du J, Joshi M, Chen D, et al. Roberta: a robustly optimized bert pretraining approach. In: ArXiv Prepr ArXiv190711692; 2019.
51. Stiennon N, Ouyang L, Wu J, Ziegler DM, Lowe R, Voss C, et al. Learning to summarize from human feedback. In: ArXiv Prepr ArXiv200901325; 2020.
52. Ziegler DM, Stiennon N, Wu J, Brown TB, Radford A, Amodei D, et al. Fine-tuning language models from human preferences. In: ArXiv Prepr ArXiv190908593; 2019.
53. Moher D, Liberati A, Tetzlaff J, Altman DG. Preferred reporting items for systematic reviews and meta-analyses: the PRISMA statement. Ann Intern Med. 2009;151:264–9.
54. Sampson M, McGowan J, Tetzlaff J, Cogo E, Moher D. No consensus exists on search reporting methods for systematic reviews. J Clin Epidemiol. 2008;61:748–54.
55. Bramer WM, Rethlefsen ML, Kleijnen J, Franco OH. Optimal database combinations for literature searches in systematic reviews: a prospective exploratory study. Syst Rev. 2017;6:245.
56. Moons KGM, Wolff RF, Riley RD, Whiting PF, Westwood M, Collins GS, et al. PROBAST: a tool to assess risk of bias and applicability of prediction model studies: explanation and elaboration. Ann Intern Med. 2019;170:W1–33.
57. Wolff RF, Moons KGM, Riley RD, Whiting PF, Westwood M, Collins GS, et al. PROBAST: a tool to assess the risk of bias and applicability of prediction model studies. Ann Intern Med. 2019;170:51–8.
58. Richards D. Handsearching still a valuable element of the systematic review. Evid Based Dent. 2008;9:85.
59. Jones E, Oliphant T, Peterson P. {SciPy}: Open source scientific tools for {Python}; 2014.

60. Pedregosa F, Varoquaux G, Gramfort A, Michel V, Thirion B, Grisel O, et al. Scikit-learn: machine learning in Python. J Mach Learn Res. 2011;12:2825–30.
61. Bird S, Klein E, Loper E. Natural language processing with Python: analyzing text with the natural language toolkit. Newton, MA: O'Reilly Media; 2009.
62. Řehůřek R. Scalability of semantic analysis in natural language processing; 2011.
63. Rehurek R, Sojka P. Software framework for topic modelling with large corpora. In: Proceedings of the Lr. 2010 Work. New challenges NLP Fram., Citeseer; 2010.
64. Chollet F. Keras: the Python deep learning library. Astrophysics Source Code Library; 2018.
65. Wolf T, Debut L, Sanh V, Chaumond J, Delangue C, Moi A, et al. HuggingFace's transformers: state-of-the-art natural language processing. ArXiv 2019:arXiv-1910.
66. Rajapakse T. Simple transformers. 2019. https://github.com/ThilinaRajapakse/simpletransformers.
67. Zhang J, Can A, Mukundan S Jr, Steigner M, Castro VM, Dligach D, et al. Morphological variables associated with ruptured middle cerebral artery aneurysms. Neurosurgery. 2019;85:75–83.
68. Karhade A V, Bongers MER, Groot OQ, Cha TD, Doorly TP, Fogel HA, et al. Development of machine learning and natural language processing algorithms for preoperative prediction and automated identification of intraoperative vascular injury in anterior lumbar spine surgery. Spine J. 2020.
69. Karhade AV, Bongers MER, Groot OQ, Kazarian ER, Cha TD, Fogel HA, et al. Natural language processing for automated detection of incidental durotomy. Spine J. 2020;20:695–700.
70. Wissel BD, Greiner HM, Glauser TA, Mangano FT, Santel D, Pestian JP, et al. Investigation of bias in an epilepsy machine learning algorithm trained on physician notes. Epilepsia. 2019;60:e93–8.
71. Senders JT, Cho LD, Calvachi P, McNulty JJ, Ashby JL, Schulte IS, et al. Automating clinical chart review: an open-source natural language processing pipeline developed on free-text radiology reports from patients with glioblastoma. JCO Clin Cancer Informatics. 2020;4:25–34.
72. Knapp M, Chua K-C, Broadbent M, Chang C-K, Fernandez J-L, Milea D, et al. Predictors of care home and hospital admissions and their costs for older people with Alzheimer's disease: findings from a large London case register. BMJ Open. 2016;6:e013591.
73. Palacios G, Noreña A, Londero A. Assessing the heterogeneity of complaints related to tinnitus and Hyperacusis from an unsupervised machine learning approach: an exploratory study. Audiol Neurotol. 2020;25:174–89.
74. Sing DC, Metz LN, Dudli S. Machine learning-based classification of 38 years of spine-related literature into 100 research topics. Spine (Phila Pa 1976). 2017;42(11):863–70. https://doi.org/10.1097/BRS.0000000000002079.
75. Danilov G, Kotik K, Shifrin M, Strunina U, Pronkina T, Potapov A. Predicting postoperative hospital stay in neurosurgery with recurrent neural networks based on operative reports. Stud Health Technol Inform. 2020;270:382–6.
76. Monsour MA, Muhlestein WE, Friedman G, Zinzuwadia A, Zachariah M, Coumans J-V, et al. Predicting discharge disposition following meningioma resection using a multiinstitutional natural language processing model. J Neurol Surg Pt B Skull Base. 2020;81:A174.
77. Campillo-Gimenez B, Garcelon N, Jarno P, Chapplain JM, Cuggia M. Full-text automated detection of surgical site infections secondary to neurosurgery in Rennes, France. Stud Health Technol Inform. 2012;192:572–5.
78. Kimia AA, Savova G, Landschaft A, Harper MB. An introduction to natural language processing: how you can get more from those electronic notes you are generating. Pediatr Emerg Care. 2015;31:536–41.
79. Khan O, Badhiwala JH, Grasso G, Fehlings MG. Use of machine learning and artificial intelligence to drive personalized medicine approaches for spine care. World Neurosurg. 2020;140:512–8.
80. Buchlak QD, Esmaili N, Leveque J-C, Bennett C, Piccardi M, Farrokhi F. Ethical thinking machines in surgery and the requirement for clinical leadership. Am J Surg. 2020;220(5):1372–4.
81. Caliskan A, Bryson JJ, Narayanan A. Semantics derived automatically from language corpora contain human-like biases. Science (80-). 2017;356:183–6.
82. Barbour K, Hesdorffer DC, Tian N, Yozawitz EG, McGoldrick PE, Wolf S, et al. Automated detection of sudden unexpected death in epilepsy risk factors in electronic medical records using natural language processing. Epilepsia. 2019;60:1209–20.
83. Buchlak QD, Yanamadala V, Leveque J-C, Sethi R. Complication avoidance with pre-operative screening: insights from the Seattle spine team. Curr Rev Musculoskelet Med. 2016;9:316. https://doi.org/10.1007/s12178-016-9351-x.
84. Honnibal M, Montani I. Spacy 2: natural language understanding with bloom embeddings. In: Convolutional neural networks and incremental parsing, vol. 7; 2017. To Appear.
85. Sievert C, Shirley K. LDAvis: A method for visualizing and interpreting topics. In: Proceedings of the workshop on interactive language learning, visualization, and interfaces; 2014. p. 63–70.
86. Manning C, Surdeanu M, Bauer J, Finkel J, Bethard S, McClosky D. The Stanford CoreNLP natural language processing toolkit. In: Proceedings of the 52nd Annual Meeting of the Association for Computational Linguistics: System Demonstrations; 2014. p. 55–60.
87. Qi P, Dozat T, Zhang Y, Manning CD. Universal dependency parsing from scratch. In: ArXiv Prepr ArXiv190110457; 2019.
88. Cunningham H, Tablan V, Roberts A, Bontcheva K. Getting more out of biomedical documents with GATE's full lifecycle open source text analytics. PLoS Comput Biol. 2013;9:e1002854.
89. Choi JD, Tetreault J, Stent A. It depends: dependency parser comparison using a web-based evaluation tool. In: Proceedings of the 53rd Annual Meeting of the Association for Computational Linguistics and the 7th International Joint Conference on Natural Language Processing (Volume 1: Long Papers). (Volume 1: Long Papers); 2015. p. 387–96.
90. Loper E, Bird S. NLTK: the natural language toolkit. In: ArXiv Prepr Cs/0205028; 2002.
91. Huang K, Altosaar J, Ranganath R. Clinicalbert: modeling clinical notes and predicting hospital readmission. In: ArXiv Prepr ArXiv190405342; 2019.
92. Qi P, Zhang Y, Zhang Y, Bolton J, Manning CD. Stanza: a Python natural language processing toolkit for many human languages. In: ArXiv Prepr ArXiv200307082; 2020.
93. Schmitt X, Kubler S, Robert J, Papadakis M, LeTraon Y. A replicable comparison study of NER Software: StanfordNLP, NLTK, OpenNLP, SpaCy, Gate. In: Sixth International conference on social networks analysis, management and security. Piscataway, NJ: IEEE; 2019. p. 338–43.
94. Castro VM, Dligach D, Finan S, Yu S, Can A, Abd-El-Barr M, et al. Large-scale identification of patients with cerebral aneurysms using natural language processing. Neurology. 2017;88:164–8.
95. Chase HS, Mitrani LR, Lu GG, Fulgieri DJ. Early recognition of multiple sclerosis using natural language processing of the electronic health record. BMC Med Inform Decis Mak. 2017;17:1–8.
96. Cohen KB, Glass B, Greiner HM, Holland-Bouley K, Standridge S, Arya R, et al. Methodological issues in predicting pediatric epilepsy surgery candidates through natural language processing and machine learning. Biomed Inform Insights. 2016;8:BII–S38308.
97. Connolly B, Matykiewicz P, Bretonnel Cohen K, Standridge SM, Glauser TA, Dlugos DJ, et al. Assessing the similarity of surface linguistic features related to epilepsy across pediatric hospitals. J Am Med Inform Assoc. 2014;21:866–70.

98. Crasto CJ, Shepherd GM. Managing knowledge in neuroscience. In: Neuroinformatics. Berlin: Springer; 2007. p. 3–21.
99. Crasto CJ, Marenco LN, Migliore M, Mao B, Nadkarni PM, Miller P, et al. Text mining neuroscience journal articles to populate neuroscience databases. Neuroinformatics. 2003;1:215–37.
100. Cui L, Sahoo SS, Lhatoo SD, Garg G, Rai P, Bozorgi A, et al. Complex epilepsy phenotype extraction from narrative clinical discharge summaries. J Biomed Inform. 2014;51:272–9.
101. Dang PA, Kalra MK, Blake MA, Schultz TJ, Stout M, Halpern EF, et al. Use of Radcube for extraction of finding trends in a large radiology practice. J Digit Imaging. 2009;22:629.
102. Danilov G, Shifrin M, Strunina Y, Kotik K, Tsukanova T, Pronkina T, et al. Semiautomated approach for muscle weakness detection in clinical texts. Stud Health Technol Inform. 2020;272:55–8.
103. Dergachyova O, Morandi X, Jannin P. Knowledge transfer for surgical activity prediction. Int J Comput Assist Radiol Surg. 2018;13:1409–17.
104. Elkins JS, Friedman C, Boden-Albala B, Sacco RL, Hripcsak G. Coding neuroradiology reports for the northern Manhattan stroke study: a comparison of natural language processing and manual review. Comput Biomed Res. 2000;33:1–10.
105. Fonferko-Shadrach B, Lacey AS, Roberts A, Akbari A, Thompson S, Ford DV, et al. Using natural language processing to extract structured epilepsy data from unstructured clinic letters: development and validation of the ExECT (extraction of epilepsy clinical text) system. BMJ Open. 2019;9:e023232.
106. Fraser KC, Meltzer JA, Graham NL, Leonard C, Hirst G, Black SE, et al. Automated classification of primary progressive aphasia subtypes from narrative speech transcripts. Cortex. 2014;55:43–60.
107. Gaebel J, Kolter T, Arlt F, Denecke K. Extraction of adverse events from clinical documents to support decision making using semantic preprocessing. Stud Health Technol Inform. 2015;216:1030.
108. Hoogenboom WS, Perlis RH, Smoller JW, Zeng-Treitler Q, Gainer VS, Murphy SN, et al. Limbic system white matter microstructure and long-term treatment outcome in major depressive disorder: a diffusion tensor imaging study using legacy data. World J Biol Psychiatry. 2014;15:122–34.
109. Lin JM, Bohland JW, Andrews P, Burns GAPC, Allen CB, Mitra PP. An analysis of the abstracts presented at the annual meetings of the Society for Neuroscience from 2001 to 2006. PLoS One. 2008;3:e2052.
110. Naud A, Usui S. Exploration of a collection of documents in neuroscience and extraction of topics by clustering. Neural Netw. 2008;21:1205–11.
111. Noorbakhsh-Sabet N, Tsivgoulis G, Shahjouei S, Hu Y, Goyal N, Alexandrov AV, et al. Racial difference in cerebral microbleed burden among a patient population in the mid-South United States. J Stroke Cerebrovasc Dis. 2018;27:2657–61.
112. Pantazatos SP, Li J, Pavlidis P, Lussier YA. Integration of neuroimaging and microarray datasets through mapping and model-theoretic semantic decomposition of unstructured phenotypes. Cancer Inform. 2009;8:CIN-S1046.
113. Pons E, Foks KA, Dippel DWJ, Hunink MGM. Impact of guidelines for the management of minor head injury on the utilization and diagnostic yield of CT over two decades, using natural language processing in a large dataset. Eur Radiol. 2019;29:2632–40.
114. Speier W, Fried I, Pouratian N. Improved P300 speller performance using electrocorticography, spectral features, and natural language processing. Clin Neurophysiol. 2013;124:1321–8.
115. Tan WK, Hassanpour S, Heagerty PJ, Rundell SD, Suri P, Huhdanpaa HT, et al. Comparison of natural language processing rules-based and machine-learning systems to identify lumbar spine imaging findings related to low back pain. Acad Radiol. 2018;25:1422–32.
116. Thirukumaran CP, Zaman A, Rubery PT, Calabria C, Li Y, Ricciardi BF, et al. Natural language processing for the identification of surgical site infections in orthopaedics. J Bone Joint Surg Am. 2019;101(24):2167–74.
117. Wissel BD, Greiner HM, Glauser TA, Holland-Bouley KD, Mangano FT, Santel D, et al. Prospective validation of a machine learning model that uses provider notes to identify candidates for resective epilepsy surgery. Epilepsia. 2020;61:39–48.
118. Xu L, Chen L, Wang S, Feng J, Liu L, Liu G, et al. Incidence and prevalence of amyotrophic lateral sclerosis in urban China: a national population-based study. J Neurol Neurosurg Psychiatry. 2020;91:520–5.
119. Yang S, Wang K, Qian C, Song Z, Pu P, Zhang A, et al. A predicted miR-27a-mediated network identifies a signature of glioma. Oncol Rep. 2012;28:1249–56.
120. Yarkoni T, Poldrack RA, Nichols TE, Van Essen DC, Wager TD. Large-scale automated synthesis of human functional neuroimaging data. Nat Methods. 2011;8:665–70.
121. Crowley RS, Castine M, Mitchell K, Chavan G, McSherry T, Feldman M. caTIES: a grid based system for coding and retrieval of surgical pathology reports and tissue specimens in support of translational research. J Am Med Inform Assoc. 2010;17:253–64.
122. Pennington J, Socher R, Manning CD. Glove: global vectors for word representation. In: Proceedings of the 2014 Conference on Empirical Methods in Natural Language Processing; 2014. p. 1532–43.
123. Zeng QT, Goryachev S, Weiss S, Sordo M, Murphy SN, Lazarus R. Extracting principal diagnosis, co-morbidity and smoking status for asthma research: evaluation of a natural language processing system. BMC Med Inform Decis Mak. 2006;6:1–9.
124. Coden A, Savova G, Sominsky I, Tanenblatt M, Masanz J, Schuler K, et al. Automatically extracting cancer disease characteristics from pathology reports into a disease knowledge representation model. J Biomed Inform. 2009;42:937–49.
125. Happe A, Pouliquen B, Burgun A, Cuggia M, Le Beux P. Automatic concept extraction from spoken medical reports. Int J Med Inform. 2003;70:255–63.
126. Le FD, Burgun A, Pouliquen B, Delamarre D, Le PB. Automatic enrichment of the unified medical language system starting from the ADM knowledge base. Stud Health Technol Inform. 1999;68:881–6.
127. Mikolov T, Chen K, Corrado G, Dean J. Efficient estimation of word representations in vector space. In: ArXiv Prepr ArXiv13013781; 2013.
128. Garla V, Re III V Lo, Dorey-Stein Z, Kidwai F, Scotch M, Womack J, et al. The Yale cTAKES extensions for document classification: architecture and application. J Am Med Inform Assoc. 2011;18:614–20.
129. Goeuriot L, Suominen H, Kelly L, Miranda-Escalada A, Krallinger M, Liu Z, et al. Overview of the CLEF eHealth Evaluation Lab 2020. In: International Conference of the Cross-Language Evaluation Forum for European Languages. Berlin: Springer; 2020. p. 255–71.
130. Ta CN, Dumontier M, Hripcsak G, Tatonetti NP, Weng C. Columbia open health data, clinical concept prevalence and co-occurrence from electronic health records. Sci Data. 2018;5:180273.
131. Ohno-Machado L, Bafna V, Boxwala AA, Chapman BE, Chapman WW, Chaudhuri K, et al. iDASH: integrating data for analysis, anonymization, and sharing. J Am Med Inform Assoc. 2012;19:196–201.
132. Aramaki E, Morita M, Kano Y, Ohkuma T. Overview of the NTCIR-11 MedNLP-2 task. NTCIR; 2014.
133. Suominen H, Zhou L, Hanlen L, Ferraro G. Benchmarking clinical speech recognition and information extraction: new data, methods, and evaluations. JMIR Med Inform. 2015;3:e19.

33 Machine Learning in Pituitary Surgery

Vittorio Stumpo, Victor E. Staartjes, Luca Regli, and Carlo Serra

33.1 Introduction

Pituitary tumors (PTs) constitute a heterogeneous group of lesions of the central nervous system (CNS) with high incidence Pituitary adenomas (PAs) are categorized by their dimension and their hormone secretion. Specific clinical features are associated with oversecretion of each hormone i.e., Cushing's disease for adrenocorticotrophic hormone (ACTH), acromegaly for growth hormone (GH), and galactorrhea/amenorrhea for prolactin [1]. Non-functioning pituitary adenomas are usually identified by sequelae of their mass effect, such as headache, visual defects (bitemporal hemianopsia), hormonal deficits, or also an incidental radiological finding [1]. Transsphenoidal surgery is recommended in symptomatic patients, In the case of prolactinomas, medical treatment is recommended [2]. Fifteen to fifty percent of functioning PA patients resolve their hormonal abnormality after surgical treatment, while 2% to 15% of patients may have new hormonal deficits [1]. Other less common pituitary lesions of neurosurgical pertinence include craniopharyngiomas, Rathke cleft cysts and pituitary carcinomas [3–5].

Machine learning (ML) is a rapidly developing field in clinical neuroscience with applications to neurosurgical disease management. Given the advent of "big data," technical improvements and widespread availability of sufficient computational power, ML algorithms have the potential to help tackle existing issues in daily clinical practice [6, 7]. A recent worldwide survey strikingly found that almost 28.5% of neurosurgeons reported using ML in their clinical practice, and 31.1% in research, most commonly for outcome and complication prediction, imaging interpretation or quantification, or patient counseling and shared decision-making [8]. A review by Senders et al. [9] systematically reviewed past studies in neurosurgery where human expert evaluation was compared to ML algorithms' performance for a variety of tasks including tumor classification and grading, surgical decision-making, segmentation and localization of epileptogenic zones, as well as outcome prediction. The authors concluded that although ML models have the potential to enhance decision-making capacity of clinicians, significant challenges remain to be addressed to switch from competitive to a collaborative human-machine paradigm. Despite the promises held by ML and artificial intelligence (AI), translation clinical practice is complex [7]. Selection of a clinical problem, the prediction of which can be relevant at the appropriate steps during therapeutic management is critical. Once a suitable clinical problem is identified, the approach needs to equally be well thought out with respect modeling strategy and data collection. Data availability is another crucial issue, as thousands of patients may be needed for proper model training and external validation, which is necessary for confirming adequate generalizability of the developed model [10]. At the same time, implementation of the model in the daily clinical practice should ideally be straightforward and not require extensive data collection. Heterogenous data sources can be selected as input variables to train a ML model such as, for example, clinical data, histopathological slides, as well as radiological images [11–14]. Importantly, a variety of technical pitfalls, including overfitting and class imbalance, need to be accurately addressed to assure reliability of the trained model [10, 15, 16].

33.2 Machine Learning Applications in Pituitary Surgery

ML learning applications in surgical specialties, and in neurosurgery specifically, are more commonly reported for diverse tasks including faster and more accurate preoperative diagnosis [17, 18], enhanced lesion characterization [19],

V. Stumpo · V. E. Staartjes (✉) · L. Regli · C. Serra
Machine Intelligence in Clinical Neuroscience (MICN) Laboratory, Department of Neurosurgery, Clinical Neuroscience Center, University Hospital Zurich, University of Zurich, Zurich, Switzerland
e-mail: victoregon.staartjes@usz.ch

V. E. Staartjes et al. (eds.), *Machine Learning in Clinical Neuroscience*, Acta Neurochirurgica Supplement 134,
https://doi.org/10.1007/978-3-030-85292-4_33

and surgical outcome [20–22], complications [13, 23] and cost prediction [24]. In this respect, pituitary surgery makes no exception, even if—compared to other diseases of neurosurgical relevance—the reported literature is less extensive [25, 26]. Past research has attempted to answer clinically relevant questions to better assist surgeons and clinicians in differential diagnosis [27, 28], pituitary tumor biology investigation before surgery [29–33], prediction of gross total resection (GTR) and recurrence [34–37], complications such as intraoperative cerebrospinal fluid (CSF) [38] and postoperative hyponatremia [39] or response to pharmacological therapy [40]. In the present chapter, we provide an overview and discuss relevant publications of ML in pituitary tumor management (Table 33.1).

Enhanced Preoperative Lesion Characterization

ML has been preliminarily investigated for presurgical tumor characterization i.e., differential diagnosis [27, 28], immunohistochemical markers prediction [31, 32], anatomical invasion of surrounding structures like cavernous sinus (CS) [30], and texture features such as tumor consistency [29, 33].

Differential Diagnosis

Already in 2009, a small-scale study evaluated the assistance of artificial neural network (ANN) in increasing radiologists' diagnostic performance regarding large sellar and suprasellar masses (rathke cleft cysts, PA, craniopharyngioma). The study showed improved accuracy and AUC with a greater improvement obtained in general radiologists which—with ANN assistance—performed as well as neuroradiologists in differentiating these lesions [27]. An imaging-based decision-making algorithm to support differential diagnosis of pituitary metastasis from immune checkpoint inhibitor-induced autoimmune hypophysitis was also recently developed by means of a random forest (RF) algorithm [28]. Other studies attempted to identify acromegalic patients with ML approaches analyzing facial features [41, 42].

Immunohistochemical Characterization of PA

Despite PAs being mostly clinically silent lesions identified on incidental imaging, a subpopulation of these tumors has a more aggressive biology, with features of local invasiveness and higher risk of recurrence after surgical removal [43]. It has been shown that a variety markers such as for example strong immunopositivity for p53 and high Ki-67 can identify lesions associated with more malignant behavior [44]. At present, such biomarker evaluation is available only postoperatively, thus preoperative prediction of lesion aggressiveness at an early stage may enable more aggressive management and follow-up indication [31]. Ugga et al. [32] evaluated 89 patients who underwent endoscopic endonasal removal of PA, whose Ki-67 labeling was investigated postoperatively and, after identifying a subset of relevant radiomic features, trained a *k* nearest neighbor (KNN) classifier to accurately identify patients' Ki-67 based on MR images. The algorithm was able to correctly discriminate patients with high versus low Ki-67 with an accuracy of 92%. A similar attempt on MRI data was pursued by Peng et al. [31] who, in a population of 235 PA patients, trained different ML models to predict immunohistochemical marker positivity (t-box pituitary transcription factor—Tpit; pituitary transcription factor 1—Pit-1; steroidogenic factor 1—SF-1). The models were trained on T1-weighted, T2-weighted and contrast-enhanced T1-weighted radiomic features. Among the trained models, SVM performed best on T2w images with an accuracy of 0.89, area under the curve (AUC) of 0.95, and high sensitivity and specificity.

CS Invasion by PA Adenoma

Tumor invasion into the CS is one of the most important determinants of subtotal pituitary adenoma resection [45, 46]. Unfortunately, distinction between CS compression and invasion preoperatively is not always possible and is ultimately established at intraoperative visualization [47]. In view of the fact that a failure to achieve GTR leads to a combination of subtotal resection and radiotherapy as a viable strategy, more accurate preoperative confirmation of CS invasion can better inform patient management decision. In particular, especially for Knosp grades 2 and 3, invasion is to be determined on a case by case basis [46]. Niu et al. [30] in a population of 194 patients with PA Knosp grade 2 and 3, split in a 50/50 ratio into training and test set, used least absolute shrinkage and selection operator (LASSO) regression to identify radiomic features predictive of invasion. They then used a support vector machine (SVM) to fit CE-T1 weighted radiomic signature, and constructed a nomogram based on clinical-radiological risk factors and radiomic signature reporting an AUC of 0.87 in the test set.

Tumor Consistency

Firm consistency—or texture—is widely recognized as a significant limiting factor in adequate PA resection [48–50]. As opposed to soft tumors, whose removal can be easily performed by means of endoscopic approach, hard fibrous tumors are associated with failure of transsphenoidal resection, and may require a second surgery or complementary treatment strategies. For this reason, prediction of tumor texture can be valuable for better planning surgical strategy and informed patient management decision. A variety of approaches have attempted to characterize PA consistency using MRI features with conflicting results [48, 51–53]. More recently, also ML applications for texture prediction have been attempted based on MR images [29, 33, 54].

Table 33.1 Selected publications exploiting ML approaches for pituitary disease classification and/or outcome prediction

Author	Year	Journal	Patients (training/ validation)	Model/ Algorithm	Outcome	Performance	Main findings
Kitajima et al.	2009	Academic Radiology	43	ANN	Classification of sellar/ suprasellar masses into PA, craniopharyngioma, and Rathke's cleft cyst	GR: General radiologists, NR: Neuroradiologists **AUC** All w/o ANN: 0.91; All w/ANN: 0.98 GR w/o ANN: 0.88; GR w/ ANN: 0.98; NR w/o ANN: 0.95; NR w/ ANN: 0.99	ANN output can significantly improve accuracy of NR and GR performance in the DD of sellar-suprasellar mass lesions using MRI. ↑ improvement for GA After ANN → GR = NR
Hollon et al.	2018	Neurosurgical Focus	400 (300/100)	NB, SVM, LR-EN, RF	Poor early post-op outcome defined as any of the following: Major medical and early surgical complications, extended LOS, ED admission, inpatient readmission, and death	**AUC-ROC**—NB: 0.79; SVM: 0.83; **RF: 0.85**; LR-EN: 0.83 **AUC-PR**—NB: 0.65; SVM: 0.67; RF: 0.67; LR-EN: **0.69** **Accuracy**—NB: 0.79; SVM: 0.83; RF: 0.85; LR-EN: 0.87 **Sensitivity**—NB: 0.24; SVM: 0.48; RF: 0.56; LR-EN: **0.68** **Specificity**—NB: **0.97**; SVM: 0.95; RF: 0.95; LR-EN: 0.93 **PPV**—NB: 0.75; SVM: 0.75; RF: 0.78; LR-EN: 0.77 **NPV**—NB: 0.79; SVM: 0.84; RF: 0.86; LR-EN: 0.90	LR-EN best predicted early postoperative outcomes of pituitary adenoma surgery testing set. The most important predictive variables were lowest perioperative sodium, age, BMI, highest perioperative sodium, and Cushing's disease
Kocak et al.	2018	European Radiology	47	KNN	Response to somatostatin analogues (SA) in acromegaly patients with growth hormone (GH)-secreting pituitary macroadenoma	Resistant: Rt; responsive: Rp **AUC**—0.847 **Sensitivity**—Rt: 0.83; Rp: 0.87 **Specificity**—Rt: 0.87; Rp: 0.83 **Precision**—Rt: 0.86; Rp: 0.84 **Recall**—Rt: 0.83; Rp: 0.87 ***F* measure**—Rt: 0.84; Rp: 0.86	ML-based quantitative texture analysis of T2-weighted MRI is a potential non-invasive tool in predicting response to SAs in patients with acromegaly and GH-secreting pituitary macroadenoma. ↑ performance than qualitative and quantitative rSI and immunohistochemical evaluation
Muhlestain et al.	2018	The Journal of Neurosurgery	15,487	Gradient boost tree ensemble	Total charges for TSS surgery	**Ensemble 1**—T RMSE: 0.45; V RMSE: 0.45 **Ensemble 2**—T RMSE: 0.52; V RMSE: 0.53	Ensemble model comprising three gradient boosted tree classifiers best predicted total charges. LOS was the strongest predictor—↑ $5000/ day. Others: Admission type, hospital region, race, post-op complication, hospital ownership type
Zhang et al.	2018	European Radiology	112 (75/37)	SVM	NFPA subtype prediction (NCAs vs. others)	**AUC**—T1: 0.80; CE-T1: 0.51 **Sensitivity**—T1: 0.81; CE-T1: 0.58 **Specificity**—T1: 0.82; CE-T1: 0.45 **Accuracy**—T1: 0.81; CE-T1: 0.54	A model developed using clinical and radiomic features achieves good performance for NFPA subtype preoperative diagnosis. CE-T1 features achieve ↓ performance that T1 features

(continued)

Table 33.1 (continued)

Author	Year	Journal	Patients (training/validation)	Model/Algorithm	Outcome	Performance	Main findings
Fan et al.	2019	European Journal of Radiology	163 (108/55)	SVM-RBF kernel	Invasive FPA remission after surgery	RS: radiomic signature; CM: clinical model; RM: radiomic model **Accuracy**—RS: 0.73; CM: 0.65; RM: 0.74 **Sensitivity**—RS: 0.77; CM: 0.65; RM: 0.61 **Specificity**—RS: 0.67; CM: 0.67; RM: 0.92 **PPV**—RS: 0.75; CM: 0.71; RM: 0.71 **NPV**—RS: 0.70; CM: 0.59; RM: 0.70 **AUC**—RS: 0.81; CM: 0.76; RM: 0.81	Radiomic-clinical data can be successfully employed to train ML models with good discrimination and calibration to predict treatment response in patients with invasive FPA
Fan et al.	2019	Frontiers in Endocrinology	163	SVR, LR	Postsurgical response in invasive functioning PA	**Radiomic model** **AUC**—0.81 **Accuracy**—0.74 **Sensitivity**—0.61 **Specificity**—0.92 **PPV**—0.70 **NPV**—0.65	7 radiomic features → radiomic signature (RS) Radiomic model (RM): RS + Knosp grade The RS and RM ↑ performance than clinical features model
Liu et al.	2019	Neuroendocrinology	354	LR, NB, DT, GBDT, RF, AdaBoost, XGBoost	12-months CD recurrence	**AUC**—DT: 0.63; **RF: 0.78**; LR: 0.68; NB: 0.61; GBDT: 0.69; AdaBoost: 0.72; XGBoost: 0.73; post-op morning cortisol: 0.63 RF—Youden's index: 0.45; sensitivity: 0.87; specificity: 0.58	AUCs of the 7 models ranged from 0.61 to 0.78. Best performance achieved by RF > LR > Post-op morning cortisol. According to the feature selection Algorithms, top 3 predictors were age, postoperative serum cortisol, and postoperative ACTH
Niu et al.	2019	European Radiology	194 (97/97)	SVM	CS invasion by PA	CR: Clinico-radiological, CE-T1; T2; CE-T1 + T2; N: Normogram **AUC**—CR: 0.83; CE-T1: 0.83; T2: 0.73; CE-T1 + T2: 0.80; N: 0.87 **Accuracy**—CR: 0.77; CE-T1: 0.80; T2: 0.68; CE-T1 + T2: 0.79; N: 0.79 **Sensitivity**—CR: 0.82; CE-T1: 0.80; T2: 0.63; CE-T1 + T2: 0.77; N: 0.86 **Specificity**—CR: 0.69; CE-T1: 0.81; T2: 0.71; CE-T1 + T2: 0.79; N: 0.76	The developed nomogram incorporating the radiomics signature and clinico-radiological risk factors performed better than clinic-radiological model and radiomics models based on CE-T1, T2, and CE-T1 and T2 images for pre-op prediction of CS invasion
Staartjes et al.	2019	Neurosurgical Focus	140 CV w/o holdout	KC, Deep NN, LR	PA GTR	**AUC**—K: 0.87; NN: **0.96**; LR: 0.86 **Accuracy**—K: 0.81; NN: **0.91**; LR: 0.82 **Sensitivity**—K: 0.92; NN: **0.94**; LR: 0.81 **Specificity**—K: 0.70; NN: **0.89**; LR: 0.83 **PPV**—K: 0.75; NN: **0.89**; LR: 0.83 **NPV**—K: 0.90; NN: **0.94**; LR: 0.81 **F1 score**—K: 0.83; NN: **0.91**; LR: 0.82	Deep neural network outperforms LR and Knosp classification in predicting GTR in PA patients

Table 33.1 (continued)

Author	Year	Journal	Patients (training/validation)	Model/Algorithm	Outcome	Performance	Main findings
Ugga et al.	2019	Neuroradiology	108 (60%/40%)	KNN	Pre-op MRI-base ki-67 proliferation index class prediction	**AUC**—0.87 **Sensitivity**—0.92 **Specificity**—0.86 **Precision**—0.92 **Matthews correlation coefficient**—0.79 ***F* score**—0.92	ML analysis of texture-derived parameters from preoperative T2 MRI is effective for prediction of pituitary macroadenomas ki-67 proliferation index class
Zeynalova et al.	2019	Neuroradiology	55	ANN	PA consistency	**AUC**—0.71 **Accuracy**—0.72 **Sensitivity**—0.66 **Specificity**—0.79 **Precision**—0.73 ***F* measure** – 0.69	ML-based histogram analysis on T2-weighted MRI has potential to predict consistency of PAs. Future large-scale studies needed
Cuocolo et al.	2020	Neuroradiology	89	Extra trees	Pituitary surgical consistency	S: soft; F: fibrous **AUC**—S, F: 0.99 **Sensitivity**—S: 0.87; F: 1.00 **PPV**—S: 1.00; F: 0.87 ***F* score**—S, F: 0.93	ML model trained on radiomic data extracted from T2w MRI had high accuracy in classification of soft and fibrous pituitary macroadenomas
Machado et al.	2020	Computers in Biology and Medicine	27	MLP, RF, SVM, LR, KNN	NFPA recurrence after surgery 2D/3D radiomic features (RF) models	3DRF **Accuracy**—MLP: 0.90; RF: 0.96; SVM: 0.93; LR: 0.89; KNN: 0.93 **Specificity**—MLP: 0.96; RF: 1.00; SVM: 1.00; LR: 1.00; KNN: 1.00 **Sensitivity**—MLP: 0.83; RF: 0.92; SVM: 0.83; LR: 0.75; KNN: 0.83 **AUC**—MLP: 0.96; RF: 0.96; SVM: 0.95; LR: 0.95; KNN: 0.94	2D and 3D RF models achieve high discrimination in predicting NFPA tumor recurrence 3D-based models achieved ↑ performances using ↓ features when compared to 2D-based models
Meng et al.	2020	Frontiers in Endocrinology	124	LDA	Acromegaly patients identification using facial features	NA	3D imaging enables quantification of facial characteristics. ML can be used for early detection of acromegalic patients
Peng et al.	2020	European Journal of Radiology	235	SVM, KNN, NB	Immunohistochemical characterization of PAs	T2w radiomic feature model—SVM: 0.89; KNN: 0.83; 0.80 **Accuracy**—Pit-1: 0.91; SF-1: 0.94; Tpit: 0.91 **Sensitivity**—Pit-1: 0.81; SF-1: 0.93; Tpit: 0.86 **Specificity**—Pit-1: 0.82; SF-1: 0.89; Tpit: 0.85	SVM model trained on radiomics features based on pre-op MR images precisely classify immunohistochemical PA subtypes. T2-w images model had a better performance compared with that from T1-w and ceT1-w images
Qiao et al.	2020	Pituitary	833	Penalized LR, SVM, GBM, NN, Ensemble	6 months endocrine remission in GH-secreting adenoma pts	Ensemble model—Partial: P; full: F **Remission based on GH** **AUC**—*P*: 0.80; *F*: 0.88; Prospective validation cohort—*P*: 0.80; *F*: 0.90 External validation cohort—*P*: 0.77; *F*: 0.87 **Remission based on GH and IGF-1** **AUC**—*P*: 0.77; *F*: 0.85; Prospective validation cohort—*P*: 0.76; *F*: 0.90	Development and validation of interpretable and applicable ML model to predict early endocrine remission after surgical resection of a GH-secreting pituitary adenoma. ↑ performance with respect TO single variables
Staartjes et al.	2020	The Journal of Neurosurgery	154 (70%/15%/15%)	NN	Intraoperative CSF leak	**AUC**—0.84 **Accuracy**—0.88 **Sensitivity**—0.83 **Specificity**—0.89 **PPV**—0.71 **NPV**—0.94 **F1 score**—0.77	Deep neural network well predicts intraoperative CSF leak High suprasellar hardy grade, prior surgery, and older age contributed most to the predictions

(continued)

Table 33.1 (continued)

Author	Year	Journal	Patients (training/ validation)	Model/ Algorithm	Outcome	Performance	Main findings
Voglis et al.	2020	Pituitary	207 (155/52)	RF, NB, bGLM, GLM	Hyponatremia within 30 days of surgery	**AUC**—RF: 0.64; NB: 0.65; bGLM: **67.1**; GLM: 59.5 **Accuracy**—RF: **0.69**; NB: 0.48; bGLM: 0.68; GLM: 0.63 **Sensitivity**—RF: 0.28; NB: **0.73**; bGLM: 0.48; GLM: 0.47 **Specificity**—RF: 0.82; NB: 0.41; bGLM: **0.74**; GLM: 0.68 **PPV**—RF: 0.32; NB: 0.27; bGLM: **0.35**; GLM: 0.31 **NPV**—RF: 0.79; NB: 0.84; bGLM: **0.82**; GLM: 0.81 **F1**—RF: 0.30; NB: 0.40; bGLM: **0.41**; GLM: 0.27	Boosted generalized linear model was able to learn the complex risk factor interactions and showed a high discriminative capability on unseen patient data to predict postoperative hyponatremia
Zhu et al.	2020	BMC Med Inform Decis Mak	374	CycleGAN DenseNet ResNet CRNN	Tumor texture classification	**Multisequence: M; T1; T2** **Accuracy**—M: 0.92; T1: 0.89: T2: 0.89 **Precision**—M: 0.90; T1: 0.87; T2: 0.87 **Recall**—M: 0.95; T1: 0.93: T2: 0.94 **F1 score**—M: 0.92; T1: 0.60: T2: 0.90	Deep NN model for determining consistency of pituitary tumors (PT). CycleGAN amplifies the PT dataset to generate multisequence samples (to solve undersampling) ResNet extracts PT features, which improve the classification efficiency of the network to some extent. Extracted PT features are fed to CRNN for classification/grading of the softness level of pituitary tumors. ↑ results than previous methods
Zoli et al.	2020	Neurosurgical Focus	151 (80%/20%)	GTR: KNN, early post-op remission: SVM; Long-term remission: GBM	Cushing disease-GTR, post-surgical remission, long-term disease control	G: GTR; E: Early remission; L: Late remission **AUC**—G: 0.99; E: 1.00; L: 0.78 **Accuracy**—G: 0.97; E: 1.00; L: 0.81 **Sensitivity**—G: 0.96; E: 1.00; L: 0.96 **Specificity**—G: 1.00; E: 1.00; L: 0.37 **PPV**—G: 1.00; E: 1.00; L: 0.81 **NPV**—G: 0.75; E: 1.00; L: 0.75 **F1 score**—G: 0.98; E: 1.00; L: 0.88 **Brier score**—G: 0.0.35; E: 0.097; L: 0.151	Demographic, radiological, and histological variables can be employed for robust ML models training and internal validation for GTR and remission prediction in CD patients

AdaBoost adaptive boosting, *ANN* artificial neural network, *AUC* area under the curve, *CD* Cushing disease, *CRNN* convolutional recurrent neural network, *CS* cavernous sinus, *CSF* cerebrospinal fluid, *CV* cross-validation, *DD* differential diagnosis, *DenseNet* densely connected convolutional networks, *ED* emergency department, *EN* elastic net, *DT* decision tree, *GAN* generative adversarial network, *GBM* gradient boosting machine, *GBDT* gradient boosting decision tree, *GLM* generalized linear model, *GTR* gross total resection, *KC* Knosp classification, *KNN* k nearest neighbor, *LDA* linear discriminant analysis, *LOS* length of stay, *NB* Naïve Bayes, *NN* neural network, *NF* non-functioning, *LDA* linear discriminant analysis, *LOS* length of stay, *LR* logistic regression, *ML* machine learning, *MR* magnetic resonance, *mos* months, *NA* not available, *NCA* null cell adenoma, *NB* Naïve Bayes, *NN* neural network, *PA* pituitary adenoma, *PPV* positive predictive value, *PR* precision recall, *Pit-1* pituitary transcription factor 1, *RBF* radial basis function, *ResNet* deep residual networks, *RF* random forest, *RMSLE* root mean square logarithmic error, *SF-1* steroidogenic factor, *SVM* support vector machine, *w/o* without, *Tpit* t-box pituitary transcription factor, *TSS* transsphenoidal surgery, *XGBoost* extreme gradient boost

Zeynalova et al. [33], after a series of processing steps, extracted first order texture features using PyRadiomics from 55 patients with PA and, after training an artificial neural network (ANN) for classifying their consistency, compared resulting AUC with that obtained using signal intensity ratio (SIR) evaluation. They found that ANN achieved a significantly higher AUC with respect to SIR. Similarly, Cuocolo et al. [29] in a population of 89 patients used an Extra Tree classifier for the same purpose. After feature stability analysis and a multistep selection, synthetic minority oversampling technique (SMOTE) was applied to counteract class imbalance. Data were split in a 80/20 ratio, with the former training group serving for hyperparameter tuning via stratified fivefold cross-validation, and the latter left as holdout set. Despite the small study population, the model achieved good discrimination confirming the hypothesis that radiomic features can in principle be exploited to predict tumor texture. Zhu et al. [54] reported use of an automatic method for pituitary tumors texture analysis starting from unbalanced MRI data using a combination of a cycleGAN, DenseNet, ResNet, and a convolutional recurrent neural network.

Surgical Outcome and Complication Prediction

Gross Total Resection

One existing issue in clinical practice consists in approximating the prediction of gross total resection (GTR) after PA surgery. A variety of factors can influence surgical outcome such as adenoma dimension, growth pattern, invasion of the dura or of the cavernous sinus (CS), surgical strategy, etc. To guide best management approaches, clinical scores have been proposed proving an estimate of GTR resection probability, among which the gold standard is represented by the Knosp classification [45, 46]. More recently, the Zurich Pituitary Score (ZPS) was introduced, the 4 grades of which are calculated by simply dividing the maximum horizontal adenoma diameter (HD) by the minimal intercarotid distance at the level of the horizontal C4 segment of the internal carotid artery (ICD) and evaluating tumor encasement of the ICA [55]. External validation of this model showed steady decrease in GTR and EOR as well as increasing RV for each step-up in ZPS grade [56]. Moreover, the model was found to have high inter-rater agreement. Computational power granted by ML is particularly attractive for evaluating surgical outcome prediction with even higher accuracy for a patient-specific tailored prognostic evaluation. GTR prediction in PA surgery by means of ML was preliminarily investigated by our group in a cohort of 140 patients who underwent endoscopic transsphenoidal surgery [36]. A deep neural network, namely a multilayer perceptron with five hidden layers, was chosen for this purpose. In this study, with limited sample size, fivefold cross-validation without holdout to assess out-of-sample performance for deep learning (DL) and logistic regression (LR) was chosen with respect to conventional holdout for model testing. This allowed to compare LR and DL approach, and both of them were compared to Knosp classification as a recognized clinical standard. The neural network trained reached optimal performance with an AUC of 0.96. Other discrimination parameters were higher with the proposed model than those obtained by conventional LR and by Knosp classification. In summary, the trained model improved GTR prediction with respect to more traditional statistical methods and the gold standard clinical classification. Of note, the improved accuracy was particularly relevant in intermediate Knosp grades—where the preoperative prediction of CS invasion is more difficult. Zoli et al. [37] also showed that a KNN algorithm trained on demographic, radiological, and histological variables achieved remarkably high AUC and accuracy in predicting GTR.

Intraoperative Cerebrospinal Fluid (CSF) Leak

CSF leaks during transsphenoidal surgery are associated with postoperative CSF fistulas and consequent patient morbidity, meningitis, increased length of stay, readmission and costs. For this reason, several publications aimed to identify factors that predict intraoperative CSF leaks [57, 58]. In a study by our group, a prospective registry of 154 patients was used to train a deep neural network (DNN) to predict CSF leaks during transsphenoidal surgery. While traditional statistics could not identify any risk factor for this complication, the ML model reached a high accuracy and high AUC. The importance of prediction of complication development resides in the possibility to adjust surgical strategy in a patient-tailored manner, for example by using lumbar drains in a targeted patient population [38, 59].

Tumor Recurrence and Endocrinological Remission

For functioning adenomas, incomplete tumor resection will lead to tumor recurrence with endocrinological manifestations. A variety of risk factors associated with recurrence have been investigated in the past by means of traditional statistical methods, including postoperative hormonal levels, with conflicting results and variable accuracy [60–64]. Some studies applied ML algorithms to predict disease recurrence after surgical treatment for functional adenomas using diverse approaches [34, 35, 37, 65]. Zoli et al. [37] showed that SVM and gradient boosting machine (GBM) algorithms can be trained to predict early and late remission in a population of 151 patients with Cushing disease (CD). The trained models achieved excellent discrimination for early remission prediction and fair discrimination for late remission. Similarly, Liu et al. [35] followed-up a population of 354 CD patients for at least 1 year, and trained different ML algorithms to predict recurrence showing that a random forest (RF) achieved best performance and outperformed traditional statistics or postoperative serum cortisol nadir, which was often evaluated in previous studies. For invasive functioning PA, a preoperative prediction can better inform patient management strategy and the relative symptom persistence, due to elevated hormone levels after surgical resection. Previous research tried to identify variables influencing prognosis. With respect to traditional investigations, ML has the potential to better integrate the ever-growing complexity of available data. Combining radiomic features extraction and ML algorithms has proved to be a viable strategy. In particular, Fan et al. [34] built a radiomic signature using a SVM algorithm in a population of invasive functional PA patients to predict treatment response preoperatively, and evaluated its performance metrics as compared with a clinical model and a radiomic model including both radiomic signature and Knosp classification.

Hyponatremia

Postoperative hyponatremia is a relevant complication occurring in 2% to 25% of patients after transsphenoidal pituitary surgery, which can lead to patient readmission. Factors predictive of hyponatremia are unclear, and associations have been described between entity of the pituitary tumor or tumor size and hyponatremia [66]. However, as delayed hyponatremia occurs mainly around the 8–10 day after surgery, routine measurement of sodium should be recommended on the day of hospital dismission [67]. Voglis et al. [39] investigated prediction of hyponatremia by means of ML. After evaluating on the training set generalized linear models (glm), boosted GLMs [glmBoost], naïve Bayes classifiers (NB), and RF, based on performance metric glmBoost was selected for validation on an unseen internal validation set. This model confirmed high discrimination with AUC of 0.84 and accuracy of 0.78.

Drug Treatment Response

Kocak et al. [40] investigated the potential of quantitative texture analysis extracted from T2-weighted MRI in predicting the response of GH-secreting pituitary macroadenomas to somatostatin analogues in a cohort of 47 patients. A KNN algorithm was shown to correctly classify 85.1% of the macroadenomas regarding response to secreting adenomas with an AUC of 0.85—significantly better than qualitative and quantitative relative signal intensity and immunohistochemical evaluation (the accuracy range of other methods was 57.4–70.2%, AUC 0.57–0.70, $p < 0.05$).

Costs

Increased interest in health care quality improvement, coupled with resource optimization and policies on reimbursement strategies led to increasing number of publications in recent years [68–70]. Muhlestein et al. [24] trained an ensemble model made up of 3 gradient boosted tree classifiers on 15,487 patients who underwent TSS to predict total hospital charges (note: different from total costs). Length of stay (LOS) was—unsurprisingly—found to be the most important predictor for charges (increasing them of 5000 dollars/day). Additional predictors identified were non-elective admission, geographic hospital location, postoperative complication and others. Measured root mean square logarithmic error was 0.446.

Limitations

Many ML publications in pituitary surgery suffer from small sample size, considerably limiting the reported findings. In order to achieve the ultimate goal of ML predictive analytics, strong methodological accuracy is required to overcome pitfalls of model training and reach sufficient generalizability. Most studies were not externally validated, making them unsuitable for clinical practice [71]. To this end, pitfalls such as class imbalance, overfitting, et cetera need to be accurately ruled out. Moreover, thorough discrimination and calibration reporting are required [10]. The swift rise of deep learning and of black box models due to their excellent performance should not come at the cost of interpretability given the ethical issues deriving from potential translation to patient management of inexplicable "black box" models—the decision-making of which is, by definition, not known [72].

Future Directions

Despite the limited current translation to the clinic of ML applications in pituitary surgery, the topic represents a paradigm of challenges to be addressed in order for this research field to reach its maximal potential. Upon selection of a clinically relevant outcome, development of a robust model by means of multicenter collaboration for data collection, external validation, implementation and impact assessment is required for improving patient management [7, 10]. Moreover, the potential of ML to include a notable number of features to achieve a performance benefit should not come at the cost of inapplicability in the clinical practice, and integration into the clinical workflow of a web-app for quick prediction estimate has been proposed as a practical strategy [13, 73, 74].

33.3 Conclusions

With respect to other neurosurgical diseases, pituitary surgery has so far received less scrutiny as target of ML and AI algorithms. Reported applications include mainly preoperative lesion characterization (immunohistochemistry, CS invasion, tumor consistency), surgical outcome and complication predictions (GTR, tumor recurrence and endocrinological remission, CSF leak, hyponatremia). ML models have shown potential for translation into the clinic, but most reports can be considered preliminary and require larger training populations and strong external validation. In order for ML to be exploited clinically, a thoughtful selection of clinically relevant and modifiable outcome of interest and application of a methodologically solid model development pipeline are required, together with accurate multicenter collaborations allowing sufficient data collection and external validation.

References

1. Molitch ME. Diagnosis and treatment of pituitary adenomas: a review. JAMA. 2017;317(5):516–24.
2. Molitch ME. Management of medically refractory prolactinoma. J Neurooncol. 2014;117(3):421–8.
3. Kaltsas GA, Nomikos P, Kontogeorgos G, Buchfelder M, Grossman AB. Diagnosis and management of pituitary carcinomas. J Clin Endocrinol Metabol. 2005;90(5):3089–99.
4. Müller HL, Merchant TE, Warmuth-Metz M, Martinez-Barbera J-P, Puget S. Craniopharyngioma. Nat Rev Dis Primers. 2019; 5(1):75.
5. Zada G. Rathke cleft cysts: a review of clinical and surgical management. Neurosurg Focus. 2011;31(1):E1.
6. Beam AL, Kohane IS. Big data and machine learning in health care. JAMA. 2018;319(13):1317.
7. Chen P-HC, Liu Y, Peng L. How to develop machine learning models for healthcare. Nat Mater. 2019;18(5):410–4.
8. Staartjes VE, Stumpo V, Kernbach JM, et al. Machine learning in neurosurgery: a global survey. Acta Neurochir. 2020;162(12):3081–91. https://doi.org/10.1007/s00701-020-04532-1.
9. Senders JT, Arnaout O, Karhade AV, Dasenbrock HH, Gormley WB, Broekman ML, Smith TR. Natural and artificial intelligence in neurosurgery: a systematic review. Neurosurgery. 2018;83(2): 181–92.
10. Kernbach JM, Staartjes VE. Machine learning-based clinical prediction modeling—a practical guide for clinicians; 2020.
11. Akeret K, Stumpo V, Staartjes VE, et al. Topographic brain tumor anatomy drives seizure risk and enables machine learning based prediction. NeuroImage Clin. 2020;28:102506.
12. Hollon TC. Near real-time intraoperative brain tumor diagnosis using stimulated Raman histology and deep neural networks. Nat Med. 2020;26:52–8.
13. Van Niftrik CHB, van der Wouden F, Staartjes VE, et al. Machine learning algorithm identifies patients at high risk for early complications after intracranial tumor surgery: registry-based cohort study. Neurosurgery. 2019;85(4):E756–64.
14. Willemink MJ, Koszek WA, Hardell C, Wu J, Fleischmann D, Harvey H, Folio LR, Summers RM, Rubin DL, Lungren MP. Preparing medical imaging data for machine learning. Radiology. 2020;295(1):4–15.
15. Srivastava N, Hinton G, Krizhevsky A, Sutskever I, Salakhutdinov R. Dropout: a simple way to prevent neural networks from overfitting. J Mach Learn Res. 2014;15(1):1929–58.
16. Staartjes VE, Schröder ML. Letter to the editor. Class imbalance in machine learning for neurosurgical outcome prediction: are our models valid? J Neurosurg Spine. 2018;29(5):611–2.
17. Anwar SM, Majid M, Qayyum A, Awais M, Alnowami M, Khan MK. Medical image analysis using convolutional neural networks: a review. J Med Syst. 2018;42(11):226.
18. Bennai MT, Guessoum Z, Mazouzi S, Cormier S, Mezghiche M. A stochastic multi-agent approach for medical-image segmentation: application to tumor segmentation in brain MR images. Artif Intell Med. 2020;110:101980.
19. Citak-Er F, Firat Z, Kovanlikaya I, Ture U, Ozturk-Isik E. Machine-learning in grading of gliomas based on multi-parametric magnetic resonance imaging at 3T. Comput Biol Med. 2018;99: 154–60.
20. Senders JT, Staples PC, Karhade AV, Zaki MM, Gormley WB, Broekman MLD, Smith TR, Arnaout O. Machine learning and neurosurgical outcome prediction: a systematic review. World Neurosurg. 2018;109:476–486.e1.
21. Siccoli A, de Wispelaere MP, Schröder ML, Staartjes VE. Machine learning–based preoperative predictive analytics for lumbar spinal stenosis. Neurosurg Focus. 2019;46(5):E5.
22. Staartjes VE, de Wispelaere MP, Vandertop WP, Schröder ML. Deep learning-based preoperative predictive analytics for patient-reported outcomes following lumbar diskectomy: feasibility of center-specific modelling. Spine J. 2018;19(5):853–61. https://doi.org/10.1016/j.spinee.2018.11.009.
23. Arvind V, Kim JS, Oermann EK, Kaji D, Cho SK. Predicting surgical complications in adult patients undergoing anterior cervical discectomy and fusion using machine learning. Neurospine. 2018;15(4):329–37.
24. Muhlestein WE, Akagi DS, McManus AR, Chambless LB. Machine learning ensemble models predict total charges and drivers of cost for transsphenoidal surgery for pituitary tumor. J Neurosurg. 2019;131(2):507–16.
25. Saha A, Tso S, Rabski J, Sadeghian A, Cusimano MD. Machine learning applications in imaging analysis for patients with pituitary tumors: a review of the current literature and future directions. Pituitary. 2020;23(3):273–93.
26. Soldozy S, Farzad F, Young S, Yağmurlu K, Norat P, Sokolowski J, Park MS, Jane JA, Syed HR. Pituitary tumors in the computational era, exploring novel approaches to diagnosis, and outcome prediction with machine learning. World Neurosurg. 2020;146: 315–321.e1.
27. Kitajima M, Hirai T, Katsuragawa S, et al. Differentiation of common large Sellar-Suprasellar masses. Acad Radiol. 2009;16(3):313–20.
28. Mekki A, Dercle L, Lichtenstein P, Nasser G, Marabelle A, Champiat S, Chouzenoux E, Balleyguier C, Ammari S. Machine learning defined diagnostic criteria for differentiating pituitary metastasis from autoimmune hypophysitis in patients undergoing immune checkpoint blockade therapy. Eur J Cancer. 2019;119:44–56.
29. Cuocolo R. Prediction of pituitary adenoma surgical consistency: radiomic data mining and machine learning on T2-weighted MRI. Neuroradiology. 2020;62(12):1649–56.
30. Niu J, Zhang S, Ma S, Diao J, Zhou W, Tian J, Zang Y, Jia W. Preoperative prediction of cavernous sinus invasion by pituitary adenomas using a radiomics method based on magnetic resonance images. Eur Radiol. 2019;29(3):1625–34.
31. Peng A, Dai H, Duan H, Chen Y, Huang J, Zhou L, Chen L. A machine learning model to precisely immunohistochemically classify pituitary adenoma subtypes with radiomics based on preoperative magnetic resonance imaging. Eur J Radiol. 2020;125:108892.
32. Ugga L, Cuocolo R, Solari D, Guadagno E, D'Amico A, Somma T, Cappabianca P. Prediction of high proliferative index in pituitary macroadenomas using MRI-based radiomics and machine learning. Neuroradiology. 2019;61(12):1365–73.
33. Zeynalova A, Kocak B, Durmaz ES, et al. Preoperative evaluation of tumour consistency in pituitary macroadenomas: a machine learning-based histogram analysis on conventional T2-weighted MRI. Neuroradiology. 2019;61(7):767–74.

34. Fan Y. Development and validation of an MRI-based radiomic signature for the preoperative prediction of treatment response in patients with invasive functional pituitary adenoma. Eur J Radiol. 2019;121:108647.
35. Liu Y, Liu X, Hong X, et al. Prediction of recurrence after transsphenoidal surgery for Cushing's disease: the use of machine learning algorithms. Neuroendocrinology. 2019;108(3):201–10.
36. Staartjes VE, Serra C, Muscas G, Maldaner N, Akeret K, van Niftrik CHB, Fierstra J, Holzmann D, Regli L. Utility of deep neural networks in predicting gross-total resection after transsphenoidal surgery for pituitary adenoma: a pilot study. Neurosurg Focus. 2018;45(5):E12.
37. Zoli M, Staartjes VE, Guaraldi F, et al. Machine learning–based prediction of outcomes of the endoscopic endonasal approach in Cushing disease: is the future coming? Neurosurg Focus. 2020;48(6):E5.
38. Staartjes VE, Zattra CM, Akeret K, Maldaner N, Muscas G, van Niftrik CH, Fierstra J, Regli L, Serra C. Neural network–based identification of patients at high risk for intraoperative cerebrospinal fluid leaks in endoscopic pituitary surgery. J Neurosurg. 2019:1–7.
39. Voglis S, van Niftrik CHB, Staartjes VE, Brandi G, Tschopp O, Regli L, Serra C. Feasibility of machine learning based predictive modelling of postoperative hyponatremia after pituitary surgery. Pituitary. 2020;23(5):543–51.
40. Kocak B, Durmaz ES, Kadioglu P, Polat Korkmaz O, Comunoglu N, Tanriover N, Kocer N, Islak C, Kizilkilic O. Predicting response to somatostatin analogues in acromegaly: machine learning-based high-dimensional quantitative texture analysis on T2-weighted MRI. Eur Radiol. 2019;29(6):2731–9.
41. Kong X, Gong S, Su L, Howard N, Kong Y. Automatic detection of acromegaly from facial photographs using machine learning methods. EBioMedicine. 2017;27:94–102.
42. Meng T, Guo X, Lian W, Deng K, Gao L, Wang Z, Huang J, Wang X, Long X, Xing B. Identifying facial features and predicting patients of acromegaly using three-dimensional imaging techniques and machine learning. Front Endocrinol. 2020;11:492.
43. Yang Q, Li X. Molecular network basis of invasive pituitary adenoma: a review. Front Endocrinol. 2019;10:7.
44. Del Basso De Caro M, Solari D, Pagliuca F, Villa A, Guadagno E, Cavallo LM, Colao A, Pettinato G, Cappabianca P. Atypical pituitary adenomas: clinical characteristics and role of ki-67 and p53 in prognostic and therapeutic evaluation. A series of 50 patients. Neurosurg Rev. 2017;40(1):105–14.
45. Knosp E, Steiner E, Kitz K, Matula C. Pituitary adenomas with invasion of the cavernous sinus space: a magnetic resonance imaging classification compared with surgical findings. Neurosurgery. 1993;33(4):610–7. discussion 617-618.
46. Micko ASG, Wöhrer A, Wolfsberger S, Knosp E. Invasion of the cavernous sinus space in pituitary adenomas: endoscopic verification and its correlation with an MRI-based classification. J Neurosurg. 2015;122(4):803–11.
47. Ahmadi J, North CM, Segall HD, Zee C-S, Weiss MH. Cavernous sinus invasion by pituitary adenomas. AJR Am J Roentgenol. 1986;146:257–62.
48. Alimohamadi M, Sanjari R, Mortazavi A, Shirani M, Moradi Tabriz H, Hadizadeh Kharazi H, Amirjamshidi A. Predictive value of diffusion-weighted MRI for tumor consistency and resection rate of nonfunctional pituitary macroadenomas. Acta Neurochir. 2014;156(12):2245–52.
49. Romano A, Coppola V, Lombardi M, et al. Predictive role of dynamic contrast enhanced T1-weighted MR sequences in presurgical evaluation of macroadenomas consistency. Pituitary. 2017;20(2):201–9.
50. Rutkowski MJ, Chang K-E, Cardinal T, et al. Development and clinical validation of a grading system for pituitary adenoma consistency. J Neurosurg. 2020:1–8.
51. Smith K, Leever J, Chamoun R. Prediction of consistency of pituitary adenomas by magnetic resonance imaging. J Neurol Surg B. 2015;76(05):340–3.
52. Thotakura AK, Patibandla MR, Panigrahi MK, Mahadevan A. Is it really possible to predict the consistency of a pituitary adenoma preoperatively? Neurochirurgie. 2017;63(6):453–7.
53. Yiping L, Ji X, Daoying G, Bo Y. Prediction of the consistency of pituitary adenoma: a comparative study on diffusion-weighted imaging and pathological results. J Neuroradiol. 2016;43(3):186–94.
54. Zhu H, Fang Q, Huang Y, Xu K. Semi-supervised method for image texture classification of pituitary tumors via CycleGAN and optimized feature extraction. BMC Med Inform Decis Mak. 2020;20(1):215.
55. Serra C, Staartjes VE, Maldaner N, Muscas G, Akeret K, Holzmann D, Soyka MB, Schmid C, Regli L. Predicting extent of resection in transsphenoidal surgery for pituitary adenoma. Acta Neurochir. 2018;160(11):2255–62. https://doi.org/10.1007/s00701-018-3690-x.
56. Staartjes VE, Serra C, Zoli M, Mazzatenta D, Pozzi F, Locatelli D, D'Avella E, Solari D, Cavallo LM, Regli L. Multicenter external validation of the Zurich pituitary score. Acta Neurochir. 2020;162(6):1287–95.
57. Patel PN, Stafford AM, Patrinely JR, Smith DK, Turner JH, Russell PT, Weaver KD, Chambless LB, Chandra RK. Risk factors for intraoperative and postoperative cerebrospinal fluid leaks in endoscopic Transsphenoidal Sellar surgery. Otolaryngol Head Neck Surg. 2018;158(5):952–60.
58. Strickland BA, Lucas J, Harris B, Kulubya E, Bakhsheshian J, Liu C, Wrobel B, Carmichael JD, Weiss M, Zada G. Identification and repair of intraoperative cerebrospinal fluid leaks in endonasal transsphenoidal pituitary surgery: surgical experience in a series of 1002 patients. J Neurosurg. 2017;129:425–9.
59. Mehta GU, Oldfield EH. Prevention of intraoperative cerebrospinal fluid leaks by lumbar cerebrospinal fluid drainage during surgery for pituitary macroadenomas. J Neurosurg. 2012;116(6):1299–303.
60. Abdelmannan D, Chaiban J, Selman WR, Arafah BM. Recurrences of ACTH-secreting adenomas after pituitary adenomectomy can be accurately predicted by perioperative measurements of plasma ACTH levels. J Clin Endocrinol Metabol. 2013;98(4):1458–65.
61. AbdMoainAbu D, Singh Ospina NM, AlaaAl N, et al. Predictors of biochemical remission and recurrence after surgical and radiation treatments of Cushing disease: a systematic review and meta-analysis. Endocr Pract. 2016;22(4):466–75.
62. Hameed N, Yedinak CG, Brzana J, Gultekin SH, Coppa ND, Dogan A, Delashaw JB, Fleseriu M. Remission rate after transsphenoidal surgery in patients with pathologically confirmed Cushing's disease, the role of cortisol, ACTH assessment and immediate reoperation: a large single center experience. Pituitary. 2013;16(4):452–8.
63. Ironside N, Chatain G, Asuzu D, Benzo S, Lodish M, Sharma S, Nieman L, Stratakis CA, Lonser RR, Chittiboina P. Earlier postoperative hypocortisolemia may predict durable remission from Cushing's disease. Eur J Endocrinol. 2018;178(3):255–63.
64. Roelfsema F, Biermasz NR, Pereira AM. Clinical factors involved in the recurrence of pituitary adenomas after surgical remission: a structured review and meta-analysis. Pituitary. 2012;15(1):71–83.
65. Qiao N, Shen M, He W, et al. Machine learning in predicting early remission in patients after surgical treatment of acromegaly:

a multicenter study. Pituitary. 2020;24(1):53–61. https://doi.org/10.1007/s11102-020-01086-4.
66. Janneck M, Burkhardt T, Rotermund R, Sauer N, Flitsch J, Aberle J. Hyponatremia after trans-sphenoidal surgery. Minerva Endocrinol. 2014;39(1):27–31.
67. Krogh J, Kistorp CN, Jafar-Mohammadi B, Pal A, Cudlip S, Grossman A. Transsphenoidal surgery for pituitary tumours: frequency and predictors of delayed hyponatraemia and their relationship to early readmission. Eur J Endocrinol. 2018;178(3):247–53.
68. Arutyunyan GG, Angevine PD, Berven S. Cost-effectiveness in adult spinal deformity surgery. Neurosurgery. 2018;83(4):597–601.
69. Leonart LP, Borba HHL, Ferreira VL, Riveros BS, Pontarolo R. Cost-effectiveness of acromegaly treatments: a systematic review. Pituitary. 2018;21(6):642–52.
70. Zygourakis CC, Kahn JG. Cost-effectiveness research in neurosurgery. Neurosurg Clin N Am. 2015;26(2):189–96, viii.
71. Staartjes VE, Kernbach JM. Significance of external validation in clinical machine learning: let loose too early? Spine J. 2020;20(7):1159–60.
72. Rudin C. Stop explaining black box machine learning models for high stakes decisions and use interpretable models instead. Nat Mach Intell. 2019;1(5):206.
73. Laws ER, Catalino MP. Editorial. Machine learning and artificial intelligence applied to the diagnosis and management of Cushing disease. Neurosurg Focus. 2020;48(6):E6.
74. Staartjes VE, Broggi M, Zattra CM, et al. Development and external validation of a clinical prediction model for functional impairment after intracranial tumor surgery. J Neurosurg. 2020:1–8.

At the Pulse of Time: Machine Vision in Retinal Videos

34

Timothy Hamann, Maximilian Wiest, Anton Mislevics, Andrey Bondarenko, and Sandrine Zweifel

34.1 Introduction

Pulsations of the central retinal vein and its branches often referred to as spontaneous venous pulsations (SVP) are a common finding in fundus biomicroscopy and have been described as far back as 1921 [1]. While the presence of SVP is a feature of a clinically normal optic disc (OD) in a healthy individual [2], its absence can be of clinical importance [3–5]. A relevant example in ophthalmology is glaucoma, one of the leading cause of blindness worldwide [6]. Here, the absence of SVP is directly correlated to a higher probability of rapid disease progression [7]. In neurology, the absence of SVP has been reported to indicate increased intracranial pressure (ICP) [4, 8, 9], with some authors reporting no observation of SVP in patients with an ICP of higher than 190 mmH_2O [4].

To date, identification of SVP is mostly performed by clinicians during biomicroscopy of the fundus. This method is observer-dependent, thereby subjective, and rarely documented. To objectify SVP findings, an automated approach is warranted. Upon review of the literature, two groups investigating this were identified.

McHugh et al. demonstrated successful detection of SVP utilizing near-infrared devices [10].

Shariflou et al. assessed SVP via a tablet-based camera approach in a cohort of 30 patients [11]. While near-infrared devices provide high-quality, stabilized black and white videos, which allow easy identification of SVP, they are of reduced availability as they are mostly cost-intensive devices used in ophthalmological institutions. Therefore, a potential approach based on visible light videos might target a broader public than an automatic assessment of SVP based on near-infrared imaging. Shariflou et al. used color videos acquired using a tablet-based camera, augmented with 28 diopter optics [11]. This represents a type of input that is more openly available, but their method requires manual segmentation of the optic nerve disc in at least one image per video, which requires a high level of ophthalmological expertise and again constitutes a non-standardized approach.

While both of these approaches show promising results, they are based on high-quality scientific data, which are not necessarily reproducible in a routine clinical practice setting. In order to introduce automated detection of SVP to clinical practice, several factors need to be addressed. First, a tool for enhancing SVP in videos of varying quality and different origins should be created. This would ease the burden of access as less training for personnel, and no specific imaging devices are required using such a tool. Second, automatic detection of SVP in the resulting imaging data should be developed.

To embrace the challenge of enhancing SVP in imaging data of various quality, we introduce a machine vision approach for SVP enhancement in grayscale videos acquired using a Zeiss FF450 plus fundus camera (Carl Zeiss Meditec AG, Jena, Germany). We aim to provide a detailed protocol of our research to present a foundation for future investigations using retinal videos for machine vision projects.

Timothy Hamann and Maximilian Wiest have contributed equally to this paper.

T. Hamann · M. Wiest · S. Zweifel (✉)
Department of Ophthalmology, University Hospital Zurich, University of Zurich, Zurich, Switzerland
e-mail: timothy.hamann@usz.ch; maximilian.wiest@usz.ch; sandrine.zweifel@usz.ch

A. Mislevics
Department of Artificial Intelligence and Systems Engineering, Riga Technical University, Riga, Latvia

C.T.Co, Riga, Latvia
e-mail: antons.mislevics@ctco.lv

A. Bondarenko
C.T.Co, Riga, Latvia

Faculty of Computer Science and Information Technology, Riga Technical University, Riga, Latvia
e-mail: andrey.bondarenko@ctco.lv

V. E. Staartjes et al. (eds.), *Machine Learning in Clinical Neuroscience*, Acta Neurochirurgica Supplement 134,
https://doi.org/10.1007/978-3-030-85292-4_34

34.2 Methods

Source Data

The dataset consists to date of 718 video sequences acquired in 523 patients. The video sequence resolution is 720 × 576 pixels; they have been recorded with a frame rate of 24 frames per second, coded in 8-bit grayscale. Videos have varying lengths ranging from roughly 8000 to 15,000 frames, which approximately corresponds to 330–625 s. The field of view of the frames is 30° displaying the OD fully or partially in one of the corners or borders with the associated retinal vasculature, and the surrounding retinal tissue. Outer limiting elements of the frames include static black areas, an artifact of the optical lens and a static bright needle which allows patients to focus during video recording (see Fig. 34.1). Challenges resulting from this data set and how to overcome them are outlined in successive order.

Non-aligned frames, further referred to as non-registered frames, were assessed with regard to translation and rotation. Medium amounts of frame translation (in worst cases, up to 200 pixels, usually less than 100 pixels) and slight rotation (less than 10°) were present within some frames. Motion-blurred frames, a result of microsaccade movements of the eye, were identified to be a major problem for successful registration. The majority of such blurry frames are standalone, meaning that nearby frames are free of blurriness. An additional blur-related problem is the shallow depth of field of the lens. Frames exploration has shown that the lens could be correctly focused on the mid-part of the frame but will lack focus on the frame edges—OD and other border areas due to the geometry of the eye. In addition to that, there are many artifacts like large blurry areas induced by the eyelashes or light-glare artifacts. Motion blur was considered as a critical problem, while other blur types such as minor ones prevented the successful registration of the frame sequences.

The varying illumination field introduced large variability even into seemingly similar frames. This was another critical problem that prevented successful registration. However, it should be noted that some registration approaches suffered more from this than the others. On the far end of this problem, there are fully or partially overexposed and underexposed frames. OD was found to be overexposed in part of the frames and have normal exposure in the other frames, which posed an additional problem on how we will be comparing such frames to detect blood vessel pulsations. Figure 34.1 shows blurry, underexposed, and partially overexposed frames.

Square regions of the frames that had slightly different gray-values distribution (color) in comparison to nearby regions were detected during workup. These artifacts were results of image correction algorithms applied by the imaging device; obviously, they were introduced to resolve some image capturing error, possibly to mask out some high-level noise or artifact introduced by the noise. Such noise is an error introduced by the measurement device, in this case, the imaging sensor. This error is highly evident in the frame's dark regions and especially obvious when frames are compared side by side. Although such type of artifacts was considered as non-critical, due to the fact that it appeared only in severely underexposed areas of the frames without any blood vessels, hence no pulsations could be potentially corrupted by such type of noise. Apart from such rare noisy regions, the background noise was observed in all of the pixels. Here, the same pixel, when compared to all its time-domain neighbors from nearby frames, displays a slight variation in its intensity, which results from the measurement error. This type of noise, given its amount, was not of critical importance for the registration procedure but turned out to be a major problem for the pulsations detection.

Pre-Processing

There are many approaches on how to deal with the above-listed problems. The main problem apart from blurriness was variability due to illumination changes and the various types

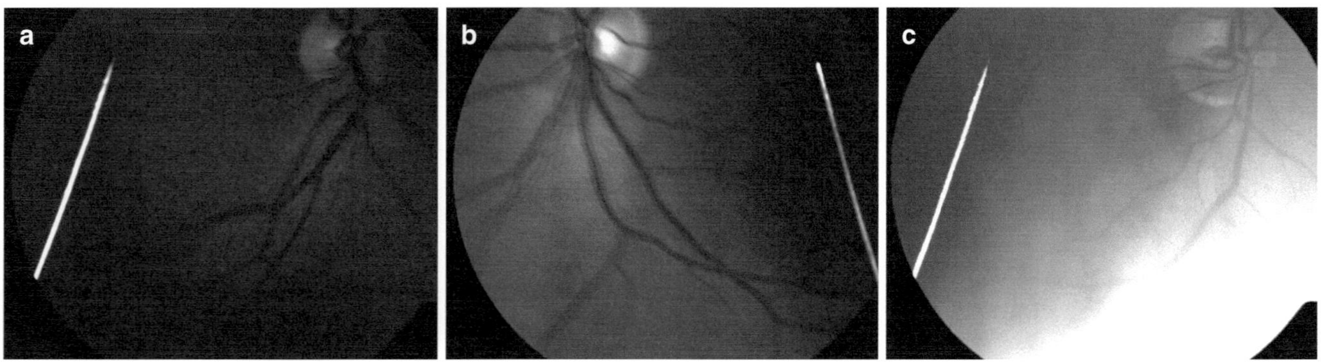

Fig. 34.1 An example of the underexposed frame (**a**), a blurry frame is showing "ghosted" blood vessels (**b**) and partially overexposed frame (**c**). In all of the frames, a static "needle" and surrounding black region is shown

of noise. Examination of the overexposed and underexposed frames have shown that they are not usable due to a large amount of noise, which became highly pronounced once image illumination was normalized.

Filters for Frames Normalization and Noise Reduction

Based on data exploration, the pre-processing routine that would suppress the retina surface and highlight blood vessels best was evaluated. Thus the aim was to reduce illumination variability and noise—ideally, a segmentation map of blood vessels without any other details would be achieved. In many cases, such a blood vessels segmentation map is frequently acquired by applying filters to the green channel of the color (red, green, blue (RGB)) frames, or application of various filters [12]. Some are coupling sophisticated filters with classifiers and perform supervised training [13, 14]. Finally, deep learning-based segmentation models are widespread [15]. Green channel-based approaches were not usable as the dataset consisted of grayscale images. A deep learning-based U-Net segmentation network trained on the available dataset was evaluated, but due to illumination variability, high variability in the extracted segmentation maps was the result.

Another problem experienced was that the U-Net model could correctly mark pixel belonging to the wall of the blood vessel on one frame and discard it on the next (aligned) slightly underexposed frame. Therefore, image processing and filtering approaches like Contrast Limited Adaptive Histogram Equalization (CLAHE) [16], Retinex filter, based on Land et al. theory of color perception [17], Sobel filters [18], which is one of the edge detection algorithms, Gaussian blurring [19], a Laplacian operator applied on a 2D image [20] in combination with regular histogram equalization and a Meijering filter [21] were investigated. We applied these operators in varying order, with varying parameters, and in varying combinations. The best registration results were acquired using the Meijering filter applied over a slightly blurred (Gaussian blur with kernel = 5 × 5) image. Images processed using this approach have highlighted blood vessels networks with suppressed background details.

Dealing with Blurry Frames

The next critical problem for the successful registration was blurry images. There are several types of blur present in our images. The most critical one is motion blur, which produced images with ghosted blood vessels pattern (see Fig. 34.1b for reference). Non-critical types of a blur for registration are out-of-focus blur due to shallow depth of focus and blur induced by eyelashes. An overview of the deblurring approaches is given by [22], where non-deep-learning-based approaches are covered. Out of the extended list of available methods, approaches like Wiener filer-based deblurring [23] and Richardson-Lucy algorithm [24] were explored, but both produced unsatisfactory results. A simple blind deblurring approach with point spread function estimation that transforms the image from the spatial domain to the frequency domain and performs operations there with subsequent backward transformation was evaluated as well. However, the deblurred images contained an extensive amount of noise, a high amount of blur and so-called "rounding" artifacts introduced by the procedure. This might be due to the high noise level present in the frames and possibly due to the used algorithm's simplicity. Instead of further experimentation, this approach was abandoned.

The deblurring approaches review would not be complete without a deep-learning-based method; for the review of deep learning-based approaches, please refer to [25]. These deblurring tools have gained huge popularity. There are several available types of algorithms, like utilization of the deep network for features extraction. The idea is to utilize a deep learning artificial neural network to come up with features that are later combined for "deblurring" kernel estimation [26]. Another approach uses a convolutional neural network for direct kernel coefficients estimation to directly perform deblurring [27]. Previously described algorithms are calculating the motion blur kernel for the whole image. At the same time, some methods are working on a patch level and are estimating motion kernel for each patch separately [28]; this allows to perform deblurring with varying kernels in different parts of the picture. The most recent techniques use an end-to-end approach where a convolutional neural network-based model is directly restoring an image. These methods were considered unsuitable because such artificial neural networks are trained to perform deblurring on high-quality RGB images, for example, photos of real-life objects. Our dataset is small, grayscale, and depicts retina; thus, available pre-trained deblurring models would produce below-average results. To circumnavigate this issue, training a new model would be required, but no sharp grayscale images are available. Another concern was that most recent and advanced end-to-end models are essentially "drawing" a new version of the image, potentially introducing some artificial data, and might prevent detection of blood vessel pulsations and correct estimation.

Therefore a blur detector approach, which would be used to drop blurry frames, was constructed. This approach turned to be viable as the exploration of the data has shown that blurry frames are standalone, and in between such frames, there are lengthy sequences of frames with acceptable quality that could be successfully registered. The simplest blur detector could be built by calculating the variance of the

Laplacian operator. A variance of Laplacian applied over the Meijering filtered masked images proved successful as a blur detector. Laplacian itself measures the second spatial derivative of the image, i.e., how fast intensity changes when moving from one pixel to its spatial neighbors. Hence blurry images will have smoother (slower) transitions in color intensities, and this will result in a smaller Laplacian variance measure; in contrast, detail-rich and sharp images will have a larger variance of Laplacian values. For blur detection, static areas (surrounding black region and "the needle") were masked out and were excluded from calculations. In initial experiments, this mask was created manually, although its creation could be automated via filters or with the help of a trained U-Net segmentation model. An example of the blur detector applied over the whole frame sequence can be seen in Fig. 34.2.

The blur detector based on a variance of Laplacian allowed detection of not only blurry images but also of underexposed, overexposed, partially overexposed images and the sharpest image, which will be used as a keyframe against which all others will be registered. Series of images with the low variance of Laplacian around frame numbers 1200–1800, 3800–4200, and 6200–6800 in Fig. 34.2 are originated due to the blinking light source applied to the retina rendering every second frame underexposed. It is worth mentioning that more sophisticated alternatives for blur detection exist [29], and some of them [30] are capable of detecting different types of blur (motion vs. out-of-focus) in different parts of the image. Finally deblurring based on deep learning (non end-to-end approach) is capable of detecting blurring kernel.

Registration

In the scope of registration (alignment), there are several aspects that should be considered when the registration algorithm is selected. The first dichotomy is feature-based vs. area-based algorithms. The feature-based approach relies on the extraction of key-points from two frames with subsequent matching and calculation of the deformation transformation needed to align images. ORB [31], SIFT [32], and SURF [33] algorithms were explored without success. This is due to the fact that such algorithms were not able to reliably detect and match key-points. The problem is that there are many patches of varying intensity (for example, junctions of blood vessels) with high similarity to one another; thus, the matching algorithm fails. This is the reason why many authors are performing registration based on the green channel of the RGB images, which is filtered to contain only blood vessels, which later on are processed to build a graph of the blood vessels. Later on, two such graphs from the pair of images are compared, and transformation is found to match these graphs [34]. Stewart et al. [35] have developed a successful implementation that extracts blood vessels junctions and, using the Iterative Closest Point (ICP) algorithm,

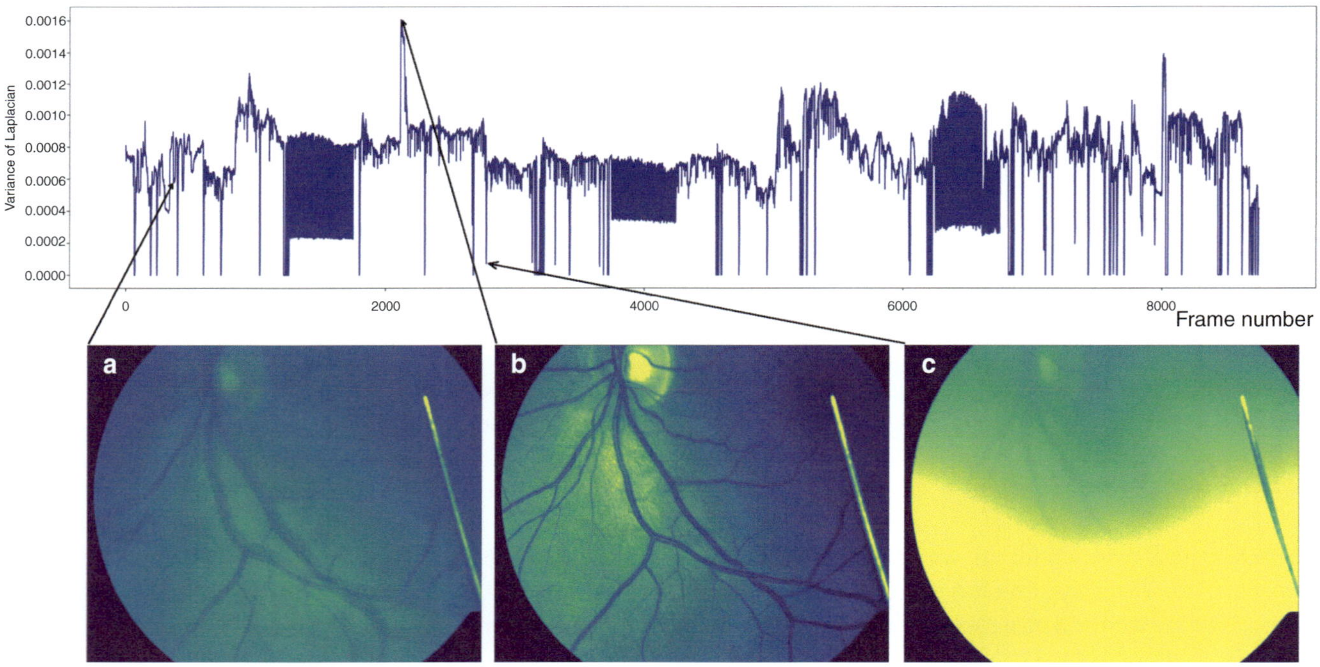

Fig. 34.2 The variance of Laplacian was calculated over the Meijering filtered, blurred and masked frames. Decrease of variance of Laplacian shows blurred frames (**a**), the highest peak denotes sharpest frame (**b**), low variance Laplacian values mark over/underexposed frames (**c**)

performs their matching. This algorithm is specifically applicable in cases when significant changes can be present in between two frames (in cases when images were taken several weeks or months apart).

The next dichotomy is transformation, i.e., deformation needed to be applied to the second frame to align it with the first (key) frame. The complexity of the deformation dictates the complexity of the problem and a registration algorithm. There are several types of deformations present in the image set: translation (shift) and rotation.

The next thing to consider is the domain in which the algorithm will be operating, i.e., spatial or frequency domain. The spatial domain is working with some sort of image similarity measure in the spatial domain, while frequency-based methods are working in the transformation domain. These methods tend to work faster but are able to find only simple transformations like scaling, rotation, and translation.

Lastly, in the case of area-based approaches, it is important to select appropriate similarity measure. In cases when images are similar intensity-based comparison like the sum of squared differences (SSD) [36, 37] is the simplest one, but in cases when images are belonging to different modalities, like CT/MRI or PET/CT, a more sophisticated similarity measure is needed, like Joint Histogram Mutual Information [38] or Mattes Mutual Information measure [39]. Mutual Information measure was relied on when experimenting with the spatial domain; this is due to the fact that the images have varying illumination and other noises.

There are a plethora of frameworks available to perform registration. It is worth mentioning the command-line toolbox Elastix [40, 41], which allows registering images. It has a set of available GUI frontends, which makes it a user-friendly solution not requiring any programming skills. But the aim is a fully automated solution. Thus, programmatic frameworks such as SimpleITK (SITK) [42], OpenCV [43], Scikit-Image [44], and PyStackReg library, which is based on the following publication [45], were explored. Only the last one worked, but this is just due to the specifics of the dataset. For different datasets, all mentioned frameworks would be a good choice for exploration. SimpleITK is a well-known registration framework with an emphasis on medical data registration, be it 2D or 3D volumes. Different sets of combinations of algorithms, similarity measures, and other parameters were evaluated without a consistent result. OpenCV was utilized to try out its optical-flow algorithms. The first one is the Lucas–Kanade algorithm, which is relying on corners detection using the Shi–Tomasi algorithm to estimate motion [46]. The second one is Dense Motion Estimation, which is calculating motion field using all pixels in the image [47], which unfortunately have failed on this dataset; again, the most probable reason was illumination variability and presence of noise in frames.

The Scikit-Image framework was utilized to explore its frequency-based algorithm, which worked well for translational deformation in images, but not good results were achieved when rotation was added. Finally, PyStackReg is a library that works in the frequency domain, so it supports only basic transformations. It allows to perform a sub-pixel level registration (like SITK and Scikit-Image) but does not support masking to exclude static regions, which should not be considered during registration (which is available in SITK and Scikit-Image for pixel-level translation-only registration). This required to crop out a rectangular sub-frame so that it will not contain nor static black region nor "needle." The problem was resolved by posing a non-convex optimization problem of finding the largest area rectangle inscribed into the non-masked area (area marked as not having static regions). For this task, the pyOpt python optimization library was successfully applied [48].

Overall image normalization and registration procedure could be seen in Fig. 34.3. The first step is static elements mask creation, then frames quality assessment, which is performed using the variance of Laplacian applied over the Meijering filtered + Gaussian (5 × 5) blurred image. This allows detecting the best quality keyframe and best quality sequence of frames. Afterward, based on the static elements mask, the largest rectangle was inscribed, which will be used to crop sub-frames for subsequent registration. Then registration is performed on rectangular sub-frames, and transformation matrices are acquired; afterward, they are used to transform full-scale frames.

Detection/Enhancement of SVP

The end goal of the whole process is the detection of blood vessels pulsations. This stage assumes normalized, denoised, and registered frames. Even though the best quality registered frame sequence was identified, there is still a great degree of noise and variation in illumination. The simplest way to deal with that is to normalize illumination across each frame separately, which can be achieved by simple calculation of the mean grayscale color of the square patch of preselected size (in this case 12 × 12 size, but the exact size has to be chosen in the scope of the overall workflow by measuring end result). This operation will produce an illumination map of reduced size (12 times smaller than the original in this case), which has to be up-scaled to the original image size and subtracted from that. This approach did not serve well as it smoothens single frame illumination, but different frames still have varying light fields. To overcome that, a better approach is to match histograms of all frames against the single frame in the sequence [49].

Once histograms are equalized, different sources of noise were still present, like minimal illumination varia-

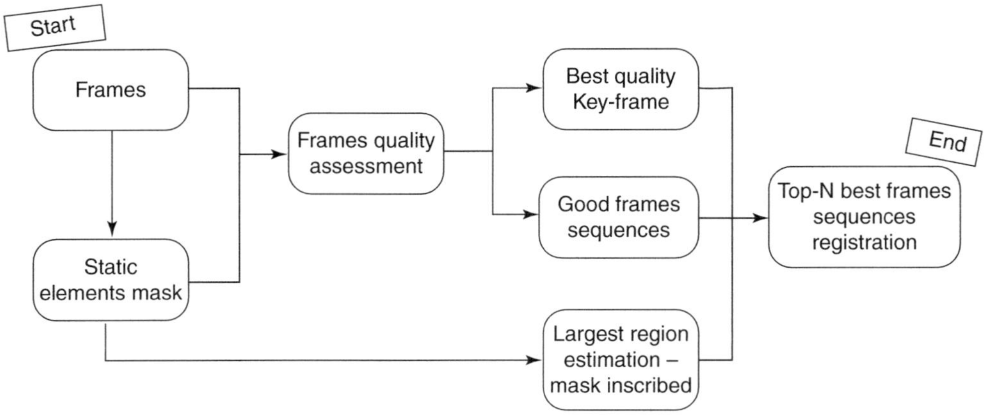

Fig. 34.3 The overall workflow of the frame sequences pre-processing and best sub-sequence registration

tions, camera sensor noise, and spontaneous eyelashes or/and blur glare artifacts. A nice overview of noise reduction methods can be found here [50]. The approaches that were readily available within the OpenCV framework and targeted at video noise reduction were explored with good results [51]. However, we have to sacrifice the first *n*-frames and last *n*-frames. Again *n* have to be chosen experimentally via the assessment of the overall workflow result.

In the introductory part, Reza et al.'s method was mentioned [52], but a manual selection of the blood vessels cross-sections was used to measure changes in blood vessels diameters, which was not acceptable.

In the scope of the pulsations detection, Morgan et al. [53] have used a video sequence that was synchronized with sound recording heartbeats, which eased the blood vessel pulsation detection. As our dataset lacked heartbeat data, a simpler approach was necessary, like principal component analysis based algorithm, which was proposed by Moret et al. [54]. It enhances images in a way that pulsations are magnified and made more pronounced. In addition, extracted principal components analysis can show areas where pulsations are present (frame sequences have to be long enough to catch up heartbeat cycle). The problem with this approach was that the images still contained large amounts of noise (as described—due to specifics of our dataset), and PCA extracted components that were describing such undesirable noises. Thus it was impossible to clearly separate pulsations from background noise.

Another viable approach is Eulerian Video Magnification [55], which works in the frequency domain and allows to select a frequency band (in which heartbeat can occur) that should be magnified. This results in pronounced movement explicitly visible after magnification is performed. The magnification factor can be changed as well. This approach tended to be useful as it allowed to magnify pulsations so that they became clearly visible and detectable by simple motion detection approaches. A simple difference-based approach, i.e., difference calculation between the first frame and every other frame, was evaluated with success. Another viable solution is blood vessels segmentation map acquisition and calculation of the union and intersection of such segmentation maps. The difference between segmentation maps union and the intersection will uncover changes in blood vessels diameters and will highlight collapse and dilation. It is important to note that just like with registration, motion detection is possible not only on a pixel level but on a sub-pixel level in case the image will be up-scaled and analyzed.

Hracho et al. [56] are using Discrete Fourier Transform to analyze each pixel values changes across the registered stack of frames, which allows applying filters to detect heartbeat by analyzing frequency power-spectrum and building a heatmap for each pixel. Overlaying such "pulsations" heatmap over the segmentation map showing blood vessels allows to see, detect, and quantify pulsations. This algorithm seems the most viable alternative to PCA and EVM approaches, as it will deal with noises and detect slightest variations in the pixels values.

34.3 Discussion

During the review of the data, it became evident that in the setting of our study, where source data was of varying quality, proper registration of images stack necessitated careful selection and pre-processing of input data. The greatest challenge was a wide range of image exposure and blurriness.

In order to perform registration, normalization of images was executed by reducing variability as far as possible. This was achieved by the application of the Meijering Filter applied as an overlay to the Gaussian blurred (5×5) image. As a result, blood vessels were highlighted, and the background with high levels of noise was suppressed, which supported performing registration on non-blurry images. Deep learning-based approaches are a topical method in enhancing image quality [57]. One major disadvantage to established deep learning algorithms, featuring pre-trained convolutional neural network learned filters for deblurring of images is training in color images, whereas our dataset consists of grayscale images. Noteworthy, the most recent end-to-end deep learning-based deblurring creates novel information during the deblurring process by essentially redrawing an image that appears sharper and cleaner to the human eye but not necessarily conserves information of the original image. For our aim, to detect the subtle changes of SVP, we depend on precise pixels intensity values. Thereby deep learning approaches were disqualified for our study. Still, due to motion blur present in some images, registration did not yield sufficient quality. Hence, an approach for blur detection was developed, which allowed us to identify and eliminate blurry frames.

After applying different methods for noise reduction and deblurring on the full extent of the dataset, we found regular occurrences of 3–4 s long image sequences of sufficient quality to be used for registration. In order to identify these frames in an efficient way, we have built a blur detector using the variance of Laplacian as a measurement for the overall sharpness and detail of any single image. This helped us to identify and exclude said images from further investigations. In conclusion, the total number of frames included for registration was reduced by a factor of 1000 (3–4 s of video instead of 330–625 s long videos), which forces us to drop some potentially useful frames, but at the same time greatly improves overall workflow execution speed.

In the next step, registration was performed. Our chosen library "Pystackreg" qualified for registration purposes as it fulfilled the requirement of sub-pixel registration, compensating for translation and rotation, thereby accounting for non-stabilization of the source data. As outlined in the methods section, static elements constituted a major challenge to image registration. To overcome this challenge, masking of these sub-regions was executed. Nevertheless, the OD, as well as the peripapillary region (the area surrounding the optic nerve head), which displays the largest retinal vessels, were not affected.

Since retinal vessel pulsation can be very subtle, we explored various mathematical methods of enhancing rhythmic changes in our dataset. While principal component analysis (PCA) allows us to highlight small pulsations, it, unfortunately, does not allow us to control the magnitude of the movement enhancement. To overcome the limitations of PCA, we turned to Eulerian Video Magnification. This method allows controlling the movement magnification. Furthermore, because it works in the frequency domain, it allows defining a range of frequencies that will be magnified. Such magnified video can then be fed into image analysis workflow that will pick up movements and quantify them.

34.4 Conclusion

In conclusion, we provide a detailed assessment of the curation of retinal videos using machine vision techniques. We showcase the tools helpful in circumventing challenges regarding video quality, registration of images, and enhancement of SVP or other pulsatile movements using frequency domain.

While our approach has certain limitations, such as the loss of information through the elimination of frames and masking of static pixels, it has been shown to be an efficient and easy method to implement for retinal imaging data.

Acknowledgments None.

Conflict of Interest The authors declare that they have no conflict of interest.

References

1. Elliot RH. The retinal pulse. Br J Ophthalmol. 1921;5:481–500. https://doi.org/10.1136/bjo.5.11.481.
2. Ford M, Sarwar M. Features of a clinically normal optic disc. Br J Ophthalmol. 1963;47:50–2. https://doi.org/10.1136/bjo.47.1.50.
3. Kahn EA, Cherry GR. The clinical importance of spontaneous retinal venous pulsation. Med Bull (Ann Arbor, Mich). 1950;16:305–8.
4. Levin BE. The clinical significance of spontaneous pulsations of the retinal vein. Arch Neurol. 1978;35:37–40. https://doi.org/10.1001/archneur.1978.00500250041009.
5. Hedges TR Jr, Baron EM, Hedges TR III, Sinclair SH. The retinal venous pulse: its relation to optic disc characteristics and choroidal pulse. Ophthalmology. 1994;101:542–7. https://doi.org/10.1016/S0161-6420(94)31302-9.
6. Flaxman SR, Bourne RRA, Resnikoff S, Ackland P, Braithwaite T, Cicinelli MV, Das A, Jonas JB, Keeffe J, Kempen JH, Leasher J, Limburg H, Naidoo K, Pesudovs K, Silvester A, Stevens GA, Tahhan N, Wong TY, Taylor HR. Global causes of blindness and distance vision impairment 1990–2020: a systematic review and meta-analysis. Lancet Glob Health. 2017;5:e1221–34. https://doi.org/10.1016/s2214-109x(17)30393-5.
7. Chan TCW, Bala C, Siu A, Wan F, White A. Risk factors for rapid Glaucoma disease progression. Am J Ophthalmol. 2017;180:151–7. https://doi.org/10.1016/j.ajo.2017.06.003.
8. Choudhari NS, Raman R, George R. Interrelationship between optic disc edema, spontaneous venous pulsation and intracranial pressure. Indian J Ophthalmol. 2009;57:404–6. https://doi.org/10.4103/0301-4738.55061.
9. D'Antona L, McHugh JA, Ricciardi F, Thorne LW, Matharu MS, Watkins LD, Toma AK, Bremner FD. Association of intracranial pressure and spontaneous retinal venous pulsation. JAMA Neurol. 2019;76(12):1502–5. https://doi.org/10.1001/jamaneurol.2019.2935.
10. McHugh JA, D'Antona L, Toma AK, Bremner FD. Spontaneous venous pulsations detected with infrared videography. J Neuroophthalmol. 2020;40:174–7. https://doi.org/10.1097/wno.0000000000000815.
11. Shariflou S, Agar A, Rose K, Bowd C, Golzan SM. Objective quantification of spontaneous retinal venous pulsations using a novel tablet-based ophthalmoscope. Transl Vis Sci Technol. 2020;9:19. https://doi.org/10.1167/tvst.9.4.19.

12. Soares JVB, Leandro JJG, Cesar RM, Jelinek HF, Cree MJ. Retinal vessel segmentation using the 2-D Gabor wavelet and supervised classification. IEEE Trans Med Imaging. 2006;25:1214–22. https://doi.org/10.1109/TMI.2006.879967.
13. Osareh A, Shadgar B. Automatic blood vessel segmentation in color images of retina. Iran J Sci Technol. 2009;33:191–206.
14. Ramachandran S, Strisciuglio N, Vinekar A, John R, Azzopardi G. U-COSFIRE filters for vessel tortuosity quantification with application to automated diagnosis of retinopathy of prematurity. Neural Comput Applic. 2020;32:12453–68. https://doi.org/10.1007/s00521-019-04697-6.
15. Ronneberger O, Fischer P, Brox T. U-Net: convolutional networks for biomedical image segmentation. In: Medical image computing and computer-assisted intervention—MICCAI. Cham: Springer International; 2015. p. 234–41.
16. Zuiderveld K. Contrast limited adaptive histogram equalization. In: Graphics gems IV. San Diego, CA: Academic Press Professional; 1994. p. 474–85.
17. Land EH, McCann JJ. Lightness and retinex theory. J Opt Soc Am. 1971;61:1–11. https://doi.org/10.1364/josa.61.000001.
18. Gonzalez R, Woods R. Digital image processing, vol. 5. Boston, MA: Addison Wesley; 1992. p. 414–28.
19. Stockman G, Shapiro LG. Computer vision. 1st ed. Hoboken, NJ: Prentice Hall PTR; 2001.
20. Haralock RM, Shapiro L. Computer and robot vision. 1991.
21. Meijering E, Jacob M, Sarria JC, Steiner P, Hirling H, Unser M. Design and validation of a tool for neurite tracing and analysis in fluorescence microscopy images. Cytometry A. 2004;58:167–76. https://doi.org/10.1002/cyto.a.20022.
22. Sada M, Mahesh G. Image deblurring techniques—a detail review. IJSRSET. 2018;4:176–88.
23. Orieux F, Giovannelli J-F, Rodet T. Bayesian estimation of regularization and point spread function parameters for wiener–hunt deconvolution. J Opt Soc Am A. 2010;27:1593–607. https://doi.org/10.1364/JOSAA.27.001593.
24. Richardson WH. Bayesian-based iterative method of image restoration*. J Opt Soc Am. 1972;62:55–9. https://doi.org/10.1364/JOSA.62.000055.
25. Sahu S, Lenka MK, Sa PK. Blind deblurring using deep learning: a survey. In: CoRR abs/1907.10128; 2019.
26. Schuler CJ, Hirsch M, Harmeling S, Schölkopf B. Learning to Deblur. In: CoRR abs/1406.7444; 2014.
27. Chakrabarti AA. Neural approach to blind motion deblurring. In: Computer vision—ECCV 2016. Cham: Springer International. p. 221–35.
28. Sun J, Wenfei C, Zongben X, Ponce J. Learning a convolutional neural network for non-uniform motion blur removal. In: 2015 IEEE Conference on Computer Vision and Pattern Recognition (CVPR), 7–12 June 2015; 2015. p. 769–77. https://doi.org/10.1109/CVPR.2015.7298677.
29. Renting L, Zhaorong L, Jiaya J. Image partial blur detection and classification. In: 2008 IEEE Conference on Computer Vision and Pattern Recognition, 23–28 June 2008; 2008. p. 1–8. https://doi.org/10.1109/CVPR.2008.4587465.
30. Su B, Lu S, Tan CL. Blurred image region detection and classification. In: Paper presented at the Proceedings of the 19th ACM International conference on multimedia, Scottsdale, Arizona, USA; 2011.
31. Rublee E, Rabaud V, Konolige K, Bradski G. ORB: an efficient alternative to SIFT or SURF. In: 2011 International Conference on Computer Vision, 6–13 November 2011; 2011. p. 2564–71. https://doi.org/10.1109/ICCV.2011.6126544.
32. Lowe DG. Distinctive image features from scale-invariant keypoints. Int J Comput Vis. 2004;60:91–110. https://doi.org/10.1023/B:VISI.0000029664.99615.94.
33. Bay H, Tuytelaars T, Van Gool L. SURF: speeded up robust features. In: Computer vision—ECCV 2006. Berlin, Heidelberg: Springer; 2006. p. 404–17.
34. Deng K, Tian J, Zheng J, Zhang X, Dai X, Xu M. Retinal fundus image registration via vascular structure graph matching. Int J Biomed Imaging. 2010;2010:906067. https://doi.org/10.1155/2010/906067.
35. Stewart CV, Tsai CL, Roysam B. The dual-bootstrap iterative closest point algorithm with application to retinal image registration. IEEE Trans Med Imaging. 2003;22:1379–94. https://doi.org/10.1109/tmi.2003.819276.
36. Ashburner J, Friston KJ. Nonlinear spatial normalization using basis functions. Hum Brain Mapp. 1999;7:254–66. https://doi.org/10.1002/(SICI)1097-0193(1999)7:4<254::AID-HBM4>3.0.CO;2-G.
37. Friston KJ, Ashburner J, Frith CD, Poline J-B, Heather JD, Frackowiak RSJ. Spatial registration and normalization of images. Hum Brain Mapp. 1995;3:165–89. https://doi.org/10.1002/hbm.460030303.
38. Gulsoy EB, Simmons JP, De Graef M. Application of joint histogram and mutual information to registration and data fusion problems in serial sectioning microstructure studies. Scr Mater. 2009;60:381–4. https://doi.org/10.1016/j.scriptamat.2008.11.004.
39. Mattes D, Haynor D, Vesselle H, Lewellyn T, Eubank W. Nonrigid multimodality image registration. In: Medical imaging 2001, vol. 4322. Bellingham, WA: SPIE; 2001.
40. Klein S, Staring M, Murphy K, Viergever MA, Pluim JP. Elastix: a toolbox for intensity-based medical image registration. IEEE Trans Med Imaging. 2010;29:196–205. https://doi.org/10.1109/tmi.2009.2035616.
41. Shamonin DP, Bron EE, Lelieveldt BP, Smits M, Klein S, Staring M. Fast parallel image registration on CPU and GPU for diagnostic classification of Alzheimer's disease. Front Neuroinform. 2013;7:50. https://doi.org/10.3389/fninf.2013.00050.
42. Beare R, Lowekamp B, Yaniv Z. Image segmentation, registration and characterization in R with SimpleITK. J Stat Softw. 2018;86:8. https://doi.org/10.18637/jss.v086.i08.
43. https://opencv.org/.
44. van der Walt S, Schönberger JL, Nunez-Iglesias J, Boulogne F, Warner JD, Yager N, Gouillart E, Yu T, The Scikit-Image C. Scikit-image: image processing in Python. Peer J. 2014;2:e453. https://doi.org/10.7717/peerj.453.
45. Thévenaz P, Ruttimann UE, Unser M. A pyramid approach to subpixel registration based on intensity. IEEE Trans Image Process. 1998;7:27–41. https://doi.org/10.1109/83.650848.
46. Lucas BD, Kanade T. An iterative image registration technique with an application to stereo vision. In: Paper presented at the Proceedings of the 7th International joint conference on artificial intelligence, Vancouver, BC, Canada, vol. 2; 1981.
47. Farnebäck G. Two-frame motion estimation based on polynomial expansion. In: Image analysis. Berlin, Heidelberg: Springer; 2003. p. 363–70.
48. Perez RE, Jansen PW, Martins JR. pyOpt: a Python-based object-oriented framework for nonlinear constrained optimization. Struct Multidiscip Optim. 2012;45:101–18. https://doi.org/10.1007/s00158-011-0666-3.
49. Masters B, Gonzalez R, Woods R. Book review: digital image processing, third edition. J Biomed Opt. 2009;14:029901.
50. Goyal B, Dogra A, Agrawal S, Sohi BS, Sharma A. Image denoising review: from classical to state-of-the-art approaches. Inform Fusion. 2020;55:220–44. https://doi.org/10.1016/j.inffus.2019.09.003.
51. Buades A, Coll B, Morel J-M. Denoising image sequences does not require motion estimation, vol. 2005; 2005. https://doi.org/10.1109/AVSS.2005.1577245.

52. Reza AM. Realization of the contrast limited adaptive histogram equalization (CLAHE) for real-time image enhancement. J VLSI Signal Process Syst. 2004;38:35–44.
53. Morgan WH, Abdul-Rahman A, Yu D-Y, Hazelton ML, Betz-Stablein B, Lind CRP. Objective detection of retinal vessel pulsation. PLoS One. 2015;10:e0116475. https://doi.org/10.1371/journal.pone.0116475.
54. Moret F, Poloschek C, Lagrèze W-D, Bach M. Visualization of fundus vessel pulsation using principal component analysis. Invest Ophthalmol Vis Sci. 2011;52:5457–64. https://doi.org/10.1167/iovs.10-6806.
55. Wu H-Y, Rubinstein M, Shih E, Guttag J, Durand F, Freeman W. Eulerian video magnification for revealing subtle changes in the world. In: ACM Transactions on Graphics—TOG, vol. 31; 2012. p. 1–8. https://doi.org/10.1145/2185520.2185561.
56. Hracho M, Kolar R, Odstrcilik J, Labounkova I, Tornow R. Automatic detection of spontaneous venous pulsations using retinal image sequences; 2018. p. 27. https://doi.org/10.1007/978-3-319-68195-5_90.
57. Tao X, Gao H, Shen X, Wang J, Jia J. Scale-recurrent network for deep image deblurring. In: CoRR abs/1802.01770. 2018.

Artificial Intelligence in Adult Spinal Deformity

35

Pramod N. Kamalapathy, Aditya V. Karhade, Daniel Tobert, and Joseph H. Schwab

35.1 Introduction

Adult spinal deformity (ASD) is a complex, heterogenous condition resulting in severe pain and functional limitations [1–3]. The burden of ASD is comparable or greater than that caused by chronic diseases such as hypertension, diabetes, or heart disease [1, 2]. The prevalence of ASD is reported to be over 65% in patients over 60 years old [4], and as the average life expectancy continues to increase, the number of patients undergoing ASD surgery will grow [5–7]. Previous studies have found that operative management is beneficial for patients with ASD, but the procedure can be complex and difficult with complication rates approaching nearly 100% (depending on the definition of complication) [6, 8–11]. While understanding of the pathophysiology of the disorder and surgical techniques have significantly improved, application of emerging technologies represents opportunities to further optimize interventions and patient outcomes [10–13].

Advancements in software and hardware as well as increasing availability of large datasets have allowed artificial intelligence (AI) to gain traction in medicine [14]. Recent studies in spine surgery, orthopedic surgery, and neurosurgery have reported several applications of this technology [15–18].

Sub-fields of AI such as computer vision and predictive analytics may improve precision medicine and optimize patient safety in ASD surgery [19]. As such, the purpose of this study was to review the current literature on the use of artificial intelligence in ASD.

35.2 Methods

A literature review of adult spinal deformity and artificial intelligence was conducted according to Preferred Reporting Items for Systematic reviews and Meta-analysis (PRISMA) guidelines to identify all articles available in PubMed from January 1st, 2015 to August 1st, 2020. Ten journals were queried: The Spine Journal, Spine, Clinical Spine Surgery, Spine Deformity, Asian Spine Journal, European Spine Journal, Journal of Neurosurgery: Spine, Global Spine Journal, Clinical Orthopaedics and Related Research, and Journal of Bone and Joint Surgery. Search syntax was built from terms related to "adult spinal deformity" and "artificial intelligence." Supplementary Fig. S1 includes specific search syntax.

Inclusion criteria for the study were any articles that involved topics of spinal deformity and artificial intelligence. Exclusion criteria includes patients less than 18 years of age, studies including spine surgery in general and not adult spinal deformity specifically (Fig. 35.1).

35.3 Results

Figure 35.2 shows the flow diagram for data collection. The initial PubMed search started with 152 articles. Of the 19 eligible studies, 13 (68%) included machine learning, four incorporated computer vision, one involved augmented reality, and one combined augmented reality and machine learning. Seventeen of 19 studies were published in the year 2018 or later. The cohort size in each study ranged from 15 to 37,852 (median = 557) subjects with variables ranging from 12 to 150 (median = 32). The data were predominantly retrospectively (n = 9, 47%) or prospectively collected (n = 8,

Supplementary Information The online version contains supplementarymaterial available at (https://doi.org/10.1007/978-3-030-85292-4_35).

P. N. Kamalapathy · A. V. Karhade · D. Tobert · J. H. Schwab (✉)
Department of Orthopedic Surgery, Orthopedic Spine Center and Orthopedic Oncology Service, Massachusetts General Hospital, Boston, MA, USA
e-mail: jhschwab@mgh.harvard.edu

V. E. Staartjes et al. (eds.), *Machine Learning in Clinical Neuroscience*, Acta Neurochirurgica Supplement 134,
https://doi.org/10.1007/978-3-030-85292-4_35

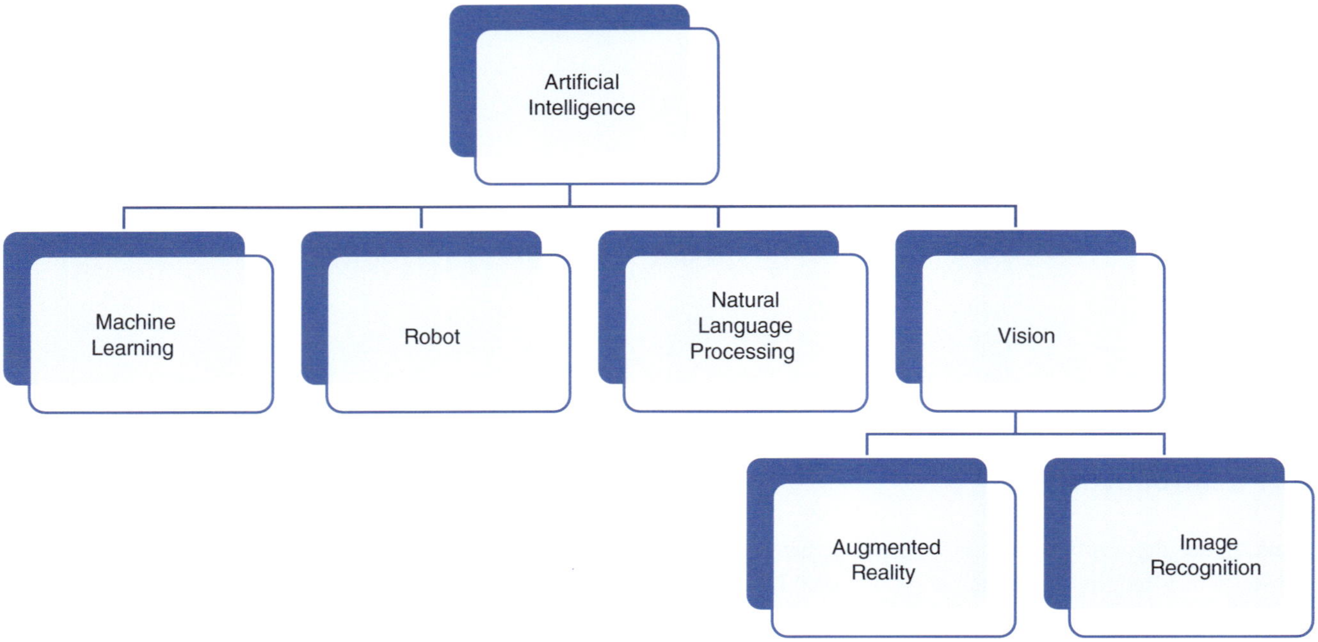

Fig. 35.1 Types of artificial intelligence

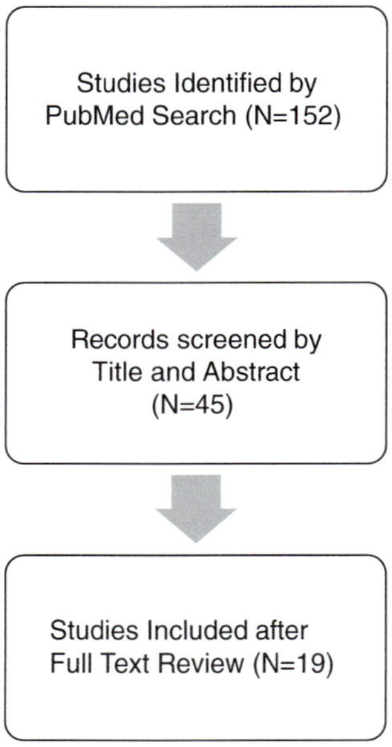

Fig. 35.2 Flow diagram of studies included

42%). One (5%) study used a large national database and one (5%) was a biomechanical study. All of the nine (47%) studies by the International Spine Study Group (ISSG) and European Spine Study Group (ESSG) were prospectively collected using multicenter databases.

The most common predictive variables of machine learning studies were intraoperative and postoperative complications following ASD and risk factor predictions. Of the 13 machine learning studies, 12 (92%) were supervised and one (8%) was clustering or unsupervised. One study (8%) reported percentages of missing values and four (31%) used multiple imputation to approximate the missing values. Common predictive analytic modeling mechanisms include tree-based algorithms, consisting of decision trees, random forest, and classification and regression trees. Nine (69%) studies reported outcomes using area under the curve and one (8%) study also reported the Brier score. Six (46%) machine learning studies included global explanation for relative variable importance and zero studies evaluated calibration or decision curve analysis as part of their results (Table 35.1).

35.4 Discussion

ASD is a debilitating condition that often causes chronic pain and disability [1–3]. AI usage is growing rapidly in healthcare for its ability to solve complex problems and without requiring simplifications such as linear assumptions for biomedical data. This study reviews the use of AI in ASD studies. There are 19 studies that were included in this review, of which 13 included machine learning or predictive analytics, four incorporated computer vision, one involved augmented reality, and one combined computer vision and machine learning over the past 5 years.

Machine Learning

The number of studies utilizing machine learning in ASD has increased rapidly over the past few years and their methodology has become more advanced. In 2018, Durand et al.

Table 35.1 Adult spinal deformity and artificial intelligence studies included

Study	Type of AI	Outcome variable	AUC	Other results
Jain (2020) [46]	Machine learning	90-day discharge, readmission, medical complication	0.65–0.77	
Cho (2020) [36]	Computer vision	Lumbar lordosis angle	0.914	86.2% accuracy
Edström (2020) [39]	Augmented reality	Pedicle screw density		PS density: Navigation 86.3% vs. free hand 74.7%
Ebrahimi S (2019) [47]	Machine learning/computer vision	Vertebral axis rotation		84% accuracy
Ames (2019) [24]	Machine learning	Catastrophic cost		$R^2 = 28.8\%–87.8\%$
Pan (2019) [35]	Computer vision	Cobb angle		Intraclass correlation coefficient: 0.854, absolute difference = 3.32°
Ames (2019) [25]	Machine learning	SRS-22R questions	0.56–0.87	
Pellisé (2019) [16]	Machine learning	Risk stratification model	0.717	Brier score = 10.1%–19.5%
Ames (2019) [26]	Machine learning	Clustering of patient types and intervention		Gap statistic $K = 0.67$
Khatri (2019) [48]	Machine learning	Pullout strength of pedicle screw		Correlation coefficient 0.96, relative absolute error 0.28
Burström (2019) [38]	Computer vision	Automatic segmentation, pedicle screw navigation		Overall accuracy 86.1%
Galbusera (2019) [37]	Computer vision	Anatomical parameters		Standard error 2.7 degrees-11.5
Yagi (2019) [49]	Machine learning	2 year major complications	0.963	84% accuracy in external dataset
Kim (2018) [50]	Machine learning	Surgical complications	0.547–0.787	
Scheer (2018) [27]	Machine learning	Oswestry disability index minimal clinically important difference		$R^2 = 20\%–45\%$, MAE = 8%–15%
Passias (2018) [28]	Machine learning	Distal junctional kyphosis	0.870	
Durand (2018) [20]	Machine learning	Blood transfusion	0.850	
Scheer (2017) [29]	Machine learning	Major complications	0.89	Accuracy = 87.6%
Scheer (2017) [30]	Machine learning	Proximal junction failure	0.89	Accuracy = 86.3%

developed a classification tree and random forest models to predict blood transfusions after ASD surgery using a retrospective database [20]. The authors employed multiple imputation for missing values and tenfold cross-validation to optimize their model. Multiple imputation can reduce bias which is created when exclusion of missing variables occurs in datasets [21]. Cross-validation is a statistical method that estimates performance and prevents overfitting of models [22, 23].

The ISSG and ESSG have used multicenter prospective databases to develop models [16, 24–30]. This may increase generalizability of findings compared to institutional databases [31–33]. Ames et al. compared eight algorithms to predict answers to the Scoliosis Research Society Questionnaire 22 [25]. Five hundred sixty-one patients and 150 variables were used to predict these responses, with testing AUC of 0.56–0.87, producing accuracy of 35%–80% [25]. While many of the machine learning studies use supervised learning, Ames et al. (AI based −2019) created AI-based hierarchical clustering of patient types and intervention categories using unsupervised learning [26]. Unsupervised learning identifies undetected patterns with no pre-existing labels and minimum human involvement. For example, supervised learning uses a labeled dataset of both outcomes and predictor variables to learn and train the model, whereas an unsupervised model draws inferences and patterns without labeled outcomes [34].

Computer Vision/Augmentation

There are four studies that utilized computer vision with respect to ASD [35–38]. The utilization of computer vision ranges from fully automating radiological analysis to integrating computer vision to the navigation system and optimize pedicle screw placement. Convolutional neural network was the most common deep learning methodology used in these studies. Cho et al. used U-Net, a well-established convolutional neural network, to automate lumbar lordosis angles [36]. The study was able to automate evaluation of radiological parameters with excellent performance—testing AUC of 0.914 and accuracy of 86.2%. Moreover, Burstrom et al. created a system to automate segmentation, pedicle identification, and pedicle screw placement with the use of a three-dimensional navigation system [38]. The technology has potential to aid surgeons in navigational planning and optimization of workflow to increase patient safety. Of note, this study was performed on cadavers without spinal deformity and future studies in ASD patients will further substantiate the promise of this technology.

Similarly, the same group investigated whether the use of augmented reality surgical navigation could impair implant density compared to the free hand technique [39]. They found that augmented reality enabled surgeons to increase pedicle screw density and minimize use of hooks during surgery without prolonging OR time. This results in robust constructs that might last longer, thereby possibly decreasing the need for revision surgery without compromising patient safety during the operation. The use of navigation in spine surgery is limited by cost and operative time, but this study showed how augmented reality surgical navigation might be used to decrease length of hospital stay and decrease blood loss [40, 41].

Future

Artificial intelligence is a continuously growing field and there is high level of optimism for the future of AI in ASD surgery. Algorithms are continuing to grow in complexity with additional techniques and modifications. Despite this promise, this review uncovered some areas in which studies may improve in the future. Studies might improve by reporting the number of missing values as well as the methodology used to handle missing data, which could potentially bias the results and the derived algorithm. Multiple imputation and cross-validation are not yet standardized, of which only six studies used multiple imputation and seven using cross-validation. Also, while many studies do report an area under the curve (AUC), formalized TRIPOD reporting would make systematic and easily comparable models [42]. The TRIPOD-ML (cite the study proposing TRIPOD-ML) have recently been proposed and adherence to these guidelines when they become available will further improve the methodological rigor of predictive studies in ASD. Until then, the standard TRIPOD criteria include calibration-in-the-large or the model intercept (A); calibration slope (B); discrimination with an AUC (C); and clinical usefulness with decision curve analysis (D). Finally, many models were created using multi-institutional, prospective databases, thereby increasing the generalizability of the data. Continued cross-institutional collaboration and work by international study groups such as ISSG and ESSG promises to improve both ASD patients' outcomes and our understanding of this pathology.

Computer vision and augmentation reality are more recent in their adaptation to healthcare and ASD, but the potential applications are extensive. Gregory et al. presented a study that showed a 3-D hologram of a patient's scapula in real time during a shoulder replacement with the use of the Microsoft HoloLens [43]. This headset allows surgeons to maintain sterility while accessing 3-D holograms and interact with others. Recently, as of June 2020, three surgeons at Johns Hopkins University performed spine surgery using head-mounted display of augmented reality. The technology provides both 2-D and 3-D views of the surgical field without the necessity to view a screen and reduce obstruction [44].

There are also applications of robotics and natural language processing that have not been published in ASD literature. Other surgical subspecialties have thus far outpaced spine surgery in the use of robotics. AI advancements can help automate procedures and help surgeons plan using the 3-D digital segmentation generated prior to surgery to personalize their techniques [19, 45]. Natural language processing is another subset of artificial intelligence that continues to grow in its application in healthcare. It can be used to automate research, but also be implemented in hospital systems to continuously survey hospital records for detection of adverse events—enhancing safety reporting and monitoring hospital quality.

35.5 Conclusion

This study shows the conscious efforts of spine surgeons to employ evolving technology to advance the field of ASD. Artificial intelligence allows surgeons to further optimize precision medicine and improve patient safety in ASD. As surgeons become familiar with this technology, the applications of AI will continue to grow in both the clinical and research settings.

Conflicts of Interest Statement The authors of this study have no financial disclosures.

References

1. Pellisé F, et al. Impact on health related quality of life of adult spinal deformity (ASD) compared with other chronic conditions. Eur Spine J. 2015;24(1):3–11. https://doi.org/10.1007/s00586-014-3542-1.
2. Bess S, et al. The health impact of symptomatic adult spinal deformity: comparison of deformity types to United States population norms and chronic diseases. Spine (Phila Pa 1976). 2016;41(3):224–33. https://doi.org/10.1097/BRS.0000000000001202.
3. Bess S, et al. Pain and disability determine treatment modality for older patients with adult scoliosis, while deformity guides treatment for younger patients. Spine (Phila Pa 1976). 2009;34(20):2186–90. https://doi.org/10.1097/BRS.0b013e3181b05146.

4. Schwab F, et al. Adult scoliosis: prevalence, SF-36, and nutritional parameters in an elderly volunteer population. Spine (Phila Pa 1976). 2005;30(9):1082–5. https://doi.org/10.1097/01.brs.0000160842.43482.cd.
5. Jain A, et al. Incidence of perioperative medical complications and mortality among elderly patients undergoing surgery for spinal deformity: analysis of 3519 patients. J Neurosurg Spine. 2017;27(5):534–9. https://doi.org/10.3171/2017.3.SPINE161011.
6. Smith C, et al. The prevalence of complications associated with lumbar and thoracic spinal deformity surgery in the elderly population: a meta-analysis. J Spine Surg. 2019;5(2):2.
7. Cheng JS, Forbes J, Wong C, Perry E. The epidemiology of adult spinal deformity and the aging population. In: Wang MY, Lu Y, Anderson DG, Mummaneni PV, editors. Minimally invasive spinal deformity surgery: an evolution of modern techniques. Vienna: Springer; 2014. p. 3–10.
8. Kelly MP, et al. Operative versus nonoperative treatment for adult symptomatic lumbar scoliosis. JBJS. 2019;101(4):338–52. https://doi.org/10.2106/JBJS.18.00483.
9. Lonergan T, Place H, Taylor P. Acute complications after adult spinal deformity surgery in patients aged 70 years and older. Clin Spine Surg. 2016;29(8):314–7. https://doi.org/10.1097/BSD.0b013e3182764a23.
10. Uribe JS, et al. Complications in adult spinal deformity surgery: an analysis of minimally invasive, hybrid, and open surgical techniques. Neurosurg Focus. 2014;36(5):E15. https://doi.org/10.3171/2014.3.FOCUS13534.
11. Zanirato A, et al. Complications in adult spine deformity surgery: a systematic review of the recent literature with reporting of aggregated incidences. Eur Spine J. 2018;27(9):2272–84. https://doi.org/10.1007/s00586-018-5535-y.
12. Emami A, Deviren V, Berven S, Smith JA, Hu SS, Bradford DS. Outcome and complications of long fusions to the sacrum in adult spine deformity: Luque-Galveston, combined iliac and sacral screws, and sacral fixation. Spine (Phila Pa 1976). 2002;27(7):776–86. https://doi.org/10.1097/00007632-200204010-00017.
13. Soroceanu A, et al. Medical complications after adult spinal deformity surgery: incidence, risk factors, and clinical impact. Spine (Phila Pa 1976). 2016;41(22):1718–23. https://doi.org/10.1097/BRS.0000000000001636.
14. Bohr A, Memarzadeh K. The rise of artificial intelligence in healthcare applications. In: Artificial intelligence in healthcare; 2020. p. 25–60. https://doi.org/10.1016/B978-0-12-818438-7.00002-2.
15. Azad TD, et al. Fostering reproducibility and generalizability in machine learning for clinical prediction modeling in spine surgery. Spine J. 2020. https://doi.org/10.1016/j.spinee.2020.10.006.
16. Pellisé F, et al. Development and validation of risk stratification models for adult spinal deformity surgery. J Neurosurg Spine. 2019:1–13. https://doi.org/10.3171/2019.3.SPINE181452.
17. Han X, et al. Safety and accuracy of robot-assisted versus fluoroscopy-assisted pedicle screw insertion in thoracolumbar spinal surgery: a prospective randomized controlled trial. J Neurosurg Spine. 2019;30:1–8. https://doi.org/10.3171/2018.10.SPINE18487.
18. Tack C. Artificial intelligence and machine learning | applications in musculoskeletal physiotherapy. Musculoskelet Sci Pract. 2019;39:164–9. https://doi.org/10.1016/j.msksp.2018.11.012.
19. Rasouli JJ, et al. Artificial intelligence and robotics in spine surgery. Global Spine J. 2020;11:556–64. https://doi.org/10.1177/2192568220915718.
20. Durand WM, DePasse JM, Daniels AH. Predictive modeling for blood transfusion after adult spinal deformity surgery: a tree-based machine learning approach. Spine (Phila Pa 1976). 2018;43(15):1058–66. https://doi.org/10.1097/BRS.0000000000002515.
21. Kang H. The prevention and handling of the missing data. Korean J Anesthesiol. 2013;64(5):402–6. https://doi.org/10.4097/kjae.2013.64.5.402.
22. Deng B-C, et al. A new strategy to prevent over-fitting in partial least squares models based on model population analysis. Anal Chim Acta. 2015;880:32–41. https://doi.org/10.1016/j.aca.2015.04.045.
23. Granholm V, Noble WS, Käll L. A cross-validation scheme for machine learning algorithms in shotgun proteomics. BMC Bioinform. 2012;13(Suppl 16):S3. https://doi.org/10.1186/1471-2105-13-S16-S3.
24. Ames CP, et al. Utilization of predictive modeling to determine episode of care costs and to accurately identify catastrophic cost nonwarranty outlier patients in adult spinal deformity surgery: a step toward bundled payments and risk sharing. Spine (Phila Pa 1976). 2020;45(5):E252–65. https://doi.org/10.1097/BRS.0000000000003242.
25. Ames CP, et al. Development of predictive models for all individual questions of SRS-22R after adult spinal deformity surgery: a step toward individualized medicine. Eur Spine J. 2019;28(9):1998–2011. https://doi.org/10.1007/s00586-019-06079-x.
26. Ames CP, et al. Artificial intelligence based hierarchical clustering of patient types and intervention categories in adult spinal deformity surgery: towards a new classification scheme that predicts quality and value. Spine (Phila Pa 1976). 2019;44(13):915–26. https://doi.org/10.1097/BRS.0000000000002974.
27. Scheer JK, et al. Development of a preoperative predictive model for reaching the Oswestry disability index minimal clinically important difference for adult spinal deformity patients. Spine Deform. 2018;6(5):593–9. https://doi.org/10.1016/j.jspd.2018.02.010.
28. Passias PG, et al. Predictive model for distal junctional kyphosis after cervical deformity surgery. Spine J. 2018;18(12):2187–94. https://doi.org/10.1016/j.spinee.2018.04.017.
29. Scheer JK, et al. Development of a preoperative predictive model for major complications following adult spinal deformity surgery. J Neurosurg Spine. 2017;26(6):736–43. https://doi.org/10.3171/2016.10.SPINE16197.
30. Scheer JK, et al. Development of validated computer-based preoperative predictive model for proximal junction failure (PJF) or clinically significant PJK with 86% accuracy based on 510 ASD patients with 2-year follow-up. Spine (Phila Pa 1976). 2016;41(22):E1328–35. https://doi.org/10.1097/BRS.0000000000001598.
31. Sanders C, Saltzstein SL, Nguyen DH, Stafford HS, Schultzel M, Sadler GR. Understanding the limits of large datasets. J Cancer Educ. 2012;27(4):664–9. https://doi.org/10.1007/s13187-012-0383-7.
32. Wild S, Fischbacher C, McKnight J. Using large diabetes databases for research. J Diabetes Sci Technol. 2016;10(5):1073–8. https://doi.org/10.1177/1932296816645120.
33. Alluri RK, Leland H, Heckmann N. Surgical research using national databases. Ann Transl Med. 2016;4(20):393. https://doi.org/10.21037/atm.2016.10.49.
34. Rajkomar A, Dean J, Kohane I. Machine learning in medicine. N Engl J Med. 2019;380(14):1347–58.
35. Pan Y, et al. Evaluation of a computer-aided method for measuring the cobb angle on chest X-rays. Eur Spine J. 2019;28(12):3035–43. https://doi.org/10.1007/s00586-019-06115-w.
36. Cho BH, et al. Automated measurement of lumbar lordosis on radiographs using machine learning and computer vision. Global Spine J. 2020;10(5):611–8. https://doi.org/10.1177/2192568219868190.
37. Galbusera F, et al. Fully automated radiological analysis of spinal disorders and deformities: a deep learning approach. Eur Spine J. 2019;28(5):951–60. https://doi.org/10.1007/s00586-019-05944-z.
38. Burström G, et al. Machine learning for automated 3-dimensional segmentation of the spine and suggested placement of pedicle screws based on intraoperative cone-beam computer tomography. J Neurosurg Spine. 2019;31(1):147–54. https://doi.org/10.3171/2018.12.SPINE181397.
39. Edström E, et al. Does augmented reality navigation increase pedicle screw density compared to free-hand technique in deformity surgery? Single surgeon case series of 44 patients. Spine

(Phila Pa 1976). 2020;45(17):E1085–90. https://doi.org/10.1097/BRS.0000000000003518.
40. Mezger U, Jendrewski C, Bartels M. Navigation in surgery. Langenbecks Arch Surg. 2013;398(4):501–14. https://doi.org/10.1007/s00423-013-1059-4.
41. Gargallo-Albiol J, Barootchi S, Salomó-Coll O, Wang H. Advantages and disadvantages of implant navigation surgery. A systematic review. Ann Anat. 2019;225:1–10. https://doi.org/10.1016/j.aanat.2019.04.005.
42. Towards better clinical prediction models: seven steps for development and an ABCD for validation. Abstract—Europe PMC. https://europepmc.org/article/PMC/4155437. Accessed 2 Mar 2020.
43. Gregory TM, Gregory J, Sledge J, Allard R, Mir O. Surgery guided by mixed reality: presentation of a proof of concept. Acta Orthop. 2018;89(5):480–3. https://doi.org/10.1080/17453674.2018.1506974.
44. Volpe KD. Heads up! Docs perform first augmented reality-guided spinal fusion. SpineUniverse. https://www.spineuniverse.com/professional/news/first-augmented-reality-guided-spinal-fusion. Accessed 6 Nov 2020.
45. Bhandari M, Zeffiro T, Reddiboina M. Artificial intelligence and robotic surgery: current perspective and future directions. Curr Opin Urol. 2020;30(1):48–54. https://doi.org/10.1097/MOU.0000000000000692.
46. Jain D, Durand W, Burch S, Daniels A, Berven S. Machine learning for predictive modeling of 90-day readmission, major medical complication, and discharge to a facility in patients undergoing long segment posterior lumbar spine fusion. Spine (Phila Pa 1976). 2020;45(16):1151–60. https://doi.org/10.1097/BRS.0000000000003475.
47. Ebrahimi S, Gajny L, Vergari C, Angelini ED, Skalli W. Vertebral rotation estimation from frontal X-rays using a quasi-automated pedicle detection method. Eur Spine J. 2019;28(12):3026–34. https://doi.org/10.1007/s00586-019-06158-z.
48. Khatri R, Varghese V, Sharma S, Kumar GS, Chhabra HS. Pullout strength predictor: a machine learning approach. Asian Spine J. 2019;13(5):842–8. https://doi.org/10.31616/asj.2018.0243.
49. Yagi M, et al. Predictive model for major complications 2 years after corrective spine surgery for adult spinal deformity. Eur Spine J. 2019;28(1):180–7. https://doi.org/10.1007/s00586-018-5816-5.
50. Kim JS, et al. Predicting surgical complications in patients undergoing elective adult spinal deformity procedures using machine learning. Spine Deform. 2018;6(6):762–70. https://doi.org/10.1016/j.jspd.2018.03.003.

Machine Learning and Intracranial Aneurysms: From Detection to Outcome Prediction

36

Vittorio Stumpo, Victor E. Staartjes, Giuseppe Esposito, Carlo Serra, Luca Regli, Alessandro Olivi, and Carmelo Lucio Sturiale

36.1 Introduction

Intracranial aneurysms (IAs) affect 3 to 5% of the general population and their incidental diagnosis has been rising due to the increased availability of diagnostic imaging performed for minor neurological symptoms [1]. Unfortunately, in most circumstances aneurysm rupture results in severe subarachnoid hemorrhage (SAH) as first clinical manifestation, which carries significant morbidity and mortality [2]. After SAH, patient prognosis is determined not only by the rupture event, but also by secondary major complications such as vasospasm, hydrocephalus, seizures, and delayed ischemic events [3]. Recent computational advancements and increased availability of epidemiological, clinical, and imaging data constitute the basis for enhanced disease detection, more informed management evaluation, and treatment planning [4, 5]. Improving the detection of unruptured IAs (uIAs) is the most effective way to prevent SAH. The evaluation of risk of rupture is at the cornerstone of management for these patients as rupture risk has to be balanced with treatment-related risk. Moreover, in the event of SAH presentation, identifying patients with higher risk for developing vasospasm, hydrocephalus, seizures, and ischemic complications could represent a significant therapeutic advantage favoring a possible outcome improvement [3, 6]. Also, functional outcome prediction has the potential to better inform patient management. In this context, machine learning (ML) and artificial intelligence (AI) constitute a rapidly rising research area in biomedical sciences that covers several applications spanning from image processing, segmentation and classification, disease detection, as well as complication and outcome prediction [7–10]. With respect to traditional statistical methods, ML algorithms have the potential to learn and improve their predictive performance when fed with large data sets without the need of being specifically programmed. The implications of such approach are several: firstly, depending of the desired ML approach, data can be presented to the algorithm categorized/processed or uncategorized/raw. A certain degree of pre-processing may be required to improve the model performance or, on the contrary, algorithms can also be trained to automatically extract certain features that are important for the resulting prediction. Many publications have already investigated ML applications in diverse pathologies of neurosurgical relevance including primary and secondary brain tumors and spinal diseases [7, 9, 11–16]. More recently ML has also been introduced in the area of IA research, especially in the subfield relating to deep learning [17]. Given the pace at which new progress is made, it is not unreasonable to expect that future developments will result in a computer-assisted working framework for more informed and transversal aneurysm patient management.

Supplementary Information The online version contains supplementary material available at (https://doi.org/10.1007/978-3-030-85292-4_36).

V. Stumpo
Machine Intelligence in Clinical Neuroscience (MICN) Laboratory, Department of Neurosurgery, Clinical Neuroscience Center, University Hospital Zurich, University of Zurich, Zurich, Switzerland

Institute of Neurosurgery, Università Cattolica del Sacro Cuore, Rome, Italy

V. E. Staartjes (✉) · G. Esposito · C. Serra · L. Regli
Machine Intelligence in Clinical Neuroscience (MICN) Laboratory, Department of Neurosurgery, Clinical Neuroscience Center, University Hospital Zurich, University of Zurich, Zurich, Switzerland
e-mail: victoregon.staartjes@usz.ch

A. Olivi
Institute of Neurosurgery, Università Cattolica del Sacro Cuore, Rome, Italy

Department of Neurosurgery, Fondazione Policlinico Universitario A. Gemelli IRCCS, Rome, Italy

C. L. Sturiale
Department of Neurosurgery, Fondazione Policlinico Universitario A. Gemelli IRCCS, Rome, Italy

V. E. Staartjes et al. (eds.), *Machine Learning in Clinical Neuroscience*, Acta Neurochirurgica Supplement 134,
https://doi.org/10.1007/978-3-030-85292-4_36

New studies in the field are reported on a daily basis, and adequate understanding of ML is required for informed clinicians to remain up-to-date on one side and to embrace and contribute to the progress in aneurysm research on the other. In the present study, we aimed to provide an overview of past studies applying ML and AI in the field of intracranial aneurysm surgery and aneurysm patient management.

36.2 Machine Learning Applications in the Management of Patients with Intracranial Aneurysms

Based on our literature review, we identified four main areas of ML and AI research applications in the field of intracranial aneurysm management.

Aneurysm Detection [18–27] (Table 36.1)

For this task, electronic health records and transcriptomic signatures have been used to identify subpopulations at higher risk of aneurysm development [20, 25]. Convolutional neural networks (CNNs) have been also exploited for image segmentation and processing to enhance detection accuracy on 3D time-of-flight magnetic resonance angiography (3D-TOF-MRI) [21, 22, 26, 27], digital subtraction angiography (DSA) [18, 19], and computed tomography angiography (CTA) [23]. Aneurysm detection studies on neurovascular imaging mostly evaluated CNN algorithms [18, 19, 21–24, 26, 27]. These studies provide evidence that automatic ML-based segmentation is not inferior to manual contouring and may result in increased sensitivity and accuracy in aneurysm detection compared with traditional image analyses [23, 24, 27]. Use of commercially available CNNs has been also reported with encouraging results [19, 27]. Concerns of excessive false positive (FP) findings have been raised by some authors, but specific solutions such as a certain degree of image processing have been successfully implemented [22, 26]. Additionally, the potential for reduced time in aneurysm detection has been highlighted [18]. When demographic, clinical, and laboratory data were used, models were trained using algorithms such as logistic regression (LR), random forest (RF), support vector machine (SVM) for aneurysm detection tasks [20, 25].

Aneurysm Rupture Risk and Stability Prediction [28–32] (Table 36.2)

Of higher clinical importance, some studies assessed the possibility to predict the risk of aneurysm rupture—a highly debated clinical topic in scientific literature intrinsically linked with the still not fully understood natural history of IAa. The reported approaches are heterogeneous and include use of demographic, clinical, and morphological features, as previously attempted by means of scores developed using traditional statistics or expert consensus [28, 33, 34]. One study recently aimed to predict the risk of rupture through the evaluation of the aneurysm wall contrast-enhancement—which is known to be associated with tissue degeneration and higher wall instability—combining geometrical features, clinical risk factors, and hemodynamic pattern [30]. Other studies tried to identify features suggestive of aneurysms stability by means of ML [29, 32]. Importantly, ML-derived model developed on a relatively limited patient population has been reported to outperform more traditional statistical approaches as well as previously developed risk scores [32]. The use of radiomic features obtained from CTA for ML model training has also been evaluated in some pilot studies showing promising results for aneurysm risk or rupture stratification and stability prediction [29, 31].

Complications and Outcome Prediction [35–43] (Table 36.3)

Several studies have attempted to accurately predict the occurrence of vasospasm and delayed cerebral ischemia (DCI) [35, 36, 38, 39]. For vasospasm prediction, either angiographic images or a variable combination of clinical and laboratory parameters were used [35, 38]. For DCI prediction, demographical, clinical, and CT images were instead employed to train different ML models [38, 39]. Functional outcome prediction after SAH has also been studied [40, 42–44]. Survival at day 1, favorable Glasgow Coma Scale (GCS) at discharge and at 6 months, and modified Rankin Score were investigated. These studies almost exclusively used demographic and clinical variables for model training [40, 42–44]. Algorithms employed included decision tree, LR ad RF [40, 42–44]. Ventriculo-peritoneal shunt dependency after SAH was also studied [36, 44]. With respect to periprocedural outcome and complications, Paliwal et al. developed a model to predict occlusion after flow-diverter (FD) treatment [37]. Finally, Staartjes et al. in a pilot study investigated ML potential to predict functional outcome, new neurological deficits, and complication after uIA microsurgery [41].

36.3 Discussion

IA Screening and Detection

Given its relatively rare incidence, screening for intracranial aneurysms is not performed except in high-risk circumstances, e.g., positive family history [45]. Several factors are

Table 36.1 Studies focusing on aneurysm development and detection

Author	Year	Journal	No. of patients (training/validation)	Analyzed	Algorithm	Outcome evaluated	Results and performance
Nakao et al.	2018	*J Magn Reson Imag*	450 300 training, 50 parameter tuning, 100 final evaluation	3D TOF-MRA	CNN, MIP	IA detection	CAD system detected 94.2% (98/104) of aneurysms with 2.9 false positives per case (FPs/case). At a sensitivity of 70% → FPs/case: 0.26
Duan et al.	2019	*BioMed Eng OnLine*	241/40	2D DSA	2-stage CNN	IA detection	**Classical DIP**—Accuracy: 62.5%; AUC: 0.69, detection time: 62.546 s **Proposed architecture**—Accuracy: 93.5%; AUC: 0.942; detection time: 0.569 s
Park et al.	2019	*JAMA Open*	818 examinations from 662 patients 328 CTAs w/1 or + IAs 490 CTAs w/o IA	CTA	3D CNN	IA detection	AI-produced segmentation predictions resulted in clinicians achieving statistically significant improvements in sensitivity, accuracy, and interrater agreement when compared with no augmentation. No significant changes in specificity and time to diagnosis
Podgorsak et al.	2019	*J Neurointerv Surg*	350 images	DSA	CNN	IA detection	CNN segmentation of IAs and surrounding vasculature from DSA images is non-inferior to manual contours of aneurysms and can be used in parametric imaging procedures IA/vasculature—Mean JI: 0.823/0.737; mean DSC: 0.903/0.849; mean AUC: 0.791/0.715
Sichtermann et al.	2019	*American Journal of Neuroradiology*	85 patients/115 aneurysms	3D TOF-MRA	CNN	IA detection	Overall sensitivity 90%–96% if diameter 3–7 mm; 100% if diameter > 7 mm. ↑ performance was in the posterior circulation. Pre- and postprocessing reduced FPs
Ueda et al.	2019	Neuroradiology	638	TOF MRA	CNN ResNet-18	IA detection	Sensitivity 91%/93% for the internal/external test data sets, respectively ↑ aneurysm detection in internal/external test data sets by 4.8%/13% respectively, compared with the initial reports
Hainc et al.	2020	*The Neuroradiology Journal*	240 patients/ 706 DSA images W/Wo aneurysm 335/371 DSAs	2D DSA	Commercial CNN	IA detection	Sensitivity: 79%, specificity: 79%, precision: 0.75, F1 score: 0.77, mean AUC: 0.76 (range 0.68–0.86)

(continued)

Table 36.1 (continued)

Author	Year	Journal	No. of patients (training/validation)	Analyzed	Algorithm	Outcome evaluated	Results and performance
Heo et al.	2020	*Scientific Reports*	426,295 controls 974 SAH or uIA 299,088 training 128,181testing	Demographic, clinical and laboratory data	LR, RF, XGB, DNN	IA development	Five risk groups obtained w/ model prediction probabilities. Incidence rate ratios between the lowest- and highest-risk groups were compared. Best prediction: XGB model w/ AUROC: 0.765; also predicted lowest incidence (3.20) in the lowest-risk group. RF model predicted highest incidence (161.34) in the highest-risk group. The incidence rate ratios between the lowest and highest risk groups were 49.85, 35.85, 34.90, and 30.26, for the XGB, LR, DNN, and RF models, respectively
Joo et al.	2020	*European Radiology*	Training/internal test: 468/ 120 + 50 w/o aneurysms external test set 56 w/ IAs, 50 w/o	TOF-MRA	3D ResNet Architecture	IA detection	**Internal test set—**Sensitivity: 87.1%; PPV: 92.8%; specificity: 92.0% **External test set—**Sensitivity: 85.7%; PPV: 91.5%; specificity: 98.0%
Poppenberg et al.	2020	*Journal of Translational Medicine*	134 patients (55 with IA, 79 IA-free controls) 94/40	Transcriptomic signatures	KNN, RF, SVM with Gaussian and Cubic kernels	IA detection	Feature selection using LASSO in the training cohort identified 37 IA-associated transcripts Max accuracy: 90% in the testing cohort The testing performance across all methods had an average area under ROC curve (AUC) = 0.97 The RF model performed best across both training and testing cohorts. Demographics and comorbidities did not affect model performance

AUC area under the curve, *CAD* computer-aided diagnosis, *CNN* convolutional neural network, *DSC* dice similarity coefficient, *DNN* deep neural network, *DSA* digital subtraction angiography, *glm* generalized linear model, *JI* Jaccard index, *KNN k* nearest neighbor, *LR* logistic regression, *IA* intracranial aneurysm, *MR* magnetic resonance, *RF* random forest, *SAH* subarachnoid hemorrhage, *SD* subspace discriminant, *SVM* support vector machine, *TOF* time-of-flight, *XGB* scalable tree boosting system, *uIA* unruptured intracranial aneurysm

Table 36.2 ML studies for prediction of rupture risk and aneurysm stability

Author	Year	Journal	No. of patients (training/validation)	Outcome	Data	Algorithm	Performance
Liu et al.	2018	*European Radiology*	594	ACOM Rupture risk	Demographic, clinical and aneurysm morphological	Two-layer feed-forward ANN	**AUC**: Training, validating, testing and overall were 0.953, 0.937, 0.928 and 0.950, respectively. Overall accuracy: 94.8%
Liu et al.	2019	*Stroke*	420 IAs in 368 pts 296 (86 unstable)/124 (38 unstable)	IA stability	Clinical and morphological	glm, ridge and lasso regression	Lasso regression—Predictors of aneurysms stability: Flatness > spherical disproportion > maximum 2D diameter slice > surface area AUC: 0.853
Lv et al.	2020	*International Journal of Computer Assisted Radiology and Surgery*	65 IAs	Aneurysm wall enhancement	Clinical, morphological, hemodynamic	RF, nnet, knn, glm, pls GBM, svmRadial, lda, mda	**AUC**—GBM: **0.98**; glm: 0.80; svmRadial: 0.77; mda: 0.73; RF: 0.71; knn: 0.71; nnet: 0.69; pls: 0.68 **Sensitivity**—RF: 0.91; nnet: 0.82; glm: 0.81; pls: 0.82; GBM: 0.82; svmRadial: 0.73; lda: 0.91; mda: 0.73; knn: 0.91 **Specificity**—RF: 0.63; nnet: 0.63; glm: 0.75; pls: 0.63; GBM: 0.75; svmRadial: 0.63; lda: 0.63; mda: 0.63; knn, 0.50
Ou et al.	2020	*European Radiology*	122 IAs rIAs ($n = 93$)	Rupture prediction	Morphological and radiomic features (CTA)	glm, lasso and ridge regression	Model A: conventional morphological parameters; Model B: morphological + radiomic shape features; Model C: morphological + radiomic shape features + first-order histogram and second-order texture features; Model D: Simplified model **AUC**—A: 0.77; B: 0.81; C: 0.88; D: 0.88 **Sensitivity**—A: 0.62; B: 0.68; C: 0.72; D: 0.70 **Specificity**—A: 0.77; B: 0.77; C: 0.88; D: 0.88 **Precision**—A: 0.39; B: 0.44; C: 0.52; D: 0.51
Zhu et al.	2020	Translational Stroke Research	1897 1539 stable 528 unstable	IA stability	Clinical, morphological	SVM, RF, and feed-forward ANN	**AUC**—RF: 0.85; SVM: 0.85; ANN: 0.86 All ML models ↑ performance than LR and PHASES score (AUC – 0.83 and 0.59, $p < 0.001$ and $p = 0.038$ respectively)

ACOM anterior communicating artery, *ANN* artificial neural network, *AUC* area under the curve, *GBM* stochastic gradient boosting machine, *glm* generalized linear model, *KNN* k nearest neighbor, *lda* linear discriminant analysis, *LR* logistic regression, *IA* intracranial aneurysm, *mda* mixture discriminant analysis, *MLP* multi-layer perceptron, *mRS* modified Rankin Scale, *nnet* neural network, *PCA* principal component analysis, *pls* partial least square, *RF* random forest, *IA* ruptured intracranial aneurysm, *SVM* support vector machine, *TOF* time-of-flight, *Tx* treatment, *XGB* scalable tree boosting system, *uIA* unruptured intracranial aneurysm

Table 36.3 ML studies for outcome prediction after uIA aneurysm treatment or SAH

Author	Year	Journal	No. of patients (training/validation)	Outcome	Data	Algorithm	Performance
De Toledo et al.	2009	IEEE Transactions on Information Technology in Biomedicine	441/193	GCS at discharge and at 6 Mos	Demographical and clinical	C4.5, fast decision tree learner, partial decision trees, repeated incremental pruning to produce error reduction, nearest neighbor with generalization, ripple down rule learner	Favorable outcome C4.5 algorithm—AUC: 0.84; TPR: 0.87; FPR: 0.25; precision: 0.85 LR AUC = 0.86
Zafar et al.	2017	Neurocritical Care	153	GCS at discharge	Clinical and laboratory	Penalized LR	Poor/good outcome prediction accuracy: 80% Intermediate outcome prediction accuracy: >70%
Hostettler et al.	2018	*The Journal of Neurosurgery*	548 329/219	Survival at day 1 GCS VP shunt	Clinical and laboratory	Decision tree	Prediction accuracy for survival on day 1: 0.75 Favorable functional outcome at all time points had a prediction accuracy of 0.71 in the training data set, with procalcitonin on day 1 being the most important differentiating factor at all time points
Paliwal et al.	2018	*Neurosurgical Focus*	84 64/20	Occlusion after FD tx (ICA aneurysms only)	Morphological, hemodynamic, and FD-based	LR, SVM with linear and Gaussian kernels, KNN, nnet.	**Training**—NN AUC: 0.97; LR AUC: 0.94; linear SVM AUC: 0.91 **Testing**—NN and Gaussian-SVM models had highest accuracy (0.90) in predicting occlusion outcome
Ramos et al.	2018	*Hemorrhagic Stroke*	317	DCI after SAH	Demographical, clinical, and CT images	LR, SVM, RFC, MLP, stacked convolutional denoising autoencoders, PCA	**LR**—AUC: 0.63; sensitivity: 0.67; specificity: 0.62 **Clinical data ML.** AUC—SVM: 0.64; RFC: 0.68; LR: 0.61; MLP: 0.63. Sensitivity—SVM: 0.67; RFC: 0.78; LR: 0.65; MLP: 0.59. Specificity—SVM: 0.64; RFC: 0.57; LR: 0.62; MLP: 0.79 **Clinical + imaging data ML.** AUC—SVM: 0.68; RFC: 0.74; LR: 0.65; MLP: 0.67. Sensitivity—SVM: 0.63; RFC: 0.67; LR: 0.65; MLP: 0.64. Specificity—SVM: 0.73; RFC: 0.75; LR: 0.69; MLP: 0.72
Rubbert et al.	2018	*European Radiology*	143	6-mos mRS	Demographical and clinical variables	RF with conditional inference trees	Accuracy—Training: 0.84; validation: 0.71 The five most important features were the modified fisher grade, age, MTT range, WFNS and early EVD.

Capoglu et al.	2019	41st Annual International Conference of the IEEE EMBC	20	Vasospasm	Angiograms	LR	AUC: 0.93
Tanioka et al.	2019	*Molecular Neurobiology*	95	DCI after SAH, Angiographic vasospasm Cerebral infarction	3 models: 1. Clinical variables on admission; 2. Only plasma levels of MCP at post-onset days 1–3; 3. Both clinical variables on admission and MCP values at days 1–3.	RF	**DCI**—Accuracy: 0.94 in model 1; 0.87 in model 2; 0.95 in model 3; sensitivity: 0.93 in model 1; 0.95 in model 2; 0.94 in model 3 **Angiographic vasospasm**—Accuracy: 0.73 in model 1; 0.73 in model 2; 0.78 in model 3; sensitivity: 0.72 in model 1; 0.81 in model 2, and 0.77 in model 3 **Cerebral infarction**—Accuracy: 0.82 in model 1; 0.79 in model 2; 0.84 in model 3; sensitivity: 0.77 in model 1; 0.84 in models 2 and 3
Muscas et al.	2020	*Acta Neurochirurgica*	386 296/90	Shunt-dependent hydrocephalus after SAH	Demographical, clinical, radiological, patient-related	Glm, distributed RF, GBM, DL	Distributed RF had best performance **Training**—AUC: 0.85; sensitivity: 0.78; specificity: 0.84; PPV: 0.50; accuracy: 0.84; φ: 0.53 **Testing**—AUC: 0.88; sensitivity: 0.73; specificity: 0.92; PPV: 0.59; accuracy: 0.90; φ: 0.59
Staartjes et al.	2020	*Acta Neurochirurgica*	156	mRS at discharge, deficits and complications after uIA surgery	Demographic and clinical variables	SVM, GAM, RF, decision trees (C5.0), glm, GBM	**Neurological outcome at discharge (GBM)** —Training set (AUC: 0.87; accuracy: 0.75); internal validation (AUC: 0.67; accuracy: 0.91; sensitivity: 0.67; specificity: 0.93) **New neurological deficits (glm)**—Training set (AUC: 0.71; accuracy: 0.82); internal validation (AUC: 0.77; accuracy: 0.78; sensitivity: 0.50; specificity: 0.80) **Surgical complications (nnet)**—Training set (AUC: 0.69; accuracy: 0.83); internal validation (AUC: 0.63; accuracy: 0.84; sensitivity: 0.0; specificity: 0.96)

DCI delayed cerebral ischemia, *DL* deep learning, *GAM* generalized additive model, *GBM* stochastic gradient boosting machine, *GCS* Glasgow Coma Scale, *glm* generalized linear model, *LR* logistic regression, *IA* intracranial aneurysm, *MCP* matricellular proteins, *MLP* multi-layer perceptron, *Mos* months; *MR* magnetic resonance, *mRS* modified Rankin Scale, *nnet* neural network, *PCA* principal component analysis, *RF* random forest, *SAH* subarachnoid hemorrhage, *SVM* support vector machine, *TOF* time-of-flight, *Tx* treatment, *XGB* scalable tree boosting system, *uIA* unruptured intracranial aneurysm, *WBC* white blood cells, *φ* correlation coefficient

thought to contribute to de novo aneurysm formation and rupture but the current evidence with respect to screening guidelines is limited [46]. ML methods are in principal ideal to identify hidden features and nonlinear associations in the data, for this reason they have been proposed as a valuable tool to be applied to electronic health care records, with the caveat that this would require external validation in different healthcare settings and that different geographical regions may need tailored algorithm development [47]. Heo et al. hypothesized that health records at population level could be used to identify a subpopulation at higher risk of aneurysm development. Among the studied algorithm, a scalable tree boosting model (XGB) was found to achieve the best AUC (0.765). Classes of risk were identified with the XGB reporting a incidence rate ratio between the lowest- and highest-risk groups of 49.85 [20]. Despite the study limitations, the possibility of identifying a group of patients as at higher risk for screening purposes based on electronic health data well exemplifies the power granted by big data analysis. The integration of high-throughput genomic and transcriptomic data with ML technologies has the potential to classify and risk-stratify different patient groups with respect to a given outcome of interest [48, 49]. Based on previous evidence that unruptured aneurysms present a specific RNA neutrophil signature, Poppenberg et al. [25] used LASSO feature selection to identify non-redundant candidate features and showed that RF algorithm outperformed other classification models in both training and test set with high AUC. Interestingly, demographic and comorbidities did not affect model performance [25, 50, 51]. Despite encouraging results, a combination of personalized medicine and ML computational power are still fully to be exploited. It is growingly common for aneurysms to be incidentally identified as neuroimaging is performed for other neurological symptoms [1, 52]. Despite this trend, image evaluation is time-consuming and aneurysm identification is not straightforward especially in an unspecific clinical context, and, moreover, reports may suffer from inter-rater variability [23, 53]. CNNs have proven extremely well-performing algorithms for detection and recognition tasks [54]. Readers are encouraged to consult Dhillon and Verma [54], Anwar et al. [55], and Yamashita et al. [56] for more organized overview on CNNs. Semi- and fully-automated machine learning approaches for aneurysm detection on neuroradiological images obtained with different modalities have been proposed employing CNNs [23, 27]. Ueda et al. trained a CNN algorithm for the automated diagnosis of cerebral aneurysms from TOF MR angiography images showing sensitivity of 91% and 93% in internal and external test data sets, respectively, and further improving detection with respect to initial radiologist report by 4.8% in the internal test data set and by 13% in the external test data set [27]. Sichtermann et al. trained a previously developed open-source CNN to detect aneurysm from TOF-MRA 3D images and could demonstrate an overall sensitivity of 90% even if this model also suffered from a high FP-to-case ratio. Importantly, some degree of processing was able to decrease FP findings. A lower sensitivity was measured for small lesions but, as these were underrepresented in the data set, the authors suggested that increased sample size may achieve optimal performance also in this setting [26]. Park et al. applied a 3D CNN to CTA exams to obtain segmentation outputs to be evaluated by clinicians. Such hybrid AI-augmented image evaluation by clinicians increased sensitivity, accuracy, and inter-rater agreement with respect to traditional evaluation [23]. Importantly, the high-computational power and extensive data availability needed to appropriately train a CNN for task such as segmentation and object detection can be overcome by employing previously developed algorithms in different setting followed by fine-tuning to accurately tailor algorithm to the requested problem-solving scenario (transfer learning) [26, 57].

While rupture status can be easily diagnosed by hemorrhage patterns on the computed tomography (CT), multiple aneurysms are a common finding. As inaccurate identification of a ruptured aneurysm can lead to re-bleeding events, accurate assessment of rupture is essential [6, 58]. Rajabzadeh-Oghaz et al. used morphological and hemodynamic data to identify bleeding aneurysm in patients with multiple aneurysms and reported increased performance of two different LR models with respect to the best associated variable they found in their study, namely size ratio [59].

Some studies make the assumption that rupture-prone aneurysms may more closely resemble ruptured ones than their unruptured stable counterparts. This is why some authors have developed models to discriminate such patient populations, speculating a possible future use in the context of rupture risk prediction (Supplementary Table S1). For example, Detmer et al. developed and externally validated a model based on morphological and hemodynamic parameters that was able to well discriminate among ruptured and unruptured aneurysms [60, 61]. Silva et al. reported training of different ML models using demographic, clinical, and radiological variables from 845 aneurysms in 615 patients (309 of which were ruptured) and could achieve good AUC in all the cases with satisfying discrimination measures [62]. CNN application has been also reported to discriminate among ruptured and unruptured aneurysms. Kim et al. applied a CNN to images of 3D DSA to evaluate the rupture status in patients with small-sized aneurysms of the anterior circulation. The algorithm was trained on a retrospective data set of 368 patients and prospectively tested in 272 patients [63].

These publications are limited by the use of models developed for rupture assessment—Only being able to differentiate unruptured cases from SAH cases on neuroimaging is of limited real-world clinical relevance. These models all being trained to discriminate among ruptured and unruptured cases, the predicted probabilities very likely only represent the model's confidence in the detection of SAH, as opposed to a true rupture risk. Predicting rupture risk would warrant longitudinal data for training and validation on unruptured aneurysms—a more difficult approach to pursue, given that once high-risk incidental aneurysms are discovered, these would receive prophylactic treatment [60, 62].

Rupture Risk and Aneurysm Stability

Once a given aneurysm is identified, the benefits granted from prophylactic treatment need to be weighed against the risks inherent to surgical or endovascular treatment. This topic is highly debated in the literature with respect to both indication for treatment and best therapeutic strategy. Several attempts were made to inform clinicians' decision-making through clinical scores weighing some of known risk factors for aneurysm rupture. Specifically, the PHASES [33] and the Tominari score [34] were developed for estimation of aneurysm rupture risk, the ELAPSS [64] and Juvela growth score [65] for assessing risk of growth which is in turn considered a surrogate of rupture risk, besides being size still considered by surgeon one of the most important parameters evaluated before clinical decision. Also an international multidisciplinary consensus established an additional score named UIATS [66] which provides distinct recommendations about management (treatment versus conservative management versus unclear indication) and a similar attempt was produced by Juvela (Juvela treatment score) [67]. Unfortunately, following initial introduction and some sparse validation attempts (mostly on retrospective studies and on ruptured aneurysm), these scores have only partially entered the clinical setting due to concerns of unreliability or insufficient validation [68, 69]. Other studies have investigated morphological characteristics and hemodynamic parameters [70, 71]. Importantly, these scores, with the exception of UIATS—the only one not based on a statistical derivation of risk factors but deriving from an expert consensus—only evaluate a limited amount of variables [66, 69]. ML unleashes the potential of including a huge variety of different data from significant number of patients. A well-trained model can in principle provide a prediction tool that is specific with respect to the outcome of interest. Given the open question on aneurysm risk of rupture evaluation for incidental aneurysm, some studies assessed this clinical issue. Despite aneurysm diameter being still considered the most important determinant for treatment decision, it is widely accepted that many ruptured aneurysms are instead of small dimension, lower than the 7 mm cut-off suggested by the ISAT trial and that these lesions are not well identified as high risk with available scores such as PHASES [69, 72, 73]. For this reason, the other clinically relevant side of risk of rupture evaluation can be considered the assessment of aneurysm "stability"—defined as an unruptured aneurysm not increasing in size at imaging follow-up and not becoming symptomatic. Instead of trying to predict which aneurysms will rupture, a specular clinical question consists in identifying variables predictive of stability, or, by means of ML, training models to recognize such features. Liu et al. automatically extracted morphological features from 719 aneurysms from PyRadiomics and identified association of some variables to aneurysm stability while also reporting hypertension can significantly alter morphology of unstable aneurysm. The authors propose a combined morphological/topographical/clinical prediction model which could reach an AUC of 0.85 [29]. Ou et al. [31] recently reported an interesting investigation where morphological and radiomic features were extracted to train progressively complex ML models. Only unruptured aneurysms parameters were used to train the model as rupture status significantly alters aneurysm morphology, but the trained model could well discriminate between aneurysms remained stable during a follow-up of at least 2 years and those that ruptured during yearly follow-up. A limited sample size and short follow-up limits the findings of the study but the methodological approach of the authors is commendable [31].

As wall enhancement in MRI has been associated with increased rupture risk, also its prediction by means of ML has been attempted. Lv et al. showed that a variety of hemodynamic factors, size ratio and PHASES score can be successfully used for training ML model to predict wall enhancement [30]. For aneurysm stability prediction, a variety of ML models like RF, SVM, and ANN trained with clinical morphological variables have been shown to outperform LR and PHASES score suggesting that this strategy may be successfully employed in the future for optimal patient management [32].

Outcome Prediction

Another relevant contribution of ML to aneurysm research can be identified in post-procedural clinical outcome prediction. Data-driven clinical predictions are an integral part of medical practice. With ML, different data sources enable to rapidly develop prediction models. With respect to inferential model development—whose study setting has often been well-controlled to mitigate potential sources of bias and confounding—recent ML applications have the risk to overlook such phenomena and for this reason sound methodology in model training and strong external validation are requested [74].

Delayed Cerebral Ischemia, Vasospasm, and Shunt-Dependent Hydrocephalus

Delayed cerebral ischemia (DCI) caused by vasospasm is a feared complication of aneurysmal SAH occurring 7 to 10 days from aneurysm rupture. Moreover, management of vasospasm is complex—from identification to treatment [6]. For these reasons, a reliable prediction of vasospasm would better inform therapeutic strategy and patient monitoring. Ramos et al. [39] demonstrated that machine learning can achieve a significantly better—even if modest—AUC than conventional logistic regression when clinical variables only are used for model training while a combination of extracted image features and clinical data can significantly improve the performance of DCI prediction [39]. Another study by Tanioka et al. [38] trained a RF model with a combination of clinical data and matricellular protein plasma levels in 95 patients and showed accurate prediction of DCI, angiographic vasospasm, and cerebral infarction—without any validation. Hydrocephalus is another relatively common SAH complication. Such manifestations can be transient and self-limiting, require external ventricular drainage or become chronic requiring permanent cerebrospinal fluid diversion with all its associated drawbacks [75]. Identification of patients at high risk for shunt-dependent hydrocephalus could result in optimized management avoiding neurological complications, increased hospital length of stay—ultimately improving functional outcome and quality of life [75]. Several predictors have been identified and clinical risk scores proposed, despite being their reliability poorly investigated [36, 75]. ML has been also employed in such setting by Muscas et al. who showed that among 4 models trained, a distributed RF model including 21 input variables predicted development of shunt-dependent hydrocephalus in a SAH patient population with high accuracy [36].

Functional Outcome Prediction

Functional outcome prediction after SAH is clinically relevant. A large number of studies have investigated predictors of poor functional and cognitive performance after aSAH while less have addressed predictions of favorable outcome [76]. A long list of prognostic scores has been proposed including but not limited to Hunt and Hess, WFNS, modified Fisher, BNI, HATCH, HAIR, FRESH, and SAFIRE scores [44, 77]. Most of these predictive tools are developed by means of traditional statistical methods and may fail to integrate the ever-growing complexity of heterogeneous data sources [44]. While no ML-based algorithm has yet entered clinical practice with this purpose, previous research is promising. Zafar et al. developed a penalized LR model that based on readily available data at SAH diagnosis could predict GCS functional outcome at discharge with accuracy >80% [43]. Rubbert et al. trained a random forest algorithm using a variety of demographical and clinical variables obtained at admission and reported fairly accurate prediction of 6-month functional outcome after SAH [40]. Another study by Hostettler et al. [44] reported similar accuracy for favorable GCS prediction at diverse timepoints using decision tree model and could also predict with an accuracy of 0.75 survival at day 1.

Periprocedural Outcome Prediction

Clipping of unruptured aneurysm has been the standard of care for decades. More recently, endovascular modalities have been added to the therapeutic armamentarium, including standard coiling, balloon and stent-assisted coiling, flow diversion [78]. Only few reports are present with respect to ML applications for periprocedural outcome prediction, whether endovascular or surgical. Paliwal et al. reported use of ML to predict aneurysm occlusion after FD treatment based on morphological and hemodynamic data. Although limited by small sample size, evaluation limited to ICA aneurysms, lack of inclusion of patient clinical and comorbidities data, they could show a 90% predictive accuracy in the internal test set. The authors also highlighted how best performance was reached when the model was trained also using variables not significantly associated with occlusion further highlighting the additional potential of ML with respect to conventional statistics [37]. With respect to post-surgical outcome, a recent pilot study by Staartjes et al. evaluated the performance metrics of machine learning-based models on data from a prospective registry to predict early clinical endpoints after microsurgery for UIAs. In the internal validation cohort, area under the curve (AUC) and accuracy values for new neurological deficit and for any complication were 0.63–0.77 and 0.78–0.91, respectively. As the study cohort included only 156 patients, larger training samples and external validation on a multi-center patient cohorts are required [41]. In the near future, the PRediction of Adverse Events after Microsurgery for Unruptured AneurysMs (PRAEMIUM) study, a multi-center collaborative effort stemming from this investigation may provide an externally validated model suitable for clinical practice.

36.4 Future Directions

ML in neuroscience—and in neurosurgery in particular—is rapidly advancing, yet relatively unexplored, and without standardized methodology. ML research remains largely heterogenous in approaches and reporting, and the clinical benefits derived so far in the field of IAs can be considered limited to non-existing. External validation is largely missing, too.

Despite extensive scientific knowledge and increased therapeutic possibilities, the management of IAs patients has so far failed to translate ML- and AI-based experimental results into the clinic. CNNs hold promise for assisting clinicians in imaging analysis and it is not unreasonable that commercial software may aid in this task already in the next future. In terms of ML-based prediction of rupture risk, stronger methodology based on longitudinal data, larger training sample size, and extensive external validation to confirm findings generalizability are required. For complication and functional outcome prediction, the ongoing PRAEMIUM study aims to translate to clinic possible application of a ML generated model in the form a web-app, like previously established for example in brain tumors to predict functional impairment [79].

36.5 Conclusions

ML approaches are increasingly reported as a viable strategy to tackle existing clinical issues in IA research. Several studies have attempted to provide reliable models for screening indication and aneurysm detection. CNN models trained with variable degree of human interaction on data obtained from diverse imaging modalities have shown high sensitivity in aneurysm detection tasks, also outperforming expert image analysis. When prediction of rupture and stability assessment were chosen as outcome, ML was preliminarily shown to achieve better performance of conventional statistical methods and existing risk scores but replication of these findings, larger training population, and stronger external validation are needed before clinical implementation. ML-based complication and functional outcome prediction in the event of SAH have been more extensively reported, in contrast to outcome investigation in unruptured IA patients. In conclusion, ML has the potential to be a major game changer in IA patient management, but currently translation of experimental results to the clinic is limited.

References

1. Etminan N, Rinkel GJ. Unruptured intracranial aneurysms: development, rupture and preventive management. Nat Rev Neurol. 2016;12(12):699–713.
2. Macdonald RL. Spontaneous subarachnoid haemorrhage. Lancet. 2017;389:12.
3. Steiner T, Juvela S, Unterberg A, Jung C, Forsting M, Rinkel G. European stroke organization guidelines for the management of intracranial aneurysms and subarachnoid haemorrhage. Cerebrovasc Dis. 2013;35(2):93–112.
4. Beam AL, Kohane IS. Big data and machine learning in health care. JAMA. 2018;319(13):1317.
5. Topol EJ. High-performance medicine: the convergence of human and artificial intelligence. Nat Med. 2019;25(1):44–56.
6. Connolly ES, Rabinstein AA, Carhuapoma JR, et al. Guidelines for the management of aneurysmal subarachnoid hemorrhage: a guideline for healthcare professionals from the American Heart Association/American Stroke Association. Stroke. 2012;43(6):1711–37.
7. Akkus Z, Galimzianova A, Hoogi A, Rubin DL, Erickson BJ. Deep learning for brain MRI segmentation: state of the art and future directions. J Digit Imaging. 2017;30(4):449–59.
8. Razzak MI, Naz S, Zaib A. Deep learning for medical image processing: overview, challenges and future, vol. 30; 2017. p. 449–59.
9. Senders JT, Staples PC, Karhade AV, Zaki MM, Gormley WB, Broekman MLD, Smith TR, Arnaout O. Machine learning and neurosurgical outcome prediction: a systematic review. World Neurosurg. 2018;109:476–486.e1.
10. Swinburne NC, Schefflein J, Sakai Y, Oermann EK, Titano JJ, Chen I, Tadayon S, Aggarwal A, Doshi A, Nael K. Machine learning for semiautomated classification of glioblastoma, brain metastasis and central nervous system lymphoma using magnetic resonance advanced imaging. Ann Transl Med. 2019;7(11):232–2.
11. Arvind V, Kim JS, Oermann EK, Kaji D, Cho SK. Predicting surgical complications in adult patients undergoing anterior cervical discectomy and fusion using machine learning. Neurospine. 2018;15(4):329–37.
12. Kim JS, Arvind V, Oermann EK, Kaji D, Ranson W, Ukogu C, Hussain AK, Caridi J, Cho SK. Predicting surgical complications in patients undergoing elective adult spinal deformity procedures using machine learning. Spine Deformity. 2018;6(6):762–70.
13. Siccoli A, de Wispelaere MP, Schröder ML, Staartjes VE. Machine learning–based preoperative predictive analytics for lumbar spinal stenosis. Neurosurg Focus. 2019;46(5):E5.
14. Staartjes VE, Serra C, Muscas G, Maldaner N, Akeret K, van Niftrik CHB, Fierstra J, Holzmann D, Regli L. Utility of deep neural networks in predicting gross-total resection after transsphenoidal surgery for pituitary adenoma: a pilot study. Neurosurg Focus. 2018;45(5):E12.
15. Staartjes VE, Zattra CM, Akeret K, Maldaner N, Muscas G, van Niftrik CH, Fierstra J, Regli L, Serra C. Neural network–based identification of patients at high risk for intraoperative cerebrospinal fluid leaks in endoscopic pituitary surgery. J Neurosurg. 2019:1–7.
16. Van Niftrik CHB, van der Wouden F, Staartjes VE, et al. Machine learning algorithm identifies patients at high risk for early complications after intracranial tumor surgery: registry-based cohort study. Neurosurgery. 2019;85(4):E756–64.
17. Shi Z, Hu B, Schoepf UJ, Savage RH, Dargis DM, Pan CW, Li XL, Ni QQ, Lu GM, Zhang LJ. Artificial intelligence in the management of intracranial aneurysms: current status and future perspectives. AJNR Am J Neuroradiol. 2020;41(3):373–9.
18. Duan H, Huang Y, Liu L, Dai H, Chen L, Zhou L. Automatic detection on intracranial aneurysm from digital subtraction angiography with cascade convolutional neural networks. Biomed Eng Online. 2019;18(1):110.
19. Hainc N, Mannil M, Anagnostakou V, Alkadhi H, Blüthgen C, Wacht L, Bink A, Husain S, Kulcsár Z, Winklhofer S. Deep learning based detection of intracranial aneurysms on digital subtraction angiography: a feasibility study. Neuroradiol J. 2020;33(4):311–7.
20. Heo J, Park SJ, Kang S-H, Oh CW, Bang JS, Kim T. Prediction of intracranial aneurysm risk using machine learning. Sci Rep. 2020;10(1):6921.
21. Joo B, Ahn SS, Yoon PH, Bae S, Sohn B, Lee YE, Bae JH, Park MS, Choi HS, Lee S-K. A deep learning algorithm may automate intracranial aneurysm detection on MR angiography with high diagnostic performance. Eur Radiol. 2020;30(11):5785–93.
22. Nakao T, Hanaoka S, Nomura Y, Sato I, Nemoto M, Miki S, Maeda E, Yoshikawa T, Hayashi N, Abe O. Deep neural network-based computer-assisted detection of cerebral aneurysms in MR angiography. J Magn Reson Imaging. 2018;47(4):948–53.

23. Park A, Chute C, Rajpurkar P, et al. Deep learning–assisted diagnosis of cerebral aneurysms using the HeadXNet model. JAMA Netw Open. 2019;2(6):e195600.
24. Podgorsak AR, Rava RA, Shiraz Bhurwani MM, Chandra AR, Davies JM, Siddiqui AH, Ionita CN. Automatic radiomic feature extraction using deep learning for angiographic parametric imaging of intracranial aneurysms. J NeuroIntervent Surg. 2020;12(4):417–21.
25. Poppenberg KE, Tutino VM, Li L, et al. Classification models using circulating neutrophil transcripts can detect unruptured intracranial aneurysm. J Transl Med. 2020;18(1):392.
26. Sichtermann T, Faron A, Sijben R, Teichert N, Freiherr J, Wiesmann M. Deep learning–based detection of intracranial aneurysms in 3D TOF-MRA. AJNR Am J Neuroradiol. 2019;40(1):25–32.
27. Ueda D, Yamamoto A, Nishimori M, et al. Deep learning for MR angiography: automated detection of cerebral aneurysms. Radiology. 2019;290(1):187–94.
28. Liu J, Chen Y, Lan L, et al. Prediction of rupture risk in anterior communicating artery aneurysms with a feed-forward artificial neural network. Eur Radiol. 2018;28(8):3268–75.
29. Liu Q, Jiang P, Jiang Y, Ge H, Li S, Jin H, Li Y. Prediction of aneurysm stability using a machine learning model based on PyRadiomics-derived morphological features. Stroke. 2019;50(9):2314–21.
30. Lv N, Karmonik C, Shi Z, Chen S, Wang X, Liu J, Huang Q. A pilot study using a machine-learning approach of morphological and hemodynamic parameters for predicting aneurysms enhancement. Int J CARS. 2020;15(8):1313–21.
31. Ou C, Chong W, Duan C-Z, Zhang X, Morgan M, Qian Y. A preliminary investigation of radiomics differences between ruptured and unruptured intracranial aneurysms. Eur Radiol. 2020;31(5):2716–25. https://doi.org/10.1007/s00330-020-07325-3.
32. Zhu W, Li W, Tian Z, Zhang Y, Wang K, Zhang Y, Liu J, Yang X. Stability assessment of intracranial aneurysms using machine learning based on clinical and morphological features. Transl Stroke Res. 2020;11(6):1287–95. https://doi.org/10.1007/s12975-020-00811-2.
33. Greving JP, Wermer MJH, Brown RD, et al. Development of the PHASES score for prediction of risk of rupture of intracranial aneurysms: a pooled analysis of six prospective cohort studies. Lancet Neurol. 2014;13(1):59–66.
34. Tominari S, Morita A, Ishibashi T, et al. Prediction model for 3-year rupture risk of unruptured cerebral aneurysms in Japanese patients: cerebral aneurysm rupture risk. Ann Neurol. 2015;77(6):1050–9.
35. Capoglu S, Savarraj JP, Sheth SA, Choi HA, Giancardo L. Representation Learning of 3D Brain Angiograms, an Application for Cerebral Vasospasm Prediction. In: 2019 41st annual international conference of the IEEE engineering in medicine and biology society (EMBC). Berlin: IEEE; 2019. p. 3394–8.
36. Muscas G, Matteuzzi T, Becattini E, et al. Development of machine learning models to prognosticate chronic shunt-dependent hydrocephalus after aneurysmal subarachnoid hemorrhage. Acta Neurochir. 2020;162(12):3093–105.
37. Paliwal N, Jaiswal P, Tutino VM, Shallwani H, Davies JM, Siddiqui AH, Rai R, Meng H. Outcome prediction of intracranial aneurysm treatment by flow diverters using machine learning. Neurosurg Focus. 2018;45(5):E7.
38. pSEED Group, Tanioka S, Ishida F, Nakano F, Kawakita F, Kanamaru H, Nakatsuka Y, Nishikawa H, Suzuki H. Machine learning analysis of Matricellular proteins and clinical variables for early prediction of delayed cerebral ischemia after aneurysmal subarachnoid hemorrhage. Mol Neurobiol. 2019;56(10):7128–35.
39. Ramos LA, van der Steen WE, Sales Barros R, et al. Machine learning improves prediction of delayed cerebral ischemia in patients with subarachnoid hemorrhage. J NeuroIntervent Surg. 2019;11(5):497–502.
40. Rubbert C, Patil KR, Beseoglu K, et al. Prediction of outcome after aneurysmal subarachnoid haemorrhage using data from patient admission. Eur Radiol. 2018;28(12):4949–58.
41. Staartjes VE, Sebök M, Blum PG, Serra C, Germans MR, Krayenbühl N, Regli L, Esposito G. Development of machine learning-based preoperative predictive analytics for unruptured intracranial aneurysm surgery: a pilot study. Acta Neurochir. 2020;162(11):2759–65. https://doi.org/10.1007/s00701-020-04355-0.
42. de Toledo P, Rios PM, Ledezma A, Sanchis A, Alen JF, Lagares A. Predicting the outcome of patients with subarachnoid hemorrhage using machine learning techniques. IEEE Trans Inform Technol Biomed. 2009;13(5):794–801.
43. Zafar SF, Postma EN, Biswal S, et al. Electronic health data predict outcomes after aneurysmal subarachnoid hemorrhage. Neurocrit Care. 2018;28(2):184–93.
44. Hostettler IC, Muroi C, Richter JK, Schmid J, Neidert MC, Seule M, Boss O, Pangalu A, Germans MR, Keller E. Decision tree analysis in subarachnoid hemorrhage: prediction of outcome parameters during the course of aneurysmal subarachnoid hemorrhage using decision tree analysis. J Neurosurg. 2018:1–12.
45. Rinkel GJ. Intracranial aneurysm screening: indications and advice for practice. Lancet Neurol. 2005;4(2):122–8.
46. Brown RD, Broderick JP. Unruptured intracranial aneurysms: epidemiology, natural history, management options, and familial screening. Lancet Neurol. 2014;13(4):393–404.
47. Rose S. Machine learning for prediction in electronic health data. JAMA Netw Open. 2018;1(4):e181404.
48. Koumakis L. Deep learning models in genomics; are we there yet? Comput Struct Biotechnol J. 2020;18:1466–73.
49. Su C, Tong J, Wang F. Mining genetic and transcriptomic data using machine learning approaches in Parkinson's disease. NPJ Parkinsons Dis. 2020;6(1):24.
50. Tutino VM, Poppenberg KE, Jiang K, et al. Circulating neutrophil transcriptome may reveal intracranial aneurysm signature. PLoS One. 2018;13(1):e0191407.
51. Tutino VM, Poppenberg KE, Li L, et al. Biomarkers from circulating neutrophil transcriptomes have potential to detect unruptured intracranial aneurysms. J Transl Med. 2018;16(1):373.
52. Renowden S, Nelson R. Management of incidental unruptured intracranial aneurysms. Pract Neurol. 2020;20(5):347–55.
53. Lubicz B, Levivier M, Francois O, Thoma P, Sadeghi N, Collignon L, Baleriaux D. Sixty-four-row multisection CT angiography for detection and evaluation of ruptured intracranial aneurysms: interobserver and Intertechnique reproducibility. Am J Neuroradiol. 2007;28(10):1949–55.
54. Dhillon A, Verma GK. Convolutional neural network: a review of models, methodologies and applications to object detection. Prog Artif Intell. 2020;9(2):85–112.
55. Anwar SM, Majid M, Qayyum A, Awais M, Alnowami M, Khan MK. Medical image analysis using convolutional neural networks: a review. J Med Syst. 2018;42(11):226.
56. Yamashita R, Nishio M, Do RKG, Togashi K. Convolutional neural networks: an overview and application in radiology. Insights Imaging. 2018;9(4):611–29.
57. Swati ZNK, Zhao Q, Kabir M, Ali F, Ali Z, Ahmed S, Lu J. Brain tumor classification for MR images using transfer learning and fine-tuning. Comput Med Imaging Graph. 2019;75:34–46.
58. Björkman J, Frösen J, Tähtinen O, et al. Irregular shape identifies ruptured intracranial aneurysm in subarachnoid hemorrhage patients with multiple aneurysms. Stroke. 2017;48(7):1986–9.
59. Rajabzadeh-Oghaz H, Wang J, Varble N, et al. Novel models for identification of the ruptured aneurysm in patients with subarachnoid hemorrhage with multiple aneurysms. AJNR Am J Neuroradiol. 2019;40:1939–46.

60. Detmer FJ, Chung BJ, Mut F, Slawski M, Hamzei-Sichani F, Putman C, Jiménez C, Cebral JR. Development and internal validation of an aneurysm rupture probability model based on patient characteristics and aneurysm location, morphology, and hemodynamics. Int J CARS. 2018;13(11):1767–79.
61. Detmer FJ, Fajardo-Jiménez D, Mut F, Juchler N, Hirsch S, Pereira VM, Bijlenga P, Cebral JR. External validation of cerebral aneurysm rupture probability model with data from two patient cohorts. Acta Neurochir. 2018;160(12):2425–34.
62. Silva MA, Patel J, Kavouridis V, et al. Machine learning models can detect aneurysm rupture and identify clinical features associated with rupture. World Neurosurg. 2019;131:e46–51.
63. Kim HC, Rhim JK, Ahn JH, et al. Machine learning application for rupture risk assessment in small-sized intracranial aneurysm. J Clin Med. 2019;8(5):683.
64. Backes D, Rinkel GJE, Greving JP, et al. ELAPSS score for prediction of risk of growth of unruptured intracranial aneurysms. Neurology. 2017;88(17):1600–6.
65. Juvela S. Scoring of growth of unruptured intracranial aneurysms. J Clin Med. 2020;9(10):3339.
66. Etminan N, Brown RD, Beseoglu K, et al. The unruptured intracranial aneurysm treatment score: a multidisciplinary consensus. Neurology. 2015;85(10):881–9.
67. Juvela S. Treatment scoring of unruptured intracranial aneurysms. Stroke. 2019;50(9):2344–50.
68. Stumpo V, Sturiale CL. Inquiring the real-world clinical performance of the unruptured intracranial aneurysm treatment score (UIATS). Neurosurg Rev. 2020;44:1–3. https://doi.org/10.1007/s10143-020-01354-8.
69. Sturiale CL, Stumpo V, Ricciardi L, Trevisi G, Valente I, D'Arrigo S, Latour K, Barbone P, Albanese A. Retrospective application of risk scores to ruptured intracranial aneurysms: would they have predicted the risk of bleeding? Neurosurg Rev. 2020;44:1655–63. https://doi.org/10.1007/s10143-020-01352-w.
70. Liu Q, Jiang P, Wu J, Li M, Gao B, Zhang Y, Ning B, Cao Y, Wang S. Intracranial aneurysm rupture score may correlate to the risk of rebleeding before treatment of ruptured intracranial aneurysms. Neurol Sci. 2019;40(8):1683–93.
71. Xiang J, Yu J, Choi H, Dolan Fox JM, Snyder KV, Levy EI, Siddiqui AH, Meng H. Rupture resemblance score (RRS): toward risk stratification of unruptured intracranial aneurysms using hemodynamic–morphological discriminants. J NeuroIntervent Surg. 2015;7(7):490–5.
72. Molyneux AJ, Kerr RSC, Yu L-M, Clarke M, Sneade M, Yarnold JA, Sandercock P. International subarachnoid aneurysm trial (ISAT) of neurosurgical clipping versus endovascular coiling in 2143 patients with ruptured intracranial aneurysms: a randomised comparison of effects on survival, dependency, seizures, rebleeding, subgroups, and aneurysm occlusion. Lancet. 2005;366:9.
73. Rutledge C, Jonzzon S, Winkler EA, Raper D, Lawton MT, Abla AA. Small aneurysms with low PHASES scores account for most subarachnoid hemorrhage cases. World Neurosurg. 2020;139:e580–4.
74. Chen JH, Asch SM. Machine learning and prediction in medicine—beyond the peak of inflated expectations. N Engl J Med. 2017;376(26):2507–9.
75. Adams H, Ban VS, Leinonen V, et al. Risk of shunting after aneurysmal subarachnoid hemorrhage: a collaborative study and initiation of a consortium. Stroke. 2016;47(10):2488–96.
76. Pegoli M, Mandrekar J, Rabinstein AA, Lanzino G. Predictors of excellent functional outcome in aneurysmal subarachnoid hemorrhage. J Neurosurg. 2015;122:414–8.
77. van Donkelaar CE, Bakker NA, Birks J, Veeger NJGM, Metzemaekers JDM, Molyneux AJ, Groen RJM, van Dijk JMC. Prediction of outcome after aneurysmal subarachnoid hemorrhage: development and validation of the SAFIRE grading scale. Stroke. 2019;50(4):837–44.
78. Flemming KD, Lanzino G. Management of unruptured intracranial aneurysms and cerebrovascular malformations. Continuum. 2017;23(1):181–210.
79. Staartjes VE, Broggi M, Zattra CM, et al. Development and external validation of a clinical prediction model for functional impairment after intracranial tumor surgery. J Neurosurg. 2020:1–8.

37 Clinical Prediction Modeling in Intramedullary Spinal Tumor Surgery

Elie Massaad, Yoon Ha, Ganesh M. Shankar, and John H. Shin

37.1 Introduction

Intramedullary spinal cord tumors (IMSCT) are challenging to diagnose and treat as they are rare lesions that can cause severe neurologic deterioration and affect quality of life [1]. Numerous IMSCT exist, of which, ependymoma, astrocytoma, and hemangioblastoma are most commonly encountered. Each type of tumor has characteristic radiographic and pathologic features and can present with variable clinical symptoms [2]. Sometimes, these lesions are found incidentally. To date, surgical resection remains the mainstay approach for diagnosis and removal of these tumors with the goal of improving neurological symptoms. In cases of invasive tumors such as astrocytoma however, complete resection is often not possible due to the absence of clear margins between the tumor and spinal cord. As such, local control for these and any type of IMSCT is a challenge, and recurrence is subject to achieving gross total resection when feasible. Adjuvant therapies including radiation therapy, systemic therapies, or a combination of both, are offered to patients with high-grade tumors, and in instances when total resection cannot be achieved to avoid progression of the disease [3]. Because the role of such adjuvant regimens is not well established, surgeons seek to refine resection strategies utilizing advances in intraoperative imaging and neuromonitoring [4].

Recent years have seen an extensive exploration of predictive analytics and machine learning algorithms (ML) to provide mathematical-based solutions to the most intricate aspects of management of spine tumors [5]. Several applications of artificial intelligence (AI) in cancer have focused on improving the accuracy of diagnostic tools, modeling the progression and treatment of diseases, risk stratification, discovering potential therapeutics, and ultimately improving quality of life [6]. Because benign and malignant intramedullary tumors represent a heterogenous group of different primary histologies, and often times respond differently to surgical, systemic, and radiation treatment, AI and high-throughput, data-intensive biomedical research assays and technologies could provide a greater understanding of pathophysiologic factors and processes that contribute to tumor behavior, and could lead to personalized approaches to the nuanced and often unique features possessed by individual patients diagnosed with IMSCT [7]. In this chapter, we review the state-of-the-art AI and ML applications in spine oncology, particularly those relevant to intramedullary tumors and forecast how spine surgery will incorporate AI in the future.

37.2 A Primer on Machine Learning and Predictive Analytics

Before getting into specific skills and tasks that could be performed using AI, there are some concepts in ML that need to be defined [8]. Machine learning strategies can be broadly split into two approaches that have different goals: (1) unsupervised and (2) supervised learning [9]. Unsupervised learning focuses on discovering underlying structure or relationships among variables in a dataset, whereas supervised learning often involves classification of an observation into 1 or more categories or outcomes (e.g., "Does this spinal cord lesion represent a high-grade or low-grade lesion?"). Supervised learning thus requires a dataset with predictor variables (features) and labeled outcomes. Predictive modeling is often performed when observations have labels such as "cases" or "controls," and these observations are paired to associated features such as age, sex, or clinical variables. In the next section of this chapter, we will look at the various

E. Massaad · G. M. Shankar · J. H. Shin (✉)
Department of Neurosurgery, Massachusetts General Hospital, Harvard Medical School, Boston, MA, USA
e-mail: shin.john@mgh.harvard.edu

Y. Ha
Department of Neurosurgery, Spine and Spinal Cord Institute, Yonsei University College of Medicine, Seoul, South Korea

V. E. Staartjes et al. (eds.), *Machine Learning in Clinical Neuroscience*, Acta Neurochirurgica Supplement 134,
https://doi.org/10.1007/978-3-030-85292-4_37

types of features that could help us predict with enough power and accuracy, the different outcomes that are of interest to both surgeons and patients. For predictive analytics to be effective, we first need to define the problem that we want to address. In the following section, we detail the most common outcomes of interest for spine surgeons treating IMSCT.

37.3 Defining Outcome Measures for Intramedullary Spinal Cord Tumors

The challenge with treating IMSCT is that though natural history without treatment may lead to neurologic and functional deterioration, surgery itself can lead to significant morbidity and mortality [2]. While the primary goal of surgery is to restore neurological function and improve functional status and quality of life, the risks associated with surgery are balanced with achieving gross total resection to decrease the chance of tumor recurrence [10–12]. Several studies showed that the extent of resection is a strong predictor of overall survival, with 90%–100% of patients showing improvement following complete resection [4, 13, 14]. However, certain characteristics like tumor infiltration, high-grade histopathology, and absence of a clear surgical plane of dissection pose significant challenges for surgeons [15]. In general, benign tumors such as ependymomas and hemangioblastomas may exhibit a plane of dissection that facilitates resection [16]. The absence of a normal spinal cord–tumor interface in infiltrative tumors such as astrocytoma often leads to subtotal resection or biopsy alone as gross total resection is often not possible [17].

Patients with IMSCTs who present with minimal or no focal neurological deficits are often faced with the decision to undergo surgical resection and risk neurological decline. Moreover, studies have showed mixed results about the effectiveness of surgery to improve neurological outcomes [11, 15]. Predictors of neurological outcomes can be measured (1) before surgery; such as the intramedullary lesion length, baseline neurological and functional status; (2) intraoperatively by assessment of somatosensory-evoked potentials (SSEP) and transcranial motor evoked potentials (TCMEPs); (3) after surgery by modeling functional progress during recovery and rehabilitation [18–21].

During surgery for IMSCT, there is risk of injury to the dorsal column, which stems from the difficulty of identifying the appropriate place of tumor resection. Intraoperative monitoring using SSEPs and TCMEPs provides increased accuracy in detecting injury to sensory and motor pathways that can help prevent postoperative neurologic dysfunction [22]. D-waves recordings directly monitor the fast motor fibers in the corticospinal tracts and are more sensitive in detecting early injury to the spine. Moreover, dorsal column mapping may be used to guide a safer resection by identifying anatomic landmarks such as the dorsal median sulcus to guide a safe midline myelotomy and maximize the extent of the resection when the tumor distorts normal anatomy [23].

Studies have shown that combining both SSEPs and TCMEPs monitoring can help predict neurological outcomes after surgery [21, 24]. Many factors like tumor location, anatomy, extent of infiltration, and the threshold for signal changes affect the sensitivity and specificity of these monitoring tools. For this reason, D-wave monitoring is recommended to monitor motor pathways to decrease false-positive results and maximize resection [25]. However, D-wave monitoring may not be available in a given hospital, so TCMEP is the workhorse modality to assess motor function intraoperatively [26].

Apart from tumor recurrence and neurological function, quality of life after surgery for IMSCT may be compromised by neuropathic pain or postsurgical myelopathy [27]. Syringomyelia associated with IMSCT is a strong predictor of neuropathic pain [28]. Other factors like older age and preoperative presence of neuropathic pain may contribute to neuropathic pain after surgery [29].

Machine learning approaches can be applied to predict and calculate each of the outcomes discussed above. Because the outcomes of interest involve highly interdependent features that stem from surgical, pathologic, genomic, biomedical imaging, and clinical data, it is important to capture and centralize this data to train models that could more accurately predict outcomes.

37.4 Available Sources of Data for Prediction Modeling in IMSCT

Clinical prediction models are emerging in spine surgery as data-driven decision-making tools. At present, clinical prediction models for IMSCT are derived from a variety of data sources, notably institutional and national databases [30]. Because primary spinal cord tumors are rare, the volume of data available to develop prediction models that are both accurate and reproducible are particularly difficult to achieve. Though survival is the most common outcome in IMSCT that researchers often seek to predict using machine learning algorithms, research groups are also interested in predicting other treatment-related outcomes such as local control, progression-free survival, readmission, revision surgery, complications, long-term opioid use, and functional outcomes [12, 31–35].

Although the aforementioned outcomes are of great interest for the spine surgeon and other specialists involved in the treatment of IMSCT, modeling clinical predictive models for these outcomes is practically limited and dependent on the availability of data. The Surveillance, Epidemiology, and End Results (SEER) registry, which serves as a source of population-based data to analyze cancer treatment outcomes, was utilized to predict survival of patients with spinal ependymoma [35]. In parallel, the MD Anderson Cancer Center and institutions from the Rare Cancer Network engaged in the curation of a more granular research database that was able to provide greater insight about the potential predictors of outcomes for IMSCT. Most studies look at demographic variables, tumor histology, disease status, and treatment modality. Achieving gross total resection (GTR) was associated with improved overall survival [35]. A nomogram to predict 5- and 10-year overall survival for Primary Intramedullary Spinal Cord Grade II/III Ependymoma (636 patients registered in SEER) was developed and included age (40–64 or ≥65), gender (female or male), marital status (unknown, married, or single), surgery (GTR, subtotal resection, or no surgery), WHO grade (grade II or grade III) [36]. The nomogram was able to accurately distinguish the prognosis in different risk groups [36], but external validation is required at this point to confirm the performance of the nomogram. The role of radiation therapy (RT) is controversial, but prospective studies may provide more evidence if adjuvant RT could benefit progression-free survival in ependymoma [35, 37–39].

As detailed above, available prediction models for IMSCT are primarily based on clinical data and do not incorporate other sources of data. For clinical prediction models to perform better, different sources of data that provide valuable information about IMSCT are required as inputs, such as imaging studies.

37.5 Imaging Features and Biomarkers to Predict Outcomes for IMSCT

As for many spinal conditions, Magnetic Resonance Imaging (MRI) is the modality of choice to evaluate a potential spinal cord tumor by delineating the spinal cord and surrounding structures. Because medical image analysis has advanced with more facilitated processes to extract quantitative features from images that reflect underlying pathophysiology, it is now more commonly used for hypothesis generation and decision support [40]. Visualization of tumor heterogeneity may prove critical in the assessment of tumor aggressiveness and prognosis. In the case of IMSCT, lesions may have well-circumscribed or infiltrative margins. Being able to characterize tumor margins on MRI is important to spine surgeons who are more likely to pursue a gross total resection in a circumscribed tumor with a well-defined surgical plane, versus a subtotal resection in an infiltrative tumor [41].

Preoperative neuroimaging assessment of a circumscribed tumor (e.g., ependymoma arising from the central canal) or an infiltrative tumor (e.g., astrocytoma arising from the cord parenchyma) can help devise the microsurgical strategy of resection or biopsy, especially given the limited accuracy (about 70%) of intraoperative frozen-section diagnosis [10]. The diagnosis of IMSCT tumors is a challenge for both radiologists and surgeons when considering the heterogenous characteristics of lesions exhibited on imaging. Though there are discerning characteristics of various tumor types, pathologic diagnosis is not currently possible by MRI alone. Imaging segmentation could help delineate tumor components and overcome intra- and inter-variability in assessing tumor characteristics. To the best of our knowledge, only one pipeline to automate the segmentation of IMSCT has been developed. Lemay et al. prepared and labeled a large number of MRI scans for three main components associated with IMSCT: enhanced and non-enhanced tumor component, liquid-filled cavities, and edema [42]. A convolutional neural network was trained to recognize these specific elements of the tumors, but the performance of the model was not perfect because the volume of imaging studies that were used to train the model to recognize cavities and edemas was limited as tumors have variable intensity patterns and ill-defined boundaries. In the future, the performance of the model can be optimized by training on larger imaging datasets that better represent the variability of the tumors.

More recently, the concept of using image data to identify physiologically distinct regions within lesions has been described [43]. In this approach, images with different acquisition parameters (e.g., contrast material-enhanced T1-weighted MR imaging, diffusion-weighted, and fluid attenuation sequences) can be combined to yield regions with specific combinations of quantitative image data. These regions are called habitats, because they represent physiologically distinct volumes, each with a specific combination of blood flow, cell density, necrosis, and edema. This approach could be of particular interest for IMSCT, as being able to extract features from these habitats could help identify unique properties of the tumors that would guide surgical treatment, response to radiation or chemotherapy, and follow-up plans.

IMSCT are a group of heterogenous tumors with several identifiable radiologic features that may suggest potential diagnoses. For instance, an intramedullary lesion at the epicenter of the central canal is most likely an ependymoma [44, 45]. Unlike ependymomas, astrocytomas tend to manifest eccentric to the central canal and may be associated with neurofibromatosis type 1 but not neurofibromatosis type 2. These account for the majority of pediatric intramedullary tumors [45, 46]. Hemangioblastoma tends to arise at the pial surface and exhibits intense T1-post contrast enhancement often associated with flow voids and vasogenic edema [47]. Both astrocytoma and ependymoma also tend to enhance at imaging with possible cystic or hemorrhagic changes. Diffuse infiltrating astrocytoma can show a range of possible enhancement patterns from a range of possible enhancement patterns from non-enhancing to homogeneously or heterogeneously enhancing that is associated with a higher-grade tumor and lower 5-year survival. For example, angiogenesis and necrosis in spinal cord glioblastoma manifest as heterogeneous enhancement that can be multicentric in location.

In addition to demonstrating tumor location and margins on conventional sequences, DTI in spinal cord tractography has also been shown to be helpful [48]. Specifically, the displacement or splaying of white matter tracts (streamlines) has a high positive predictive value for a circumscribed tumor, including ependymomas in adults and pilocytic astrocytomas in children [49]. The depiction of disrupted or traversing white matter tracts is nonspecific and can be seen in circumscribed or infiltrative tumors. Traversing streamlines can also be seen in inflammatory lesions [50].

Clearly, radiomics could offer a nearly limitless supply of imaging biomarkers that could potentially improve diagnosis and prognosis accuracy, and prognosis accuracy. These data can be combined with clinical data and other patient data like genomics (Fig. 37.1). In the following section, we will discuss studying genomics markers to understand IMSCT biology and improve prediction of treatment outcomes.

37.6 Genetic Biomarkers of IMSCT

In recent years, genomics has emerged as an innovative area of research that could potentially transform our understanding of tumor biology and response to treatment. Advances in genetic sequencing could provide new insights into understanding the pathobiology of IMSCT and their tumor microenvironment. The ultimate goal is to identify biomarkers that could objectively differentiate among different groups of microscopically indistinguishable IMSCT and more accurately predict prognosis. At present, large-scale genomic efforts that systematically profile IMSCT are limited, due to the rarity of the lesions and small size of the lesion that limits availability of tissue for research purposes. To start, next generation sequencing revealed that IMSCT may be different than their brain counterparts [51]. Because reviewing all genetic markers for IMSCT is beyond the scope of this chapter, we will focus more on molecular targets that were reported to have prognostic and treatment value.

Ependymoma

Investigation of the PI3K signaling pathway in pediatric ependymomas indicates that upregulation of protein kinase B (PKB or Akt protein kinase) and PI3K correlates with poor progression-free survival. Although both PKB and PI3K are potential therapeutic targets, their expression is lower in spinal ependymomas, which could potentially limit their usefulness in treatments of these tumors. Upregulated expression of epidermal growth factor receptor (EGFR) in intracranial ependymomas correlates with poor prognosis; this association was further demonstrated by targeted inhibition of EGFR with gefitinib and with AEE788, which reduced tumor proliferation in an in vivo model [52, 53]. These results sug-

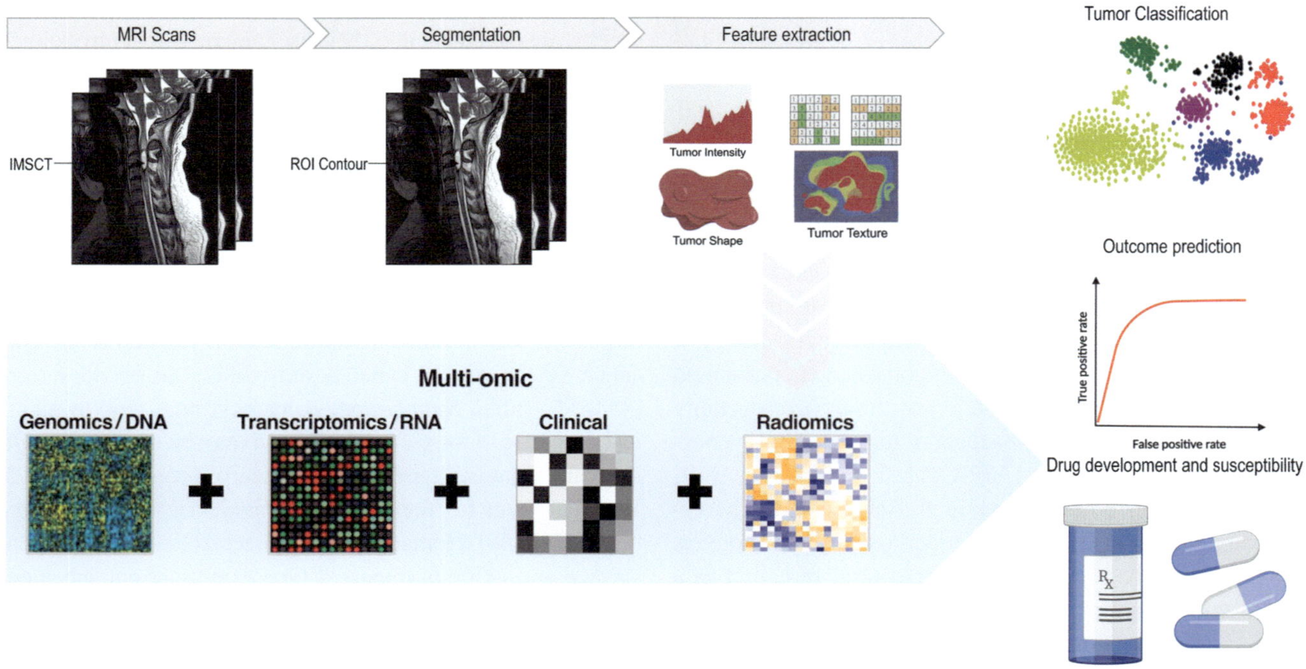

Fig. 37.1 Standard pipeline of the radiomics analysis and integration of genomics, transcriptomics, and clinical data for classification of tumor biology, prediction of clinical outcomes, and development of targeted therapies

gest that inhibition of EGFR may prove beneficial in spinal ependymomas, should it be validated as a tumor driver. Targeted therapy for spinal ependymomas is also scarcely described in the literature, although a report of a PDGF-expressing tumor that responded to treatment with imatinib suggests that this medication may have a potential for treating such tumors [54].

Astrocytoma

Although many studies have investigated the genetics of intracranial astrocytomas, fewer studies have probed the genetics of astrocytomas occurring in the spinal cord. Some common mutations observed in cranial GBMs are also noted in spinal astrocytomas, including mutations in the *p16* gene, the phosphatase and tensin homolog *(PTEN)*gene, the B-Raf proto-oncogene *(BRAF)*, *p53*, and the replication-independent histone 3 variant H3.3 gene (H3F3A). Importantly, numerous downstream targets from PTEN have been identified, such as mTOR and Akt, and several chemical antagonists of these effector proteins are currently under clinical investigation for managing cranial astrocytoma, which may offer the possibility of expanding treatments to spinal astrocytoma.

The *BRAF* gene has been observed to contain mutations in spinal astrocytomas, namely the *BRAF-KIAA1549* fusion gene and $BRAF^{V600E}$ mutation. *KIAA1549–BRAF* was seen in higher frequency than *BRAFV600E* or other genetic aberrations in pediatric spinal low-grade gliomas and experienced lower death rates compared to *KIAA1549–BRAF* negative patients, although this was not statistically significant [55]. This further supports that BRAF mutations may be useful in prognostication and could provide information for therapy choice as more targeted therapies are being studied.

In parallel, high-grade spinal astrocytomas are rare. The so-called H3-K27M-mutant which was classified in a separate entity in the 2016 World Health Organization (WHO) was found to be associated with survival and prognosis in glioma. However, studies showed inconsistent results concerning the prognostic role of H3-K27M mutation in glioma [56, 57].

Hemangioblastoma

Approximately 25% of hemangioblastoma patients have evidence of familial von Hippel-Lindau (VHL) disease characterized by the *VHL* mutation. The impact of *VHL* mutations on spinal hemangioblastoma has not been extensively studied, but 1 study reported that spinal hemangioblastomas were strongly associated with the VHL syndrome (in 88% of cases) but occurred less frequently in sporadic cases (21%) and often were associated with significant VHL expression in multilevel disease [58]. Overall, the understanding of the role of mutated genes other than *VHL* in spinal hemangioblastoma remains limited.

37.7 Genome-Wide Association Studies

Machine learning methods have been applied in genome-wide association studies (GWAS) to discover genetic variants underlying complex human diseases and to dissect the biological basis of diseases, develop new drugs, and to advance precision medicine. At present, GWAS are more prevalent to brain than to spine tumors. GWAS have been successful in identifying germline variants associated with glioma susceptibility. Traditionally, the risk of glioma is recognized to be associated with a number of Mendelian cancer predisposition syndromes, notable neurofibromatosis (NF1 and NF2), Li–Fraumeni, and Turcot. More fruitful have been efforts over the past decade to investigate the contribution of small-effect variants that are common in the general population to many traits including glioma through GWAS. The combination of technological advancements and collaborative efforts in establishment of consortia such as the Glioma International Case–Control (GICC) [59] study has enabled genotyping of hundreds of thousands of variants in thousands of glioma cases and controls. It is now recognized that a substantial component of glioma genetic risk is explained by combinations of common polymorphisms of modest effect, with 27 loci in total identified so far from glioma GWAS. Many studies have explored GWAS in intracranial tumors, but data regarding their spinal counterparts remain scarce, likely because of the rarity of the IMSCT. Because it is well established that GWAS improves understanding of disease etiology, a model collaboration program that includes various centers of excellences around the world that treat IMSCT is needed to collect genomic and clinical data to study genetic variants of the disease.

37.8 Discovery of Biomarkers and Prediction of Therapeutic Responses

Many therapies enter clinical trials for potential treatment, but a very small proportion of these targeted therapies gain approval for clinical use. The problem becomes particularly challenging for cancers that are not associated with strong targetable genetic drivers. Biomarkers are needed to develop targeted therapies and predict a drug response. Since cancers without these known drivers lack clear biomarkers with which to stratify drug response, A better basic understanding of the molecular pathways governing drug sensitivity would help greatly in determining which patients should be treated and with which drugs. There has recently been a great deal of interest in applying advances in artificial intelligence, including machine learning and deep learning, to classic problems in biomedicine. Whereas popular applications include disease diagnosis from biomedical images and interpretation of electronic medical records, machine learning models are also of high interest in predicting drug responses.

37.9 Conclusion

The potential areas of application of machine learning extend far beyond the analyses of clinical data to include several areas of artificial intelligence, such as genomics and computer vision. Integration of various sources of data and application of advanced analytical approaches could improve risk assessment for intramedullary tumors. Although recent years have seen great interest in the development of prediction models in spine oncology, there remains uncertainty over whether use of any of the models in clinical practice actually improves surgical and patient-reported outcomes. For now, collaborations are needed to integrate molecular and radiographic features in clinical prediction tools. Ultimately, we must continue the difficult work of identifying the best strategies for collecting data and implementing these tools in practice to help decision-making and shared treatment discussions with patients.

References

1. Shao J, Jones J, Ellsworth P, et al. A comprehensive epidemiological review of spinal astrocytomas in the United States. J Neurosurg Spine. 2020:1–7.
2. Samartzis D, Gillis CC, Shih P, O'Toole JE, Fessler RG. Intramedullary spinal cord tumors: part I-epidemiology, pathophysiology, and diagnosis. Glob Spine J. 2015;5(5):425–35.
3. Abd-El-Barr MM, Huang KT, Moses ZB, Iorgulescu JB, Chi JH. Recent advances in intradural spinal tumors. Neuro Oncol. 2018;20(6):729–42.
4. Garcés-Ambrossi GL, McGirt MJ, Mehta VA, Sciubba DM, Witham TF, Bydon A, Wolinksy J-P, Jallo GI, Gokaslan ZL. Factors associated with progression-free survival and long-term neurological outcome after resection of intramedullary spinal cord tumors: analysis of 101 consecutive cases. J Neurosurg Spine. 2009;11(5):591–9.
5. Massaad E, Fatima N, Hadzipasic M, Alvarez-Breckenridge C, Shankar GM, Shin JH. Predictive analytics in spine oncology research: first steps, limitations, and future directions. Neurospine. 2019;16(4):669–77.
6. Perez-Breva L, Shin JH. Artificial intelligence in neurosurgery: a comment on the possibilities. Neurospine. 2019;16(4):640–2.
7. Nam KH, Kim DH, Choi BK, Han IH. Internet of things, digital biomarker, and artificial intelligence in spine: current and future perspectives. Neurospine. 2019;16(4):705–11.
8. Beam AL, Kohane IS. Big data and machine learning in health care. JAMA. 2018;319(13):1317–8.
9. Beaulieu-Jones B, Finlayson SG, Chivers C, Chen I, McDermott M, Kandola J, Dalca AV, Beam A, Fiterau M, Naumann T. Trends and focus of machine learning applications for Health Research. JAMA Netw Open. 2019;2(10):e1914051.
10. Hongo H, Takai K, Komori T, Taniguchi M. Intramedullary spinal cord ependymoma and astrocytoma: intraoperative frozen-section diagnosis, extent of resection, and outcomes. J Neurosurg Spine. 2018;30(1):133–9.
11. Li D, Hao S-Y, Wu Z, Jia G-J, Zhang L-W, Zhang J-T. Intramedullary medullocervical ependymoma—surgical treatment, functional recovery, and long-term outcome. Neurol Med Chir (Tokyo). 2013;53(10):663–75.
12. Weber DC, Wang Y, Miller R, et al. Long-term outcome of patients with spinal myxopapillary ependymoma: treatment results from the MD Anderson Cancer Center and institutions from the rare cancer network. Neuro Oncol. 2015;17(4):588–95.
13. Abdullah KG, Lubelski D, Miller J, Steinmetz MP, Shin JH, Krishnaney A, Mroz TE, Benzel EC. Progression free survival and functional outcome after surgical resection of intramedullary ependymomas. J Clin Neurosci. 2015;22(12):1933–7.
14. Tobin MK, Geraghty JR, Engelhard HH, Linninger AA, Mehta AI. Intramedullary spinal cord tumors: a review of current and future treatment strategies. Neurosurg Focus. 2015;39(2):E14.
15. Karikari IO, Nimjee SM, Hodges TR, et al. Impact of tumor histology on resectability and neurological outcome in primary intramedullary spinal cord tumors: a single-center experience with 102 patients. Neurosurgery. 2015;76(Suppl 1):S4–13; discussion S13.
16. Hoshimaru M, Koyama T, Hashimoto N, Kikuchi H. Results of microsurgical treatment for intramedullary spinal cord ependymomas: analysis of 36 cases. Neurosurgery. 1999;44(2):264–9.
17. Constantini S, Miller DC, Allen JC, Rorke LB, Freed D, Epstein FJ. Radical excision of intramedullary spinal cord tumors: surgical morbidity and long-term follow-up evaluation in 164 children and young adults. J Neurosurg. 2000;93(2 Suppl):183–93.
18. Aarabi B, Sansur CA, Ibrahimi DM, Simard JM, Hersh DS, Le E, Diaz C, Massetti J, Akhtar-Danesh N. Intramedullary lesion length on postoperative magnetic resonance imaging is a strong predictor of ASIA impairment scale grade conversion following decompressive surgery in cervical spinal cord injury. Neurosurgery. 2017;80(4):610–20.
19. Cheng JS, Ivan ME, Stapleton CJ, Quinones-Hinojosa A, Gupta N, Auguste KI. Intraoperative changes in transcranial motor evoked potentials and somatosensory evoked potentials predicting outcome in children with intramedullary spinal cord tumors. J Neurosurg Pediatr. 2014;13(6):591–9.
20. Ghadirpour R, Nasi D, Iaccarino C, Romano A, Motti L, Sabadini R, Valzania F, Servadei F. Intraoperative neurophysiological monitoring for intradural extramedullary spinal tumors: predictive value and relevance of D-wave amplitude on surgical outcome during a 10-year experience. J Neurosurg Spine. 2018;30(2):259–67.
21. Lakomkin N, Mistry AM, Zuckerman SL, Ladner T, Kothari P, Lee NJ, Stannard B, Vasquez RA, Cheng JS. Utility of intraoperative monitoring in the resection of spinal cord tumors: an analysis by tumor location and anatomical region. Spine. 2018;43(4):287–94.
22. Verla T, Fridley JS, Khan AB, Mayer RR, Omeis I. Neuromonitoring for intramedullary spinal cord tumor surgery. World Neurosurg. 2016;95:108–16.
23. Mehta AI, Mohrhaus CA, Husain AM, Karikari IO, Hughes B, Hodges T, Gottfried O, Bagley CA. Dorsal column mapping for intramedullary spinal cord tumor resection decreases dorsal column dysfunction. J Spinal Disord Tech. 2012;25(4):205–9.
24. Barzilai O, Lidar Z, Constantini S, Salame K, Bitan-Talmor Y, Korn A. Continuous mapping of the corticospinal tracts in intramedullary spinal cord tumor surgery using an electrified ultrasonic aspirator. J Neurosurg Spine. 2017;27(2):161–8.

25. Costa P, Peretta P, Faccani G. Relevance of intraoperative D wave in spine and spinal cord surgeries. Eur Spine J. 2013;22(4):840–8.
26. Morota N, Deletis V, Constantini S, Kofler M, Cohen H, Epstein FJ. The role of motor evoked potentials during surgery for intramedullary spinal cord tumors. Neurosurgery. 1997;41(6):1327–36.
27. Nakamura M, Tsuji O, Iwanami A, Tsuji T, Ishii K, Toyama Y, Chiba K, Matsumoto M. Central neuropathic pain after surgical resection in patients with spinal intramedullary tumor. J Orthop Sci. 2012;17(4):352–7.
28. Klekamp J. Spinal ependymomas. Part 1: Intramedullary ependymomas. Neurosurg Focus. 2015;39(2):E6.
29. McGirt MJ, Chaichana KL, Atiba A, Attenello F, Yao KC, Jallo GI. Resection of intramedullary spinal cord tumors in children: assessment of long-term motor and sensory deficits. J Neurosurg Pediatr. 2008;1(1):63–7.
30. Schwartz JT, Gao M, Geng EA, Mody KS, Mikhail CM, Cho SK. Applications of machine learning using electronic medical records in spine surgery. Neurospine. 2019;16(4):643–53.
31. Arima H, Naito K, Yamagata T, Kawahara S, Ohata K, Takami T. Quantitative analysis of near-infrared Indocyanine green Videoangiography for predicting functional outcomes after spinal intramedullary Ependymoma resection. Oper Neurosurg. 2019;17(5):531–9.
32. Eroes CA, Zausinger S, Kreth F-W, Goldbrunner R, Tonn J-C. Intramedullary low grade astrocytoma and ependymoma. Surgical results and predicting factors for clinical outcome. Acta Neurochir. 2010;152(4):611–8.
33. Jin MC, Ho AL, Feng AY, Zhang Y, Staartjes VE, Stienen MN, Han SS, Veeravagu A, Ratliff JK, Desai AM. Predictive modeling of long-term opioid and benzodiazepine use after intradural tumor resection. Spine J. 2020.
34. Karhade AV, Vasudeva VS, Dasenbrock HH, Lu Y, Gormley WB, Groff MW, Chi JH, Smith TR. Thirty-day readmission and reoperation after surgery for spinal tumors: a National Surgical Quality Improvement Program analysis. Neurosurg Focus. 2016;41(2):E5.
35. Ryu SM, Lee S-H, Kim E-S, Eoh W. Predicting survival of patients with spinal Ependymoma using machine learning algorithms with the SEER database. World Neurosurg. 2019;124:e331–9.
36. Wang C, Yuan X, Zuo J. Individualized prediction of overall survival for primary intramedullary spinal cord grade II/III Ependymoma. World Neurosurg. 2020;143:e149–56.
37. Akyurek S, Chang EL, Yu T-K, Little D, Allen PK, McCutcheon I, Mahajan A, Maor MH, Woo SY. Spinal myxopapillary ependymoma outcomes in patients treated with surgery and radiotherapy at M.D. Anderson cancer center. J Neurooncol. 2006;80(2):177–83.
38. Brown DA, Goyal A, Takami H, Graffeo CS, Mahajan A, Krauss WE, Bydon M. Radiotherapy in addition to surgical resection may not improve overall survival in WHO grade II spinal ependymomas. Clin Neurol Neurosurg. 2020;189:105632.
39. Lee S-H, Chung CK, Kim CH, Yoon SH, Hyun S-J, Kim K-J, Kim E-S, Eoh W, Kim H-J. Long-term outcomes of surgical resection with or without adjuvant radiation therapy for treatment of spinal ependymoma: a retrospective multicenter study by the Korea spinal oncology research group. Neuro Oncol. 2013;15(7):921–9.
40. Kim M, Yun J, Cho Y, Shin K, Jang R, Bae H-J, Kim N. Deep learning in medical imaging. Neurospine. 2019;16(4):657–68.
41. Mack WJ. In: Winn HR, editor. Youmans and Winn neurological surgery. Amsterdam: Elsevier; 2018. p. 4320 pages, $839.99 print+ ebook, ISBN 9780323287821.
42. Lemay A, Gros C, Zhuo Z, Zhang J, Duan Y, Cohen-Adad J, Liu Y. Multiclass spinal cord tumor segmentation on MRI with deep learning. In: ArXiv Prepr. ArXiv201212820; 2020.
43. Gatenby RA, Grove O, Gillies RJ. Quantitative imaging in cancer evolution and ecology. Radiology. 2013;269(1):8–15.
44. Herbrecht A, Messerer M, Parker F. Development of a lateralization index for intramedullary astrocytomas and ependymomas. Neurochirurgie. 2017;63(5):410–2.
45. Shih RY, Koeller KK. Intramedullary masses of the spinal cord: radiologic-pathologic correlation. Radiographics. 2020;40(4):1125–45.
46. Patronas NJ, Courcoutsakis N, Bromley CM, Katzman GL, MacCollin M, Parry DM. Intramedullary and spinal canal tumors in patients with neurofibromatosis 2: MR imaging findings and correlation with genotype. Radiology. 2001;218(2):434–42.
47. Xu D, Feng M, Suresh V, Wang G, Wang F, Song L, Guo F. Clinical analysis of syringomyelia resulting from spinal hemangioblastoma in a single series of 38 consecutive patients. Clin Neurol Neurosurg. 2019;181:58–63.
48. Setzer M, Murtagh RD, Murtagh FR, Eleraky M, Jain S, Marquardt G, Seifert V, Vrionis FD. Diffusion tensor imaging tractography in patients with intramedullary tumors: comparison with intraoperative findings and value for prediction of tumor resectability. J Neurosurg Spine. 2010;13(3):371–80.
49. Choudhri AF, Whitehead MT, Klimo P, Montgomery BK, Boop FA. Diffusion tensor imaging to guide surgical planning in intramedullary spinal cord tumors in children. Neuroradiology. 2014;56(2):169–74.
50. Egger K, Hohenhaus M, Van Velthoven V, Heil S, Urbach H. Spinal diffusion tensor tractography for differentiation of intramedullary tumor-suspected lesions. Eur J Radiol. 2016;85(12):2275–80.
51. Korshunov A, Neben K, Wrobel G, Tews B, Benner A, Hahn M, Golanov A, Lichter P. Gene expression patterns in ependymomas correlate with tumor location, grade, and patient age. Am J Pathol. 2003;163(5):1721–7.
52. Meco D, Servidei T, Lamorte G, Binda E, Arena V, Riccardi R. Ependymoma stem cells are highly sensitive to temozolomide in vitro and in orthotopic models. Neuro Oncol. 2014;16(8):1067–77.
53. Mendrzyk F, Korshunov A, Benner A, Toedt G, Pfister S, Radlwimmer B, Lichter P. Identification of gains on 1q and epidermal growth factor receptor overexpression as independent prognostic markers in intracranial ependymoma. Clin Cancer Res. 2006;12(7 Pt 1):2070–9.
54. Fakhrai N, Neophytou P, Dieckmann K, Nemeth A, Prayer D, Hainfellner J, Marosi C. Recurrent spinal ependymoma showing partial remission under Imatimib. Acta Neurochir. 2004;146(11):1255–8.
55. Grob ST, Nobre L, Campbell KR, et al. Clinical and molecular characterization of a multi-institutional cohort of pediatric spinal cord low-grade gliomas. Neuro Oncol Adv. 2020;2(1):vdaa103.
56. Chai R-C, Zhang Y-W, Liu Y-Q, Chang Y-Z, Pang B, Jiang T, Jia W-Q, Wang Y-Z. The molecular characteristics of spinal cord gliomas with or without H3 K27M mutation. Acta Neuropathol Commun. 2020;9:119. https://doi.org/10.1186/s40478-020-00913-w.
57. Yi S, Choi S, Shin DA, et al. Impact of H3.3 K27M mutation on prognosis and survival of Grade IV spinal cord glioma on the basis of new 2016 World Health Organization classification of the central nervous system. Neurosurgery. 2019;84(5):1072–81.
58. Takai K, Taniguchi M, Takahashi H, Usui M, Saito N. Comparative analysis of spinal hemangioblastomas in sporadic disease and Von Hippel-Lindau syndrome. Neurol Med Chir (Tokyo). 2010;50(7):560–7.
59. Amirian ES, Armstrong GN, Zhou R, et al. The glioma international case-control study: a report from the genetic epidemiology of glioma international consortium. Am J Epidemiol. 2016;183(2):85–91.

Radiomic Features Associated with Extent of Resection in Glioma Surgery

38

Giovanni Muscas, Simone Orlandini, Eleonora Becattini, Francesca Battista, Victor E. Staartjes, Carlo Serra, and Alessandro Della Puppa

38.1 Introduction

Gliomas consist of a heterogeneous pathology characterized by diverse anatomic-pathological and molecular features. This aspect has been stressed in 2016 WHO classification of brain tumors by introducing molecular profiles as a requested hallmark to categorize gliomas better and to understand their behavior and prognosis in a more precise way [1]. Besides tumor-specific features, gliomas harbor individual genetic and molecular traits that confer every tumor a characteristic signature, ultimately translating in an intrinsic difficulty to predict tumor behavior and prognosis reliably [2, 3].

In recent years, radiomics has undergone a significant development also in the field of neuro-oncology. Radiomics defines a set of techniques that extracts and quantifies digital medical data from digitalized radiological exams in a reproducible way to detect features possibly related to a clinical dilemma such as, for instance, the definition of the histological tumor grading, identification of tumor infiltration zones, disease stratification and prognosis, survival prediction, presence of specific molecular markers, and others [4–6]. Such features are otherwise either subject to a descriptive and individual interpretation, thereby lacking a precise recognition and quantification, or cannot be detected by a medical investigator.

Due to the high volume of features investigated, to select and incorporate them in a reproducible model to answer a clinical question, the knowledge and use of machine learning techniques are essential in radiomics [7, 8].

In this chapter, we aim at reviewing the fundamental concepts of radiomics and the critical steps of model creation with a focus on neurosurgical tasks. Next, a short review of recent applications in the field of neuro-oncology and specifically of gliomas will be carried through. Finally, the identification of radiomic features able to improve the extent of surgical resection will follow.

38.2 Basic Workflow in Radiomics

The goal of radiomics is to generate quantitative data from medical imaging and create reproducible and generalizable models for a specific task. Every kind of imaging scan can be investigated, like computed tomography (CT), magnetic resonance imaging (MRI), and positron emission tomography (PET). However, a considerable amount of information in brain tumors has been extracted from MRI due to its common application for diagnosing and following-up of brain gliomas [9, 10]. The specific features of different MR sequences exploit and highlight the pathological features of the tumor differently: radiomics performs an automated features extraction and creates algorithms that incorporate the most informative features to predict a specific event like, for instance, overall survival, response to treatment, and MGMT methylation [9, 11]. This is based on the hypothesis that tumor imaging reflects pathological anatomy and physiology of small-scale phenomena that cannot be detected on the mesoscopic scale of clinical, radiological evaluation [12].

G. Muscas (✉) · S. Orlandini · E. Becattini · F. Battista
A. Della Puppa
Neurosurgery Clinic, Department of Neuroscience, Psychology, Pharmacology and Child Health, Careggi University Hospital and University of Florence, Florence, Italy
e-mail: muscasgi@aou-careggi.toscana.it

V. E. Staartjes · C. Serra
Klinik für Neurochirurgie, University Hospital Zurich and University of Zurich, Zurich, Switzerland

Machine Intelligence in Clinical Neuroscience (MICN) Laboratory, Department of Neurosurgery, University Hospital Zurich, Clinical Neuroscience Centre, University of Zurich, Zurich, Switzerland

V. E. Staartjes et al. (eds.), *Machine Learning in Clinical Neuroscience*, Acta Neurochirurgica Supplement 134,
https://doi.org/10.1007/978-3-030-85292-4_38

Image Post-Processing and Tumor Segmentation

In clinical routine, data are acquired from different scans with different acquisition protocols, limiting the generalizability and reproducibility of models. A few steps are required to overcome these limits before extracting data from the scans to correct inter-subjects and pathology-related inhomogeneities, signal noise, and differences among machines and acquisition parameters. The goal is to obtain standardized intensity ranges for each imaging modality across all subjects and generate well-defined inputs for quantitative feature extraction [4, 13]. The critical steps include, but are not limited to, intensity normalization, spatial smoothing, spatial resampling, noise reduction, and corrections of MRI field inhomogeneities [14] and can be achieved through different methods [4, 15–17]. Smoothing and intensity normalization and decomposition can be executed by applying filters, dividing each voxel intensity by the standard deviation of the whole-brain value, or performing the *z*-score transformation to whole-brain images [5, 18]. An alternative approach excluded the top 0.1% intensity voxels on both non-contrast- and contrast-enhanced T1-weighted images and reallocated the remaining voxels in 256 grayscale [11]. Eventually, different correction methods can be used, whose in-depth discussion is beyond this chapter's purposes and is reviewed here [19].

Consequently, an operator manually selects the region of interest (ROI) from which data shall be extracted (i.e., visual characteristics should be quantified) by masking the region's contour. Since the ROIs ultimately influence the radiomic analysis results, semiautomatic segmentation has been recently developed to aid dedicated machine learning algorithms [13, 18, 20]. Important to mention, different aspects can be investigated, like the contrast-enhancing lesion, the necrotic core, or the perilesional edema [14].

Radiomic Features

Radiomic features can be extracted from different sequences after post-processing [16]. This is an automated process for which different methods and dedicated software have been used, whose detailed description can be found elsewhere [4, 11, 13, 16–18, 21, 22]. Two approaches can be used to extract features, namely the computational or the biologically inspired [12]: the first select and compute visual characteristics within the ROIs (i.e., tumor, edema, or specific regions within it), whereas the latter is based on specific biological hypotheses that quantify the recognized radiological knowledge. Biologically inspired features can be disease-specific and dependent on the MR sequence being used (for example, the measured extracellular space per unit of tissue volume [23], local contrast enhancement, edema, or cellularity [24]). In contrast, computational features are shared among different diseases and divided into two main subgroups: local-level and global-level features [12]. Local-level features compare a given pixel with its immediate neighbors and detect characteristics that may not be detectable to the medical investigator. In contrast, global-level features investigate the ROI features as a whole and concentrate on their shape and overall appearance [12]. A different way to classify radiomic features describes different groups [4, 13, 22]: first-order statistics; second-order statistics (or textural features); shape- and size-based features; wavelet features (see Table 38.1 for a partial summary of commonly extracted features).

Feature Selection and Model Creation

The extraction of features for a specific task in radiomics brings to the identification of hundreds of items, of which only a part is relevant to build a valuable radiomic model. Some features may be redundant, correlated, irrelevant, or duplicated, thereby producing an overfitting model [14, 22]. To avoid this, scanning high-volume databases and feature selection through either supervised or unsupervised machine learning algorithms is essential before creating the model [14]. These techniques can be synthetically defined as methods that do not consider class labels and remove redundant features (unsupervised methods, like principal component and cluster analysis) [13], against those examining the feature's relationship with the investigated class or their contribution to the correct classification. There are three main subtypes of supervised algorithms [14]: filter or univariate methods, which investigate the relationship of each feature with the outcome but ignore the correlations within the different features (for instance, the Wilcoxon rank-sum test, the Fisher score, the Chi-squared score, the Student's t-test, or the minimum redundancy maximum relevance) [25]; wrapper or multivariate methods, that take into account the relationships between features by scoring how different subsets of features influence the predictive performance and include forward feature selection, backward feature elimination, complete feature selection, or bidirectional search [25, 26]; embedded methods, which select the most appropriate features during the training of the predictive machine learning models: compared to wrapper methods, these are less computationally demanding and less prone to overfitting. Commonly used embedded methods are ridge regression, tree-based algorithms like random forest classifiers, or the least absolute shrinkage and selection operator (LASSO) [14].

After feature selection, different algorithms are granted to train a model to predict a specific task. The detailed

Table 38.1 Summary of some of commonly used radiomic features and their description [12–14, 18, 20, 22]

Feature group	Definition	Examples	Description
First-order statistics	Quantitative statistical description of the distribution of signal intensities in an ROI regardless of spatial relationships	*Entropy*	Measures the inherent randomness in the gray-level intensities of an image or ROI
		Uniformity	Measures the homogeneity of gray-level intensities within an image or ROI
		Kurtosis	The degree of intensities histogram sharpness
		Maximum	Maximum intensity value
		Mean	Mean intensity value
		Median	Median intensity value
		Range	Range of intensity values
		Skewness	The degree of the intensities histogram asymmetry around the mean
		Standard deviation and variance	Measures of the histogram dispersion, that is, a measure of how much the gray levels differ from the mean
Second-order statistics or textural features	Statistical relationships between intensity levels of neighboring pixels or voxels or groups of pixels or voxels. Reflect tumor heterogeneity	*Gray-level co-occurrence matrix*	Represents the number of times that two intensity levels occur in neighboring pixels or voxels within a specific distance along a fixed direction
		Neighborhood Gray-level different matrix	The difference of intensity levels between one voxel and its 26 neighbors in three dimensions
		Short runs emphasis	Measures distributions of short runs. Higher values indicate fine textures
		Long runs emphasis	Measures distribution of long runs. Higher values indicate course textures
		Gray-level non-uniformity	Measures the distribution of runs over the gray values. Lower value indicates higher similarity in intensity values
		Coarseness	Quantitative measure of local uniformity
		Busyness	Rapid intensity changes of neighborhoods in a given ROI
		Local binary pattern	Quantifies local pixel structures through a binary coding scheme. Measures tumor microenvironment
		Histogram of oriented gradients	Computes block-wise histogram gradients with multiple orientations
Shape- and size-based features	Descriptors of the three-dimensional size and shape of the tumor region	*Volume*	Determined by counting the number of pixels in the tumor region and multiplying this value by the voxel size
		Maximum 3D diameter	The maximum three-dimensional tumor diameter
		Surface area	The surface area can be calculated by triangulation (i.e., dividing the surface into connected triangles)
		Surface to volume ratio	Describes how elongated the shape of the tumor is
		Sphericity	Describes how spherical the shape of the tumor is
High-order statistics or wavelet features	Extracted by applying filters or mathematical transforms to images for the identification of repeating patterns, noise suppression, edge enhancement, histogram-oriented gradients, or local binary patterns	*After decomposition, each first- or second-order statistic can be further computed*	

discussion of each model definition and mechanisms is beyond this chapter's purposes and can be found elsewhere [27]. The selection of the best model for a specific task follows an established pipeline in machine learning, which is described in detail in other chapters and will be only summarized here. Briefly, the dataset is split into two groups, of which one is used to training the model (train set, i.e., to select the best algorithm and its parameter using the previously selected features) and the other, the test set to evaluate the model performances. Ideally, a third dataset is created at the beginning to further validate the model efficacy in performing a specific task on previously unseen data.

38.3 Applications in Neuro-Oncology

A considerable amount of efforts in radiomics research has been put in recent years in the field of high-grade gliomas, the ultimate goal being to predict overall survival, a possible response to treatment or tumor histology, and grading and pathological features.

Many studies have found a consistent association between textural heterogeneity described as the spatial distribution of gray levels in an ROI and higher glioma grades on T1-weighted, FLAIR sequences, and diffusion-weighted imaging (DWI) through apparent diffusion coefficient

(ADC) [28–31]. With the 2016 update to the WHO classification of brain tumors and the growing role of molecular profiles in the diagnosis of gliomas, the research for a noninvasive identification through radiomics of specific biomolecular patterns has gained further attention. For instance, identifying IDH mutation and MGMT promoter methylation [11, 32] could be done successfully. Specifically, the use of diffusional kurtosis imaging, together with texture analysis, has proved to be a valid method to discriminate IDH-mutant from IDH-wildtype tumors and grade II from grade III gliomas [33]. Similarly, the presence of 1p/19q co-deletion could be successfully predicted using decisional three-based algorithms and features extracted from contrast-enhanced T1-weighted, T2-weighted, and FLAIR sequences with an accuracy as high as 96% [34, 35].

However, a considerable amount of research concentrated on identifying the most accurate composition of features (so-called "radiomic signature") to identify the tumor response to treatment or the tumor behavior regardless of the presence of any particular biomolecular feature. For example, Liu et al. [18] created a radiomic signature composed of 9 features correlated with progression-free survival in low-grade gliomas in both training and validation sets, independent of any clinicopathological factor. Similarly, a survival estimate before treatment was also possible in patients with glioblastoma by identifying different radiomic profiles describing different tumor heterogeneity grades based on T1, T2, FLAIR sequences, and ADC [5, 13], and also independently from other clinicopathological factors [4, 6]. Alternatively, radiomic profiles can be integrated into the knowledge of the tumor molecular profile and histology to improve disease stratification and prognosis, without an explicit dependency of radiomic features to the tumor characteristics being demonstrated [16, 17].

Also, radiomic research has focused on the discrimination between gliomas and other entities with similar radiologic manifestations on MR imaging. For instance, radiomics have shown encouraging results in diagnosing glioblastoma versus brain metastasis [36] or recognizing treatment-related changes in suspected disease relapse [37–40].

38.4 Features Associated with Extent of Resection in Brain Glioma

The role of radiomics in brain gliomas surgery holds promise to support decision making for planning surgical strategies, post-surgical therapy, and follow-up. The main factor influencing these three phases is the amount of residual tumor after surgical exeresis, which, as previously demonstrated, correlates with the patient's prognosis [41]. Therefore, the earlier and the most accurate the identification or the estimate of the residual tumor, the more appropriate the planned therapeutic strategies will be, aiming at precision treatment on an individual basis beyond shared protocols and algorithms with their intrinsic limitations.

Radiomic models can influence the treatment strategy by creating maps of tumoral infiltration to guide the surgeon in tumor removal and enhance the extent of resection [42, 43]; by searching for preoperative features that could predict tumor remnants [6]; or by detecting early postoperative tumor residuals, identifying areas at the need for further treatment and replacing the qualitative and operator-dependent definitions of "gross total," "subtotal," "partial resection" [44].

Different information on the presence of tumoral cells can be extracted from different MRI sequences. For instance, T1-weighted contrast-enhanced sequences depict alterations in regional angiogenesis and integrity of the blood-brain barrier in the tumor; T2-weighted and FLAIR sequences assess extracellular fluid in brain parenchyma; diffusion tensor imaging (DTI) informs about the water molecules diffusion in the brain, which affected in part by tumor cells architecture and density; dynamic susceptibility contrast-enhanced (DSC)-MRI techniques reflect aspects of perfusion in the brain and of regional microvasculature and hemodynamics.

All these aspects can be altered by infiltrating tumor cells and, individually, may not be sufficiently specific to define tumor infiltration areas. Recent studies dealing with the correct identification of tumoral extension have variably combined the information gained from these different methods to offer reliable radiomic models.

For example, Akbari et al. [42] proposed a model based on supporting vector machine (SVM) combining features extracted from T1, T2-weighted and FLAIR sequences, diffusion tensor imaging (DTI; specifically: fractional anisotropy [FA], radial diffusivity [RAD], axial diffusivity [AX], and trace [TR]), and perfusion. They were able to identify three categories of features used for estimating the infiltration pattern: a first group describing signal intensity from contrast- and non-contrast-enhanced T1, T2-weighted and FLAIR sequences; a second group consisting of statistics from features derived from diffusion tensor DTI; and a third group relating to tissue vascularization, perfusion, and permeability of blood vessels, identified through principal component analysis (PCA). Despite a satisfactory ability to topographically identify areas of tumor recurrence with an AUC of 0.84, sensitivity of 91%, and specificity of 93%, and recurrence odds ratio estimates of 9.29 for tissue predicted to be infiltrated, the retrospective nature of the study and the absence of histological specimen confirmations requires caution before clinical application.

Rathore et al. [6] produced an estimates map of glioblastoma recurrence based on preoperative MRIs. To do this, they analyzed preoperative pre- and post-contrast T1-weighted, T2, FLAIR, DTI, and DSC-MRI. They identified five types of radiomic features from peritumoral zones on a voxel-wise basis: intensity features, distance (from the tumor) features, statistical features (or first-order features), textural features, and temporal perfusion dynamics. SVM was used to assign each voxel a probability score, and then a comparison was made between the estimated infiltration map and post-surgical MRIs of patients with and without actual tumor recurrence. The model's predictive power was described by the area under the receiver operating characteristic curve (AUC) of 0.83 and 0.91 for the training and validation sets, respectively. Interestingly, they found tumor recurrence areas to be characterized by higher cellularity and vascularity and lower signal intensities on T2 and FLAIR, suggesting lower water concentration than areas without recurrence. The exciting results of this work may further benefit from multicenter validation.

Attempts to purposefully distinguish peritumoral edema from real tumor infiltration have been made with different approaches [45], like extracting first-, second-, and high-order statistics from peritumoral edema in patients with glioblastoma and meningioma. Features were selected with a LASSO method. The best performances to predict tumor infiltration in glioblastomas in perilesional edema (AUC 0.99) were obtained from GLCM difference entropy on contrast-enhanced T1-weighted imaging after post-processing normalization. The main limitation of this study, however, was the small cohort involved.

In their recent work, Yan et al. [46] developed convolutional neural networks with 112 features among first- and second-order features to predict tumor recurrence areas after surgery, with the most distinctive features being gained from contrast-enhanced T1 sequences and ADC. The overall sensitivity and specificity were 80% and 97.7%, respectively.

Future Perspectives

Different radiomics-based models to identify tumor infiltration zones in gliomas share some features despite studies being conducted with diverse methodologies. The most recent studies concentrated on identifying tumor recurrence areas, early or delayed, within anatomic zones usually deemed as either perilesional edema or unaffected brain tissue with conventional radiological examinations. Overall, radiomic features that measure cellularity and histological irregularities, as well as features describing irregularities in the diffusion of water molecules, seem to provide a reliable means to spot tumor infiltration, mainly through first- and second-order features. On the other hand, shape- and size-based features have gained less attention concerning this specific aspect of neuro-oncology.

However, incorporating and validating size- and shape-related features could be interesting to test some fascinating biological hypotheses concerning gliomas behavior. For instance, a larger tumor would represent an advanced stage of the disease with a higher chance of presenting infiltration zones. The field of fractal analysis, defined as a mathematical tool to assess and quantify natural objects' morphological features [22], has obtained limited attention regarding this task.

38.5 Conclusions

Radiomics has proven to offer significant advantages over conventional radiological analysis, and benefits seem to be granted in the future for the field of neuro-oncology.

To further influence surgery and improve patients' prognosis, correct identification of tumor borders beyond the limits identified by conventional radiological techniques and more precise identification of areas at risk for disease relapse should be sought more extensively.

Although some patterns seem to emerge from the studies that have dealt with the issue, research is still open to fully exploiting the support provided by radiomics and possibly discovering new strategies for a more precise measurement of radiological data.

Conflicts of Interest The authors declare that they have no conflicts of interest to disclose.

References

1. Louis DN, Perry A, Reifenberger G, von Deimling A, Figarella-Branger D, Cavenee WK, Ohgaki H, Wiestler OD, Kleihues P, Ellison DW. The 2016 World Health Organization classification of tumors of the central nervous system: a summary. Acta Neuropathol. 2016;131:803–20. https://doi.org/10.1007/s00401-016-1545-1.
2. Bozdag S, Li A, Riddick G, Kotliarov Y, Baysan M, Iwamoto FM, Cam MC, Kotliarova S, Fine HA. Age-specific signatures of glioblastoma at the genomic, genetic, and epigenetic levels. PLoS One. 2013;8:e62982. https://doi.org/10.1371/journal.pone.0062982.
3. Patel VN, Gokulrangan G, Chowdhury SA, Chen Y, Sloan AE, Koyuturk M, Barnholtz-Sloan J, Chance MR. Network signatures of survival in glioblastoma multiforme. PLoS Comput Biol. 2013;9:e1003237. https://doi.org/10.1371/journal.pcbi.1003237.
4. Kickingereder P, Neuberger U, Bonekamp D, Piechotta PL, Gotz M, Wick A, Sill M, Kratz A, Shinohara RT, Jones DTW, Radbruch A, Muschelli J, Unterberg A, Debus J, Schlemmer HP, Herold-Mende C, Pfister S, von Deimling A, Wick W, Capper D, Maier-Hein KH, Bendszus M. Radiomic subtyping improves disease stratification beyond key molecular, clinical, and standard imaging characteristics in patients with glioblastoma. Neuro Oncol. 2018;20:848–57. https://doi.org/10.1093/neuonc/nox188.
5. McGarry SD, Hurrell SL, Kaczmarowski AL, Cochran EJ, Connelly J, Rand SD, Schmainda KM, LaViolette PS. Magnetic resonance imaging-based radiomic profiles predict patient prognosis in newly diagnosed glioblastoma before therapy. Tomography. 2016;2:223–8. https://doi.org/10.18383/j.tom.2016.00250.

6. Rathore S, Akbari H, Doshi J, Shukla G, Rozycki M, Bilello M, Lustig R, Davatzikos C. Radiomic signature of infiltration in peritumoral edema predicts subsequent recurrence in glioblastoma: implications for personalized radiotherapy planning. J Med Imaging (Bellingham). 2018;5:021219. https://doi.org/10.1117/1.JMI.5.2.021219.
7. Seow P, Wong JHD, Ahmad-Annuar A, Mahajan A, Abdullah NA, Ramli N. Quantitative magnetic resonance imaging and radiogenomic biomarkers for glioma characterisation: a systematic review. Br J Radiol. 2018;91:20170930. https://doi.org/10.1259/bjr.20170930.
8. Vaidya T, Agrawal A, Mahajan S, Thakur MH, Mahajan A. The continuing evolution of molecular functional imaging in clinical oncology: the road to precision medicine and radiogenomics (part II). Mol Diagn Ther. 2019;23:27–51. https://doi.org/10.1007/s40291-018-0367-3.
9. Baid U, Rane SU, Talbar S, Gupta S, Thakur MH, Moiyadi A, Mahajan A. Overall survival prediction in glioblastoma with radiomic features using machine learning. Front Comput Neurosci. 2020;14:61. https://doi.org/10.3389/fncom.2020.00061.
10. Thust SC, Heiland S, Falini A, Jäger HR, Waldman AD, Sundgren PC, Godi C, Katsaros VK, Ramos A, Bargallo N, Vernooij MW, Yousry T, Bendszus M, Smits M. Glioma imaging in Europe: a survey of 220 centres and recommendations for best clinical practice. Eur Radiol. 2018;28:3306–17. https://doi.org/10.1007/s00330-018-5314-5.
11. Sasaki T, Kinoshita M, Fujita K, Fukai J, Hayashi N, Uematsu Y, Okita Y, Nonaka M, Moriuchi S, Uda T, Tsuyuguchi N, Arita H, Mori K, Ishibashi K, Takano K, Nishida N, Shofuda T, Yoshioka E, Kanematsu D, Kodama Y, Mano M, Nakao N, Kanemura Y. Radiomics and MGMT promoter methylation for prognostication of newly diagnosed glioblastoma. Sci Rep. 2019;9:14435. https://doi.org/10.1038/s41598-019-50849-y.
12. Zhou M, Scott J, Chaudhury B, Hall L, Goldgof D, Yeom KW, Iv M, Ou Y, Kalpathy-Cramer J, Napel S, Gillies R, Gevaert O, Gatenby R. Radiomics in brain tumor: image assessment, quantitative feature descriptors, and machine-learning approaches. AJNR Am J Neuroradiol. 2018;39:208–16. https://doi.org/10.3174/ajnr.A5391.
13. Kickingereder P, Burth S, Wick A, Götz M, Eidel O, Schlemmer HP, Maier-Hein KH, Wick W, Bendszus M, Radbruch A, Bonekamp D. Radiomic profiling of glioblastoma: identifying an imaging predictor of patient survival with improved performance over established clinical and radiologic risk models. Radiology. 2016;280:880–9. https://doi.org/10.1148/radiol.2016160845.
14. Lohmann P, Galldiks N, Kocher M, Heinzel A, Filss CP, Stegmayr C, Mottaghy FM, Fink GR, Jon Shah N, Langen KJ. Radiomics in neuro-oncology: basics, workflow, and applications. Methods. 2020;188:112–21. https://doi.org/10.1016/j.ymeth.2020.06.003.
15. Avants BB, Tustison NJ, Song G, Cook PA, Klein A, Gee JC. A reproducible evaluation of ANTs similarity metric performance in brain image registration. Neuroimage. 2011;54:2033–44. https://doi.org/10.1016/j.neuroimage.2010.09.025.
16. Bae S, Choi YS, Ahn SS, Chang JH, Kang SG, Kim EH, Kim SH, Lee SK. Radiomic MRI phenotyping of glioblastoma: improving survival prediction. Radiology. 2018;289:797–806. https://doi.org/10.1148/radiol.2018180200.
17. Park JE, Kim HS, Jo Y, Yoo RE, Choi SH, Nam SJ, Kim JH. Radiomics prognostication model in glioblastoma using diffusion- and perfusion-weighted MRI. Sci Rep. 2020;10:4250. https://doi.org/10.1038/s41598-020-61178-w.
18. Liu X, Li Y, Qian Z, Sun Z, Xu K, Wang K, Liu S, Fan X, Li S, Zhang Z, Jiang T, Wang Y. A radiomic signature as a non-invasive predictor of progression-free survival in patients with lower-grade gliomas. Neuroimage Clin. 2018;20:1070–7. https://doi.org/10.1016/j.nicl.2018.10.014.
19. Song S, Zheng Y, He Y. A review of methods for bias correction in medical images. Biomed Eng Rev. 2017;1(1). https://doi.org/10.18103/bme.v3i1.1550.
20. Chaddad A, Kucharczyk MJ, Daniel P, Sabri S, Jean-Claude BJ, Niazi T, Abdulkarim B. Radiomics in glioblastoma: current status and challenges facing clinical implementation. Front Oncol. 2019;9:374. https://doi.org/10.3389/fonc.2019.00374.
21. Chaddad A. Automated feature extraction in brain tumor by magnetic resonance imaging using Gaussian mixture models. Int J Biomed Imaging. 2015;2015:868031. https://doi.org/10.1155/2015/868031.
22. Jang K, Russo C, Di Ieva A. Radiomics in gliomas: clinical implications of computational modeling and fractal-based analysis. Neuroradiology. 2020;62:771–90. https://doi.org/10.1007/s00234-020-02403-1.
23. Yun TJ, Park CK, Kim TM, Lee SH, Kim JH, Sohn CH, Park SH, Kim IH, Choi SH. Glioblastoma treated with concurrent radiation therapy and temozolomide chemotherapy: differentiation of true progression from pseudoprogression with quantitative dynamic contrast-enhanced MR imaging. Radiology. 2015;274:830–40. https://doi.org/10.1148/radiol.14132632.
24. Zhou M, Hall L, Goldgof D, Russo R, Balagurunathan Y, Gillies R, Gatenby R. Radiologically defined ecological dynamics and clinical outcomes in glioblastoma multiforme: preliminary results. Transl Oncol. 2014;7:5–13. https://doi.org/10.1593/tlo.13730.
25. Kuhn M, Johnson K. Applied predictive modeling. New York: Springer; 2013. https://doi.org/10.1007/978-1-4614-6849-3.
26. Parekh V, Jacobs MA. Radiomics: a new application from established techniques. Expert Rev Precis Med Drug Dev. 2016;1:207–26. https://doi.org/10.1080/23808993.2016.1164013.
27. Cleophas TJ, Zwinderman AH. Machine learning in medicine—a complete overview. 2nd ed. New York: Springer; 2015.
28. Bahrami N, Hartman SJ, Chang Y-H, Delfanti R, White NS, Karunamuni R, Seibert TM, Dale AM, Hattangadi-Gluth JA, Piccioni D, Farid N, McDonald CR. Molecular classification of patients with grade II/III glioma using quantitative MRI characteristics. J Neurooncol. 2018;139:633–42. https://doi.org/10.1007/s11060-018-2908-3.
29. Darbar A, Waqas M, Enam SF, Mahmood SD. Use of preoperative apparent diffusion coefficients to predict brain tumor grade. Cureus. 2018;10:e2284. https://doi.org/10.7759/cureus.2284.
30. Ditmer A, Zhang B, Shujaat T, Pavlina A, Luibrand N, Gaskill-Shipley M, Vagal A. Diagnostic accuracy of MRI texture analysis for grading gliomas. J Neurooncol. 2018;140:583–9. https://doi.org/10.1007/s11060-018-2984-4.
31. Skogen K, Schulz A, Dormagen JB, Ganeshan B, Helseth E, Server A. Diagnostic performance of texture analysis on MRI in grading cerebral gliomas. Eur J Radiol. 2016;85:824–9. https://doi.org/10.1016/j.ejrad.2016.01.013.
32. Yang D, Rao G, Martinez J, Veeraraghavan A, Rao A. Evaluation of tumor-derived MRI-texture features for discrimination of molecular subtypes and prediction of 12-month survival status in glioblastoma. Med Phys. 2015;42:6725–35. https://doi.org/10.1118/1.4934373.
33. Bisdas S, Shen H, Thust S, Katsaros V, Stranjalis G, Boskos C, Brandner S, Zhang J. Texture analysis- and support vector machine-assisted diffusional kurtosis imaging may allow in vivo gliomas grading and IDH-mutation status prediction: a preliminary study. Sci Rep. 2018;8:6108. https://doi.org/10.1038/s41598-018-24438-4.
34. Lu C-F, Hsu F-T, Hsieh KL-C, Kao Y-CJ, Cheng S-J, Hsu JB-K, Tsai P-H, Chen R-J, Huang C-C, Yen Y, Chen C-Y. Machine learning–based radiomics for molecular subtyping of gliomas. Clin Cancer Res. 2018;24:4429–36. https://doi.org/10.1158/1078-0432.Ccr-17-3445.

35. Zhou H, Chang K, Bai HX, Xiao B, Su C, Bi WL, Zhang PJ, Senders JT, Vallières M, Kavouridis VK, Boaro A, Arnaout O, Yang L, Huang RY. Machine learning reveals multimodal MRI patterns predictive of isocitrate dehydrogenase and 1p/19q status in diffuse low- and high-grade gliomas. J Neurooncol. 2019;142:299–307. https://doi.org/10.1007/s11060-019-03096-0.
36. Chen C, Ou X, Wang J, Guo W, Ma X. Radiomics-based machine learning in differentiation between glioblastoma and metastatic brain tumors. Front Oncol. 2019;9:806. https://doi.org/10.3389/fonc.2019.00806.
37. Hu X, Wong KK, Young GS, Guo L, Wong ST. Support vector machine multiparametric MRI identification of pseudoprogression from tumor recurrence in patients with resected glioblastoma. J Magn Reson Imaging. 2011;33:296–305. https://doi.org/10.1002/jmri.22432.
38. Kim JY, Park JE, Jo Y, Shim WH, Nam SJ, Kim JH, Yoo R-E, Choi SH, Kim HS. Incorporating diffusion- and perfusion-weighted MRI into a radiomics model improves diagnostic performance for pseudoprogression in glioblastoma patients. Neuro Oncol. 2018;21:404–14. https://doi.org/10.1093/neuonc/noy133.
39. Peng L, Parekh V, Huang P, Lin DD, Sheikh K, Baker B, Kirschbaum T, Silvestri F, Son J, Robinson A, Huang E, Ames H, Grimm J, Chen L, Shen C, Soike M, McTyre E, Redmond K, Lim M, Lee J, Jacobs MA, Kleinberg L. Distinguishing true progression from radionecrosis after stereotactic radiation therapy for brain metastases with machine learning and radiomics. Int J Radiat Oncol Biol Phys. 2018;102:1236–43. https://doi.org/10.1016/j.ijrobp.2018.05.041.
40. Zhang Z, Yang J, Ho A, Jiang W, Logan J, Wang X, Brown PD, McGovern SL, Guha-Thakurta N, Ferguson SD, Fave X, Zhang L, Mackin D, Court LE, Li J. A predictive model for distinguishing radiation necrosis from tumour progression after gamma knife radiosurgery based on radiomic features from MR images. Eur Radiol. 2018;28:2255–63. https://doi.org/10.1007/s00330-017-5154-8.
41. Molinaro AM, Hervey-Jumper S, Morshed RA, Young J, Han SJ, Chunduru P, Zhang Y, Phillips JJ, Shai A, Lafontaine M, Crane J, Chandra A, Flanigan P, Jahangiri A, Cioffi G, Ostrom Q, Anderson JE, Badve C, Barnholtz-Sloan J, Sloan AE, Erickson BJ, Decker PA, Kosel ML, LaChance D, Eckel-Passow J, Jenkins R, Villanueva-Meyer J, Rice T, Wrensch M, Wiencke JK, Oberheim Bush NA, Taylor J, Butowski N, Prados M, Clarke J, Chang S, Chang E, Aghi M, Theodosopoulos P, McDermott M, Berger MS. Association of Maximal Extent of resection of contrast-enhanced and non–contrast-enhanced tumor with survival within molecular subgroups of patients with newly diagnosed glioblastoma. JAMA Oncol. 2020;6:495–503. https://doi.org/10.1001/jamaoncol.2019.6143.
42. Akbari H, Macyszyn L, Da X, Bilello M, Wolf RL, Martinez-Lage M, Biros G, Alonso-Basanta M, O'Rourke DM, Davatzikos C. Imaging surrogates of infiltration obtained via multiparametric imaging pattern analysis predict subsequent location of recurrence of glioblastoma. Neurosurgery. 2016;78:572–80. https://doi.org/10.1227/NEU.0000000000001202.
43. Sloan AE, Shukla G, Rathore S, Akbari H, Gondi V, Davatzikos C. Radiomics-based identification of peritumoral infiltration in de novo glioblastoma imaging presents targets amenable for potential targeted extended resection: a neurosurgical survey. J Clin Oncol. 2019;37:e13573. https://doi.org/10.1200/JCO.2019.37.15_suppl.e13573.
44. Scherer M, Jungk C, Gotz M, Kickingereder P, Reuss D, Bendszus M, Maier-Hein K, Unterberg A. Early postoperative delineation of residual tumor after low-grade glioma resection by probabilistic quantification of diffusion-weighted imaging. J Neurosurg. 2018:1–9. https://doi.org/10.3171/2018.2.JNS172951.
45. Florez E, Nichols T, Parker EE, Seth TL, Howard CM, Fatemi A. Multiparametric magnetic resonance imaging in the assessment of primary brain tumors through radiomic features: a metric for guided radiation treatment planning. Cureus. 2018;10:e3426. https://doi.org/10.7759/cureus.3426.
46. Yan JL, Li C, van der Hoorn A, Boonzaier NR, Matys T, Price SJ. A neural network approach to identify the Peritumoral invasive areas in glioblastoma patients by using MR Radiomics. Sci Rep. 2020;10:9748. https://doi.org/10.1038/s41598-020-66691-6.

39 Machine Learning in Neuro-Oncology, Epilepsy, Alzheimer's Disease, and Schizophrenia

Mason English, Chitra Kumar, Bonnie Legg Ditterline, Doniel Drazin, and Nicholas Dietz

39.1 Introduction

Machine learning (ML) involves dynamic evaluation of healthcare data by artificial intelligence that may be applied to diagnostic and therapeutic medical interventions [1–3]. Analysis for pattern extraction aids to classify and design an algorithm to predict outcomes from a trained dataset while mitigating bias [4]. Advances in the neurosciences—including diagnostic imaging, genetic correlates, and improved understanding of neural circuits—have enhanced application of machine learning to gain new insight into disease and optimize identification and treatment that account for complex interactions of clinical, environmental, and genetic variables [5, 6]. Machine learning may aid physician diagnosis and decision-making in treatment plans by analyzing complex variable interactions (i.e., clinical, genetic, environmental) for peak performance. Practically, these algorithms may aid in determining an individual's candidacy for surgery or optimizing intraoperative identification for retrieval of cancerous tissue. Predictive algorithms are a current metric for healthcare utilization to anticipate a patient's hospital stay, payments, and readmission [7, 8].

Mason English and Chitra Kumar have contributed equally to this work.

M. English · C. Kumar
Department of Neurological Surgery, University of Louisville, Louisville, KY, USA

B. L. Ditterline · N. Dietz (✉)
Department of Neurological Surgery, University of Louisville, Louisville, KY, USA

Kentucky Spinal Cord Injury Research Center, University of Louisville, Louisville, KY, USA
e-mail: nick.dietz@uoflhealth.org

D. Drazin
Evergreen Hospital Neuroscience Institute, Kirkland, WA, USA

Algorithms (e.g., decision trees, support vector machine (SVM), random forest, and gradient boosting models, among others) that have been applied to medical translational research are classified as supervised learning, unsupervised learning, or reinforcement learning [9]. Machine learning in the neurosciences primarily utilizes supervised learning models for their optimal ability to account for and integrate complex and dynamic models [10–22]. The most frequently used model for neurological pathologies is SVM due to its flexibility to represent complex relationships and moderate nonlinearities for classification, regression, and outlier detection [23–25]. Glaser et al. propose four specific areas in which machine learning can be categorized: (1) solving engineering problems, (2) identifying predictive variables, (3) benchmarking simple models, and (4) serving as a model for the brain [24]. Machine learning has been utilized to predict neural activity related to seizures [24, 26, 27]. Depending on the engineered algorithm, its flexibility attempts to reflect reality to accurately evaluate and correlate multiple variables for optimal function [24, 28]. The most accurate model of ganglion cell activity currently is a deep learning algorithm that demonstrates the present deficiencies in the biological model [14]. Deep learning neural networks demonstrate parallels to the neural network of our brains not only in terms of structure but also activation patterns which can be valuable in gaining a better understanding of sensory cortical processing or behavior prediction [24, 29].

In the present review, we discuss the landscape of ML in schizophrenia, epilepsy, Alzheimer's disease, and neuro-oncology as those neurological disorders are some of the most cited in association with artificial intelligence [11, 19, 23]. Additionally, multifactorial risk factors and vague clinical presentations often complicate diagnoses in absence of biomarkers for certain conditions such as Alzheimer's disease—ML may benefit surgical decision-making by utilizing predictive modeling to aid management and approach.

V. E. Staartjes et al. (eds.), *Machine Learning in Clinical Neuroscience*, Acta Neurochirurgica Supplement 134,
https://doi.org/10.1007/978-3-030-85292-4_39

39.2 Materials and Methods

Data Extraction

We framed 4 searches to identify machine learning studies across some of the fields in neuroscience richest in machine learning. A PICOS model (Participants, Intervention, Comparison, Outcomes, Study Design) was used to define the usage of machine learning algorithms in the diagnosis and treatment of epilepsy, neuro-oncology, schizophrenia, and Alzheimer's cases. We analyzed the articles that focused primarily on the use of machine learning algorithms in an adult population including systematic reviews and comparative studies.

PICOS Outline

Participants: Adult patients ≥18 years of age.

Intervention: Diagnosis and/or treatment for Alzheimer's, epilepsy, brain tumors, or schizophrenia.

Comparison: Performance of machine learning algorithms to the current diagnostic and treatment options.

Outcomes: Area under the curve (AUC) or percent accuracy in utilizing a machine learning algorithm.

Study Design: Inclusive of systematic reviews and retrospective studies.

Search Criteria

For this review, we conducted the search on January 5th, 2021 using the PubMed Databases between 2015 to 2020 [30]. Further, studies needed to report a standardized evaluation metric of accuracy with the inclusion of the area under the curve (AUC) or quantitative statistics. Additional articles used in the references were incorporated from the references of those articles identified in the searches. We used Keyword and MeSH terms for predictive outcomes to include the following terms with numbered iterations for the two databases as follows:

1. Pubmed: Neuro-oncology AND machine learning: 85 articles; 13 included.
2. Pubmed: Schizophrenia AND machine learning: 388 articles; 10 included.
3. Pubmed: Epilepsy AND machine learning: 508 articles; 11 included.
4. Pubmed: Alzheimer's AND machine learning: 967 articles: 12 included.

Risk of bias evaluation: Assessment of conflict of interest, funding for study and study design were assessed according to QUADAS criteria.

Inclusion and Exclusion Criteria

Inclusion criteria involved studies with adult patients ≥18 years of age with Alzheimer's, epilepsy, brain tumor, or schizophrenia. Randomized controlled trials, prospective, retrospective, and systematic review studies were included. Exclusion criteria involved studies with nonhuman subjects, pediatric population, language other than English, and those studies without full text. Studies that did not use a machine learning algorithm or those that did use one but did not validate their algorithm were excluded. Final selection of articles was also based on author discretion for relative impact to the field and unique purpose or methods to bring light to recent advancements.

39.3 Results

Neuro-Oncology

We identified 13 studies between 2015 and 2020 that utilized machine learning in the treatment and diagnosis of brain tumors (Table 39.1). Neuro-oncology studies reported the success of their algorithms with area under the curve (AUC) measures, accuracy percentages, similarity coefficient, concordance index, or mean absolute predicted error. Accuracy of ML algorithms ranged from AUC 0.80 to 0.85, underscoring their predictive ability in determining the location and extent of the tumor. The percent accuracy reported ranged from 61% to 99%. Studies reported sample sizes ranging from 18 to 45,814 patients. Results were verified using a subset of cross-validation. In general, studies utilized a leave-one-out cross-validation approach, possibly since it's recognized to be unbiased. However, five- and tenfold cross-validation approaches were also utilized by four studies possibly as that method has decreased variability [31].

Epilepsy

In our review of ML and epilepsy, we found support vector machine algorithm to be the most utilized in epilepsy research (Table 39.2). These studies presented with AUC ranging from 0.84 to 0.91. Others reported their results with accuracy percentages ranging from 43% to 95%. Studies reported sample sizes ranging from 20 to 519. Interestingly, studies with larger sample sizes (over 200) tended to use five- or tenfold cross-validation instead of the leave-one-out method. This could be because the leave-one-out method would be more time consuming and has more variance when handling a larger sample size [20]. From the 11 articles identified related to neurosurgery for epilepsy, seven attempted to create an algorithm to identify patients that were seizure free post-surgery (Table 39.2) [10, 12, 15, 17, 18, 32, 33]. Of the

Table 39.1 Machine learning and neuro-oncology

Title	Publication	Variables	Purpose	Machine learning algorithms	Sample size	Accuracy	Validation method
Predicting inpatient length of stay after brain tumor surgery: developing machine learning ensembles to improve predictive performance	*Neurosurgery*	Preoperative patient characteristics	Predict LOS following craniotomy	Two gradient boosted trees and SVM	45,814	RMSLE 0.555 on internal validation	Cross-validation
Machine learning assisted intraoperative assessment of brain tumor margins using HRMAS NMR spectroscopy	*PLoS Computational Biology*	HRMAS NMR	Predicting micro-scale tissue with leftover tumor during surgery	Random forest-based approach, CNN, PLS-DA	565	AUC 85.6%	Eightfold cross-validation
Raman spectroscopy to differentiate between fresh tissue samples of glioma and normal brain: a comparison with 5-ALA-induced fluorescence-guided surgery	*Journal of Neurosurgery*	Raman spectroscopy	Differentiate between Raman spectroscopy and 5ALA induced fluorescence guided surgery	Principal component analysis (PCA); linear discriminant analysis (LDA)	73	Accuracy: 0.99	Leave-one-sample-out cross-validation
Serum microRNA is a biomarker for post-operative monitoring in glioma	*Journal of Neuro-Oncology*	Serum microRNA	Find a biomarker for longitudinal monitoring	Random forest analysis	108	Accuracy: 99.8%	Monte-Carlo based validation approach
Next for neuro-radiosurgery: A fully automatic approach for necrosis extraction in brain tumor MRI using an unsupervised machine learning technique	*International Journal of Imaging Systems and Technology*	MRI	Delineates necrotic regions of tissue	NeXT, unsupervised machine learning algorithm	32	Similarity coefficient 95.93%	N/A
Integration of machine learning and mechanistic models accurately predicts variation in cell density of glioblastoma using multiparametric MRI	*Scientific Reports*	MRI	Identify tumor cell invasion	Hybrid model of proliferation-invasion (PI) with imaging data-driven graph-based model	18	Mean absolute predicted error (MAPE) of 0.106	Leave-one-patient-out cross-validation
Radiogenomics of glioblastoma: machine learning–based classification of molecular characteristics by using multiparametric and multiregional mr imaging features	*Radiology*	MRI	Association of MRI imaging features with molecular characteristics in patients	Gradient boosting, random forest, penalized logistic regression classifiers	152	Accuracy: (63% EGFR, 61% RTK II	Tenfold cross-validation
Overall survival prediction in glioblastoma multiforme patients from volumetric, shape and texture features using machine learning	*Surgical Oncology*	MRI	Survival prediction	SVM	163	Accuracy: 98.7% (2-class), 88.95% (3-class)	Fivefold cross-validation

(continued)

Table 39.1 (continued)

Title	Publication	Variables	Purpose	Machine learning algorithms	Sample size	Accuracy	Validation method
An online calculator for the prediction of survival in glioblastoma patients using classical statistics and machine learning	*Neurosurgery*	13 demographic, socioeconomic, clinical, and radiographic features	Personalized survival curves	Decision trees, random forests, linear models, etc. (15 total)	20,821	Concordance index = 0.70	Fivefold cross-validation
Imaging surrogates of infiltration obtained via multiparametric imaging pattern analysis predict subsequent location of recurrence of glioblastoma	*Neurosurgery*	MRI	Delineate areas of tumor infiltration and predict early recurrence	SVM	65	AUC: 0.84	Leave-one-patient-out cross-validation
Deep learning-based framework for in vivo identification of glioblastoma tumor using hyperspectral images of human brain	*Sensors*	Hyperspectral imaging	Delineate location of tumor in vivo	SVM and deep learning	16	AUC: 80%	Leave-one-patient-out cross-validation framework
Prediction of pseudoprogression versus progression using machine learning algorithm in glioblastoma	*Nature*	MRI	Post-surgical progression for glioblastoma	Convolutional neural network (CNN) and long short-term memory (LSTM)	78	AUC: 0.83	Tenfold cross validation
Radiomics-based machine learning in differentiation between glioblastoma and metastatic brain tumors	*Frontiers in Oncology*	MRI	Differentiate glioblastomas from metastatic brain tumors	LDA, SVM, random forest etc. (6 total)	134	AUC of 0.80 for two models	

remaining four, three publications utilized ML to determine patient candidacy for surgical intervention and one attempted to diagnose and localize the epileptic zone for surgery resection [20–22, 34]. Six publications utilized the SVM algorithm for analysis, possibly because it is often used for research, is resistant to overfitting, and performs well with high-dimensional data [15, 17, 18, 32–34]. Other models included the extreme gradient boosting algorithm, random forest, natural language processing, and linear discriminant analysis function with certain papers analyzing multiple algorithms for comparison [10, 12, 18, 20–22, 34].

Alzheimer's Disease

Of the 12 studies published between 2015 and 2020, two measured clinical variables, one measured specific serum markers in body fluid (e.g., micro-RNA), eight measured different anatomical regions with either PET or MRI scans, and one measured electroencephalography (EEG) response after scopolamine administration (Table 39.3). Accuracy of these studies is often greater than 90%. However, among studies for which the outcome was diagnosis of Alzheimer's disease, there was no consistent dependent variable investigated (in contrast to studies utilizing ML in schizophrenia, below).

Schizophrenia

Of the 10 studies identified, a majority (eight) used SVM algorithm to analyze the data. Accuracy and AUC measurements were frequently demonstrated to be greater than 0.80 and SVM was frequently the most accurate algorithm, occasionally yielding accuracies greater than 90%, when comparing ML methodologies within the same dataset (Table 39.4). Current research into ML and schizophrenia primarily focuses on imaging modalities such as MRI to identify abnormally anatomical patterns [35]. Of ten articles published within the last 5 years, nine utilize MRI measurements of cortical volume or thickness and one uses brain fractional anisotropy [36–45].

Table 39.2 Epilepsy and Machine Learning

Title	Publication	Variables	Purpose	Machine learning algorithm	Sample size	Accuracy	Validation method
Machine learning-XGBoost analysis of language networks to classify patients with epilepsy	*Brain Informatics*	fMRI	Diagnosis and localization for surgery	Extreme Gradient Boosting (XGBoost algorithm)	55	AUC: 91 ± 5%	Nested cross-validation scheme with an outer Monte Carlo cross-validation
Structural brain network abnormalities and the probability of seizure recurrence after epilepsy surgery	*Neurology*	MRI + clinical data	Post-surgical outcome	SVM	80	AUC: 0.84 ± 0.06	Nested cross-validation
Temporal lobe epilepsy surgical outcomes can be inferred based on structural connectome hubs: a machine learning study	*Annals of Neurology*	MRI	Post-surgical outcome	SPSS	168	AUC: 0.88	Cross-validation using independent multi-set data
Localization of the epileptogenic zone using Interictal MEG and Machine learning in a large cohort of drug-resistant epilepsy patients	*Frontiers in Neurology*	MEG recordings	Post-surgical outcome	SVM and random forest	94	SVM: 43.77% accuracy random forest: 49.03%	Leave-one-out cross validation
Investigation of bias in an epilepsy machine learning algorithm trained on physician notes	*Epilepsia*	Clinical notes	Surgical eligibility	NLP	443	AUC was 0.94	Tenfold cross-validation
Methodological issues in predicting pediatric epilepsy surgery candidates through natural language processing and machine learning	*Biomedical Informatics Insights*	Clinical notes	Surgical candidacy	SVM, Naive Bayes Classifier	200	*F*-measures: 0.71 to 0.82	Tenfold cross-validation
Multimodal data and machine learning for surgery outcome prediction in complicated cases of mesial temporal lobe epilepsy	*Computers in Biology and Medicine*	MRI and demographical data	Post-surgical outcome	LS-SVM	20	95.0%	Leave-one-out cross-validation
Prospective validation of a machine learning model that uses provider notes to identify candidates for resective epilepsy surgery	*Epilepsia*	Clinical notes	Surgical candidacy	NLP	519	AUC: 0.90 ± 0.04	Tenfold cross-validation
The impact of epilepsy surgery on the structural connectome and its relation to outcome	*Neuroimage: Clinical*	MRI	Post-surgical outcome	SVM	53	79% accuracy	Leave-one-out cross-validation
Evaluation of machine learning algorithms for treatment outcome prediction in patients with epilepsy based on structural connectome data	*NeuroImage*	MRI and chart review data	Post-surgical outcome	SVM	118	70% accuracy	Tenfold cross-validation
Magnetic resonance imaging pattern learning in temporal lobe epilepsy: Classification and prognostics	*Annals of Neurology*	MRI	Post-surgical outcome	LDA	114	92% accuracy	Leave-one-out cross-validation

Table 39.3 Alzheimer's disease and machine learning

Title	Publication	Variables	Purpose	Machine learning algorithm	Sample size	Accuracy	Validation method
Machine learning to detect Alzheimer's Disease from circulating non-coding RNAs	*Genomics, Proteomics and Bioinformatics*	sncRNA/ miRNA	Diagnosis	Gradient boosted tree model	465	AUC 87.6% and 83.5% (# of controls)	Tenfold cross-validation
Machine learning for comprehensive forecasting of Alzheimer's Disease progression	*Scientific Reports*	44 clinical variables	Disease progression	Conditional Restricted Boltzmann Machine (CRBM)	1909	AUC 0.5	Fivefold cross-validation
Optimizing machine learning methods to improve predictive models of Alzheimer's Disease	*Journal of Alzheimer's Disease*	MRI, demographics, APOE4	Diagnosis & Disease Progression	Decision trees, support vector machines, K-nearest neighbor, ensemble linear discriminant, boosted trees, and random forests	1329	Cognitively normal vs. AD 92.8% Future conversion—6, 12, 24, 36, & 48 months (63.8%, 68.9%, 74.9%, 75.3%, 77.0%)	Tenfold cross-validation
Machine learning based hierarchical classification of frontotemporal dementia and Alzheimer's disease	*NeuroImage: Clinical*	MRI	Diagnosis	Hierarchical classifier	50 AD, 146 CN	CN vs. dementia 0.917 AD vs. FTD 0.955	Tenfold cross-validation
A deep learning model to predict a diagnosis of Alzheimer Disease by using 18F-FDG PET of the brain	*Radiology*	18F-FDG PET	Diagnosis	Adam: first-order gradient-based stochastic optimization algorithm	899	AUC 0.92	Tenfold cross-validation
Machine learning identified an Alzheimer's disease-related FDG-PET pattern which is also expressed in Lewy body dementia and Parkinson's disease dementia	*Scientific Reports*	FDG-PET	Diagnosis	General linear model (GLM), subprofile modeling (SSM)13, and support vector machine (SVM)	346	AUC 0.945	Tenfold cross-validation
Using high-dimensional machine learning methods to estimate an anatomical risk factor for Alzheimer's disease across imaging databases	*NeuroImage*	MRI and cognitive assessment	Diagnosis	Elastic net regularized logistic regression (EN-RLR) classifier	359		Tenfold cross-validation
Hybrid multivariate pattern analysis combined with extreme learning machine for Alzheimer's dementia diagnosis using multi-measure rs-fMRI spatial patterns	*PLoS One*	rs-fMRI	Diagnosis	Support vector machine (SVM)	460	98.86%	Leave-one-out and tenfold cross-validation

Table 39.3 (continued)

Title	Publication	Variables	Purpose	Machine learning algorithm	Sample size	Accuracy	Validation method
Identification of Alzheimer's disease and mild cognitive impairment using multimodal sparse hierarchical extreme learning machine	*Human Brain Mapping*	MRI, FDG-PET, CSF	Diagnosis	Multi-modal sparse hierarchical extreme leaning	202	97.12%	Tenfold cross-validation
EEG machine learning for accurate detection of cholinergic intervention and Alzheimer's disease	*Scientific Reports*	EEG	Diagnosis	Elastic net logistic regression	158	92%	Tenfold cross-validation
A clinically-translatable machine learning algorithm for the prediction of Alzheimer's disease conversion in individuals with mild and premild cognitive impairment	*Journal of Alzheimer's Disease*	Demographics	Diagnosis	16 tested. Best results from SVM	184	AUC 0.962	Leave-pair-out-cross-validation
Machine learning-based individual assessment of cortical atrophy pattern in Alzheimer's disease spectrum: Development of the classifier and longitudinal evaluation	*Scientific Reports*	MRI	Diagnosis	Non-specific individual-level machine learning algorithm	1342	Sensitivity and specificity of 87.1% and 93.3%	Tenfold cross-validation

39.4 Discussion

Neuro-Oncology

Traditionally, one of the treatment hurdles of neuro-oncology is overcoming penetration of the blood–brain barrier that prevents systemic chemotherapy and immunotherapy [46, 47]. Often, surgical resection is necessary in cases of neurological impairment, resistance to medical therapy, dominant metastatic lesion, and/or prognosis [48, 49]. Depending on the location and type of tumor, gross total resection may not be achievable or come at the expense of vital neurovascular structure or eloquent regions [49, 50]. Machine learning may serve as a tool to maximize total resection of lesions, choose approaches or navigation equipment, predict outcomes, and/or monitor the patient postoperatively [13, 16, 51–56].

Patient samples reported therein ranged from eight patients to 45,000. Dependent variables included preoperative patient characteristics, Nuclear Magnetic Resonance spectroscopy, MRIs, and serum micro-RNA. In contrast to the epilepsy studies, more variability was observed in the type of ML algorithms to assist with treatment and diagnosis of brain tumors. Most studies did not use SVM, for instance, and the techniques utilized range from simple (e.g., random forest analysis) to complex hybrid ML analyses (e.g., semi-supervised learning model with proliferation-invasion imaging). The objectives of these studies were also different than those investigating ML in epilepsy: in neuro-oncology ML was used to delineate the borders of the tumor for better surgical outcomes, predict individual survival statistics, or aid in post-surgical follow-up, while ML was used to predict surgical candidacy or post-surgical seizure activity for epilepsy patients.

Morokoff et al. conducted a study in 2020 to compare serum micro-RNA profiles of 91 glioma patients with 17 healthy controls utilizing a random forest analysis and Monte-Carlo ML algorithm to discover a biomarker for longitudinal monitoring of glioma patients [16]. Gaw et al. conducted a study in 2019 to precisely identify the borders of tumor cell invasion using 82 preoperative biopsies from 18 glioblastoma patients [57]. Instead of using a simple ML algorithm, this study combined a proliferation-invasion model with a semi-supervised machine learning model (SSL) to combine the strengths of each algorithm. Semi-supervised

Table 39.4 Schizophrenia and machine learning

Title	Publication	Variables	Purpose	Machine learning algorithm	Sample size	Accuracy	Validation method
Classification of schizophrenia using feature-based morphometry	*Journal of Neural Transmission*	MRI	Diagnosis	SVM	108	84.1%	Leave-one-out cross validation
Using multivariate machine learning methods and structural MRI to classify childhood onset schizophrenia and healthy controls	*Front Psychiatry*	MRI	Diagnosis	Random Forest	197	73.7%	None
Clinical utility of machine-learning approaches in schizophrenia: Improving diagnostic confidence for translational neuroimaging	*Frontiers in Psychiatry*	MRI	Diagnosis	SVM	39	69.1%–77%	Leave-one-subject-out cross validation
Support vector machine-based classification of first episode drug-naïve schizophrenia patients and healthy controls using structural MRI	*Schizophrenia Research*	MRI	Diagnosis	SVM	326	81.8–85.0%	Tenfold cross-validation
Discriminative analysis of schizophrenia using support vector machine and recursive feature elimination on structural MRI images	*Medicine (Baltimore)*	MRI	Diagnosis	SVM with recursive feature elimination (RFE) classifier	83	88.4%	Leave-one-out cross-validation
Using deep belief network modelling to characterize differences in brain morphometry in schizophrenia	*Scientific Reports*	MRI	Diagnosis	Deep belief network (DBN-DNN) and SVM	258	73.6% (DBN) vs. 68.1 (SVM)	Threefold cross-validation
Decreased resting-state interhemispheric functional connectivity correlated with neurocognitive deficits in drug-naive first-episode adolescent-onset schizophrenia	*International Journal of Neuropsychopharmacology*	fMRI	Diagnosis (specific drug naive)	SVM & voxel-mirrored homotopic connectivity (VMHC)	79	94.93%	Leave-pair-out cross-validation
Shared atypical default mode and salience network functional connectivity between autism and schizophrenia	*Autism Research*	fMRI	Diagnosis	Multivariate pattern analysis (MVPA)	109	83.3%	Leave-one-out cross-validation
Multimodal discrimination of schizophrenia using hybrid weighted feature concatenation of brain functional connectivity and anatomical features with an extreme learning machine	*Frontiers in Neuroinformatics*	fMRI	Diagnosis	SVM, linear extreme learning machine (ELM), LDA, and random forest bagged tree classifier	144	99.3%	Nested 10-by-tenfold cross-validation
Machine learning classification of first-episode schizophrenia spectrum disorders and controls using whole brain white matter fractional anisotropy	*BMC Psychiatry*	Brain fractional anisotropy	Diagnosis	SVM	154	62.34%	77-fold cross-validation

machine learning has been successfully applied in previous studies that contain unlabeled data, which proved useful in this study as the authors placed a voxel in multiple cross-sections of unlabeled MRIs for analysis. Additionally, a graph-based algorithm was chosen in the supervised machine learning model as it was previously determined to accurately predict new glioblastoma patients from the trained model [57]. The proliferation-invasion model is useful as it can handle more biological information such as the intuition from patient-specific parameters. This publication indicates the usefulness of combining ML algorithms with other data analysis models.

Some studies utilize multiple ML algorithms to determine the most accurate model. Kickingereder et al. conducted a retrospective chart review in 2016 to determine associations between characteristics seen on MRI with molecular biomarkers in patients with glioblastoma [13]. The study applied three ML methods appropriate for binary classification: stochastic gradient boosting machine, random forest, and penalized logistic regression classifiers. Each classifier was then subjected to a tenfold cross-validation resampling procedure. Interestingly, whereas the penalized logistic regression model achieved the highest accuracy for predicting epidermal growth family receptor status, the gradient boosting and random forest model had the highest accuracy for predicting the receptor tyrosine kinase II status. Similarly, Senders et al. used 15 machine learning algorithms, including boosted decision trees, random forests, and naïve Bayes, among others, to create personalized survival cures based on 13 patient characteristics [56]. Through inferential analyses, the accelerated time algorithm demonstrated the highest accuracy in predicting overall and 1-year survival probability for glioblastoma patients [56]. Chen et al. conducted a study in 2019 to investigate if a ML model could differentiate between glioblastomas and metastatic brain tumors [58]. This study utilized 30 diagnostic models using five selection methods and six classification algorithms. The two models with the most promising results were (1) distance correlation with a linear discriminant analysis and (2) distance correlation with a logistic regression as both algorithms had a diagnostic ability with an AUC of 0.80 [58]. This study revealed the discrepancy in choice of algorithm and sample size as SVM performs better for sample size of 50–60 patients, whereas linear discriminant analysis or logistic regression are more suitable for a larger sample size (>100) [58].

Deep learning is a subset of machine learning that uses artificial neural networks to learn from a dataset. Fabelo et al. conducted a study in 2019 to create a framework for processing hyperspectral images of brain tissue in vivo to identify the location of a tumor and aid a surgeon in resection during operation [52]. The thematic map created with the deep learning framework had an AUC of 80%, significantly higher than that of a typical SVM map. Further exploration into deep learning models has the potential to improve care of individuals with brain tumors.

Epilepsy

Epilepsy affects around 50 million individuals worldwide, with anti-epileptic drugs benefitting up to 70% of patients [59]. As many as 33% of patients with epilepsy may be medication-resistant and possibly require surgical intervention to resect epileptic foci or receive placement of responsive neurostimulation or vagal nerve stimulator [60–62]. Such situations require many factors to be considered before reaching a decision. For example, surgery has variable benefits—closely analyzing a patient's medical history to determine their surgical candidacy is crucial. It is also important to localize the area for resection and ensure it will not affect any eloquent structures or major neural white matter tracts. Machine learning algorithms may be incorporated to map imaging and demographic characteristics that may aid surgical decision-making.

In 2019, Wissel et al. investigated the natural language processing algorithm to select surgical candidates from a cohort of 443 patients with epilepsy [22]. Because the algorithm had to be trained to analyze physician notes, using a model that could deconstruct and interpret human language such as natural language processing proved to be useful. Torlay et al. conducted a study in 2017 that used the extreme gradient boosting algorithm to discriminate between patients who did and did not have epilepsy, and to identify atypical patterns of language networks in fMRI to determine potential locations for surgical resection [20]. The extreme gradient boosting algorithm is a type of ensemble-based, supervised learning: multiple ML models that, individually, are poor predictors are combined, producing a more accurate analysis. Extreme gradient boosting creates decision trees to determine outcomes and builds this framework sequentially—i.e., each tree is built from the previous tree. The benefit of this algorithm model is that it has fast computation with high accuracy, can scale data, and can learn to improve from previous decisions [20].

Most studies used cross-validation to investigate ML in epilepsy [10, 12, 17, 18, 20, 32, 33]. Gleichgerrcht et al. conducted a retrospective study in 2020 utilizing preoperative MRI images from 121 patients with drug resistant temporal lobe epilepsy to create a neural network classification model [12]. This model was then cross-validated on 47 different patients with known outcomes to assess its predictive value. Taylor et al. conducted a study in 2018 of an SVM algorithm on diffusion MRI to predict surgical outcome [33]. Data were divided into test and training sets with a "leave-one-out" cross-validation scheme. In this approach, one data point is omitted, and the remaining data points are used to train the model. The omitted data point is then used to validate the model. The process is repeated, and new data points are omitted and subsequently used for validation.

Wissel et al. conducted a study utilizing the natural language processing algorithm to assign epilepsy surgery candidacy scores based on provider notes [21]. The training dataset of roughly 519 patients had an AUC of 0.90 and the prospective AUC for 4211 patients was 0.79. Both the sensitivity and specificity of this algorithm were calculated by comparing the algorithm's given scores to known patient outcomes. The sensitivity was 0.80 and the specificity was 0.77. The model assigned surgical candidacy scores without bias, considering the various aspects of a patient's case. Nissen et al. conducted a study analyzing magnetoencephalography recordings from 94 patients to localize epileptogenic zone for surgery by comparing delta power, low-to-high-frequency power ratio, and functional connectivity [18]. The SVM algorithm discriminated between resection and non-resection areas with 59.94% accuracy, while the random forest algorithm discriminates with 60.34% accuracy. Neither, however, could discriminate seizure-free from not seizure-free patients [18]. This underscores the necessity of analyzing and modifying the metrics utilized for the machine learning algorithm and serves as a reminder of the importance of evaluating the accuracy of the models.

Alzheimer's Disease

In 2017, Simpraga et al. attempted to identify a neural substrate or biological signature of disease state for Schizophrenia using EEG and cholinergic profiles [63]. As a selective muscarinic receptor antagonist, scopolamine is commonly regarded as the ideal study tool to induce cholinergic-dependent cognitive deficits similar to Alzheimer's disease. It was demonstrated that ML determines the peak scopolamine condition which, otherwise, would be too difficult to measure given innate variability between days. After utilizing ML to determine cholinergic profiles, measurement of electroencephalography response improved allowing for construction of a response curve to better assess an index of Alzheimer's disease state [64].

Standardized structures for cortical thickness or volume measurement in Alzheimer's disease is not present and such elucidation in the field is ongoing. One study by Kim et al., however, uniquely utilized a preprocessing algorithm to develop a frequency measurement of cortical thicknesses mapped across an oscillation map, not only bypassing the lack of a specific measurement target but improving measurement of generalized cortical atrophy [65]. Through this technique, a variety of targets were proposed for further distinguishing dementia, frontotemporal dementia, and Alzheimer's disease.

While SVM is considered one of the better algorithms in the field of neuroscience [35], the algorithms utilized in studies for Alzheimer's disease reported herein are varied. Other algorithms utilized include gradient boosted tree model, conditional restricted Boltzmann machine, K-nearest neighbor, ensemble linear discriminant, boosted tree, random forest, general linear model, multi-modal sparse hierarchical extreme leaning machine, and elastic net regularized logistic regression as well as a few proprietary algorithms.

Current publications regarding ML in Alzheimer's disease do not appear to have a targeted dependent variable such as that seen with MRI and schizophrenia; rather, studies reporting on Alzheimer's disease investigate structures with varied levels of success. A ML analysis to incorporate these disparate measurements would likely yield a better guide and provide framework for future research.

Schizophrenia

Schizophrenia is a psychiatric disorder that affects 100,000 new individuals annually [66]. Clinical diagnosis is based on the American Psychiatric Association definition given in the Diagnostic and Statistical Manual of Mental Disorders V [67], characterized by cognitive impairment, positive symptoms (i.e., delusions, hallucinations, and/or loss of reality), and negative symptoms (i.e., anhedonia, avolition, logia, and/or flat affect). Classically, while environmental and genetic factors play a role in phenotypic expression of the disease, diagnosis is clinical because objective biomarkers that may standardize diagnosis are yet unknown.

Two studies focused on larger datasets of cortical volume to assess its viability as a primary basis for diagnosis [37, 40]. Liu et al. and Chen et al. used 240 and 255 distinct volume areas, respectively, to better power their ML model to assess functional connectivity, hypothesizing that functional connectivity would be reduced in patients with schizophrenia [40, 64, 68]. The other seven studies utilize targeted measurements across a variety of structures: cortical thickness measurements include the frontal, temporal, parietal, and occipital lobes, while volume measurements include the lateral ventricle, thalamus, hippocampus, and dorsolateral prefrontal cortex.

39.5 Conclusions

Current applications of ML in medicine are far-reaching, including implementation for drug creation in pharmaceutical development, diagnostics, surgical planning, outcome prediction, and intraoperative assistance [69]. Supervised learning models appear to be the most commonly incorporated algorithm models for machine learning across the reviewed neuroscience disciplines with primary aim of diagnosis.

Accuracy ranges are from 63% to 99% across algorithms. As certain neurological diseases such as Alzheimer's disease and schizophrenia are classically influenced by multiple clinical and environmental factors, ML may offer unique insight into weighted influences of variables. Early identification of disease may allow early intervention and management. Machine learning contributions to diagnostic and therapeutic opportunities may enhance current medical best practices in the neurosciences while also broadening our understanding of the brain. As neural networks and deep learning models continue to grow, future directions and studies may harness big data and interdisciplinary management of complex disease states.

Funding No funding sources, grants, or other financial reports were used in the present study.

Conflict of Interest The authors have no conflicts of interests to disclose.

References

1. Hey T, Butler K, Jackson S, Thiyagalingam J. Machine learning and big scientific data. Philos Trans A Math Phys Eng Sci. 2020;378:20190054. https://doi.org/10.1098/rsta.2019.0054.
2. Nichols JA, Herbert Chan HW, Baker MAB. Machine learning: applications of artificial intelligence to imaging and diagnosis. Biophys Rev. 2019;11:111–8. https://doi.org/10.1007/s12551-018-0449-9.
3. Richards BA, Lillicrap TP, Beaudoin P, Bengio Y, Bogacz R, Christensen A, Clopath C, Costa RP, de Berker A, Ganguli S, Gillon CJ, Hafner D, Kepecs A, Kriegeskorte N, Latham P, Lindsay GW, Miller KD, Naud R, Pack CC, Poirazi P, Roelfsema P, Sacramento J, Saxe A, Scellier B, Schapiro AC, Senn W, Wayne G, Yamins D, Zenke F, Zylberberg J, Therien D, Kording KP. A deep learning framework for neuroscience. Nat Neurosci. 2019;22:1761–70. https://doi.org/10.1038/s41593-019-0520-2.
4. LeCun Y, Bengio Y, Hinton G. Deep learning. Nature. 2015;521:436–44. https://doi.org/10.1038/nature14539.
5. Marblestone AH, Wayne G, Kording KP. Toward an integration of deep learning and neuroscience. Front Comput Neurosci. 2016;10:94. https://doi.org/10.3389/fncom.2016.00094.
6. Vu MT, Adali T, Ba D, Buzsaki G, Carlson D, Heller K, Liston C, Rudin C, Sohal VS, Widge AS, Mayberg HS, Sapiro G, Dzirasa K. A shared vision for machine learning in neuroscience. J Neurosci. 2018;38:1601–7. https://doi.org/10.1523/JNEUROSCI.0508-17.2018.
7. Dietz N, Sharma M, Alhourani A, Ugiliweneza B, Wang D, Drazin D, Boakye M. Evaluation of predictive models for complications following spinal surgery. J Neurol Surg A Cent Eur Neurosurg. 2020;81:535–45. https://doi.org/10.1055/s-0040-1709709.
8. Stromblad CT, Baxter-King RG, Meisami A, Yee SJ, Levine MR, Ostrovsky A, Stein D, Iasonos A, Weiser MR, Garcia-Aguilar J, Abu-Rustum NR, Wilson RS. Effect of a predictive model on planned surgical duration accuracy, patient wait time, and use of Presurgical resources: a randomized clinical trial. JAMA Surg. 2021;156(4):315–21. https://doi.org/10.1001/jamasurg.2020.6361.
9. Jordan MI, Mitchell TM. Machine learning: trends, perspectives, and prospects. Science. 2015;349:255–60. https://doi.org/10.1126/science.aaa8415.
10. Bernhardt BC, Hong SJ, Bernasconi A, Bernasconi N. Magnetic resonance imaging pattern learning in temporal lobe epilepsy: classification and prognostics. Ann Neurol. 2015;77:436–46. https://doi.org/10.1002/ana.24341.
11. Celtikci E. A systematic review on machine learning in neurosurgery: the future of decision-making in patient care. Turk Neurosurg. 2018;28:167–73. https://doi.org/10.5137/1019-5149.JTN.20059-17.1.
12. Gleichgerrcht E, Keller SS, Drane DL, Munsell BC, Davis KA, Kaestner E, Weber B, Krantz S, Vandergrift WA, Edwards JC, McDonald CR, Kuzniecky R, Bonilha L. Temporal lobe epilepsy surgical outcomes can be inferred based on structural connectome hubs: a machine learning study. Ann Neurol. 2020;88:970–83. https://doi.org/10.1002/ana.25888.
13. Kickingereder P, Bonekamp D, Nowosielski M, Kratz A, Sill M, Burth S, Wick A, Eidel O, Schlemmer HP, Radbruch A, Debus J, Herold-Mende C, Unterberg A, Jones D, Pfister S, Wick W, von Deimling A, Bendszus M, Capper D. Radiogenomics of glioblastoma: machine learning-based classification of molecular characteristics by using multiparametric and multiregional MR imaging features. Radiology. 2016;281:907–18. https://doi.org/10.1148/radiol.2016161382.
14. Maheswaranathan N, Kastner DB, Baccus SA, Ganguli S. Inferring hidden structure in multilayered neural circuits. PLoS Comput Biol. 2018;14:e1006291. https://doi.org/10.1371/journal.pcbi.1006291.
15. Memarian N, Kim S, Dewar S, Engel J Jr, Staba RJ. Multimodal data and machine learning for surgery outcome prediction in complicated cases of mesial temporal lobe epilepsy. Comput Biol Med. 2015;64:67–78. https://doi.org/10.1016/j.compbiomed.2015.06.008.
16. Morokoff A, Jones J, Nguyen H, Ma C, Lasocki A, Gaillard F, Bennett I, Luwor R, Stylli S, Paradiso L, Koldej R, Paldor I, Molania R, Speed TP, Webb A, Infusini G, Li J, Malpas C, Kalincik T, Drummond K, Siegal T, Kaye AH. Serum microRNA is a biomarker for post-operative monitoring in glioma. J Neurooncol. 2020;149:391–400. https://doi.org/10.1007/s11060-020-03566-w.
17. Munsell BC, Wee CY, Keller SS, Weber B, Elger C, da Silva LA, Nesland T, Styner M, Shen D, Bonilha L. Evaluation of machine learning algorithms for treatment outcome prediction in patients with epilepsy based on structural connectome data. Neuroimage. 2015;118:219–30. https://doi.org/10.1016/j.neuroimage.2015.06.008.
18. Nissen IA, Stam CJ, van Straaten ECW, Wottschel V, Reijneveld JC, Baayen JC, de Witt Hamer PC, Idema S, Velis DN, Hillebrand A. Localization of the epileptogenic zone using Interictal MEG and machine learning in a large cohort of drug-resistant epilepsy patients. Front Neurol. 2018;9:647. https://doi.org/10.3389/fneur.2018.00647.
19. Staartjes VE, Stumpo V, Kernbach JM, Klukowska AM, Gadjradj PS, Schroder ML, Veeravagu A, Stienen MN, van Niftrik CHB, Serra C, Regli L. Machine learning in neurosurgery: a global survey. Acta Neurochir. 2020;162:3081–91. https://doi.org/10.1007/s00701-020-04532-1.
20. Torlay L, Perrone-Bertolotti M, Thomas E, Baciu M. Machine learning-XGBoost analysis of language networks to classify patients with epilepsy. Brain Inform. 2017;4:159–69. https://doi.org/10.1007/s40708-017-0065-7.
21. Wissel BD, Greiner HM, Glauser TA, Holland-Bouley KD, Mangano FT, Santel D, Faist R, Zhang N, Pestian JP, Szczesniak RD, Dexheimer JW. Prospective validation of a machine learning model that uses provider notes to identify candidates for resective epilepsy surgery. Epilepsia. 2020;61:39–48. https://doi.org/10.1111/epi.16398.
22. Wissel BD, Greiner HM, Glauser TA, Mangano FT, Santel D, Pestian JP, Szczesniak RD, Dexheimer JW. Investigation of bias in

an epilepsy machine learning algorithm trained on physician notes. Epilepsia. 2019;60:e93–8. https://doi.org/10.1111/epi.16320.
23. Buchlak QD, Esmaili N, Leveque JC, Farrokhi F, Bennett C, Piccardi M, Sethi RK. Machine learning applications to clinical decision support in neurosurgery: an artificial intelligence augmented systematic review. Neurosurg Rev. 2020;43:1235–53. https://doi.org/10.1007/s10143-019-01163-8.
24. Glaser JI, Benjamin AS, Farhoodi R, Kording KP. The roles of supervised machine learning in systems neuroscience. Prog Neurobiol. 2019;175:126–37. https://doi.org/10.1016/j.pneurobio.2019.01.008.
25. Noble WS. What is a support vector machine? Nat Biotechnol. 2006;24:1565–7. https://doi.org/10.1038/nbt1206-1565.
26. Abbasi B, Goldenholz DM. Machine learning applications in epilepsy. Epilepsia. 2019;60:2037–47. https://doi.org/10.1111/epi.16333.
27. Usman SM, Usman M, Fong S. Epileptic seizures prediction using machine learning methods. Comput Math Methods Med. 2017;2017:9074759. https://doi.org/10.1155/2017/9074759.
28. Lebedev AV, Westman E, Van Westen GJ, Kramberger MG, Lundervold A, Aarsland D, Soininen H, Kloszewska I, Mecocci P, Tsolaki M, Vellas B, Lovestone S, Simmons A, Alzheimer's Disease Neuroimaging I, The AddNeuroMed Consortium. Random Forest ensembles for detection and prediction of Alzheimer's disease with a good between-cohort robustness. Neuroimage Clin. 2014;6:115–25. https://doi.org/10.1016/j.nicl.2014.08.023.
29. Yamins DL, DiCarlo JJ. Using goal-driven deep learning models to understand sensory cortex. Nat Neurosci. 2016;19:356–65. https://doi.org/10.1038/nn.4244.
30. Moher D, Liberati A, Tetzlaff J, Altman DG, Group P. Preferred reporting items for systematic reviews and meta-analyses: the PRISMA statement. J Clin Epidemiol. 2009;62:1006–12. https://doi.org/10.1016/j.jclinepi.2009.06.005.
31. Browne MW. Cross-validation methods. J Math Psychol. 2000;44:108–32. https://doi.org/10.1006/jmps.1999.1279.
32. Sinha N, Wang Y, Moreira da Silva N, Miserocchi A, McEvoy AW, de Tisi J, Vos SB, Winston GP, Duncan JS, Taylor PN. Structural brain network abnormalities and the probability of seizure recurrence after epilepsy surgery. Neurology. 2020;96(5):e758–71. https://doi.org/10.1212/WNL.0000000000011315.
33. Taylor PN, Sinha N, Wang Y, Vos SB, de Tisi J, Miserocchi A, McEvoy AW, Winston GP, Duncan JS. The impact of epilepsy surgery on the structural connectome and its relation to outcome. Neuroimage Clin. 2018;18:202–14. https://doi.org/10.1016/j.nicl.2018.01.028.
34. Cohen KB, Glass B, Greiner HM, Holland-Bouley K, Standridge S, Arya R, Faist R, Morita D, Mangano F, Connolly B, Glauser T, Pestian J. Methodological issues in predicting pediatric epilepsy surgery candidates through natural language processing and machine learning. Biomed Inform Insights. 2016;8:11–8. https://doi.org/10.4137/BII.S38308.
35. de Filippis R, Carbone EA, Gaetano R, Bruni A, Pugliese V, Segura-Garcia C, De Fazio P. Machine learning techniques in a structural and functional MRI diagnostic approach in schizophrenia: a systematic review. Neuropsychiatr Dis Treat. 2019;15:1605–27. https://doi.org/10.2147/NDT.S202418.
36. Castellani U, Rossato E, Murino V, Bellani M, Rambaldelli G, Perlini C, Tomelleri L, Tansella M, Brambilla P. Classification of schizophrenia using feature-based morphometry. J Neural Transm (Vienna). 2012;119:395–404. https://doi.org/10.1007/s00702-011-0693-7.
37. Chen H, Uddin LQ, Duan X, Zheng J, Long Z, Zhang Y, Guo X, Zhang Y, Zhao J, Chen H. Shared atypical default mode and salience network functional connectivity between autism and schizophrenia. Autism Res. 2017;10:1776–86. https://doi.org/10.1002/aur.1834.
38. Greenstein D, Malley JD, Weisinger B, Clasen L, Gogtay N. Using multivariate machine learning methods and structural MRI to classify childhood onset schizophrenia and healthy controls. Front Psych. 2012;3:53. https://doi.org/10.3389/fpsyt.2012.00053.
39. Iwabuchi SJ, Liddle PF, Palaniyappan L. Clinical utility of machine-learning approaches in schizophrenia: improving diagnostic confidence for translational neuroimaging. Front Psych. 2013;4:95. https://doi.org/10.3389/fpsyt.2013.00095.
40. Liu Y, Guo W, Zhang Y, Lv L, Hu F, Wu R, Zhao J. Decreased resting-state interhemispheric functional connectivity correlated with neurocognitive deficits in drug-naive first-episode adolescent-onset schizophrenia. Int J Neuropsychopharmacol. 2018;21:33–41. https://doi.org/10.1093/ijnp/pyx095.
41. Lu X, Yang Y, Wu F, Gao M, Xu Y, Zhang Y, Yao Y, Du X, Li C, Wu L, Zhong X, Zhou Y, Fan N, Zheng Y, Xiong D, Peng H, Escudero J, Huang B, Li X, Ning Y, Wu K. Discriminative analysis of schizophrenia using support vector machine and recursive feature elimination on structural MRI images. Medicine (Baltimore). 2016;95:e3973. https://doi.org/10.1097/MD.0000000000003973.
42. Mikolas P, Hlinka J, Skoch A, Pitra Z, Frodl T, Spaniel F, Hajek T. Machine learning classification of first-episode schizophrenia spectrum disorders and controls using whole brain white matter fractional anisotropy. BMC Psychiatry. 2018;18:97. https://doi.org/10.1186/s12888-018-1678-y.
43. Pinaya WH, Gadelha A, Doyle OM, Noto C, Zugman A, Cordeiro Q, Jackowski AP, Bressan RA, Sato JR. Using deep belief network modelling to characterize differences in brain morphometry in schizophrenia. Sci Rep. 2016;6:38897. https://doi.org/10.1038/srep38897.
44. Qureshi MNI, Oh J, Cho D, Jo HJ, Lee B. Multimodal discrimination of schizophrenia using hybrid weighted feature concatenation of brain functional connectivity and anatomical features with an extreme learning machine. Front Neuroinform. 2017;11:59. https://doi.org/10.3389/fninf.2017.00059.
45. Xiao Y, Yan Z, Zhao Y, Tao B, Sun H, Li F, Yao L, Zhang W, Chandan S, Liu J, Gong Q, Sweeney JA, Lui S. Support vector machine-based classification of first episode drug-naive schizophrenia patients and healthy controls using structural MRI. Schizophr Res. 2019;214:11–7. https://doi.org/10.1016/j.schres.2017.11.037.
46. Ferraris C, Cavalli R, Panciani PP, Battaglia L. Overcoming the blood-brain barrier: successes and challenges in developing nanoparticle-mediated drug delivery systems for the treatment of brain tumours. Int J Nanomedicine. 2020;15:2999–3022. https://doi.org/10.2147/IJN.S231479.
47. Kumari S, Ahsan SM, Kumar JM, Kondapi AK, Rao NM. Overcoming blood brain barrier with a dual purpose Temozolomide loaded Lactoferrin nanoparticles for combating glioma (SERP-17-12433). Sci Rep. 2017;7:6602. https://doi.org/10.1038/s41598-017-06888-4.
48. Hatiboglu MA, Wildrick DM, Sawaya R. The role of surgical resection in patients with brain metastases. Ecancermedicalscience. 2013;7:308. https://doi.org/10.3332/ecancer.2013.308.
49. Lara-Velazquez M, Al-Kharboosh R, Jeanneret S, Vazquez-Ramos C, Mahato D, Tavanaiepour D, Rahmathulla G, Quinones-Hinojosa A. Advances in brain tumor surgery for glioblastoma in adults. Brain Sci. 2017;7:166. https://doi.org/10.3390/brainsci7120166.
50. Yaeger KA, Nair MN. Surgery for brain metastases. Surg Neurol Int. 2013;4:S203–8. https://doi.org/10.4103/2152-7806.111297.
51. Cakmakci D, Karakaslar EO, Ruhland E, Chenard MP, Proust F, Piotto M, Namer IJ, Cicek AE. Machine learning assisted intraoperative assessment of brain tumor margins using HRMAS NMR spectroscopy. PLoS Comput Biol. 2020;16:e1008184. https://doi.org/10.1371/journal.pcbi.1008184.
52. Fabelo H, Halicek M, Ortega S, Shahedi M, Szolna A, Pineiro JF, Sosa C, O'Shanahan AJ, Bisshopp S, Espino C, Marquez M,

Hernandez M, Carrera D, Morera J, Callico GM, Sarmiento R, Fei B. Deep learning-based framework for in vivo identification of glioblastoma tumor using hyperspectral images of human brain. Sensors (Basel). 2019;19:920. https://doi.org/10.3390/s19040920.
53. Fan Y, Chen C, Zhao F, Tian Z, Wang J, Ma X, Xu J. Radiomics-based machine learning technology enables better differentiation between glioblastoma and anaplastic Oligodendroglioma. Front Oncol. 2019;9:1164. https://doi.org/10.3389/fonc.2019.01164.
54. Livermore LJ, Isabelle M, Bell IM, Edgar O, Voets NL, Stacey R, Ansorge O, Vallance C, Plaha P. Raman spectroscopy to differentiate between fresh tissue samples of glioma and normal brain: a comparison with 5-ALA-induced fluorescence-guided surgery. J Neurosurg. 2020:1–11. https://doi.org/10.3171/2020.5.JNS20376.
55. Muhlestein WE, Akagi DS, Davies JM, Chambless LB. Predicting inpatient length of stay after brain tumor surgery: developing machine learning ensembles to improve predictive performance. Neurosurgery. 2019;85:384–93. https://doi.org/10.1093/neuros/nyy343.
56. Senders JT, Staples P, Mehrtash A, Cote DJ, Taphoorn MJB, Reardon DA, Gormley WB, Smith TR, Broekman ML, Arnaout O. An online calculator for the prediction of survival in glioblastoma patients using classical statistics and machine learning. Neurosurgery. 2020;86:E184–92. https://doi.org/10.1093/neuros/nyz403.
57. Gaw N, Hawkins-Daarud A, Hu LS, Yoon H, Wang L, Xu Y, Jackson PR, Singleton KW, Baxter LC, Eschbacher J, Gonzales A, Nespodzany A, Smith K, Nakaji P, Mitchell JR, Wu T, Swanson KR, Li J. Integration of machine learning and mechanistic models accurately predicts variation in cell density of glioblastoma using multiparametric MRI. Sci Rep. 2019;9:10063. https://doi.org/10.1038/s41598-019-46296-4.
58. Chen C, Ou X, Wang J, Guo W, Ma X. Radiomics-based machine learning in differentiation between glioblastoma and metastatic brain tumors. Front Oncol. 2019;9:806. https://doi.org/10.3389/fonc.2019.00806.
59. WHO. Epilepsy. Geneva: World Health Organization; 2019.
60. Ben-Menachem E. Vagus-nerve stimulation for the treatment of epilepsy. Lancet Neurol. 2002;1:477–82. https://doi.org/10.1016/s1474-4422(02)00220-x.
61. Skarpaas TL, Jarosiewicz B, Morrell MJ. Brain-responsive neurostimulation for epilepsy (RNS((R)) system). Epilepsy Res. 2019;153:68–70. https://doi.org/10.1016/j.eplepsyres.2019.02.003.
62. Tang F, Hartz AMS, Bauer B. Drug-resistant epilepsy: multiple hypotheses, few answers. Front Neurol. 2017;8:301. https://doi.org/10.3389/fneur.2017.00301.
63. Renner UD, Oertel R, Kirch W. Pharmacokinetics and pharmacodynamics in clinical use of scopolamine. Ther Drug Monit. 2005;27:655–65. https://doi.org/10.1097/01.ftd.0000168293.48226.57.
64. Simpraga S, Alvarez-Jimenez R, Mansvelder HD, van Gerven JMA, Groeneveld GJ, Poil SS, Linkenkaer-Hansen K. EEG machine learning for accurate detection of cholinergic intervention and Alzheimer's disease. Sci Rep. 2017;7:5775. https://doi.org/10.1038/s41598-017-06165-4.
65. Kim JP, Kim J, Park YH, Park SB, Lee JS, Yoo S, Kim EJ, Kim HJ, Na DL, Brown JA, Lockhart SN, Seo SW, Seong JK. Machine learning based hierarchical classification of frontotemporal dementia and Alzheimer's disease. Neuroimage Clin. 2019;23:101811. https://doi.org/10.1016/j.nicl.2019.101811.
66. Health NIoM. 2015. https://www.nimh.nih.gov/health/topics/schizophrenia/raise/fact-sheet-first-episode-psychosis.shtml. 2021.
67. American Psychiatric Association, American Psychiatric Association, DSM-5 Task Force. Diagnostic and statistical manual of mental disorders: DSM-5. 5th ed. Washington, DC: American Psychiatric Association; 2013.
68. Sheffield JM, Kandala S, Tamminga CA, Pearlson GD, Keshavan MS, Sweeney JA, Clementz BA, Lerman-Sinkoff DB, Hill SK, Barch DM. Transdiagnostic associations between functional brain network integrity and cognition. JAMA Psychiat. 2017;74:605–13. https://doi.org/10.1001/jamapsychiatry.2017.0669.
69. Valliani AA, Ranti D, Oermann EK. Deep learning and neurology: a systematic review. Neurol Ther. 2019;8:351–65. https://doi.org/10.1007/s40120-019-00153-8.

MIX
Papier aus verantwortungsvollen Quellen
Paper from responsible sources
FSC® C105338

If you have any concerns about our products,
you can contact us on
ProductSafety@springernature.com

In case Publisher is established outside the EU,
the EU authorized representative is:
Springer Nature Customer Service Center GmbH
Europaplatz 3, 69115 Heidelberg, Germany

Printed by Libri Plureos GmbH
in Hamburg, Germany